Statistics for Biology and Health

Series Editors
M. Gail, K. Krickeberg, J. Samet, A. Tsiatis, W. Wong

Statistics for Biology and Health

Borchers/Buckland/Zucchini: Estimating Animal Abundance: Closed Populations.
Burzykowski/Molenberghs/Buyse: The Evaluation of Surrogate Endpoints.
Everitt/Rabe-Hesketh: Analyzing Medical Data Using S-PLUS.
Ewens/Grant: Statistical Methods in Bioinformatics: An Introduction, 2nd ed.
Gentleman/Carey/Huber/Irizarry/Dudoit: Bioinformatics and Computational Biology Solutions using R and Bioconductors.
Hougaard: Analysis of Multivariate Survival Data.
Keyfitz/Caswell: Applied Mathematical Demography, 3rd ed.
Klein/Moeschberger: Survival Analysis: Techniques for Censored and Truncated Data, 2nd ed.
Kleinbaum/Klein: Survival Analysis: A Self-Learning Text.
Kleinbaum/Klein: Survival Analysis: A Self-Learning Text, 2nd ed.
Kleinbaum/Klein: Logistic Regression: A Self-Learning Text, 2nd ed.
Lange: Mathematical and Statistical Methods for Genetic Analysis, 2nd ed.
Manton/Singer/Suzman: Forecasting the Health of Elderly Populations.
Martinussen/Scheike: Dynamic Regression Models for Survival Data.
Moyé: Multiple Analyses in Clinical Trials: Fundamentals for Investigators.
Nielsen: Statistical Methods in Molecular Evolution.
Parmigiani/Garrett/Irizarry/Zeger: The Analysis of Gene Expression Data: Methods and Software.
Salsburg: The Use of Restricted Significance Tests in Clinical Trials.
Simon/Korn/McShane/Radmacher/Wright/Zhao: Design and Analysis of DNA Microarray Investigations.
Sorensen/Gianola: Likelihood, Bayesian, and MCMC Methods in Quantitative Genetics.
Stallard/Manton/Cohen: Forecasting Product Liability Claims: Epidemiology and Modeling in the Manville Asbestos Case.
Therneau/Grambsch: Modeling Survival Data: Extending the Cox Model.
Vittinghoff/Glidden/Shiboski/McCulloch: Regression Methods in Biostatistics: Linear, Logistic, Survival, and Repeated Measures Models.
Zhang/Singer: Recursive Partitioning in the Health Sciences.

Torben Martinussen
Thomas H. Scheike

Dynamic Regression Models for Survival Data

With 75 Illustrations

Springer

Torben Martinussen
Department of Natural Sciences
Royal Veterinary and Agricultural
  University
1871 Fredriksberg C
Denmark
torbenm@dina.kvl.dk

Thomas H. Scheike
Department of Biostatistics
University of Copenhagen
2200 Copenhagen N
Denmark
ts@biostat.ku.dk

Series Editors
M. Gail
National Cancer Institute
Rockville, MD 20892
USA

K. Krickeberg
Le Chatelet
F-63270 Manglieu
France

J. Samet
Department of
  Epidemiology
School of Public Health
Johns Hopkins
  University
615 Wolfe Street
Baltimore, MD
  21205-2103
USA

A. Tsiatis
Department of Statistics
North Carolina State
  University
Raleigh, NC 27695
USA

W. Wong
Sequoia Hall
Department of Statistics
Stanford University
390 Serra Mall
Stanford, CA 94305-4065
USA

Library of Congress Control Number: 2005930808

ISBN-10: 0-387-20274-9
ISBN-13: 978-0387-20274-7

Printed on acid-free paper.

© 2006 Springer Science+Business Media, Inc.
All rights reserved. This work may not be translated or copied in whole or in part without the written permission of the publisher (Springer Science + Business Media, Inc., 233 Spring Street, New York, NY 10013, USA), except for brief excerpts in connection with reviews or scholarly analysis. Use in connection with any form of information storage and retrieval, electronic adaptation, computer software, or by similar or dissimilar methodology now known or hereafter developed is forbidden.
The use in this publication of trade names, trademarks, service marks, and similar terms, even if they are not identified as such, is not to be taken as an expression of opinion as to whether or not they are subject to proprietary rights.

Printed in the United States of America.   (MVY)

9 8 7 6 5 4 3 2 1

springer.com

To Rasmus, Jeppe, Mie and Ida
To Anders, Liva and Maria

Preface

This book studies and applies flexible models for survival data. Many developments in survival analysis are centered around the important Cox regression model, which we also study. A key issue in this book, however, is extensions of the Cox model and alternative models with most of them having the specific aim of dealing with *time-varying* effects of covariates in regression analysis. One model that receives special attention is the additive hazards model suggested by Aalen that is particularly well suited for dealing with time-varying covariate effects as well as simple to implement and use.

Survival data analysis has been a very active research field for several decades now. An important contribution that stimulated the entire field was the counting process formulation given by Aalen (1975) in his Berkeley Ph.D. thesis. Since then a large number of fine text books have been written on survival analysis and counting processes, with some key references being Andersen et al. (1993), Fleming & Harrington (1991), Kalbfleisch & Prentice (2002), Lawless (1982). Of these classics, Andersen et al. (1993) and Fleming & Harrington (1991) place a strong emphasis on the counting process formulation that is becoming more and more standard and is the one we also use in this monograph. More recently, there have been a large number of other fine text books intended for different audiences, a quick look in a library data base gives around 25 titles published from 1992 to 2002. Our monograph is primarily aimed at the biostatistical community with biomedical application as the motivating factor. Other excellent texts for the same audience are, for example, Klein & Moeschberger (1997) and Therneau & Grambsch (2000). We follow the same direction as Therneau

& Grambsch (2000) and try to combine a rather detailed description of the theory with an applied side that shows the use of the discussed models for practical data. This should make it possible for both theoretical as well as applied statisticians to see how the models we consider can be used and work. The practical use of models is a key issue in biomedical statistics where the data at hand often are motivating the model building and inferential procedures, but the practical use of the models should also help facilitate the basic understanding of the models in the counting process framework.

The practical aspects of survival analysis are illustrated with a set of worked examples where we use the R program. The standard models are implemented in the `survival` package in R written by Terry Therneau that contains a broad range of functions needed for survival analysis. The flexible regression models considered in this monograph have been implemented in an R package `timereg` whose manual is given in Appendix C. Throughout the presentation of the considered models we give worked examples with the R code needed to produce all output and figures shown in the book, and the reader should therefore be able to reproduce all our output and try out essentially all considered models.

The monograph contains 11 chapters, and 10 of these chapters deal with the analysis of counting process data. The last chapter is on longitudinal data and presents a link between the counting process data and longitudinal data that is called marked point process data in the stochastic processes world. It turns out that the models from both fields are strongly related.

We use a special note-environment for additional details and supplementary material. These notes may be skipped without loss of understanding of the key issues. Proofs are also set in a special environment indicating that these may also be skipped. We hope that this will help the less mathematically inclined reader in maneuvering through the book.

We have intended to include many of the mathematical details needed to get a complete understanding of the theory developed. However, after Chapter 5, the level of detail decreases as many of the arguments thereafter will be as in the preceding material. A simple clean presentation has here been our main goal.

We have included a set of exercises at the end of each chapter. Some of these give additional important failure time results. Others are meant to provide the reader with practice and insight into the suggested methods.

Acknowledgments

We are deeply grateful for the support and help of colleagues and friends. Martin Jacobsen introduced us to counting processes and martingale calculus and his teaching has been of great inspiration ever since. Some of the exercises are taken from teaching material coming from Martin. Our interest for this research field was really boosted with the appearance of the book Andersen et al. (1993). We are grateful to these authors for the effort and interest they have put into this field. We have interacted particularly with the Danes of these authors: Per Kragh Andersen and Niels Keiding. Odd Aalen, Per Kragh Andersen, Ørnulf Borgan, Mette Gerster Harhoff, Kajsa Kvist, Yanqing Sun, Mei-Jie Zhang and some reviewers have read several chapters of earlier drafts. Their comments have been very useful to us and are greatly appreciated. Finally, we would like to thank our co-authors Mei-Jie Zhang, Christian Pipper and Ib Skovgaard of work related to this monograph for sharing their insight with us.

Copenhagen
November 2005

Torben Martinussen
Thomas H. Scheike

Contents

Preface   vii

1 Introduction   1
    1.1 Survival data 1
    1.2 Longitudinal data 14

2 Probabilistic background   17
    2.1 Preliminaries 17
    2.2 Martingales 20
    2.3 Counting processes 23
    2.4 Marked point processes 30
    2.5 Large-sample results 34
    2.6 Exercises 44

3 Estimation for filtered counting process data   49
    3.1 Filtered counting process data 49
    3.2 Likelihood constructions 62
    3.3 Estimating equations 70
    3.4 Exercises 74

4 Nonparametric procedures for survival data   81
    4.1 The Kaplan-Meier estimator 81
    4.2 Hypothesis testing 86
       4.2.1 Comparisons of groups of survival data 86

		4.2.2 Stratified tests	93
	4.3	Exercises	95

5 Additive Hazards Models — 103
5.1	Additive hazards models	108
5.2	Inference for additive hazards models	116
5.3	Semiparametric additive hazards models	126
5.4	Inference for the semiparametric hazards model	135
5.5	Estimating the survival function	146
5.6	Additive rate models	149
5.7	Goodness-of-fit procedures	151
5.8	Example	159
5.9	Exercises	165

6 Multiplicative hazards models — 175
6.1	The Cox model	181
6.2	Goodness-of-fit procedures for the Cox model	193
6.3	Extended Cox model with time-varying regression effects	205
6.4	Inference for the extended Cox model	213
6.5	A semiparametric multiplicative hazards model	218
6.6	Inference for the semiparametric multiplicative model	224
6.7	Estimating the survival function	226
6.8	Multiplicative rate models	227
6.9	Goodness-of-fit procedures	228
6.10	Examples	234
6.11	Exercises	240

7 Multiplicative-Additive hazards models — 249
7.1	The Cox-Aalen hazards model		251
	7.1.1	Model and estimation	252
	7.1.2	Inference and large sample properties	255
	7.1.3	Goodness-of-fit procedures	260
	7.1.4	Estimating the survival function	266
	7.1.5	Example	270
7.2	Proportional excess hazards model		273
	7.2.1	Model and score equations	274
	7.2.2	Estimation and inference	276
	7.2.3	Efficient estimation	280
	7.2.4	Goodness-of-fit procedures	283
	7.2.5	Examples	284
7.3	Exercises		290

8 Accelerated failure time and transformation models — 293
8.1	The accelerated failure time model	294
8.2	The semiparametric transformation model	298

	8.3	Exercises	309

9 Clustered failure time data — 313
9.1 Marginal regression models for clustered failure time data . 314
    9.1.1 Working independence assumption 315
    9.1.2 Two-stage estimation of correlation 327
    9.1.3 One-stage estimation of correlation 330
9.2 Frailty models 334
9.3 Exercises 338

10 Competing Risks Model — 347
10.1 Product limit estimator 351
10.2 Cause specific hazards modeling 356
10.3 Subdistribution approach 361
10.4 Exercises 370

11 Marked point process models — 375
11.1 Nonparametric additive model for longitudinal data 380
11.2 Semiparametric additive model for longitudinal data 389
11.3 Efficient estimation 393
11.4 Marginal models 397
11.5 Exercises 408

A Khmaladze's transformation — 411

B Matrix derivatives — 415

C The Timereg survival package for R — 417

Bibliography — 453

Index — 467

1
Introduction

The intention with this chapter is to introduce the reader to the most important issues dealt with in this monograph. As mentioned in the Preface we aim at highly flexible models for survival data with special focus on time-varying covariate effects having a statistical regression setup in mind. This chapter should give some intuition into the main ideas underlying the suggested methodology, and also a flavor of the use of the developed R-functions implementing the models that we study.

1.1 Survival data

Survival analysis or failure time data analysis means the statistical analysis of data, where the response of interest is the time T^* from a well-defined time origin to the occurrence of some given event (end-point). In biomedicine the key example is the time from randomization to a given treatment for some patients until death occurs leading to the observation of survival times for these patients. In behavioral studies in agricultural science, one often observes the time from when a domestic animal has received some stimulus until it responds with a given type of action. Returning to the survival data, the objective may be to compare different treatment effects on the survival time possibly correcting for information available on each patient such as age and disease progression indicators. This leaves us with a statistical regression analysis problem. Standard methods will, however, often be inappropriate because survival times are frequently incompletely

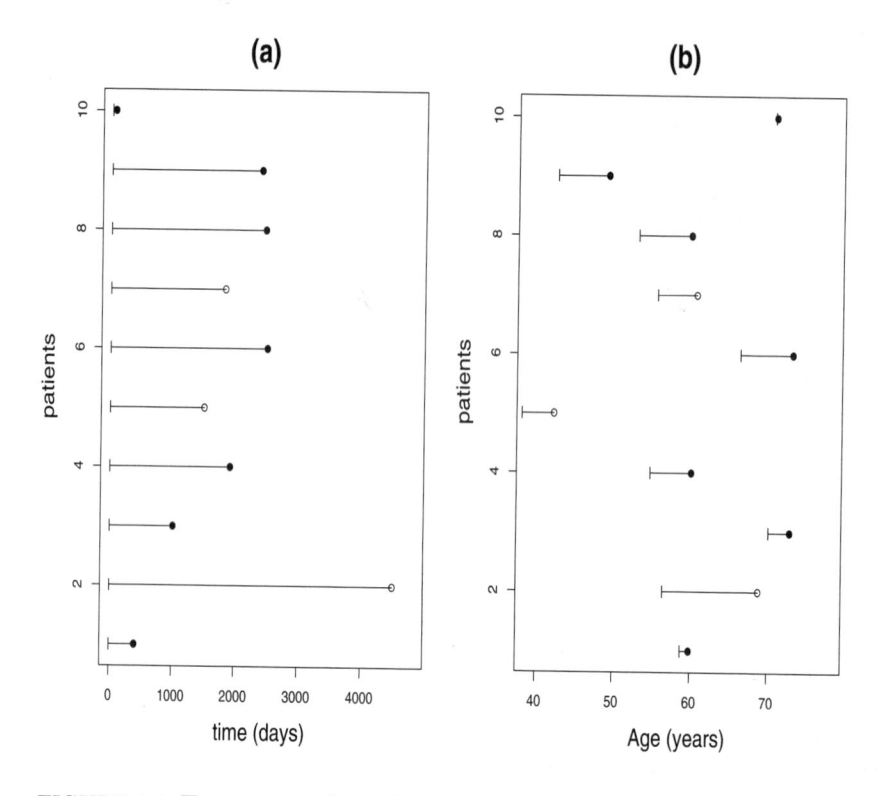

FIGURE 1.1: Ten patients from the PBC study on follow-up time scale (left panel) and on age scale (right panel)

observed with the most common example being *right censoring*. The survival time T^* is said to be right censored if it is only known that T^* is larger than an observed right censoring value. This may be because the patient is still alive at the point in time where the study is closed and the data are to be analyzed, or because the subject is lost for follow-up due to other reasons. If T^* is the time to death from a given cause, then death from another cause may also be regarded as a censored observation (competing risks). Other types of incompleteness can also occur, which are described in a general framework in Chapter 3. Below is a study used repeatedly in this book.

Example 1.1.1 (PBC data)

The PBC dataset described in Fleming & Harrington (1991) originates from a Mayo Clinic trial in primary biliary cirrhosis (PBC) of the liver and was conducted between 1974 and 1984. A total of 418 patients are included in the dataset and were followed until death or censoring. In addition to time at risk and censoring indicator, 17 covariates are recorded for this study.

1.1 Survival data

These include a treatment variable, patient age, sex and clinical, biochemical and histologic measurements made at the time of randomization to one of the two treatments. For a detailed description of all the covariates, see Fleming & Harrington (1991). Below is a printout for the first 10 patient of the dataset giving the information on the time to death (in days), whether the recorded time is censored or not, and information on five explanatory variables that are found to be important by Fleming & Harrington (1991).

```
> library(survival)
> data(pbc)
> attach(pbc)
> cbind(time,status,age,edema,alb,bili,protime)[1:10,]
      time status     age edema  alb bili protime
 [1,]  400      1 58.7652     1 2.60 14.5    12.2
 [2,] 4500      0 56.4463     0 4.14  1.1    10.6
 [3,] 1012      1 70.0726     1 3.48  1.4    12.0
 [4,] 1925      1 54.7406     1 2.54  1.8    10.3
 [5,] 1504      0 38.1054     0 3.53  3.4    10.9
 [6,] 2503      1 66.2587     0 3.98  0.8    11.0
 [7,] 1832      0 55.5346     0 4.09  1.0     9.7
 [8,] 2466      1 53.0568     0 4.00  0.3    11.0
 [9,] 2400      1 42.5079     0 3.08  3.2    11.0
[10,]   51      1 70.5599     1 2.74 12.6    11.5
```

The first patient has a lifetime (from time of randomization of treatment) of 400 days. For the second patient, which is a censored case, we only know that the lifetime is beyond 4500 (days), and so on.

We use a slightly modified version of these data where all ties are randomly broken in the remainder of the book. We also center all continuous covariates around their respective averages such that for example log(Bilirubin) is a centered version of log(Bilirubin).

Figure 1.1 shows the survival times on two different time-scales. Figure 1.1 left panel is on follow-up time-scale, which is the time-scale of interest in this study since we wish to study the lifetimes after inclusion in the study, where a specific treatment is given. Age is of course an important factor when studying the lifetimes and should therefore be corrected for in a subsequent analysis of the importance of potential risk factors. The starting point for all observations on the follow-up time-scale is zero, and those censored later on are indicated with an open ball, whereas those that are observed to die during the study are marked with a filled ball.

Figure 1.1 right panel shows the similar survival times on the age time-scale. If age was used as the time-scale for the analysis, the data would have delayed entry because the patient entered the study at different ages and are alive at inclusion, and this must be dealt with in a subsequent analysis. Otherwise there is a risk that long lifetimes will be over-represented (long lifetimes have a higher probability of being sampled), which is referred to

4   1. Introduction

as length-bias. Working on the age time-scale, such data are also called left-truncated since the subjects are sampled subject to being alive. □

One goal of an analysis of right-censored survival data could be to estimate regression parameters that relate to the mortality and examine various hypotheses about the impact of various risk factors. It is not clear at first sight how to incorporate the censored observations into such a statistical analysis. Basing the statistical analysis on only the complete data may give biased results, so the censored observations need to be taken into account. It turns out that handling of censoring and other types of incomplete survival data is surprisingly easy when basing the analysis on models for the so-called *intensity function* (given that censoring fulfills a certain condition). The intensity function is closely related to the *hazard function*. Suppose that the distribution of the lifetime T^* has density f and let $S(t) = P(T^* > t)$ denote the *survival function*. The hazard function is defined as

$$\alpha(t) = \frac{f(t)}{S(t)} = \lim_{h \downarrow 0} \frac{1}{h} P(t \leq T^* < t+h \mid T^* \geq t),$$

which may be interpreted as the instantaneous failure rate among those at risk. The survival function may be calculated from the hazard function by

$$S(t) = \exp(-\int_0^t \alpha(s)\, ds). \qquad (1.1)$$

The density, survival and hazard function provide alternative but equivalent characterizations of the distribution of T^*.

To illustrate how easy it is to estimate the hazard function even when data are observed subject to right censoring consider the simplest possible case where the hazard originates from an exponential waiting time distribution, which we return to in Example 3.2.4.

Example 1.1.2 (Exponential distribution)

If the survival time T^* has constant hazard function $\alpha(t) = \alpha$, then T^* is *exponentially* distributed with mean $1/\alpha$, see (1.1). Assume we observe in the time interval $[0, \tau]$ and that the observation is right-censored at time $U = u \wedge \tau$. We here consider U as fixed to avoid a more detailed discussion of the censoring mechanisms at this stage. We then observe $T = T^* \wedge U$ and $\Delta = I(T^* \leq U)$.

Based on n i.i.d. replicates from this model, the likelihood function may be written as

$$\prod_{i=1}^n \alpha^{\Delta_i} \exp(-\int_0^{T_i} \alpha\, ds) = \alpha^{\Delta_\cdot} \exp(-T_\cdot \alpha),$$

where $\Delta. = \sum_i \Delta_i$ is the total number of observed deaths and $T. = \sum_i T_i$ is the total risk time. The maximum likelihood estimator for the mortality rate α is thus

$$\hat{\alpha} = \frac{\Delta.}{T.}.$$

Hence, right censoring is no problem when we estimate the intensity; we should just relate the number of observed occurrences to the total amount of risk time. □

If the focus is on the cumulative hazard function ($\int_0^t \alpha(s)ds$) or the survival function, then these can be estimated non-parametrically using the Nelson-Aalen estimator and the Kaplan-Meier estimator, respectively. These classical procedures are described in Chapter 4.

It turns out that a convenient representation of the data is by the *counting process*

$$N(t) = I(T^* \leq t),$$

which is zero until t passes T^*, where it jumps to unity. A counting process has a (unique) *compensator* $\Lambda(t)$ so that

$$M(t) = N(t) - \Lambda(t)$$

is a martingale, which can be thought of as an error process. The intensity process $\lambda(t)$ is defined by

$$\Lambda(t) = \int_0^t \lambda(s)\, ds,$$

and it turns out that $\lambda(t) = Y(t)\alpha(t)$, where

$$Y(t) = I(t \leq T^*)$$

is called the at-risk process; it is one as long as the individual is at risk meaning that T^* has yet not occurred. The intensity process of $N(t)$ and the hazard function are hence closely linked with the latter being the deterministic (model) part of the former. By this representation of the data we have

$$N(t) = \Lambda(t) + M(t),$$

which can be thought of as

$$\text{observation} = \text{model} + \text{error},$$

and indeed there is a central limit theorem for martingales, which facilitates asymptotic description of the behavior of specific estimators and test statistics. The above representation of data is further convenient when we only observe incomplete data. Suppose for example that T^* is right-censored by U so the observed data are

$$(T, \Delta),$$

where $T = T^* \wedge U$ denotes the minimum of the true lifetime and censoring time and $\Delta = I(T^* \leq U)$ is an indicator telling us whether we observe T^* or U. That is, we observe the smallest value of the lifetime and the censoring time, and which of the two that has the smallest value. It turns out (under independent censoring, Chapter 3) that the intensity process of the observed counting process

$$N(t) = I(T \leq t, \Delta = 1),$$

which jumps only if the lifetime is observed, is

$$\lambda(t) = I(t \leq T)\alpha(t),$$

so $I(t \leq T^*)$ is replaced by the observed at risk indicator $I(t \leq T)$. The multiplicative structure of the intensity is thus preserved with the deterministic part still being the hazard function. The at risk indicator $Y(t)$ is as mentioned changed to $I(t \leq T)$ so the subject is at risk (for observing the specific event of interest) as long as the event or censoring has not yet occurred. The multiplicative structure of the intensity for right-censored (and more generally filtered) data is a key observation since martingale methods can then still be applied.

In many studies, as for example the PBC study, the main interest will be to evaluate different explanatory variables effect on the lifetimes taking into account that some of the lifetimes are censored (or otherwise incomplete). Suppose we observe n i.i.d. (T_i, Δ_i, X_i), where T_i is the right-censored lifetime, Δ_i is the indicator telling us whether T_i is un-censored or censored, and X_i is a (vector) of explanatory variables. As argued above it is convenient to build a regression model using the (conditional) hazard function as target function. A very popular model is the proportional hazards model (Chapter 6) of Cox (1972):

$$\alpha_i(t) = \alpha_0(t) \exp(X_i^T \beta),$$

where β denotes the unknown regression parameters and $\alpha_0(t)$ is the baseline hazard function (the hazard function for an individual with $X = 0$) that is left unspecified. The model is thus semiparametric. The regression parameters can be estimated as the zero solution to the Cox score function

$$U(\beta) = \sum_{i=1}^{n} (X_i - E(\beta, T_i))\Delta_i,$$

where

$$E(\beta, t) = \frac{\sum_{i=1}^{n} Y_i(t) X_i \exp(X_i^T \beta)}{\sum_{i=1}^{n} Y_i(t) \exp(X_i^T \beta)}$$

with $Y_i(t) = I(t \leq T_i)$, $i = 1, \ldots, n$. The Cox score function can also be written as $U(\beta, \infty)$, where

$$U(\beta, t) = \sum_{i=1}^{n} \int_0^t (X_i - E(\beta, s))dN_i(s),$$

which, evaluated at the true regression parameter β_0, is a martingale! One can show (under some regularity conditions) that the estimator $\hat{\beta}$ is asymptotically normal around the true value β_0 using the martingale central limit theorem. The theory of counting processes and martingales is described in Chapter 2.

The nonparametric element, $\alpha_0(t)$, of the Cox model makes the model flexible since no specific distribution is assumed for the baseline group (defined by $X = 0$). Owing to this, the easy interpretation of the regression parameters as (log)-relative risks:

$$\frac{\alpha(t, X_1 = 1, X_2)}{\alpha(t, X_1 = 0, X_2)} = \exp(\beta_1), \quad (1.2)$$

where X_1 is one-dimensional and $X = (X_1, X_2^T)^T$, and the availability of software to perform estimation and inference in the model, the Cox model has had tremendous success in applied work. In some applications, however, the relative risks may not take the simple form (1.2) and there is therefore a need for alternative models. A typical deviation from the Cox model is that the covariate effects change with time. In a randomized trial that aims to evaluate the effect of a new treatment, it may take some time before it has an effect, or the treatment may have an effect initially, which is then weakened with time. More generally, some risk factors will have a strong prognostic effect right after being recorded but will gradually loose their predictive power. We illustrate this by considering the TRACE study.

Example 1.1.3 (The TRACE study of AMI)

The TRACE study group, see Jensen et al. (1997), studied the prognostic importance of various risk factors on mortality for approximately 6600 patients with acute myocardial infarction (AMI). The TRACE data included in the `timereg` package is a random sample of 2000 of these patients.

The recorded risk factors are age, sex (female=1), clinical heart failure (chf) (present=1), ventricular fibrillation (vf) (present=1), and diabetes (present=1). It is well known that patients with vf present are at a much higher risk of dying soon after being admitted.

To illustrate this point we fitted a standard Cox regression model with the factors vf and sex, and compared the survival predictions with those based on a completely non-parametric modeling (four Kaplan-Meier curves). These estimates are shown in Figure 1.2 (a). We note that the constant relative risk characterization is not consistent with the data. The Cox model gives a poor fit to the data for subjects with the vf condition. The difference in survival between males and females is captured well by the Cox model. Figure 1.2 (b) shows similar predictions based on the additive hazards model with time-varying effects of vf and sex (explained below). These predictions much better describe the mortality pattern since the model captures that the effect of vf changes with time.

8   1. Introduction

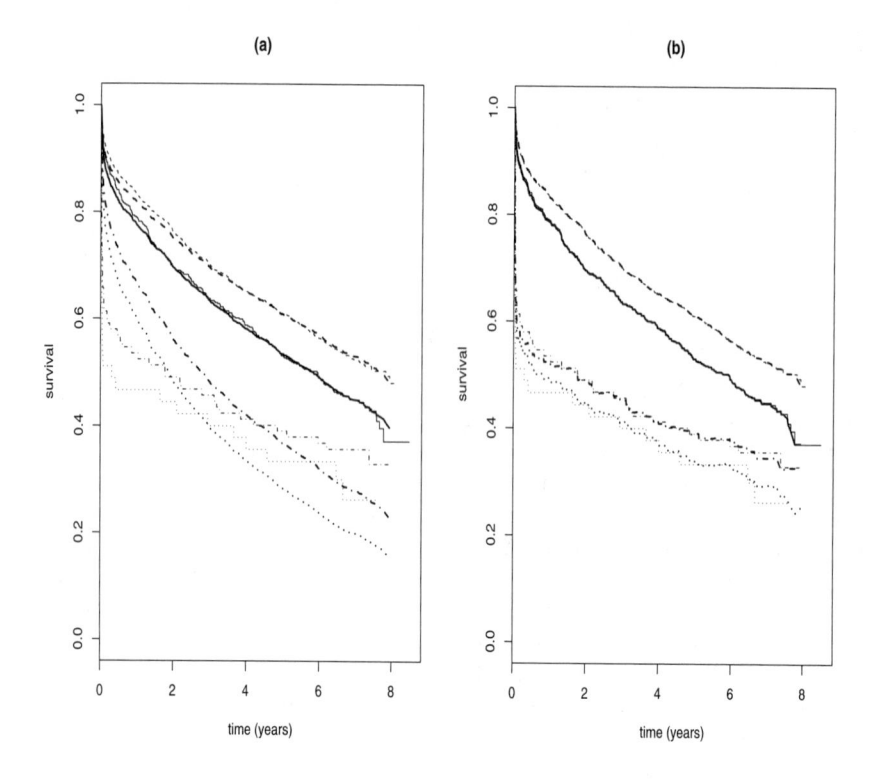

FIGURE 1.2: (a) Survival predictions based on Cox regression model compared with non-parametric (Kaplan-Meier) estimates (step functions) for four groups based on status of vf and sex. Full line (without vf, male), broken line (without vf, female), dotted line (with vf, female), and broken-dotted (with vf, male). (b) Survival predictions based on additive hazards model with time-varying effects compared with non-parametric (Kaplan-Meier) estimates for four groups. Full line (without vf, male), broken line (without vf, female), dotted line (with vf, female), and broken-dotted (with vf, male).

The additive hazards model assumes that the hazard for a subject can be written in the form

$$\alpha(t) = \beta_0(t) + X_1\beta_1(t) + X_2\beta_2(t),$$

where X_1 and X_2 are indicators of the presence of vf and sex, respectively. Figure 1.3 shows estimates with 95% pointwise confidence intervals of the cumulative regression functions of the model:

$$\int_0^t \beta_j(s)ds, \quad j = 0, 1, 2.$$

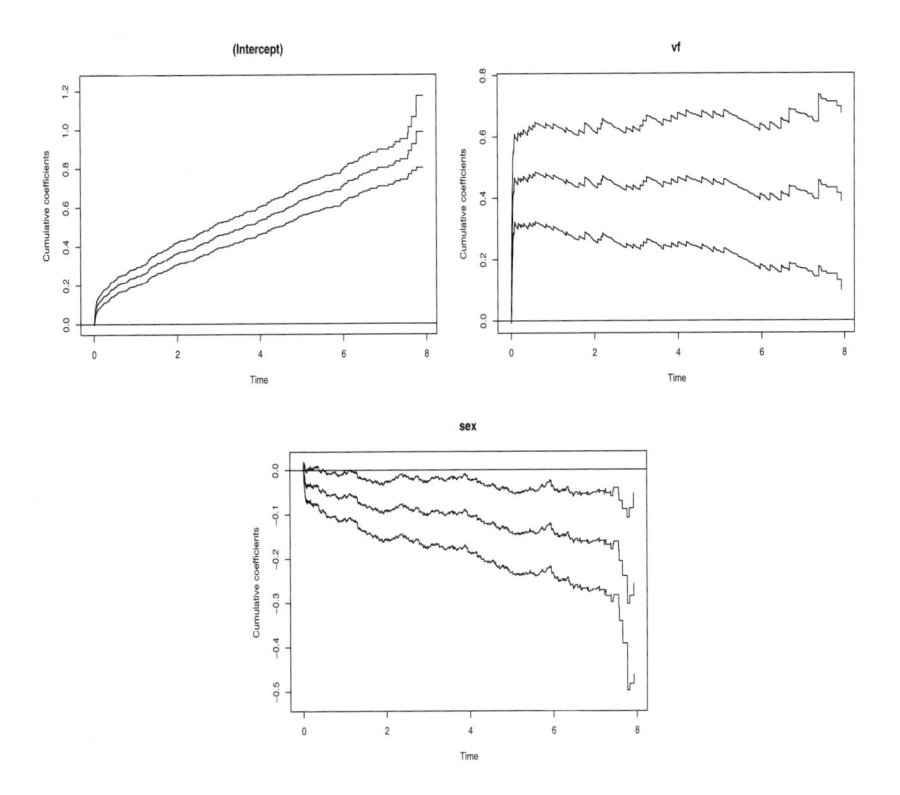

FIGURE 1.3: Effects of vf and sex (female=1) based on time-varying additive hazard model with 95% pointwise confidence intervals.

The regression function estimates are thus the slopes of the cumulative estimates, and note that, for this model, these can be interpreted as leading to excess risk of dying. It is relatively easy to see from the figure that vf has a strong effect initially and that its effect vanishes after approximately 3 months with the cumulative regression function estimate being essentially constant. Females are seen to have a constant lower risk than males. □

The TRACE study demonstrates the need for survival models that are flexible enough to deal with time-varying dynamics of covariate effects. One obvious extension of the Cox model that can accommodate this is

$$\alpha_i(t) = \alpha_0(t) \exp(X_i^T \beta(t)), \quad (1.3)$$

where the regression coefficients $\beta(t)$ are allowed to depend on time. A natural question to ask then is whether in fact all these coefficients need to depend on time or whether a treatment effect, for example, is reasonably well described by the relative-risk measure. This leads to the submodel

$$\alpha_i(t) = \alpha_0(t) \exp(X_i^T \beta(t) + Z_i \gamma), \quad (1.4)$$

where some of the covariates (X) have time-varying effect and others (Z) have constant effect. Estimation and inference for these extended Cox models, (1.3) and (1.4), are described in detail in Chapter 6. These multiplicative models are very useful but there are also other models that are simple to use and may be well suited to deal with time-varying effects.

A model class with an alternative structure is Aalen's additive hazard regression models, where it is assumed that

$$\alpha_i(t) = X_i^T \beta(t),$$

that is the effect of the covariates acts on an absolute scale rather than on a relative scale. The effect of the covariates is also allowed to change with time. This particular aspect is very easy to handle for this model because it fits nicely into the linear model structure of the counting process representation of the data:

$$N(t) = \Lambda(t) + M(t).$$

Suppose we have n i.i.d. observations from the Aalen model and let $N(t) = (N_1(t), \ldots, N_n(t))^T$, $M(t) = (M_1(t), \ldots, M_n(t))^T$, and $X(t)$ the $n \times p$-matrix with ith row

$$Y_i(t)(X_{i1}(t), \ldots, X_{ip}(t))$$

consisting of the at-risk indicator multiplied onto the p observed covariates for the ith subject. Writing the model in differential form

$$dN(t) = X(t)dB(t) + dM(t),$$

where

$$B(t) = \int_0^t \beta(s)\,ds$$

is the cumulative coefficients, immediately suggests that a reasonable (un-weighted) estimator of $B(t)$ is

$$\hat{B}(t) = \int_0^t (X(s)^T X(s))^{-1} X(s)^T dN(s)$$

since the error term, $dM(t)$, indeed has zero mean. The estimator in the last display looks complicated but is in fact nothing but a sum. It also turns out (asymptotically) that

$$n^{1/2}(\hat{B}(t) - B(t)) = n^{1/2} \int_0^t (X(s)^T X(s))^{-1} X(s)^T dM(s),$$

which is a martingale, and therefore large sample results may be derived using again the central limit theorem for martingales. As for the extended

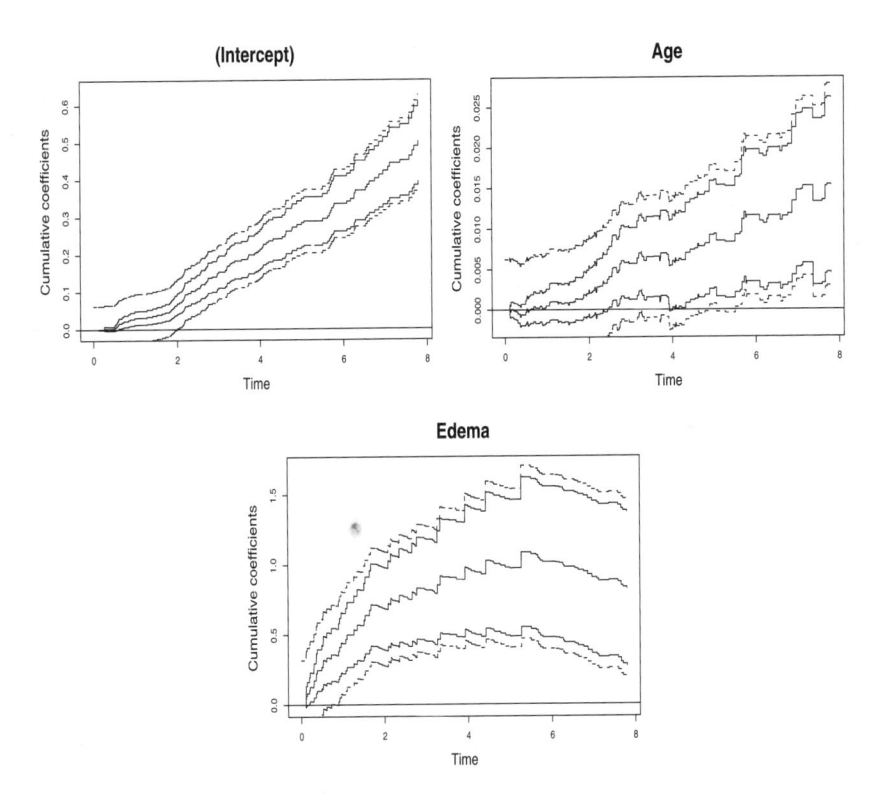

FIGURE 1.4: PBC data. Aalen-model with intercept, age centered around its mean and edema (present). Estimated cumulative regression functions with 95% pointwise confidence intervals (full lines) and 95% uniform confidence bands (broken lines).

Cox model, it is of interest to investigate whether in fact we have time-varying effect of a given covariate, X_1, say. That is, we wish to investigate the hypothesis

$$H_0 : \beta_1(t) = \gamma_1,$$

This is indeed possible using again martingale calculus. Let us see how it works for the PBC data.

Example 1.1.4 (PBC data)

For ease of interpretation lets consider only the effect of age and edema on survival. The Aalen model may be fitted in R using the package `timereg` in the following manner. Before fitting the model, age is centered around its mean and edema is scored 1 for edema present and 0 otherwise. The function `aalen` fits the model, where below we restrict attention to the first 8 years after start of the study. We see from Figure 1.4 that the regression coefficient associated with edema seems to change with time (the cumulative does not seem to be a straight line) whereas the one associated with age appears to be constant with time. The curves along with the shown estimates are 95% pointwise confidence limits (inner curves) and 95% uniform Hall-Wellner bands (outer curves). The Hall-Wellner band is introduced in Chapter 2. The intercept curve corresponds to the cumulative hazard function for a subject with average age (in the sample) and without edema.

```
> data(pbc); attach(pbc)
> Age<-age-mean(age); Edema<-edema
> fit<-aalen(Surv(time/365,status)~Age+Edema,pbc,max.time=8)
Nonparametric Additive Risk Model
Simulations start N= 1000
> plot(fit,hw.ci=2);
> summary(fit)
Additive Aalen Model

Test for nonparametric terms

Test for non-significant effects
            sup| hat B(t)/SD(t) | p-value H_0: B(t)=0
(Intercept)              9.32                0.000
Age                      3.19                0.027
Edema                    4.78                0.000
Test for time invariant effects
            sup| B(t) - (t/tau)B(tau)| p-value H_0: B(t)=b t
(Intercept)              0.06840              0.120
Age                      0.00237              0.943
Edema                    0.56700              0.000

            int (B(t)-(t/tau)B(tau))^2dt p-value H_0: B(t)=b t
(Intercept)              1.44e-02              0.052
Age                      1.34e-05              0.794
Edema                    1.32e+00              0.000
```

Based on the depicted curves it would seem natural to estimate the effect of age by a constant, and we therefore start by testing whether the effect of age is constant. This test (and the test for the other effects) is obtained using the summary function on the fitted object called fit, and we see indeed that there is no reason to believe that the effect of age should change with time while the same hypothesis concerning the effect of edema is clearly rejected. Actually two types of tests are performed: a supremum and an integrated squared test. It is described in Chapter 5 how these are constructed and what their properties are. It is thus natural to go on with the simplified model assuming constant effect of age. This model is fitted below and stored in the object fit.semi and we see that constant effect of age is estimated as 0.0018 with an estimated standard error of 0.000584, giving a clearly significant Wald test. The hypothesis of constant effect of edema is again clearly rejected. This test is now performed in the simplified model where the effect of age is set to be time-invariant.

```
> fit.semi<-aalen(Surv(time/365,status)~const(Age)+Edema,pbc,
+ max.time=8)
Semiparametric Additive Risk Model
Simulations start N= 1000
> summary(fit.semi)
Additive Aalen Model

Test for nonparametric terms

Test for non-significant effects
            sup| hat B(t)/SD(t) | p-value H_0: B(t)=0
(Intercept)           13.5                  0
Edema                  4.7                  0
Test for time invariant effects
            sup| B(t) - (t/tau)B(tau)| p-value H_0: B(t)=b t
(Intercept)           0.0667                  0.001
Edema                 0.5610                  0.000

            int (B(t)-(t/tau)B(tau))^2dt p-value H_0: B(t)=b t
(Intercept)           0.014                    0.001
Edema                 1.260                    0.000


Parametric terms :
            Coef.    SE Robust SE      z   P-val
const(Age) 0.00178 0.000584  0.000582  3.05 0.00226
```

The additive Aalen model and its semiparametric version along with goodness-of-fit and inference tools are described in Chapter 5.

Although the extended Cox model and the additive Aalen model are very flexible (they are first-order Taylor expansions, around the zero covariate, of fully nonparametric log-hazard and hazard functions, respectively), there will sometimes be a need for other models. In Chapter 7 we consider combinations of multiplicative and additive hazard models. These models can also be fitted in R using the timereg package.

Accelerated failure time and transformation models are described briefly in Chapter 8. These are regression models that are developed from another perspective than when one focuses on the hazard function, but they do of course have a hazard function representation. They may represent good alternatives to both the Cox and Aalen models, and will lead to other useful

14   1. Introduction

summary measures. These models are difficult, however, to extend to deal with time-varying effects.

Chapter 9 contains a brief and selective description of clustered survival data, again with special emphasis on how to deal with time-varying effects and how the time-varying dynamic regression models discussed in the previous chapters can be implemented for this type of data. Finally, for survival data, we have included a brief discussion in Chapter 10 on competing risks models, again with special emphasis on models that are able to deal with time-varying covariate effects.

1.2 Longitudinal data

The final chapter is on longitudinal data, which is somewhat different compared to the rest of the material of this book. It is included, however, to show that many of the same techniques used for survival analysis may in fact also be applied to longitudinal data analysis. Longitudinal data for a given subject (the ith) can be represented as

$$(T_i^k, Z_i^k, X_i(t))$$

where T_i^k is the time-point for the kth measurement Z_i^k of the longitudinal response variable, and $X_i(t)$ is a possibly time-dependent covariate vector ($q \times 1$) associated with the ith subject. We study time-varying additive models where the conditional mean $m_i(t)$ at time t of the response variable given what is observed so far is

$$m_i(t) = \beta_0(t) + \beta_1(t)X_{i1}(t) + \cdots + \beta_q(t)X_{iq}(t), \qquad (1.5)$$

where $\beta_0(t), \ldots, \beta_q(t)$ are unspecified time-dependent regression functions. For this model and a corresponding marginal model, we will show how one can estimate the cumulative regression coefficient functions $B(t) = \int_0^t \beta(s)ds$. It turns out that

$$\sum_k Z_i^k I(T_i^k \leq t) = \int_0^t \alpha(s) Y_i(s) X_i^T(s) \, dB(s) + \text{martingale}, \qquad (1.6)$$

where

$$X_i^T(t) = (1, X_{i1}(t), \ldots, X_{iq}(t))$$

and with $\alpha(t)$ the conditional measurement intensity. We see that (1.6) has the same structure as what was obtained for survival models, especially the Aalen additive model. Indeed, a natural estimator of $B(t)$ is easily constructed from the above representation, and large-sample properties and inference may be studied using martingale calculus again. The left-hand side of (1.6) is called a marked point process integral, which is introduced in Chapter 2. Let us close this section with an application showing the use of the techniques developed for longitudinal data.

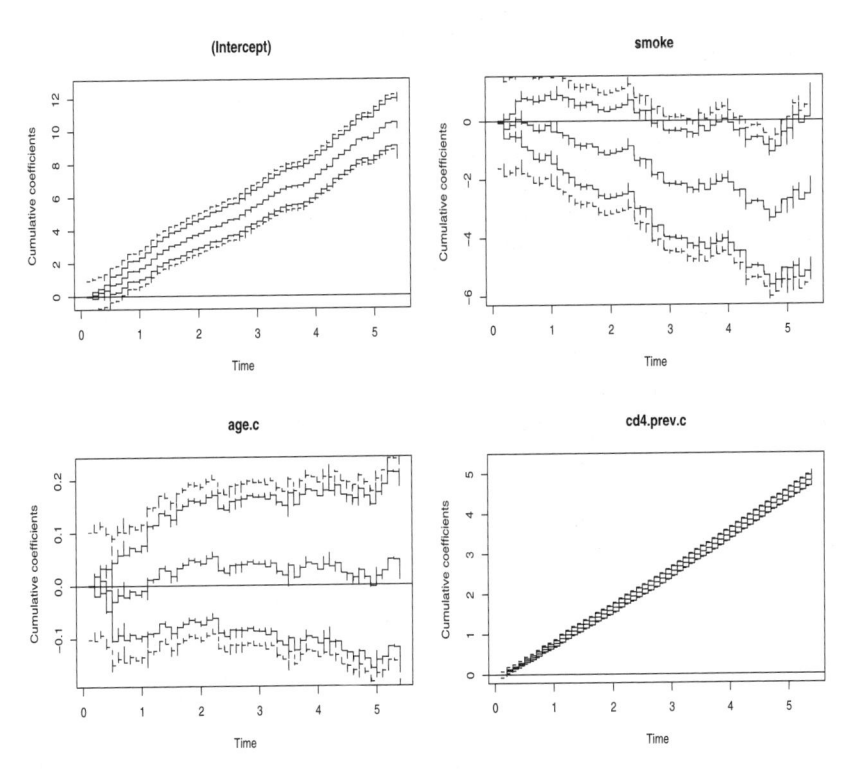

FIGURE 1.5: Estimated cumulative coefficients functions for the baseline CD4 percentage and the effects of smoking, age and previous response. Curves are shown along with 95% pointwise confidence limits and 95% Hall-Wellner bands

Example 1.2.1 (CD4 data)

The AIDS dataset described in Huang et al. (2002) is a subset from the Multicenter AIDS Cohort Study. The data include the repeated measurements of CD4 cell counts and percentages of 283 homosexual men who became HIV-positive between 1984 and 1991. Details about the design, methods and medical implications of the study can be found in Kaslow et al. (1987). All individuals were scheduled to have their measurements made at semi-annual visits, but, because many individuals missed some of their scheduled visits and the HIV infections happened randomly during the study, there are unequal numbers of repeated measurements and different measurement times per individual. We consider the model

$$m_i(t) = \beta_0(t) + \beta_1(t)X_{i1} + \beta_2(t)X_{i2} + \beta_3(t)X_{i3}(t),$$

where X_1 is smoking, X_2 is age at HIV-infection and $X_3(t)$ is the at-time-t previous measured response. Both X_2 and X_3 were centered around their respective averages. The model (1.5) can be fitted in timereg using the function dynreg as illustrated below.

```
> age.c<-age-mean(age)
> cd4.prev.c<-cd4.prev-mean(cd4.prev)
> indi<-rep(1,length(cd4$lt))
> fit.cd4<-dynreg(cd4~smoke+age.c+cd4.prev.c,data=cd4,
+ Surv(lt,rt,indi)~+1,start.time=0,max.time=5.5,id=cd4$id,
+ n.sim=500,bandwidth=0.15,meansub=1)
> plot(fit.cd4,hw.ci=2)
```

The above plot command gives the estimated cumulative regression effects associated with the included covariates along with 95% pointwise confidence limits and 95% uniform Hall-Wellner bands, Figure 1.5. Judging from the figure, it seems that the effect of all the included covariates is constant. This can be pursued with statistical tests as also illustrated before with the Aalen additive model for survival data. This is described in Chapter 11. □

2
Probabilistic background

2.1 Preliminaries

Event time data, where one is interested in the time to a specific event occurs, are conveniently studied by the use of certain stochastic processes. The data itself may be described as a so-called counting process, which is simply a random function of time t, $N(t)$. It is zero at time zero and constant over time except that it jumps at each point in time where an event occurs, the jumps being of size 1.

Figure 2.1 shows two counting processes. Figure 2.1 (a) shows a counting process for survival data where one event is observed at time 7 at the time of death for a patient. Figure 2.1 (b) illustrates the counting process for recurrent events data where an event is observed multiple times, such as the times of dental cavities, with events at times 3, 4 and 7.

Why is this useful one could ask. Obviously, it is just a mathematical framework to represent timings of events, but a nice and useful theory has been developed for counting processes. A counting process $N(t)$ can be decomposed into a model part and a random noise part

$$N(t) = \Lambda(t) + M(t),$$

referred to as the compensator $\Lambda(t)$ and the martingale $M(t)$ of the counting process. These two parts are also functions of time and stochastic. The strength of this representation is that a central limit theorem is available for martingales. This in turn makes it possible to derive large sample properties of estimators for rather general nonparametric and semiparametric models

18   2. Probabilistic background

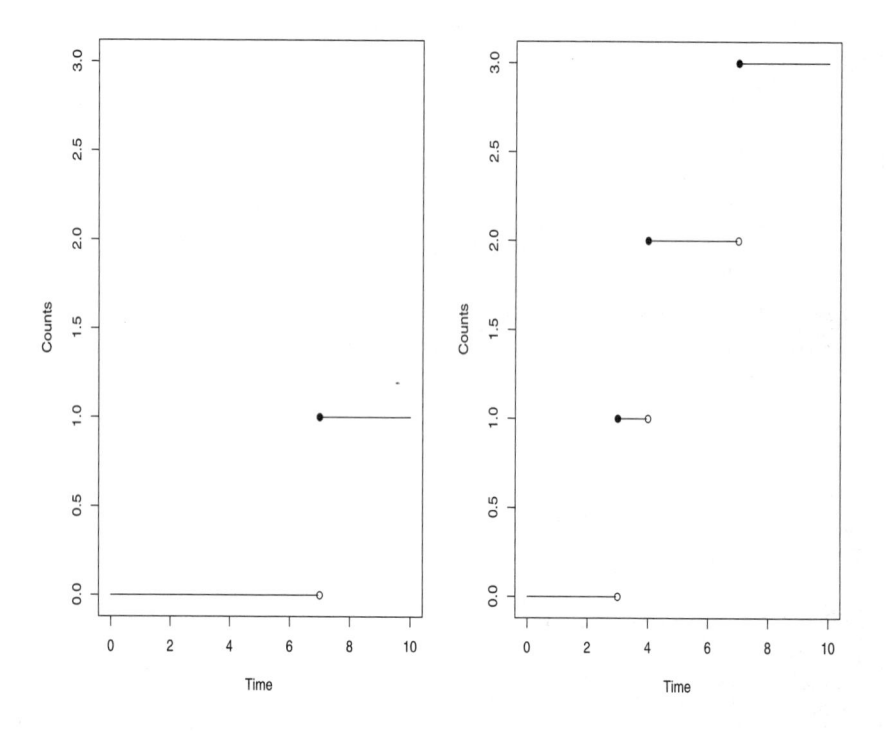

FIGURE 2.1: (a) Counting process for survival data with event time at time 7. (b) Counting process for recurrent events data, with event times at 3,4 and 7.

for such data. One chief example of this is the famous Cox model, which we return to in Section 6.1. To read more about counting processes and their theory we refer to Brémaud (1981), Jacobsen (1982), Fleming & Harrington (1991) and Andersen et al. (1993).

When assumptions are weakened, sometimes the decomposition will not result in an error term that is a martingale but only a zero-mean stochastic process, and in this case asymptotic properties can be developed using empirical process theory; see, for example, van der Vaart & Wellner (1996).

We shall also demonstrate that similar flexible models for longitudinal data may be studied fruitfully by the use of martingale methods. The key to this is that longitudinal data may be represented by a so-called marked point process, a generalization of a counting process. A marked point process is a mathematical construction to represent timing of events and their corresponding marks, and this is precisely the structure of longitudinal data where responses (marks) are collected over time. As for counting processes, a theory has been developed that decomposes a marked point process into a model part (compensator) and a random noise part (martingale). As a consequence of this, the analysis of longitudinal data therefore has many parallels with counting process data, and martingale methods may be invoked when studying large sample properties of concrete estimators. Some key references for additional reading about marked point processes are Brémaud (1981) and Last & Brandt (1995).

Before giving the definitions and properties of counting processes, marked point processes and martingales, we need to introduce some concepts from general stochastic process theory.

Behind all theory to be developed is a measurable space $(\Omega, \mathcal{F}, P)$, where $\mathcal{F}$ is a σ-field and P is probability measure defined on $\mathcal{F}$. A *stochastic process* is a family of random variables indexed by time $(X(t) : t \geq 0)$. The mapping $t \to X(t, \omega)$, for $\omega \in \Omega$, is called a sample path. The stochastic process X induces a family of increasing sub-σ-fields by

$$\mathcal{F}_t^X = \sigma\{X(s) : 0 \leq s \leq t\}$$

called the *internal history* of X. Often when formulating models we will condition on events that occurred prior in time. We could for example, at time t, condition on the history generated by the process X up to time t. In many applications, however, we will need to condition on further information than that generated by only one stochastic process. To this end we therefore define more generally a *history* $(\mathcal{F}_t; t \geq 0)$ as a family of sub-σ-fields such that, for all $s \leq t$, $\mathcal{F}_s \subset \mathcal{F}_t$, which means $A \in \mathcal{F}_s$ implies $A \in \mathcal{F}_t$. A history is also called a *filtration*. Sometimes information (filtrations) are combined and for two filtrations $\mathcal{F}_t^1$ and $\mathcal{F}_t^2$ we let $\mathcal{F}_t^1 \vee \mathcal{F}_t^2$ denote the smallest filtration that contains both $\mathcal{F}_t^1$ and $\mathcal{F}_t^2$. A stochastic process X is *adapted* to a filtration $\mathcal{F}_t$ if, for every $t \geq 0$, $X(t)$ is $\mathcal{F}_t$-measurable, and in this case $\mathcal{F}_t^X \subset \mathcal{F}_t$. We shall often be dealing with stochastic processes with sample paths that, for almost all ω, are right-continuous and with left-hand limits. Such processes are called *cadlag* (continu à droite, limité à gauche). For a function f we define the right-hand limit $f(t+) = lim_{s \to t, s > t} f(s)$ and the left-hand limit $f(t-) = lim_{s \to t, s < t} f(s)$.

A nonnegative random variable T is called a *stopping time* with respect to $\mathcal{F}_t$ if $(T \leq t) \in \mathcal{F}_t$, for all $t \geq 0$. For a stochastic process X and a stopping time T, the stopped process X^T is defined by $X(t) = X(t \wedge T)$, where $a \wedge b$ denotes the minimum of a and b. A localizing sequence is a sequence of stopping times T_n that is nondecreasing and satisfies $T_n \to \infty$ as $n \to \infty$. A property of a stochastic process X is said to hold locally if there exists a localizing sequence (T_n) such that, for each n, the stopped process X^{T_n} has the property.

2.2 Martingales

Martingales play an important role in the statistical applications to be presented in this monograph. Often we shall see that estimating functions (evaluated at true parameter values) and the difference between estimators and true values are (up to a lower-order term) martingales. Owing to the existence of the celebrated central limit theorem for martingales of Rebolledo (1980), there is an elegant and simple approach to derive a complete asymptotic description of the suggested estimators. In the following we give the definition of a martingale.

A martingale with respect to a filtration $\mathcal{F}_t$ is a right-continuous stochastic process M with left-hand limits that, in addition to some technical conditions:

(i) M is adapted to $\mathcal{F}_t$, and (ii) $E|M(t)| < \infty$ for all t,

possesses the key martingale property

$$\text{(iii)} \quad E(M(t)\,|\,\mathcal{F}_s) = M(s) \quad \text{for all } s \leq t, \tag{2.1}$$

thus stating that the mean of $M(t)$ given information up to time s is $M(s)$ or, equivalently,

$$E(dM(t)\,|\,\mathcal{F}_{t-}) = 0 \quad \text{for all } t > 0, \tag{2.2}$$

where $\mathcal{F}_{t-}$ is the smallest σ-algebra containing all $\mathcal{F}_s$, $s < t$ and $dM(t) = M((t+dt)-) - M(t-)$. A martingale thus has zero-mean increments given the past, and without conditioning. Condition (ii) above is referred to as M being *integrable*. A martingale may be thought of as an error process in the following sense.

- Since $E(M(t)) = E(M(0))$, a martingale has constant mean as a function of time, and if the martingale is zero at time zero (as will be the case in our applications), the mean will be zero. Such a martingale is also called a zero-mean martingale.

- Martingales have uncorrelated increments, that is, for a martingale M it holds that

$$\text{Cov}(M(t) - M(s), M(v) - M(u)) = 0 \tag{2.3}$$

for all $0 \leq s \leq t \leq u \leq v$.

If M satisfies

$$E(M(t)\,|\,\mathcal{F}_s) \geq M(s) \quad \text{for all } s \leq t, \tag{2.4}$$

instead of condition (2.1), then M is a submartingale. A martingale is called *square integrable* if $\sup_t E(M(t)^2) < \infty$. A *local martingale* M is a process such that there exist a localizing sequence of stopping times (T_n) such that, for each n, M^{T_n} is a martingale. If, in addition, M^{T_n} is a square integrable martingale, then M is said to be a *local square integrable martingale*.

To be able to formulate the crucial *Doob-Meyer* decomposition we need to introduce the notion of a predictable process. Loosely speaking, a predictable process is a process whose value at any time t is known just before t. Here is one characterization: a process X is predictable if and only if $X(T)$ is $\mathcal{F}_{T-}$-measurable for all stopping times T. The principal class of a predictable processes is the class of $\mathcal{F}_t$-adapted left-continuous processes.

Let X be a cadlag adapted process. Then A is said to be the *compensator* of X if A is a predictable, cadlag and *finite variation* process such that $X - A$ is a local zero-mean martingale. If a compensator exists, it is unique. A process A is said to be of finite variation if for all $t > 0$ (P-a.s.)

$$\int_0^t |dA(s)| = \sup_{\mathcal{D}} \sum_{i=1}^K |A(t_i) - A(t_{i-1})| < \infty,$$

where $\mathcal{D}$ ranges over all subdivisions of $[0,t]$: $0 = t_0 < t_1 < \cdots < t_K = t$.

One version of the Doob-Meyer decomposition as formulated in Andersen et al. (1993) is as follows.

Theorem 2.2.1 *The cadlag adapted process X has a compensator if and only if X is the difference of two local submartingales.*

An important simple consequence of the theorem is that, if the cadlag adapted process X is a local submartingale, then it has a compensator since the constant process 0 is a local submartingale.

Let M and $\tilde{M}$ be local square integrable martingales. By Jensen's inequality, M^2 is a local submartingale since

$$E(M^2(t) \mid \mathcal{F}_s) \geq (E(M(t) \mid \mathcal{F}_s))^2 = M^2(s)$$

and hence, by the Doob-Meyer decomposition, it has a compensator. This compensator is denoted by $\langle M, M \rangle$, or more compactly $\langle M \rangle$, and is termed the *predictable variation process* of M. By noting that $M\tilde{M} = \frac{1}{4}(M+\tilde{M})^2 - \frac{1}{4}(M-\tilde{M})^2$, it is similarly derived that $M\tilde{M}$ has a compensator, written $\langle M, \tilde{M} \rangle$, and termed the *predictable covariation process* of M and $\tilde{M}$.

The predictable covariation process is symmetric and bilinear like an ordinary covariance. If $\langle M, \tilde{M} \rangle = 0$, then M and $\tilde{M}$ are said to be *orthogonal*. The predictable covariation process is used to identify asymptotic covariances in the statistical applications to follow later on. This is partly explained by the relationship

$$\mathrm{Cov}(M(s), \tilde{M}(t)) = E(\langle M, \tilde{M} \rangle)(t), \quad s \leq t. \tag{2.5}$$

Estimation of the asymptotic covariances on the other hand may be carried out by use of the quadratic covariation process. This process is defined even when M and $\tilde{M}$ are just local martingales. When M and $\tilde{M}$ further are of finite variation (as will be the case in our applications), the *quadratic covariation process* of M and $\tilde{M}$, denoted by $[M,\tilde{M}]$, has the explicit form

$$[M,\tilde{M}](t) = \sum_{s\leq t} \Delta M(s)\Delta \tilde{M}(s). \tag{2.6}$$

In the case where $\tilde{M}=M$, (2.6) is written $[M](t)$ and called the *quadratic variation process* of M. The two processes $[M]$ and $[M,\tilde{M}]$ are also called the *optional variation process* and *optional covariation process*, respectively.

For the process $[M]$, it holds that $M^2 - [M]$ is a local martingale as was also the case with $\langle M \rangle$. An important distinction between the two processes, however, is that $[M]$ may not be predictable; in our applications it will never be! In the applications, the predictable variation process $\langle M \rangle$ will be determined by the model characteristics of the particular model studied while the quadratic variation process $[M]$ may be computed from the data at hand and therefore qualifies as a potential estimator.

Another useful characterization of $[M]$ is the following. When $[M]$ is locally integrable, then M will be locally square integrable and $\langle M \rangle$ will be the compensator of $[M]$! Similarly, $\langle M,\tilde{M} \rangle$ will be the compensator of $[M,\tilde{M}]$. This observation together with (2.6) enable us to compute both the quadratic and predictable covariation process.

In the statistical applications, stochastic integrals will come natural into play. Since we shall be dealing only with stochastic integrals where we integrate with respect to a finite variation process, all the considered stochastic integrals are ordinary pathwise Lebesgue-Stieltjes integrals, see Fleming & Harrington (1991) (Appendix A) for definitions. Of special interest are the integrals where we integrate with respect to a martingale. Such process integrals have nice properties as stated in the following.

Theorem 2.2.2 *Let M and $\tilde{M}$ be finite variation local square integrable martingales, and let H and K be locally bounded predictable processes. Then $\int H\,dM$ and $\int K\,d\tilde{M}$ are local square integrable martingales, and the quadratic and predictable covariation processes are*

$$\left[\int H\,dM, \int K\,d\tilde{M}\right] = \int HK\,d[M,\tilde{M}],$$
$$\left\langle\int H\,dM, \int K\,d\tilde{M}\right\rangle = \int HK\,d\langle M,\tilde{M}\rangle.$$

The quadratic and predictable variation processes of, for example, $\int H\,dM$ are seen to be

$$\left[\int H\,dM\right] = \int H^2\,d[M], \quad \left\langle\int H\,dM\right\rangle = \int H^2\,d\langle M\rangle.$$

The matrix versions of the above formulae for the quadratic and predictable covariation processes read

$$\left[\int H\,dM, \int K\,d\tilde{M}\right] = \int H\,d[M,\tilde{M}]K^T, \qquad (2.7)$$

$$\left\langle \int H\,dM, \int K\,d\tilde{M}\right\rangle = \int H\,d\langle M,\tilde{M}\rangle K^T, \qquad (2.8)$$

where M and $\tilde{M}$ are two vectors, and H and K are two matrices with dimensions such that the expressions make sense. In this case $[M,\tilde{M}]$ and $\langle M,\tilde{M}\rangle$ should be calculated componentwise.

2.3 Counting processes

Before giving the definition of a counting process we first describe one key example where counting processes have shown their usefulness.

Example 2.3.1 (Right-censored survival data)

Let T^* and C be two nonnegative, independent random variables. The random variable T^* denotes the time to the occurrence of some specific event. It could be time to death of an individual, time to blindness for a diabetic retinopathy patient or time to pregnancy for a couple. In many such studies the exact time T^* may never be observed because it may be censored at time C, that is, one only observes the minimum $T = T^* \wedge C$ of T^* and C, and whether it is the event or the censoring that has occurred, recorded by the indicator variable $\Delta = I(T^* \leq C)$. One simple type of censoring that is often encountered is that a study is closed at some point in time before all subjects have experienced the event of interest. In the counting process formulation the observed data (T, Δ) are replaced with the pair $(N(t), Y(t))$ of functions of time t, where $N(t) = I(T \leq t, \Delta = 1)$ is the counting process jumping at time T^* if $T^* \leq C$ (Figure 2.2), and $Y(t) = I(t \leq T)$ is the so-called *at risk indicator* being one at time t if neither the event nor the censoring has happened before time t. Assume that T^* has density f and let $S(t) = P(T^* > t)$ denote the *survival function*. A key concept in survival analysis is the *hazard function*

$$\alpha(t) = \frac{f(t)}{S(t)} = \lim_{h \downarrow 0} \frac{1}{h} P(t \leq T^* < t+h \mid T^* \geq t), \qquad (2.9)$$

which may also be interpreted as the instantaneous failure rate. □

The formal definition of a counting process is as follows. A *counting process* $\{N(t)\}$ is stochastic process that is adapted to a filtration $(\mathcal{F}_t)$,

24   2. Probabilistic background

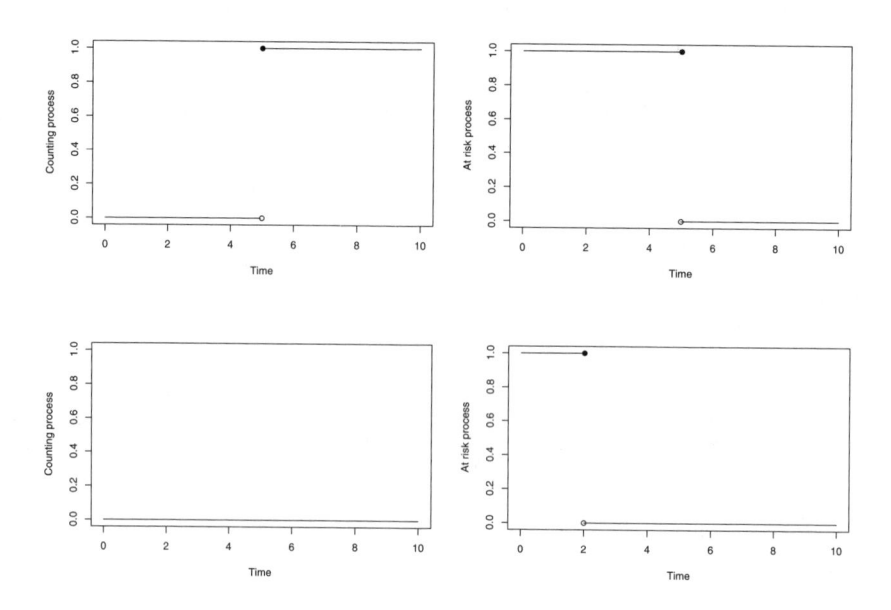

FIGURE 2.2: The counting process $N(t) = I(T \leq t, \Delta = 1)$ with $T^* = 5$ and $C > T^*$ (upper left panel) and corresponding at risk process (upper right panel). The counting process $N(t) = I(T \leq t, \Delta = 1)$ with $T^* > C$ and $C = 2$ (lower left panel) and corresponding at risk process (lower right panel).

cadlag, with $N(0) = 0$ and $N(t) < \infty$ a.s., and whose paths are piecewise constant with jumps of size 1.

A counting process N is a local submartingale and therefore has compensator, Λ, say. The process Λ is nondecreasing and predictable, zero at time zero, and such that

$$M = N - \Lambda$$

is a local martingale with respect to $\mathcal{F}_t$. In fact, M is a local square integrable martingale (Exercise 2.5). It also holds that

$$EN(t) = E\Lambda(t),$$

and further, if $E\Lambda(t) < \infty$, that M is a martingale (Exercise 2.6).

We shall only deal with the so-called *absolute continuous case*, where the above compensator has the special form

$$\Lambda(t) = \int_0^t \lambda(s)\,ds,$$

where the *intensity process* $\lambda(t)$ is a predictable process. The counting process N is then said to have intensity process λ.

By (2.6) is seen that the quadratic variation process of M is

$$[M] = N,$$

and, since it is locally integrable, the predictable variation process of M is

$$\langle M \rangle = \Lambda$$

by the uniqueness of the compensator.

A *multivariate counting process*

$$N = (N_1, \ldots N_k)$$

is a vector of counting processes such that no two components jump simultaneously. It follows that

$$\langle M_j, M_{j'} \rangle = [M_j, M_{j'}] = 0, \quad j \neq j',$$

where the M_j's are the associated counting process martingales.

Example 2.3.2 (Continuation of Example 2.3.1)

Let the history be given by

$$\mathcal{F}_t = \sigma\{I(T \leq s, \Delta = 0), I(T \leq s, \Delta = 1) : s \leq t\}.$$

As noted above, the counting process $N(t)$ has a compensator $\Lambda(t)$. It turns out that the compensator is

$$\Lambda(t) = \int_0^t Y(s)\alpha(s)\, ds, \tag{2.10}$$

and hence that $N(t)$ has intensity process

$$\lambda(t) = Y(t)\alpha(t).$$

This may be shown rigorously, see for example Fleming & Harrington (1991). A heuristic proof of the martingale condition is as follows. Since (2.10) is clearly $\mathcal{F}_t$-adapted and left-continuous, it is predictable. By the independence of T^* and C, $dN(t)$ is a Bernoulli variable with conditional probability $Y(t)\alpha(t)\, dt$ of being one given $\mathcal{F}_{t-}$, see also Exercise 2.7. Thus,

$$E(dN(t) \mid \mathcal{F}_{t-}) = Y(t)\alpha(t)\, dt = d\Lambda(t) = E(d\Lambda(t) \mid \mathcal{F}_{t-}),$$

which justify the martingale condition (2.2) for $M = N - \Lambda$. □

Let us see how the decomposition of a counting process into its compensator and martingale parts may be used to construct estimators.

Example 2.3.3 (The Nelson-Aalen estimator)

Let (T_i^*, C_i), $i = 1, \ldots, n$, be n i.i.d. replicates from the model described in Example 2.3.2. Put $N_i(t) = I(T_i \leq t, \Delta_i = 1)$ and $Y_i(t) = I(t \leq T_i)$ with $T_i = T_i^* \wedge C_i$ and $\Delta_i = I(T_i^* \leq C_i)$. Let $\mathcal{F}_t^i$ be defined similarly as $\mathcal{F}_t$ in Example 2.3.1 and 2.3.2 and let $\mathcal{F}_t = \bigvee_i \mathcal{F}_t^i$. Let further

$$N_\cdot(t) = \sum_{i=1}^n N_i(t), \quad Y_\cdot(t) = \sum_{i=1}^n Y_i(t).$$

The counting process $N_\cdot(t)$ is seen to have compensator

$$\Lambda(t) = \int_0^t Y_\cdot(s)\alpha(s)\,ds,$$

and, hence,

$$M_\cdot(t) = N_\cdot(t) - \Lambda(t)$$

is a local square integrable martingale with respect to $\mathcal{F}_t$. In the last display, $M_\cdot(t) = \sum_{i=1}^n M_i(t)$ with $M_i(t) = N_i(t) - \Lambda_i(t)$, $i = 1, \ldots, n$.

Now, decomposing the counting process into its compensator and a martingale term gives

$$N_\cdot(t) = \int_0^t Y_\cdot(s)\alpha(s)\,ds + M_\cdot(t)$$

and since $dM_\cdot(t)$ is a zero-mean process, this motivates the estimating equation

$$Y_\cdot(t)dA(t) = dN_\cdot(t),$$

where $A(t) = \int_0^t \alpha(s)\,ds$. This leads to the *Nelson-Aalen estimator*

$$\hat{A}(t) = \int_0^t \frac{J(s)}{Y_\cdot(s)}dN_\cdot(s) \tag{2.11}$$

of the integrated hazard function $A(t)$, where $J(t) = I(Y_\cdot(t) > 0)$, and where we use the convention that $0/0 = 0$. Notice that the Nelson-Aalen estimator is nothing but a simple sum:

$$\hat{A}(t) = \sum_{T_i \leq t} \frac{\Delta_i}{Y_\cdot(T_i)}.$$

One may decompose $\hat{A}(t)$ as

$$\hat{A}(t) = \int_0^t J(s)dA(s) + \int_0^t \frac{J(s)}{Y_\cdot(s)}dM_\cdot(s).$$

By Theorem 2.2.2, it is seen that the second term on the right-hand side of the above decomposition is a local square integrable martingale. Thus, $\hat{A}(t)$ is an unbiased estimator of

$$\int_0^t \alpha(s) P(Y.(s) > 0)\, ds,$$

which already indicates that the Nelson-Aalen estimator will have sound large-sample properties (under appropriate conditions). One consequence of this is that $E(\hat{A}(t)) \leq A(t)$, and that the estimator will be close to unbiased if there are subjects at risk at all times with high probability.

As we shall see later on, a lot more than (asymptotical) unbiasedness can be said by use of the central limit theorem for martingales.

The Nelson-Aalen estimator may be formulated in the more general context of *multiplicative intensity models* where, for a counting process $N(t)$, it is assumed that the intensity process $\lambda(t)$ has a multiplicative structure

$$\lambda(t) = Y(t)\alpha(t),$$

where $\alpha(t)$ is a nonnegative deterministic function (being locally integrable) while $Y(t)$ is a locally bounded predictable process. The extension thus allows $Y(t)$ to be something else than an at risk indicator and is useful to deal with a number of different situations. The Nelson-Aalen estimator is then

$$\hat{A}(t) = \int_0^t \frac{J(s)}{Y(s)} dN(s),$$

where $J(t) = I(Y(t) > 0)$. The estimator $\hat{A}(t)$ was introduced for counting process models by Aalen (1975, 1978b) and it generalizes the estimator proposed by Nelson (1969, 1972). □

The concept of a filtration $\mathcal{F}_t$ may seem rather technical. It is important, however, as it corresponds to what information we are given, which in turn is used when specifying models. Sometimes we may be interested in conditioning on more information than that carried by $\mathcal{F}_t$. This additional information may give rise to a new filtration, $\mathcal{G}_t$ say, such that $\mathcal{F}_t \subseteq \mathcal{G}_t$, for all t. Assume that the counting process $N(t)$ is adapted to both $\mathcal{F}_t$ and $\mathcal{G}_t$, and that $N(t)$ has intensity $\lambda(t)$ with respect to $\mathcal{G}_t$. The intensity with respect to the smaller filtration $\mathcal{F}_t$ is then

$$\tilde{\lambda}(t) = \mathrm{E}(\lambda(t) \mid \mathcal{F}_{t-}), \qquad (2.12)$$

which will generally be different from $\lambda(t)$ as we condition on less information. The above result is the so-called *innovation theorem*.

The following two examples of counting process models, illustrates how the innovation theorem can be used to adjust models to the amount of available information.

28   2. Probabilistic background

Example 2.3.4 (Clustered survival data)

Consider the situation where we are interested in studying the time to the occurrence of some event. Suppose in addition that there is some cluster structure in the data. An example could be the time to onset of blindness in patients with diabetic retinopathy, see Lin (1994). Patients were followed over several years and the pair of waiting times to blindness in the left and right eyes, respectively, were observed. In such a study one should expect some correlation between the waiting times within clusters. One approach to model such data is to use a random effects model, where the random effect accounts for possible (positive) correlation within the clusters. For ease of notation we describe the model in the situation where there is no censoring. Let T_{ik} denote the ith waiting time in the kth cluster, and put $N_{ik}(t) = I(T_{ik} \leq t)$, $Y_{ik}(t) = I(t \leq T_{ik})$, $i = 1, \ldots, n$, $k = 1, \ldots, K$. Assume that $T_k = (T_{ik}, \ldots, T_{nk})$, $k = 1, \ldots, K$ are i.i.d. random variables such that T_{ik} and T_{jk} ($i \neq j$) are independent given the random effect Z_k. Let $\mathcal{F}_t^{ik}$ be the internal history of N_{ik}, $\mathcal{F}_t^k = \bigvee_i \mathcal{F}_t^{ik}$ and $\mathcal{F}_t = \bigvee_k \mathcal{F}_t^k$. The Clayton-Oakes model (Clayton (1978); Oakes (1982)) is obtained by assuming that $N_{ik}(t)$ has intensity

$$\lambda_{ik}(t) = Y_{ik}(t) Z_k \alpha(t)$$

with respect to the enlarged filtration $\mathcal{G}_t$, where

$$\mathcal{G}_t = \bigvee_k \mathcal{G}_t^k; \quad \mathcal{G}_t^k = \mathcal{F}_t^k \vee \sigma(Z_k);$$

and by assuming that the Z_k's are i.i.d. gamma distributed with expectation 1 and variance η^{-1}. The random effect Z_k is also referred to as a frailty variable, see Chapter 9. Besides carrying the information generated by the counting processes, $\mathcal{G}_t$ also holds the information generated by the random effects. The filtration $\mathcal{G}_t$ is not fully observed due to the unobserved random effects. The observed filtration is $\mathcal{F}_t$, and we now find the $\mathcal{F}_t$-intensities using the innovation theorem. One may show that

$$\mathrm{E}(Z_k \mid \mathcal{F}_{t-}) = \frac{\eta + N_{\cdot k}(t-)}{\eta + \int_0^t Y_{\cdot k}(s) \alpha(s)\, ds},$$

where $N_{\cdot k}(t) = \sum_{i=1}^n N_{ik}(t)$ and $Y_{\cdot k}(t) = \sum_{i=1}^n Y_{ik}(t)$, $k = 1 \ldots, K$. The $\mathcal{F}_t$-intensity is hence

$$\tilde{\lambda}_{ik}(t) = Y_{ik}(t) \left(\frac{\eta + N_{\cdot k}(t-)}{\eta + \int_0^t Y_{\cdot k}(s) \alpha(s)\, ds} \right) \alpha(t).$$

Estimation of $A(t) = \int_0^t \alpha(s)\, ds$ in this context may be carried out by use of the EM-algorithm, which was originally suggested by Gill (1985) and further developed by Klein (1992) and Nielsen et al. (1992), see also Andersen et al. (1993).

The above approach could be called *conditional* in the sense that the intensity of $N_{ik}(t)$ is modeled conditional on Z_k. An alternative approach that avoids joint modeling of data is the so-called *marginal approach* where the intensity of $N_{ik}(t)$ is only specified with respect to the marginal filtration $\mathcal{F}_t^{ik}$. It is assumed that $N_{ik}(t)$ has $\mathcal{F}_t^{ik}$-intensity

$$Y_{ik}(t)\alpha(t), \qquad (2.13)$$

whereas it is *not* assumed that the $\mathcal{F}_t$-intensity is governed by (2.13) because that would correspond to assuming independence between subjects within each cluster, which obviously would be wrong with data like those mentioned in the beginning of this example. Estimation of $A(t)$ using the marginal approach is done by the usual Nelson-Aalen estimator ignoring the cluster structure of the data. Standard error estimates, however, should be computed differently. We return to clustered survival data in Chapter 9.

□

Example 2.3.5 (The additive hazards model and filtrations)

Consider the survival of a subject with covariates $X = (X_1, ..., X_p, X_{p+1})$ and assume that the corresponding counting process of the subject, $N(t)$, has intensity on the additive hazards form

$$\lambda^{p+1}(t) = Y(t)\left(\sum_{j=1}^{p+1} X_j \alpha_j(t)\right)$$

with respect to the history $\mathcal{F}_t^N \vee \sigma(p+1)$, where $\mathcal{F}_t^N$ is the internal history of N and $\sigma(i) = \sigma(X_1, ..., X_i)$ for $i = 1, ..., p+1$ the σ-fields generated by different sets of the covariates, In the above display, $Y(t)$ is an at risk indicator and $\alpha_j(t)$, $j = 1, ..., p+1$, are locally integrable deterministic unknown functions.

If only the p first covariates are known, or used, in the model the intensity changes, by the innovation theorem, to

$$\lambda^p(t) = E(\lambda^{p+1}(t)|\mathcal{F}_t^N \vee \sigma(p))$$
$$= \sum_{i=1}^{p} Y(t)X_j\alpha_j(t) + Y(t)\alpha_{p+1}(t)E(X_{p+1}|Y(t)=1, X_1, ..., X_p).$$

The last conditional mean of X_{p+1} given that the subject is at risk (has survived), and the observed covariates can be computed (under regularity conditions) to be minus the derivative of $\log(f(t))$, where

$$f(t) = E(\exp(-\int_0^t \alpha_{p+1}(s)ds X_{p+1})|X_1, ..., X_p)$$

is the conditional Laplace transform of X_{p+1} evaluated at $\int \alpha_{p+1}$. Under certain assumptions, such as independence between the covariates, it is seen that the additive structure of the intensity is preserved, see Exercise 5.1. This example was given by Aalen (1989) □

2.4 Marked point processes

Later on we shall describe how nonparametric and semiparametric models for regression data and longitudinal data may be analyzed fruitfully by the use of martingale calculus. A key notion in this treatment is a generalization of counting processes, or point processes, to marked point processes, which will be introduced in the following. To a large extent we follow the exposition of marked point processes given by Brémaud (1981), see also the recent Last & Brandt (1995).

The idea is that instead of just recording the time points T_k at which specific events occur (as for the counting processes) we also observe an additional variable Z_k (the response variable in the longitudinal data setting) at each time point T_k. To make things precise we fix a measurable space $(E, \mathcal{E})$, called the mark space, and assume that

(i) $(Z_k, k \geq 1)$ is a sequence of random variables in E,

(ii) the sequence $(T_k, k \geq 1)$ constitutes a counting process

$$N(t) = \sum_k I(T_k \leq t).$$

The double sequence (T_k, Z_k) is called a *marked point process* with (Z_k) being the marks. To each $A \in \mathcal{E}$ is associated a counting process

$$N_t(A) = \sum_k I(T_k \leq t)I(Z_k \in A),$$

that counts the number of jumps before time t with marks in A. The marked point process is also identified with its associated counting measure defined by

$$p((0,t] \times A) = N_t(A), \qquad t > 0,\ A \in \mathcal{E}.$$

A marked point process counting measure thus accumulates information over time about the jump times and marks just as in the simpler counting process situation where there are no marks. Just as for counting processes it is also useful to consider integrals with respect to the marked point process. A *marked point process integral* has the following simple interpretation:

$$\int_0^t \int_E H(s,z) p(ds \times dz) = \sum_k H(T_k, Z_k) I(T_k \leq t).$$

The internal history of the marked point process is defined by

$$\mathcal{F}_t^p = \sigma(N_s(A) : 0 \leq s \leq t, A \in \mathcal{E}),$$

and we let $\mathcal{F}_t$ be any history of p, that is, $\mathcal{F}_t^p \subset \mathcal{F}_t$. If, for each $A \in \mathcal{E}$, $N_t(A)$ has intensity $\lambda_t(A)$ (predictable with respect to $\mathcal{F}_t$), we then say that $p(dt \times dz)$ admits the *intensity kernel* $\lambda_t(dz)$. We let $\lambda_t = \lambda_t(E)$ and assume that λ_t is locally integrable. A probability measure on $(E, \mathcal{E})$ is then defined by

$$F_t(dz) = \frac{\lambda_t(dz)}{\lambda_t}.$$

The pair $(\lambda_t, F_t(dz))$ is called the *local characteristics* of $p(dt \times dz)$. If the history $\mathcal{F}_t$ has the special form $\mathcal{F}_t = \mathcal{F}_0 \vee \mathcal{F}_t^p$, we have the following

$$F_{T_k}(A) = P(Z_k \in A \mid \mathcal{F}_{T_k-}) \quad \text{on } \{T_k < \infty\},$$

where

$$\mathcal{F}_{T_k-} = \sigma(T_j, Z_j; 1 \leq k-1; T_k)$$

is the history generated by the occurrence times and marks obtained before time T_k, and by T_k itself. The important above characterization of the second term of the local characteristics as the distribution of the current mark given past history and the time of the current mark is proved in Brémaud (1981).

Let $\mathcal{F}_t$ be a history of $p(dt \times dz)$ and let $\tilde{\mathcal{P}}(\mathcal{F}_t)$ be the history generated by the mappings

$$H(t, z) = C(t) 1_A(z),$$

where C is a $\mathcal{F}_t$-predictable process and $1_A(z)$ is the indicator of z being in A, $A \in \mathcal{E}$. Any mapping $H : (0, \infty) \times \Omega \times E \to \mathbf{R}$, which is $\tilde{\mathcal{P}}(\mathcal{F}_t)$-measurable is called an $\mathcal{F}_t$-predictable process indexed by E. Let p have intensity kernel $\lambda_t(dz)$ and let H be a $\mathcal{F}_t$-predictable process indexed by E. We shall now consider the measure

$$q(dt \times dz) = p(dt \times dz) - \lambda_t(dz) dt \tag{2.14}$$

obtained by compensating the marked point process measure by its intensity kernel. One may show, for all $t \geq 0$, that

$$M(t) = \int_0^t \int_E H(s, z) q(ds \times dz) \tag{2.15}$$

is a locally square integrable martingale (with respect to $\mathcal{F}_t$) if and only if

$$\int_0^t \int_E H^2(s, z) \lambda_s(dz) ds < \infty \qquad P - a.s.$$

32   2. Probabilistic background

We now turn to the computation of the quadratic variation and predictable variation process of M given by (2.15). Since (2.15) is of finite variation, the optional variation process is

$$[M](t) = \sum_{s \leq t} \Delta M(s)^2 = \int_0^t \int_E H^2(s,z) p(ds \times dz).$$

The predictable variation process $\langle M \rangle$ is the compensator of $[M]$, and by the uniqueness of the compensator, we hence have

$$\langle M \rangle(t) = \int_0^t \int_E H^2(s,z) \lambda_s(dz) ds.$$

Let $p_1(dt \times dz)$ and $p_2(dt \times dz)$ be two marked point processes with intensity kernels $\lambda_t(dz)$ and $\mu_t(dz)$, respectively. Let H_j, $j = 1, 2$, be $\mathcal{F}_t$-predictable processes indexed by E where $\mathcal{F}_t \supset \mathcal{F}_t^{p_1} \vee \mathcal{F}_t^{p_2}$, and assume that

$$\int_0^t \int_E H_1^2(s,z) \lambda_s(dz) ds < \infty, \quad \int_0^t \int_E H_2^2(s,z) \mu_s(dz) ds < \infty \quad P - a.s.$$

Write $M_j(t) = \int_0^t \int_E H_j(s,z) q_j(ds \times dz)$, $j = 1, 2$. Assume that the two induced counting process, $N_1(t)$ and $N_2(t)$, have no jumps in common. Proceeding as above one may then derive that $[M_1, M_2] = 0$ and hence $\langle M_1, M_2 \rangle = 0$. Also,

$$[\int_0^t \int_E H_1 q_1(ds \times dz), \int_0^t \int_E H_2 q_1(ds \times dz)] = \int_0^t \int_E H_1 H_2 p_1(ds \times dz),$$

and

$$\langle \int_0^t \int_E H_1 q_1(ds \times dz), \int_0^t \int_E H_2 q_1(ds \times dz) \rangle = \int_0^t \int_E H_1 H_2 \lambda_s(dz) ds,$$

where the dependence of the integrands on s and z has been suppressed.

The following example illustrates how i.i.d. regression data may be put into the marked point process framework. Note how the techniques in the example closely parallel the similar development of the Nelson-Aalen estimator in the counting process setup.

Example 2.4.1 (Regression data)

Consider a sample (T_i, Z_i), $i = 1, \ldots, n$, of n i.i.d. regression data with Z_i being the (one-dimensional) response and T_i the (one-dimensional) regressor. Let

$$E(Z_i \mid T_i = t) = \phi(t)$$

2.4 Marked point processes

and assume that T_i has an absolute continuous distribution on $[0, \infty)$ with hazard function $\alpha(t)$. For simplicity we further assume for the moment that this distribution is known, that is, the hazard function is assumed to be known. Assume also that $\int_0^t \alpha(s)\phi(s)\,ds < \infty$ for all t. Each (T_i, Z_i) constitutes a marked point process p_i and with

$$\int_0^t \int_E z p_i(ds \times dz) = Z_i I(T_i \leq t),$$

we have the decomposition

$$\int_0^t \int_E z p_i(ds \times dz) = \int_0^t Y_i(s)\alpha(s)\phi(s)\,ds + \int_0^t \int_E z q_i(ds \times dz),$$

where the second term on the right-hand side of this display is a martingale with respect to the internal filtration $\mathcal{F}_t^{p_i}$. Writing the above equation in differential form and summing over all subjects gives

$$\sum_{i=1}^n \int_E z p_i(dt \times dz) = Y_\cdot(t)\alpha(t)\,d\Phi(t) + \sum_{i=1}^n \int_E z q_i(dt \times dz), \quad (2.16)$$

where $Y_\cdot(t) = \sum_{i=1}^n Y_i(t)$ and $\Phi(t) = \int_0^t \phi(s)\,ds$. Assume that $\inf_t \alpha(t) > 0$. Since α is known, (2.16) suggests the following estimator of $\Phi(t)$:

$$\hat{\Phi}(t) = \sum_{i=1}^n \int_0^t \int_E \frac{z}{Y_\cdot(s)\alpha(s)} p_i(ds \times dz)$$

$$= \sum_{i=1}^n \frac{Z_i}{Y_\cdot(T_i)\alpha(T_i)} I(T_i \leq t). \quad (2.17)$$

For this estimator we have

$$\hat{\Phi}(t) = \int_0^t J(s)\,d\Phi(s) + M(t),$$

where $J(t) = I(Y_\cdot(t) > 0)$ and

$$M(t) = \sum_{i=1}^n \int_0^t \int_E \frac{J(s)z}{Y_\cdot(s)\alpha(s)} q_i(ds \times dz),$$

which is seen to be a martingale with respect to the filtration spanned by all the $\mathcal{F}_t^{p_i}$'s. This implies that

$$E(\hat{\Phi}(t)) = \int_0^t P(Y_\cdot(t) > 0)\,d\Phi(s)$$

just as in the Nelson-Aalen estimator case. The estimator will thus be close to unbiased if there is a high probability that subjects are at risk at all times. If $\phi(t)$ is positive, then $E(\hat{\Phi}(t)) \leq \Phi(t)$. $\square$

2.5 Large-sample results

As mentioned earlier, one of the strengths of representing the data as either a counting process or a marked point process is that we get martingales into play and that a central limit theorem for martingales is available. This theorem will be the main tool when we derive asymptotic results for concrete estimators. The theorem is stated below.

We shall consider a sequence of $\mathbb{R}^k$-valued local square integrable martingales $(M^{(n)}(t) : t \in \mathcal{T})$ with either

$$\mathcal{T} = [0, \infty) \text{ or } \mathcal{T} = [0, \tau]$$

with $\tau < \infty$. For $\epsilon > 0$, we let $M_\epsilon^{(n)}$ be the $\mathbb{R}^k$-valued local square integrable martingale where $M_{\epsilon l}^{(n)}$ contains all the jumps of $M_l^{(n)}$ larger in absolute value than ϵ, $l = 1, \ldots k$, i.e.,

$$M_{\epsilon l}^{(n)}(t) = \sum_{s \leq t} \Delta M_l^{(n)}(s) I(|\Delta M_l^{(n)}(s)| > \epsilon), \quad l = 1, \ldots, k.$$

Note, that for counting process martingales of the form

$$\tilde{M}(t) = \int_0^t H(s) dM(s)$$

with $M(t) = N(t) - \Lambda(t)$ then

$$\tilde{M}_{\epsilon j}(t) = \sum_l \int_0^t H_{jl}(s) I(|H_{jl}(s)| > \epsilon) dM_l(s).$$

A *Gaussian martingale* is an $\mathbb{R}^k$-valued martingale U such that $U(0) = 0$ and the distribution of any finite family $(U(t_1), \ldots, U(t_j))$ is Gaussian. Write $V(t)$ for the variance-covariance matrix of $U(t)$. It follows that

(i) $\langle U \rangle(t) = V(t)$ for $t \geq 0$;

(ii) $V(t) - V(s)$ is positive semidefinite for $s \leq t$;

(iii) $U(t) - U(s)$ is independent of $(U(r); r \leq s)$ for $s \leq t$.

A stochastic process U with the only requirement that is has continuous sample paths and normal distributed finite dimensional distributions is said to be a *Gaussian process*.

We may then state one form of the martingale central limit theorem.

Theorem 2.5.1 *(CLT for martingales).* *Let $(M^{(n)}(t) : t \in \mathcal{T})$ be a sequence of $\mathbb{R}^k$-valued local square integrable martingales. Assume that*

$$\langle M^{(n)} \rangle(t) \xrightarrow{P} V(t) \quad \text{for all } t \in \mathcal{T} \text{ as } n \to \infty, \tag{2.18}$$

$$\langle M_{\epsilon l}^{(n)} \rangle(t) \xrightarrow{P} 0 \quad \text{for all } t \in \mathcal{T}, l \text{ and } \epsilon > 0 \text{ as } n \to \infty. \tag{2.19}$$

Then

$$M^{(n)} \xrightarrow{\mathcal{D}} U \text{ in } (D(\mathcal{T}))^k \text{ as } n \to \infty, \qquad (2.20)$$

where U is a Gaussian martingale with covariance function V. Moreover, $\langle M^{(n)} \rangle$ and $[M^{(n)}]$ converge uniformly on compact subsets of $\mathcal{T}$, in probability, to V.

The theorem is due to Rebolledo (1980). The result (2.20) says that we have weak convergence of the process $M^{(n)}$ to U on the space $(D(\mathcal{T}))^k$ that consists of cadlag functions on $\mathcal{T}$ into $\mathbb{R}^k$ and is endowed with the Skorokhod topology, see e.g. Fleming & Harrington (1991) for definitions.

The condition (2.19) states that the jumps of $M^{(n)}$ should become negligible as $n \to \infty$ (see (2.25)), which makes sense if $M^{(n)}$ shall converge towards a process with continuous sample paths. Condition (2.18) says that the (predictable) variation process of $M^{(n)}$ becomes deterministic and approaches the variance function of the limit process as $n \to \infty$, which also makes sense in light of (2.5).

To illustrate the use of the martingale central limit theorem, we consider the Nelson-Aalen estimator (Example 2.3.3), and the i.i.d. regression set-up (Example 2.4.1).

Example 2.5.1 (The Nelson-Aalen estimator)

Consider the situation with n possibly right-censored survival times as described in Example 2.3.3. It was seen there that the Nelson-Aalen estimator of the cumulative hazard function $A(t) = \int_0^t \alpha(s)\,ds$ takes the form

$$\hat{A}(t) = \int_0^t \frac{J(s)}{Y_\cdot(s)} dN_\cdot(s),$$

where $J(t) = I(Y_\cdot(t) > 0)$,

$$N_\cdot(t) = \sum_{i=1}^n N_i(t), \quad Y_\cdot(t) = \sum_{i=1}^n Y_i(t),$$

with $N_i(t) = I(T_i \leq t, \Delta_i = 1)$ and $Y_i(t) = I(t \leq T_i)$, $i = 1, \ldots, n$, the basic counting processes and the at risk indicators, respectively. With

$$A^*(t) = \int_0^t J(s) dA(s),$$

it was also seen that

$$\hat{A}(t) - A^*(t) = \int_0^t \frac{J(s)}{Y_\cdot(s)} dM_\cdot(s).$$

is a local square integrable martingale. Recall that $M.(t) = \sum_{i=1}^{n} M_i(t)$ with $M_i(t) = N_i(t) - \int_0^t Y_i(s)\alpha(s)\,ds$. By writing

$$n^{1/2}(\hat{A}(t) - A(t)) = n^{1/2}\big((A^*(t) - A(t)) + (\hat{A}(t) - A^*(t))\big)$$
$$= n^{1/2} \int_0^t (J(s) - 1)\alpha(s)\,ds + n^{1/2} \int_0^t \frac{J(s)}{Y.(s)} dM.(s), \quad (2.21)$$

we see that under regularity conditions the asymptotic distribution of the Nelson-Aalen estimator on $[0,t]$, $t \in \mathcal{T}$ is a Gaussian martingale if it can be shown that the second term in (2.21) converges to a Gaussian martingale and that the first term in (2.21) converges to zero uniformly in probability.

We assume that $\int_0^t \alpha(s)\,ds < \infty$ for all $t \in \mathcal{T}$, and that there exists a function $y(s)$ such that

$$\sup_{s \in [0,t]} |n^{-1} Y.(s) - y(s)| \xrightarrow{P} 0; \quad \inf_{s \in [0,t]} y(s) > 0. \quad (2.22)$$

It may now be shown that (Exercise 2.8)

$$\sup_{s \in [0,t]} \left| n^{1/2} \int_0^s (J(u) - 1)\alpha(u)\,du \right| \xrightarrow{P} 0,$$

and we may hence concentrate on the martingale term

$$M(s) = n^{1/2}(\hat{A}(s) - A^*(s)).$$

We see that, for $s \leq t$,

$$\langle M \rangle(s) = \int_0^s \frac{J(u)}{n^{-1} Y.(u)} \alpha(u)\,du \xrightarrow{P} \int_0^s \frac{\alpha(u)}{y(u)}\,du$$

and

$$\langle M_\epsilon \rangle(s) = \int_0^s \frac{J(u)}{n^{-1} Y.(u)} \alpha(u) I\left(n^{1/2} \frac{J(u)}{Y.(u)} > \epsilon\right) du \xrightarrow{P} 0$$

(Exercise 2.8). Thus,

$$n^{1/2}(\hat{A}(s) - A(s)) \xrightarrow{D} U(s)$$

in $\mathcal{D}[0,t]$, $t \in \mathcal{T}$, where U is a Gaussian martingale with variance function

$$V(s) = \int_0^s \frac{\alpha(u)}{y(u)}\,du.$$

Moreover, a uniformly consistent estimator of the variance function is given by the quadratic variation process

$$[M](s) = n \int_0^s \frac{J(u)}{(Y.(u))^2}\,dN.(u).$$

In the case of simple random censorship, that is, the C_i's are i.i.d. with distribution function F_C, say, (2.22) is fulfilled provided that $F_C(t-) < 1$, which says that the censoring must not be too heavy. In this case, $y(s) = (1 - F_{T*}(s))(1 - F_C(s))$, where F_{T*} denotes the distribution function of the survival times. □

Example 2.5.2 (Regression data)

Consider the i.i.d. regression setup of Example 2.4.1 where we observe i.i.d. regression data where
$$Z_i = \phi(T_i) + e_i$$
and the residual terms $e_1, \ldots, e_n$ are independent with zero mean such that $E(Z_i|T_i = t) = \phi(t)$. As noted there an estimator of $\Phi(t) = \int_0^t \phi(s)ds$ was given by
$$\hat{\Phi}(t) = \sum_{i=1}^n \int_0^t \int_E \frac{z}{Y.(s)\alpha(s)} p_i(ds \times dz),$$
which may be rewritten as
$$\hat{\Phi}(t) = \int_0^t J(s)d\Phi(s) + M(t),$$
where $J(t) = I(Y.(t) > 0)$ and
$$M(t) = \sum_{i=1}^n \int_0^t \int_E \frac{J(s)z}{Y.(s)\alpha(s)} q_i(ds \times dz),$$
the latter being a martingale with respect to the filtration spanned by all the $\mathcal{F}_t^{p_i}$'s. By imposing appropriate conditions we may show that
$$n^{1/2}(\hat{\Phi}(t) - \Phi(t)) = n^{1/2}M(t) + o_p(1),$$
uniformly in t, and the asymptotic distribution of $\hat{\Phi}(t)$ may hence be derived by use of the martingale central limit theorem. We have, for all $s \le t$,
$$\langle n^{1/2}M \rangle(s) = \int_0^s \frac{J(u)\psi(u)}{n^{-1}Y.(u)\alpha(u)} du \xrightarrow{P} \int_0^s \frac{\psi(u)}{y(u)\alpha(u)} du,$$
where
$$\psi(s) = E(Z_i^2 | T_i = s)$$
and $y(s)$ is the limit in probability of $n^{-1}Y.(t)$ assuming that $\inf_{t \in \mathcal{T}} y(t) > 0$. Assume also that $\psi(t) < \infty$ for all t. The martingale containing the jumps of absolute size larger than ϵ is
$$(n^{1/2}M)_\epsilon(s) = n^{1/2}\sum_{i=1}^n \int_0^s \int_E \frac{J(u)|z|}{Y.(u)\alpha(u)} I\left(n^{1/2}\frac{J(u)|z|}{Y.(u)\alpha(u)} > \epsilon\right) q_i(du \times dz)$$

and hence

$$\langle M_\epsilon \rangle(s) = \int_0^s \frac{J(u)}{n^{-1}Y.(u)\alpha(u)} E\left(Z^2 I\left(n^{1/2}\frac{J(u)|Z|}{Y.(u)\alpha(u)} > \epsilon\right) \bigg| T = u\right) du \xrightarrow{P} 0,$$

Exercise 2.11. Thus,

$$n^{1/2}(\hat{\Phi}(s) - \Phi(s)) \xrightarrow{D} U(s)$$

in $\mathcal{D}[0, t]$, $t > 0$, where U is a Gaussian martingale with variance function

$$V(s) = \int_0^s \frac{\psi(u)}{y(u)\alpha(u)} du.$$

A uniformly consistent estimator of the variance function is given by the quadratic variation process

$$[n^{1/2}M](s) = n \sum_{i=1}^n \int_0^s \int_E \frac{J(u)z^2}{(Y.(u)\alpha(u))^2} p_i(du \times dz)$$

$$= n \sum_{i=1}^n \frac{J(T_i)Z_i^2}{(Y.(T_i)\alpha(T_i))^2} I(T_i \leq s).$$

□

Once we have established convergence of our estimator as in the previous two examples, we can use their large-sample properties for hypothesis testing and construction of confidence bands and intervals. Consider, for example, the estimator $\hat{\Phi}(t)$ in the previous example that converged towards a Gaussian martingale $U(t)$. Suppose that the limit process $U(t)$ is $\mathbb{R}$-valued and has variance process $V(t)$. Then a $(1-\alpha)$ pointwise confidence interval for $\Phi(t) = \int_0^t \phi(s)ds$, for fixed t, is

$$\left[\hat{\Phi}(t) - c_{\alpha/2}\hat{\Sigma}(t)^{1/2}, \hat{\Phi}(t) + c_{\alpha/2}\hat{\Sigma}(t)^{1/2}\right]$$

where $n\hat{\Sigma}(t)$ is an (uniformly consistent) estimator of $V(t)$, like the one based on the quadratic variation process, and $c_{\alpha/2}$ is the $(1-\alpha/2)$-quantile of the standard normal distribution. Since we often will be interested in the behavior of $\phi(t)$, or, $\Phi(t)$, as function of t, inferences based on confidence bands may be more informative than pointwise confidence limits. One type of such confidence bands are the so-called Hall-Wellner bands (Hall & Wellner, 1980). These bands are uniform for some interval of interest that we here denote as $[0, \tau]$. Since

$$U(t)V(\tau)^{1/2}[V(\tau) + V(t)]^{-1}$$

is distributed as

$$B^0\left(\frac{V(t)}{V(\tau) + V(t)}\right),$$

where B^0 is the standard Brownian bridge (see Exercise 2.2), it follows that approximate $100(1-\alpha)\%$ confidence bands for $\Phi(t)$ are given by

$$\left[\hat{\Phi}(t) - d_\alpha \hat{\Sigma}(\tau)^{1/2}\left(1 + \frac{\hat{\Sigma}(t)}{\hat{\Sigma}(\tau)}\right), \hat{\Phi}(t) + d_\alpha \hat{\Sigma}(\tau)^{1/2}\left(1 + \frac{\hat{\Sigma}(t)}{\hat{\Sigma}(\tau)}\right)\right],$$

where d_α is the $(1-\alpha)$-quantile in the distribution of

$$\sup_{t \in [0,1/2]} |B^0(t)|,$$

see also Exercise 2.3. Tables of d_α may be found in Schumacher (1984); here we list some of the most used ones: $d_{0.01} = 1.55$, $d_{0.05} = 1.27$ and $d_{0.1} = 1.13$. Likewise, the hypothesis

$$H_0 : \phi(t) = \phi_0(t) \quad \text{for all } t$$

may be tested by use of a *Kolmogorov-Smirnov test* that rejects at level α if

$$\sup_{t \leq \tau} |(\hat{\Phi}(t) - \Phi_0(t))\hat{\Sigma}(\tau)^{1/2}[\hat{\Sigma}(\tau) + \hat{\Sigma}(t)]^{-1}| \geq d_\alpha, \tag{2.23}$$

where $\Phi_0(t) = \int_0^t \phi_0(u)\,du$. The *Cramér-von Mises test* rejects at level α if

$$\int_0^\tau \left(\frac{(\hat{\Phi}(t) - \Phi_0(t))/\hat{\Sigma}^{1/2}(\tau)}{1 + \hat{\Gamma}(t)}\right)^2 d\left(\frac{\hat{\Gamma}(t)}{1 + \hat{\Gamma}(t)}\right) \geq e_\alpha \tag{2.24}$$

where e_α is the $(1-\alpha)$-quantile in the distribution of $\int_0^{1/2} B^0(u)^2\,du$ and $\hat{\Gamma}(t) = \hat{\Sigma}(t)/\hat{\Sigma}(\tau)$. For reference: $e_{0.01} = 0.42$, $e_{0.05} = 0.25$ and $e_{0.1} = 0.19$; a detailed table of e_α may be found in Schumacher (1984).

Example 2.5.3

We here present a small simulation study to illustrate the use of confidence bands and the performance of the Kolmogorov-Smirnov and Cramér-von Mises tests. We generated data from the model described in Example 2.4.1 with T being exponential with mean one. The response variable is normal distributed with mean $\phi(t)$ and standard deviation $1/3$. The true regression function is $\phi(t) = 1/(1+t)$ resulting in the cumulative regression function $\Phi(t) = \log(1+t)$. The sample size was first set to $n = 100$ and we then generated 500 datasets. Figure 2.3 (a) shows the true $\Phi(t)$ (thick full line), a randomly chosen estimate (thin dotted line) and the average of the 500 estimators (thick dotted line), which is almost indistinguishable from the true $\Phi(t)$. A slight bias is seen towards the end of the shown interval, which has upper limit equal to 4.6 corresponding to the 99%-quantile of the exponential distribution with mean one. According to the derived formulae

40   2. Probabilistic background

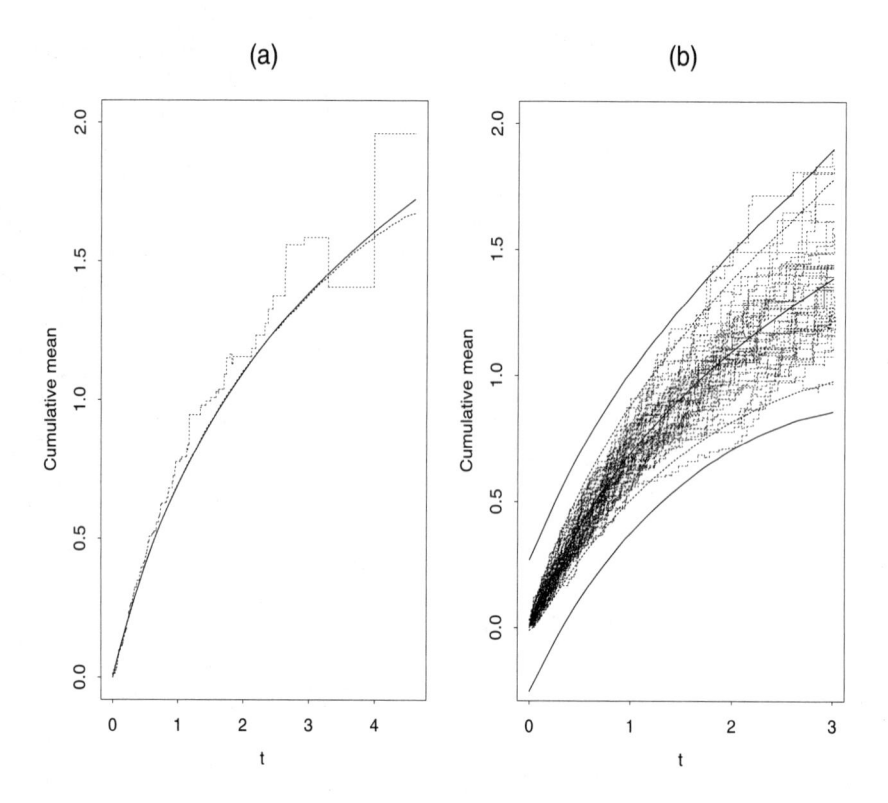

FIGURE 2.3: (a) True cumulative regression function $\Phi(t)$ (thick full line); average of 500 estimates of the cumulative regression function (thick dotted line); a typical estimator of the cumulative regression function (thin dotted line). (b) True cumulative regression function (thick full line) together with 95% pointwise confidence limits (thick dotted lines) and 95% Hall-Wellner confidence bands (thick full lines); and 40 randomly chosen estimates of the cumulative regression function (thin dotted lines).

this bias is due to the probability of being at risk towards the end of the interval deviating slightly from 1. We notice that the estimator $\hat{\Phi}(t)$, which is given by (2.17), is a step function (like the Nelson-Aalen estimator) with jumps at the observed values of t. Figure 2.3 (b) shows the true $\Phi(t)$ (thick full line), 40 randomly chosen estimates (thin dotted lines), 95% pointwise confidence limits (thick dotted lines) and 95% Hall-Wellner bands (thick full lines) with $\tau = 3$, which corresponds to 95% quantile of the considered exponential distribution. We see that the estimators are contained within the confidence bands with the exception of one or two estimators.

We also look at the performance of the Kolmogorov-Smirnov test and the Cramér-von Mises test under the null. We generated data as described above with sample size $n = 100, 400$ and computed the rejection probabilities for the two tests at level $\alpha = 1\%, 5\%, 10\%$. These are shown in Table 2.1, where each entry is based on 10000 repetitions.

n	Test statistic	$\alpha = 1\%$	$\alpha = 5\%$	$\alpha = 10\%$
100	KS	0.9	3.3	6.8
	CM	1.0	5.1	10.2
400	KS	0.8	3.9	8.1
	CM	0.9	4.9	10.6

TABLE 2.1: Rejection probabilities for the Kolmogorov-Smirnov test (KS) and the Cramér-von Mises test (CM) computed at levels $\alpha = 1\%, 5\%, 10\%$

It is seen from Table 2.1 that the Cramér-von Mises test has the correct level already at sample size $n = 100$. The Kolmogorov-Smirnov test is somewhat conservative for $n = 100$ but approaches the correct level for $n = 400$. □

A useful result is the so-called *Lenglart's inequality*, see Andersen et al. (1993), which, in the special case of a local square integrable martingale M, says that

$$P(\sup_{[0,\tau]} |M| > \eta) \leq \frac{\delta}{\eta^2} + P(\langle M \rangle(\tau) > \delta) \tag{2.25}$$

for any $\eta > 0$ and $\delta > 0$. Hence $\sup_{[0,\tau]} |M| \xrightarrow{P} 0$ if $\langle M \rangle(\tau) \xrightarrow{P} 0$. A typical application of (2.25) is the following. Suppose that H_n is a sequence locally bounded predictable stochastic processes such that

$$\sup_{[0,\tau]} |H_n| \xrightarrow{P} 0,$$

and that M_n is a sequence of local square integrable martingales such that $\langle M_n \rangle(t) = O_p(1)$. We then have

$$\sup_{[0,\tau]} \left| \int_0^t H_n dM_n \right| \xrightarrow{P} 0, \tag{2.26}$$

since

$$\langle \int H_n dM_n \rangle(\tau) \xrightarrow{P} 0.$$

In some applications, however, we may not have that the H_n's are predictable. A useful result, due to Spiekerman & Lin (1998), says that (2.26) is still true provided that

$$\int_0^\tau |dH_n(t)| = O_p(1),$$

that is, H_n is of bounded variation. The result can be further relaxed by noticing that the proof of Spiekerman & Lin (1998) remains valid if M_n is some process that converges in distribution to some zero-mean process with continuous limits M. This extended version does not require any martingales, and is used in a couple of places in the proofs and is referred to as the Lemma by Spiekerman & Lin (1998); see also Lin et al. (2000) and Lin & Ying (2001).

Often we wish to conclude that

$$\int_0^t X^{(n)}(s)\,ds \xrightarrow{P} \int_0^t f(s)\,ds \quad \text{as } n \to \infty, \tag{2.27}$$

where we know that $X^{(n)}(t) \xrightarrow{P} f(t)$ for almost all $t \in [0, \tau]$ and $\int_0^\tau |f(t)|\,dt < \infty$. A result by Gill (1983) says that (2.27) holds uniformly in t if, for all $\delta > 0$, there exists a k_δ with $\int_0^\tau k_\delta(t)\,dt < \infty$ such that

$$\liminf_{n \to \infty} P(|X^{(n)}(s)| \leq k_\delta(s) \text{ for all } s) \geq 1 - \delta. \tag{2.28}$$

We refer to (2.28) as *Gill's condition*.

A related dominated convergence theorem says that with $0 \leq X_n(s) \leq Y_n(s)$ for $s \in [0, \tau]$ and with ν a measure such that

$$Y_n(s) \xrightarrow{P} Y(s), \quad X_n(s) \xrightarrow{P} Y(s)$$

for ν almost all s and

$$\int Y_n(s)d\nu \xrightarrow{P} \int Y(s)d\nu < \infty \text{ (a.e)}$$

then

$$\int X_n(s)d\nu \xrightarrow{P} \int X(s)d\nu.$$

The *delta-method* and its equivalent functional version are very useful for deriving the asymptotic distribution in the case where a function (functional) is applied to a random-vector (process) that converges in distribution.

The simple version states that if the p-dimensional random vector's X_n, X and fixed μ satisfy that

$$n^{1/2}(X_n - \mu) \xrightarrow{D} X,$$

then if f is differentiable ($f : \mathbb{R}^p \to \mathbb{R}^q$) at μ with derivative $\dot{f}(\mu)$ (a $p \times q$ matrix function), it follows that

$$n^{1/2}(f(X_n) - f(\mu)) \xrightarrow{D} \dot{f}(\mu)X.$$

This can be extended to functional spaces by the concept of Hadamard differentiability (Andersen et al., 1993). Consider the functional spaces $B =$

$D[0,\tau]^p$ and $B' = D[0,\tau]^q$ and let $f : B \to B'$ with derivative $\dot{f}(\mu)$ at μ (a continuous linear map, $\dot{f}(\mu) : B \to B'$) such that

$$a_n(f(\mu + a_n^{-1}h_n) - f(\mu)) \to \dot{f}(\mu) \cdot h$$

for all real sequences $a_n \to \infty$ and all convergent sequences $h_n \to h$ in B. The mapping f is then said to be Hadamard differentiable at μ. If X_n and X are processes in B, μ is a fixed point in B and f is Hadamard differentiable at μ, it then follows that

$$n^{1/2}(f(X_n) - f(\mu)) \xrightarrow{D} \dot{f}(\mu) \cdot X.$$

The *functional delta theorem* can obviously be defined for all Banach spaces and one typical application is one where the p-dimensional process B_n and the q-dimensional vector θ_n jointly converge such that

$$n^{1/2}(B_n - b, \theta_n - \mu) \xrightarrow{D} (X_1, X_2)$$

and then

$$n^{1/2}(f(B_n, \theta_n) - f(b, \mu)) \xrightarrow{D} \dot{f}(b, \mu) \cdot (X_1, X_2)$$

for differentiable f.

We close this section by briefly mentioning the *conditional multiplier central limit theorem*. Suppose that $X_1, \cdots, X_n$ are i.i.d. real-valued random variables and $G_1, \cdots, G_n$ are independent standard normals independent of $X_1, \cdots, X_n$. Then if

$$n^{-1/2} \sum_{i=1}^{n} X_i \xrightarrow{D} U$$

it follows from the *conditional multiplier central limit theorem* that also

$$n^{-1/2} \sum_{i=1}^{n} G_i X_i \xrightarrow{D} U,$$

under suitably conditions (van der Vaart & Wellner, 1996) given almost every sequence of $X_1, \cdots, X_n$.

One practical use of this is that when X_i are the residuals from some regression model then it will often also be true that

$$n^{-1/2} \sum_{i=1}^{n} G_i \hat{X}_i \xrightarrow{D} U,$$

where $\hat{X}_i$ are estimated based on the data, and this result can also be expanded to functional cases where for example X_i is a residual process on $D[0,\tau]$. We will use this approach to approximate the asymptotic distribution for many estimators as suggested in the counting process situation by Lin et al. (1993).

2.6 Exercises

2.1 (Poisson process) A Poisson process $N(t)$ with intensity $\lambda(t)$ is a counting process with

- independent increments and such that
- $N(t) - N(s)$ follows a Poisson distribution with parameter $\int_s^t \lambda(u)\,du$ for all $0 \le s \le t$.

(a) Find the compensator Λ of N and put $M = N - \Lambda$. Show by a direct calculation that $E(M(t) \,|\, \mathcal{F}_s) = M(s)$, where $\mathcal{F}_t$ is the internal history N. Is M a local square integrable martingale?

(b) Find the compensator of M^2.

2.2 (Brownian motion and Brownian bridge) The Brownian motion or the Wiener process is the Gaussian process B such that $EB(t) = 0$ and $\mathrm{Cov}(B(s), B(t)) = s \wedge t$ for $s, t \ge 0$.

(a) Show that B has independent increments. Show that B is a martingale and find the compensator of B^2.

The Brownian bridge (tied down Wiener process) $B^0(t)$ with $t \in [0,1]$ is the Gaussian process such that $EB^0(t) = 0$ and $\mathrm{Cov}(B^0(s), B^0(t)) = s(1-t)$ for $0 \le s \le t \le 1$.

(b) Show that the processes $B^0(t)$ and $B(t) - tB(1)$ have the same distribution on $[0,1]$.

(c) Show that the processes $B(t)$ and $(1+t)B^0(t/(1+t))$ have the same distribution on $[0, \infty)$.

2.3 (Hall-Wellner bands) Consider the time interval $[0, \tau]$. Let $U(t)$ be a Gaussian martingale with covariance process $V(t)$, $t \in [0, \tau]$. Show that

$$U(t)V(\tau)^{1/2}[V(\tau) + V(t)]^{-1}$$

has the same distribution as

$$B^0\left(\frac{V(t)}{V(\tau) + V(t)}\right),$$

where B^0 is the standard Brownian bridge.

2.6 Exercises

2.4 Let M_1 and M_2 be the martingales associated with the components of the multivariate counting process $N = (N_1, N_2)$ with continuous compensators. Show that

$$\langle M_1, M_2 \rangle = [M_1, M_2] = 0.$$

2.5 Let $M = N - \Lambda$ be the counting process local martingale. It may be shown that Λ is locally bounded Meyer (1976), Theorem IV.12.

(a) Show that N is a local submartingale with localizing sequence

$$T_n = n \wedge \sup\{t : N(t) < n\}.$$

(b) Show that M is a local square integrable martingale using the below cited optional stopping theorem.

Theorem. *Let M be a $\mathcal{F}_t$-martingale and let T be an $\mathcal{F}_t$-stopping time. Then $(M(t \wedge T) : t \geq 0)$ is a martingale.*

2.6 Let $M = N - \Lambda$ be the counting process local martingale.

(a) Show that $EN(t) = E\Lambda(t)$ (hint: use the monotone convergence theorem).

(b) If $E\Lambda(t) < \infty$, then show that M is a martingale by verifying the martingale conditions.

(c) If $\sup_t E\Lambda(t) < \infty$, then show that M is a square integrable martingale.

2.7 Let $N(t) = (N_1(t), \ldots, N_k(t))$, $t \in [0, \tau]$, be a multivariate counting process with respect to $\mathcal{F}_t$. It holds that the intensity

$$\lambda(t) = (\lambda_1(t), \ldots, \lambda_k(t))$$

of $N(t)$ is given (heuristically) as

$$\lambda_h(t) = P(dN_h(t) = 1 \,|\, \mathcal{F}_{t-}), \tag{2.29}$$

where $dN_h(t) = N_h((t+dt)-) - N_h(t-)$ is the change in N_h over the small time interval $[t, t+dt)$.

(a) Let T^* be a lifetime with hazard $\alpha(t)$ and define $N(t) = I(T^* \leq t)$. Use the above (2.29) to show that the intensity of $N(t)$ with respect to the history $\sigma\{N(s) : s \leq t\}$ is

$$\lambda(t) = I(t \leq T^*)\alpha(t).$$

(b) Let T^* be a lifetime with hazard $\alpha(t)$ that may be right-censored at time C. We assume that T^* and C are independent. Let $T = T^* \wedge C$, $\Delta = I(T^* \leq C)$ and $N(t) = I(T \leq t, \Delta = 1)$. Use the above (2.29) to show that the intensity of $N(t)$ with respect to the history

$$\sigma\{I(T \leq s, \Delta = 0), I(T \leq s, \Delta = 1) : s \leq t\}$$

is

$$\lambda(t) = I(t \leq T)\alpha(t).$$

2.8 Let $M(s)$ and $M_\epsilon(s)$ denote the martingales introduced in Example 2.5.1.

(a) Verify the expressions for $\langle M \rangle(s)$, $[M](s)$ and $\langle M_\epsilon \rangle(s)$ given in that example and show that they converge in probability as $n \to \infty$ verifying Gill's condition (2.28).

(b) From the same example, show that:

$$\sup_{s \in [0,t]} |n^{1/2} \int_0^s (J(u) - 1)\alpha(u)\, du| \xrightarrow{P} 0.$$

2.9 (Asymptotic results for the Nelson-Aalen estimator) Let $N^{(n)}(t)$ be a counting process satisfying the multiplicative intensity structure $\lambda(t) = Y^{(n)}(t)\alpha(t)$ with $\alpha(t)$ being locally integrable. The Nelson-Aalen estimator of $\int_0^t \alpha(s)\, ds$ is

$$\hat{A}^{(n)}(t) = \int \frac{1}{Y^{(n)}(s)} dN^{(n)}(s).$$

Define $A^*(t) = \int_0^t J^{(n)}(s)\alpha(s)\, ds$ where $J^{(n)}(t) = I(Y^{(n)}(t) > 0)$.

(a) Show that $A^{(n)}(t) - A^*(t)$ is a local square integrable martingale.

(b) Show that, as $n \to \infty$

$$\sup_{s \leq t} |\hat{A}^{(n)}(t) - A(t)| \xrightarrow{P} 0$$

provided that

$$\int_0^t \frac{J^{(n)}(s)}{Y^{(n)}(s)} \alpha(s)\, ds \xrightarrow{P} 0 \quad \text{and} \quad \int_0^t (1 - J^{(n)}(s))\alpha(s)\, ds \xrightarrow{P} 0,$$

as $n \to \infty$.

(c) Show that the two conditions given in (b) are satisfied provided that

$$\inf_{s \leq t} Y^{(n)}(t) \xrightarrow{P} \infty, \quad \text{as } n \to \infty.$$

Define $\sigma^2(s) = \int_0^s \frac{\alpha(u)}{y(u)} du$, where y is a non-negative function so that α/y is integrable over $[0, t]$.

(d) Let $n \to \infty$. If, for all $\epsilon > 0$,

$$n \int_0^s \frac{J^{(n)}(u)}{Y^{(n)}(u)} \alpha(u) I\left(\left| n^{1/2} \frac{J^{(n)}(u)}{Y^{(n)}(u)} \right| > \epsilon \right) du \xrightarrow{P} 0,$$

$$n^{1/2} \int_0^s (1 - J^{(n)}(u)) \alpha(u) \, du \xrightarrow{P} 0 \quad \text{and} \quad n \int_0^s \frac{J^{(n)}(u)}{Y^{(n)}(u)} \alpha(u) \, du \xrightarrow{P} \sigma^2(s)$$

for all $s \leq t$, then show that

$$n^{1/2}(\hat{A}^{(n)} - A) \xrightarrow{D} U$$

on $D[0, t]$, where U is a Gaussian martingale with variance function σ^2.

2.10 (Right-censoring by the same stochastic variable) Let $T_1^*, \ldots, T_n^*$ be n i.i.d. positive stochastic variables with hazard function $\alpha(t)$. The observed data consist of $(T_i, \Delta_i)_{i=1,\ldots,n}$, where $T_i = T_i^* \wedge U$, $\Delta_i = I(T_i = T_i^*)$. Here, U is a positive stochastic variable with hazard function $\mu(t)$, and assumed independent of the T_i^*'s. Define

$$N_\cdot(t) = \sum_{i=1}^n N_i(t), \quad Y_\cdot(t) = \sum_{i=1}^n Y_i(t)$$

with $N_i(t) = I(T_i \leq t, \Delta_i = 1)$ and $Y_i(t) = I(t \leq T_i)$, $i = 1, \ldots, n$.

(a) Show that $\hat{A}(t) - A^*(t)$ is a martingale, where

$$\hat{A}(t) = \int_0^t \frac{1}{Y_\cdot(s)} dN_\cdot(s), \quad A^*(t) = \int_0^t J(s) \alpha(s) \, ds.$$

(b) Show that

$$\sup_{s \leq t} |\hat{A}(s) - A^*(s)| \xrightarrow{P} 0$$

if $P(T_i \leq t) > 0$.

(c) Is it also true that $\hat{A}(t) - A(t) \xrightarrow{P} 0$?

2.11 Consider again Example 2.5.2.

(a) Verify the expressions for $(n^{1/2}M)_\epsilon(s)$ and $\langle M_\epsilon\rangle(s)$.

(b) Show that $\langle M_\epsilon\rangle(s) \xrightarrow{P} 0$ using Gill's condition and that

$$\lim_{n\to\infty} \int_{A_n} X dP = 0,$$

where X is a random variable with $E|X| < \infty$, A_n is measurable and $A_n \searrow \emptyset$.

2.12 (Simulations from Example 2.5.3) Consider the simulations in Example 2.5.3. Work out the asymptotic bias for the simulations as a function of time and compare with Figure 2.3.

2.13 (Counting process with discrete compensator) Let N be a counting process with compensator Λ that may have jumps. Put $M = N - \Lambda$.

(a) Show by a direct calculation that

$$[M](t) = N(t) - 2\int_0^t \Delta\Lambda(s)dN(s) + \int_0^t \Delta\Lambda(s)d\Lambda(s),$$

where $\Delta\Lambda(t)$ denotes the jumps of $\Lambda(t)$.

(b) Show that

$$\langle M\rangle(t) = \Lambda(t) - \int_0^t \Delta\Lambda(s)d\Lambda(s).$$

3
Estimation for filtered counting process data

One particularly important aspect of counting process data is that the processes will often be observed subject to certain restrictions. For both recurrent events data and failure time data, these restrictions are most often that the failure times are observed subject to right-censoring and/or left truncation. These concepts will be explained in detail in this chapter, and we also briefly mention other types of observation schemes that generally lead to more complicated analysis. Right-censoring and left-truncation in the form that we consider here do not constitute much difficulty in terms of the analysis when the object of interest is the intensity. The key to this is that, when the right-censoring and left-truncation are unrelated to the counting process of interest, the intensity is unaffected for subjects at risk.

We start our discussion by introducing various observation schemes including right-censoring and left-truncation and give conditions under which these do not constitute any problems. Following this we take a look at the likelihood function for counting process data to see how maximum likelihood estimation may be carried out. Finally, we discuss how estimating equations may be established for counting process data.

3.1 Filtered counting process data

For failure time data one of the most common types of incompleteness is *right-censoring*, meaning that for some of the failure times we only know

Example 3.1.1 (Melanoma data)

For the melanoma data the interest lies in studying the effect of various prognostic risk factors on time to death of malignant melanoma after removal of tumor. The study was closed at the end of 1977 and the number of deaths caused by malignant melanoma in the considered period was 57. The rest of the 205 patients study did not experience the event of interest in the study period but were right-censored mostly because they were still alive at the end of 1977. Data from two patients are shown below.

```
days status sex age year thick ulc
204    1    1  28  1971  4.84  1
 35    2    1  41  1977  1.34  0
```

The first of these two patients, a 28 year old man, was enrolled in 1971 and died (status=1) from the disease 204 days after removal of tumor. The second, a 41 year old man, was enrolled in 1977 and was still alive (status=2) when the study closed 35 days after his operation. Actually, a few patients were censored because they died of something not related to the disease of interest. Formally speaking, the correct framework for considering this type of data is the competing risks model; see Chapter 10.
□

The ultimate goal of an analysis of right-censored counting process data, and as a special case survival data, is to estimate the parameters that describe the intensity and perhaps also to examine various hypotheses. It is not clear at first how to incorporate the censored observations into the statistical analysis. Obviously basing the statistical analysis on only the complete data can give biased results, so the censored observations need to be taken into account. It turns out that handling of censoring and other types of incomplete failure time data is easy when basing the analysis on models for the intensity, at least if the censoring, and more generally filtering, is so-called independent. Below we introduce the concept of filtered counting processes and give the definition of independent filtering, that is the class of filters that do not change the intensities for subjects at risk at any point in time. This includes as a special case the definition of independent right-censoring, a concept for which there exist various definitions in the literature. Our treatment restricts attention to the case of independent counting processes, although all the concepts can be defined more generally.

Consider a multivariate counting process $N^*(t) = (N_1^*(t), \ldots, N_n^*(t))$ adapted to the filtration $(\mathcal{F}_t^*)$ and defined on a probability space $(\Omega, \mathcal{F}, P)$. We assume that the counting processes $N_i^*(t)$ are independent such that

the information accumulated over time
$$\mathcal{F}_t^* = \vee_{i=1}^n \mathcal{F}_t^{i*}$$
is made up of independent pieces of information $\mathcal{F}_t^{i*}$ for the subjects. The basic model is that N_i^* has $\mathcal{F}_t^{i*}$-compensator Λ_i^*, where
$$\Lambda_i^*(t,\theta) = \int_0^t \lambda_i^*(s,\theta)\, ds \qquad (3.1)$$
with θ being some parameter of interest. Note that the filtration $(\mathcal{F}_t^{i*})$ may carry information about covariates, which may be reflected in the compensator (3.1). As argued above, N^* will typically not be fully observable, but only an incomplete version will be available. The observable part of $N_i^*(t)$ may often be expressed as
$$N_i(t) = \int_0^t C_i(s)\, dN_i^*(s),$$
where $C_i(t)$ denotes the ith so-called filtering process
$$C_i(t) = I(t \in A_i).$$
We require, for simplicity, that the filtering processes are independent across subjects. The principal example of filtering is right-censoring, where $A_i = [0, U_i]$ with U_i some random censoring time, that is,
$$C_i(t) = I(t \le U_i). \qquad (3.2)$$
In this case, $N_i^*(t)$ is observed only up to the censoring time U_i, and is unknown thereafter.

The filtration $\mathcal{F}_t^*$ contains the information on which we want to build our model. Unfortunately we cannot observe $\mathcal{F}_t^*$ fully due to various kinds of incompleteness as, for example, right-censoring. What we do observe is recorded by the observed filtration denoted by $\mathcal{F}_t$. The objective is now to find the observed intensity, that is, the intensity $\lambda_i(t)$ of $N_i(t)$ with respect to the observed filtration $\mathcal{F}_t$, and making requirements such that the parameters of the intensity of interest can still be estimated consistently. We define independent filtering as the situation where the intensity of the filtered counting process is equivalent to the intensity of the underlying counting process that is not fully observed, or phrased more explicitly, that $\lambda^*(t) = \lambda(t)$ when $C(t) = 1$. Our definition is very general and encompasses the cases of primary interest, namely right-censoring and left-truncation as well as repeated combinations of these.

Definition 3.1.1 (Independent filtering) Let N^* be a multivariate counting process with compensator Λ^* with respect to a filtration $\mathcal{F}_t^*$, and let C be a filtering process. The filtering of N^* leading to the observed $N = \int CdN^*$ generated by C is said to be independent if the compensator of N with respect to the observed filtration $\mathcal{F}_t$ is $\int_0^t C(s)\lambda^*(s)ds$. □

The above definition implicitly assumes that $C(t)\lambda^*(t)$ is predictable with respect to the observed filtration. Note that the expression "the observed compensator" refers to the probability measure with respect to which things are considered (observed); we denote this measure by $P_\mathcal{O}$. The condition of independent filtering, for the individual processes, can also be written as

$$C_i(t)P(dN_i^*(t) = 1 \mid \mathcal{F}_{t-}^*) = P_\mathcal{O}(dN_i(t) = 1 \mid \mathcal{F}_{t-}). \tag{3.3}$$

The condition states that the probability of a jump for the unobserved counting processes given full information and the observed counting processes are equivalent and thus are unaltered by the filtering, that is, those subjects at risk and under observation are representative for the entire sample had there been no filtering.

Example 3.1.2 (Left-truncation)

In the case of left-truncated survival data we observe the lifetime T^* (assuming no censoring) and the truncation variable V only if $T^* > V$, and then have $P_\mathcal{O}(\cdot) = P(\cdot \mid T^* > V)$. Assume that T^* has hazard $\alpha(t)$ and let $N^*(t) = I(T^* \leq t)$ and $C(t) = I(V < t)$. The observed counting process is thus

$$N(t) = \int_0^t C(s)dN^*(s) = I(V < T^* \leq t).$$

Define

$$\mathcal{F}_t = \sigma(V, N(s) : V \leq s \leq V + t),$$

which corresponds to the observed filtration given that $T^* > V$. It may be shown, assuming for example that T^* and V are independent, that $N(t)$ has compensator $\Lambda(t) = \int_0^t C(s)I(s \leq T^*)\alpha(s)\,ds$ with respect to $\mathcal{F}_t$ and computed under $P_\mathcal{O}$, the filtering thus being independent. See Exercise 3.5 for further results. □

Independent right-censoring is defined as independent filtering, where the filtering processes are of the form

$$C_i(t) = I(t \leq U_i)$$

with U_i, $i = 1, ..., n$, positive random variables.

To check in specific situations whether a given type of filtering is independent, one needs to compute the intensity of N with respect to the observed filtration $\mathcal{F}_t$. A useful tool is the innovation theorem, which may be thought of as a projection of an intensity from one filtration to another contained within the first one. Since $\mathcal{F}_t \subseteq \mathcal{F}_t^*$ does not hold, we cannot project from $\mathcal{F}_t^*$. We therefore define an enlarged history $\mathcal{G}_t^* = \vee_{i=1}^n \mathcal{G}_t^{i*}$ containing both the relevant information $\mathcal{F}_t^*$ and the filtering processes. We also make the requirement that the filtering processes are predictable with respect to $\mathcal{G}_t^*$. In the case of right-censoring one may take

$$\mathcal{G}_t^* = \mathcal{F}_t^* \vee \sigma(C(s+); 0 \leq s \leq t) \tag{3.4}$$

with $C(t) = (C_1(t), \ldots, C_n(t))$ given by (3.2) since these processes are left-continuous. In most cases we will then have that $\mathcal{F}_t \subseteq \mathcal{G}_t^*$, but, if this is not the case, we redefine $\mathcal{G}_t^*$ so that it also holds the information carried by $\mathcal{F}_t$. The relations between the different filtrations are thus

$$\mathcal{F}_t^* \subseteq \mathcal{G}_t^* \supseteq \mathcal{F}_t,$$

but neither $\mathcal{F}_t \subseteq \mathcal{F}_t^*$ nor $\mathcal{F}_t^* \subseteq \mathcal{F}_t$ hold. This construction ties in with the definition of independent right-censoring given by Andersen et al. (1993) (ABGK) cited below. One may try to generalize the ABGK definition to filtering in an obvious way, but as we shall see later this may lead to undesired classifications.

ABGK definition of independent right-censoring: Let N^* be a multivariate counting process with compensator Λ^* with respect to a filtration $\mathcal{F}_t^*$, and let C be a right-censoring process predictable with respect to a filtration $\mathcal{G}_t^* \supseteq \mathcal{F}_t^*$. The right-censoring of N^* leading to the observed N generated by C is said to be independent if the compensator of N^* with respect to the enlarged filtration $\mathcal{G}_t^*$ is also Λ^*.

The ABGK condition for independent right-censoring can also be written as

$$P(dN_i^*(t) = 1 \mid \mathcal{F}_{t-}^*) = P(dN_i^*(t) = 1 \mid \mathcal{G}_{t-}^*), \tag{3.5}$$

saying that the probability of a jump in the next small time interval is unaltered by the extra information about the filtering processes in the case where we have full information available about the counting processes. This definition refers solely to the underlying unobserved counting processes, and requires that the filtering process does not carry any extra information about the timing of the jumps of the counting process of interest. We give some examples below to illustrate the use of the definition in terms of its consequences for the observed processes. The ABGK definition is rather indirect as it does not directly say anything about the intensity of the observed counting process. Of course something has been said as one can use the innovation theorem to compute the observed intensity. Below, in Proposition 3.1.1, we show that, if $C_i(t)\lambda_i^*(t)$ is predictable with respect to $\mathcal{F}_t$, then the ABGK condition implies independent filtering as defined in Definition 3.1.1.

54   3. Estimation for filtered counting process data

Proposition 3.1.1 *If $C_i(t)\lambda_i^*(t)$ is predictable with respect to the observed history $\mathcal{F}_t$, then the ABGK definition of independent right-censoring implies independent filtering.*

PROOF. We have the decomposition

$$N_i^*(t) = \Lambda_i^*(t) + M_i^*(t),$$

where $M_i^*(t)$ is a local square integrable martingale with respect to $\mathcal{G}_t^*$ (ABGK condition), and therefore

$$N_i(t) = \int_0^t C_i(s)\lambda_i^*(s)\,ds + \int_0^t C_i(s)\,dM_i^*(s)$$
$$= \int_0^t \lambda_i(s)\,ds + M_i(t),$$

where $M_i(t) = \int_0^t C_i(s)\,dM_i^*(s)$ is a local square integrable martingale with respect to $\mathcal{G}_t^*$ since $C_i(t)$ is $\mathcal{G}_t^*$-predictable and bounded. From this, it is seen that $N_i(t)$ has the intensity process $C_i(t)\lambda_i^*(t)$ with respect to $\mathcal{G}_t^*$, and therefore also with respect to $\mathcal{F}_t$ by the innovation theorem (2.12) since $C_i(t)\lambda_i^*(t)$ is assumed predictable with respect to $\mathcal{F}_t$. □

Filtering processes that are independent of the underlying counting processes may not lead to independent filtering as seen in the following example. If the ABGK definition is generalized to general filtering (replace right-censoring by filtering in their definition), this may lead to an undesired classification as in the below example.

Example 3.1.3 (Dependence on the past)

Consider a counting process $N^*(t)$ with intensity $\lambda^*(t) = \max(N^*(t-), 5)$. We filter the process by the indicator $C(t) = I(t \geq V)$ where V is a stochastic variable independent of N^*. Owing to the assumed independence, this type of filtering is independent according to the ABGK definition (generalized to filtering). However, whether or not it is classified as independent filtering according to Definition 3.1.1 depends on the observed filtration. Consider two types of possible recorded information

$$\mathcal{F}_t = \sigma(V, N^*(s) - N^*(V), N^*(V); V \leq s \leq V + t), \qquad (3.6)$$
$$\mathcal{F}_t = \sigma(V, N^*(s) - N^*(V); V \leq s \leq V + t). \qquad (3.7)$$

the difference being that in (3.6) we observe $N^*(V)$ while this is not recorded by (3.7). The intensity of the observed counting process $N(t) = \int_0^t C(s)dN^*(s)$ can be computed using the innovation theorem:

$$\lambda(t) = E(C(t)\lambda^*(t)|\mathcal{F}_{t-}),$$

and is equal to $C(t)\lambda^*(t)$ if (3.6) is the actually recorded information. If, however, (3.7) is the recorded information, so we do not observe $N^*(V)$, then the observed intensity differs from $C(t)\lambda^*(t)$ and we do not have independent filtering in that case! So when the intensity depends on the past of the counting process (or possibly covariates), this type of filtering may lead to an observed intensity different from the one of the underlying counting processes N^*. We also refer the reader to the discussion in Andersen et al. (1993), p. 163. □

We now consider the special case of right-censored survival data in the following example.

Example 3.1.4 (Right-censored survival data)

Let T^* denote the survival time of interest and put $N^*(t) = I(T^* \leq t)$. Assume that the distribution of T^* is absolutely continuous with hazard function $\alpha^\theta(t)$. As we have seen earlier the counting process N^* then satisfies the Aalen multiplicative intensity model

$$\lambda^*(t,\theta) = \alpha^\theta(t) Y^*(t)$$

with respect to $\mathcal{F}_t^* = \mathcal{F}_t^{N^*}$, where $Y^*(t) = I(t \leq T^*)$ is the at risk indicator. Let U denote the censoring time, which is assumed independent of the failure time. If the filtration $\mathcal{F}_t^*$ also contains information about covariates, then one may relax the above independence assumption to a conditional independence assumption given the covariates. We only observe the failure time T^* if it exceeds the corresponding censoring time U, and information about this. We thus observe

$$T = T^* \wedge U \quad \text{and} \quad \Delta = I(T \leq U).$$

The independent censoring condition of ABGK (3.5) then reads

$$P(t \leq T^* < t + dt \,|\, T^* \geq t) = P(t \leq T^* < t + dt \,|\, T^* \geq t, U \geq t) \quad (3.8)$$

and is equivalent to (3.3), which is seen to hold due to the assumed independence. By the way, condition (3.8) is often taken as the definition of independent right-censoring; see, for example, Fleming & Harrington (1991) p. 27. The observed filtration under the considered filtering is given by

$$\mathcal{F}_t = \sigma((N(s), Y(s+)); 0 \leq s \leq t),$$

$Y(t) = C(t) Y^*(t)$ and $C(t) = I(t \leq U)$. Since we have independent filtering, the observed counting process $N(t)$ has intensity process

$$\lambda(t,\theta) = \alpha^\theta(t) Y(t) \tag{3.9}$$

with respect to $\mathcal{F}_t$. It is seen from (3.9) that the multiplicative intensity structure is preserved and the deterministic part is unchanged. The only difference is that the at risk indicator $Y^*(t) = I(t \leq T)$ is replaced by the observed at risk indicator $Y(t) = C(t)Y^*(t) = I(t \leq T \wedge C)$. Therefore, as we shall see in the subsequent section, to do maximum likelihood estimation for right-censored survival data, assuming that the right-censoring does not carry information about the parameters of interest, one should simply use the observed intensity in the computations. □

The right-censoring may depend on covariates as long as the condition is satisfied conditional on these covariates. We give the details for this in the case of independent survival data for simplicity.

Example 3.1.5 (Right-censoring depending on covariates)

A somewhat surprising result is that censoring depending on covariate values is independent as long as the covariate(s) influencing the censoring is included in the statistical model. That is, we use a filtration also carrying the information generated by the covariate(s). In the melanoma example, it would for instance be independent censoring to censor each year the oldest patient still at risk as long as we include age in our model, as was also pointed out in Andersen et al. (1993). We now give a formal proof assuming for ease of notation that the covariate is one-dimensional. Assume we have n independent subjects and let X_i denote a one-dimensional bounded covariate (age at entry) for the ith subject, $i = 1, \ldots, n$. Further, let $N^*(t) = (N_1^*(t), \ldots, N_n^*(t))$ where $N_i^*(t) = I(T_i^* \leq t)$, and let $\mathcal{F}_t^{N^*} = \sigma(N^*(s); 0 \leq s \leq t)$ and $\mathcal{F}^x = \sigma((X_1, \ldots, X_n))$. We assume that N^* has $\mathcal{F}_t^* = (\mathcal{F}_t^{N^*} \vee \mathcal{F}^x)$-compensator Λ^*, where

$$\Lambda_i^*(t) = \int_0^t \lambda_i^*(s, \theta) \, ds$$

with

$$\lambda_i^*(t, \theta) = Y_i^*(t) \alpha_i^\theta(t, X_i), \quad Y_i^*(t) = I(t \leq T_i).$$

Define $U_i = \min\{j \in \mathbb{N} : Y_i(j)(X_i + j) = \max_k(Y_k(j)(X_k + j))\}$, where $Y_i(t) = I(t \leq T_i \wedge U_i)$, that is, the ith patient is censored the first year he or she is the oldest among those still at risk. Let $\mathcal{G}_t^* = \mathcal{F}_t^* \vee \mathcal{F}_t^u$ where $\mathcal{F}_t^u = \sigma(C(s+); 0 \leq s \leq t)$, $C(t) = (C_1(t), \ldots, C_n(t))$ with $C_i(t) = I(t \leq U_i)$. Since the censoring is deterministic when we have conditioned on $(X_1, \ldots, X_n)$ there is no extra randomness in $\mathcal{G}_t^*$ compared with $\mathcal{F}_t^*$ and therefore the compensator of $N_i^*(t)$ with respect to $\mathcal{G}_t^*$ is also $\Lambda_i^*(t)$. Since $C_i(t)\lambda_i^*(t, \theta) = Y_i(t)\alpha_i^\theta(t, X_i)$ is predictable with respect to the observed filtration, it follows that the filtering induced by this type of right-censoring is independent. Note, using the innovation theorem, that the intensity with respect to $\mathcal{F}_t^{N^*}$ (omit conditioning on the covariate) is:

$$E(\lambda_i^*(t, \theta) \mid \mathcal{F}_t^{N^*}) = Y_i^*(t) E(\alpha_i^\theta(t, X_i) \mid T_i > t) = Y_i^*(t) \alpha(t),$$

say. The intensity of $N_i(t)$ with respect to the observed filtration $\tilde{\mathcal{F}}_t$ that does not hold information about the covariate is

$$E(C_i(t)\lambda_i^*(t,\theta) \mid \tilde{\mathcal{F}}_t) = Y_i(t)E(\alpha_i^\theta(t,X_i) \mid T_i > t, U_i > t) \qquad (3.10)$$

using that the censoring fulfills the ABGK-condition of independent censoring when we do condition on the covariate. Since the censoring carries information about the covariates, (3.10) differs from $Y_i(t)\alpha(t)$, and the censoring is therefore dependent if we do not include the covariate in the model! □

Example 3.1.6 (Simple and progressive type I censoring)

Simple type I censoring where all U_i are equal to a deterministic fixed time point u_0 is independent since no extra randomness is introduced by the censoring, leaving the compensator unchanged. Progressive type I censoring refers to a situation often encountered in clinical studies where patients are enrolled over (calendar) time with separate entry times W_i. At entry a treatment is applied and the life time T_i *since entry* is then of interest. Suppose the study is closed at time t_0 such that we only observe, for each subject, $T_i \wedge U_i$, $I(T_i \leq U_i)$ with $U_i = t_0 - W_i$. This is called progressive type I censoring. If we include the entry times in the filtration, then this censoring is deterministic and therefore independent. If the entry times are not included in the filtration but have an impact on the failure times, this censoring is dependent. □

Example 3.1.7 (Missing covariates. Complete case analysis)

We consider n independent subjects and let $X_i(t) = (X_{i1}(t), \ldots, X_{ip}(t))$, $i = 1, \ldots, n$, denote a p-vector of bounded covariates for the ith subject. The covariate processes are assumed to be right-continuous and we put $\mathcal{F}_t^x = \sigma((X_1(s), \ldots, X_n(s)); 0 \leq s \leq t)$. Let $N^*(t) = (N_1^*(t), \ldots, N_n^*(t))$ denote a multivariate counting process where $N_i^*(t) = I(T_i^* \leq t)$. Assume that N^* has $(\mathcal{F}_t^{N^*} \vee \mathcal{F}_t^x)$-compensator Λ^*, where

$$\Lambda_i^*(t,\theta) = \int_0^t \lambda_i^*(s,\theta)\,ds$$

with

$$\lambda_i^*(t,\theta) = Y_i^*(t)\alpha_i^\theta(t, X_i(t-)), \quad Y_i^*(t) = I(t \leq T_i).$$

Suppose that some of the covariates may be missing from a certain point in time and onwards, and that the individual is withdrawn from the study if that happens, that is, the individual is censored at that point in time. One may ask whether or not this "complete case analysis" leads to independent censoring. The answer is that the generation of missing values in the covariates is allowed to depend on the past and present but not on the future. The result is formulated below in the case where we assume that no additional censoring takes place, but can also be obtained in the case where we also have ordinary independent right-censoring.

Let
$$H_{ij}(t) = I(X_{ij}(t) \text{ is available}), \quad j = 1, \ldots, p,$$
and
$$H_{i0}(t) = I(H_{ij}(t) = 1 \text{ for all } j = 1, \ldots, p).$$

Define right-censoring times U_i caused by the incomplete covariate measurements by
$$U_i = \inf\{t \geq 0 : H_{i0}(t) = 0 \text{ and } Y_i(t) = 1\},$$
with the convention $\inf\{\emptyset\} = \infty$. The probability of missing some components of X_i (say X_i^*) is allowed to depend on X_i^*, so-called non-ignorable non-response (NINR); see Little & Rubin (1987). Let
$$C^u(t) = (C_1^u(t), \ldots, C_n^u(t))$$
denote the filtering process defined by $C_i^u(t) = I(t \leq U_i)$, and let
$$\mathcal{F}_t^u = \sigma(C^u(s+); 0 \leq s \leq t).$$

It may be shown (Martinussen, 1997) that the right-censoring caused by C^u is independent if the following conditional independence condition is fulfilled:

$$\forall B \in \mathcal{F}_t^u : \quad P(B \mid \mathcal{F}_\infty^{N^*} \vee \mathcal{F}_\infty^x) = P(B \mid \mathcal{F}_t^{N^*} \vee \mathcal{F}_t^x) \quad \text{a.s.} \qquad (3.11)$$

on $D_t^i = (T_i \geq t)$, $i = 1, \ldots, n$. The intuition behind (3.11) is that the generation of missing values in the covariates is allowed to depend on the past and present but not on the future as mentioned earlier.

If the covariate is time-independent and one-dimensional we have
$$U_i = \begin{cases} 0 & \text{if } X_i \text{ is missing} \\ +\infty & \text{otherwise} \end{cases}$$
and the censoring corresponding to the complete case analysis is hence independent if
$$P(U_i = 0 \mid T_i, X_i) = p(X_i; \phi),$$
for some parameter ϕ. Therefore, despite that X_i may be missing NINR, the parameters describing the relationship between the failure time and the covariate are estimated consistently when the probability of having missing covariate information only depends on the covariates themselves. An underlying assumption is of course that it is possible to estimate consistently in a complete data analysis (full covariate information), that is, the model should be correctly specified in the first place. □

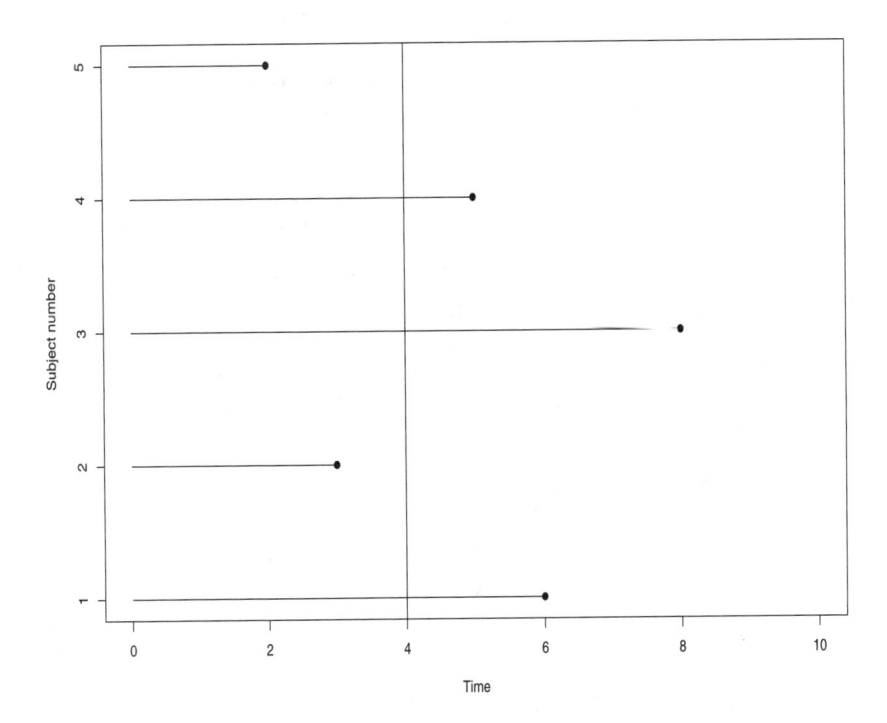

FIGURE 3.1: Left-truncation: Subject 1, 3 and 4 are at risk from time $V = 4$ and onwards. Subject 2 and 5 are never included in the sample since only individuals with event times larger than V are included. Left-censoring: Subject 1, 3 and 4 are at risk from time $V = 4$ and onwards. For individual 2 and 5 it is only known that the event time is smaller than V.

The second most important type of incomplete information for counting processes data, and failure time data in particular, is left-truncation. A failure time T^* is said to be *left-truncated* by the (possibly random) V if we only observe T^* *conditionally* on $T^* > V$, see Figure 3.1. If time to miscarriage is to be studied and a sample of pregnant women is recruited at a certain point in time (the period that they have been pregnant may vary from woman to woman) and followed on in time, then we have a sample of left-truncated waiting times as it is known for these women that the time to miscarriage (if it ever happens) is beyond the period they have been pregnant at the sampling date. We define left-truncation for counting process data similarly, but for the concept to be of value and leading to independent filtering one needs to condition on past performance of the counting process. This simplifies for the failure time data case with time-invariant covariates, where the past information about the counting process reduces to information about the subject being still at risk, whereas in the general counting process case one needs to condition on all relevant parts of the history to obtain independent filtering.

We define left-truncation as filtering with respect to the observed probability measure that is conditional on past information and with filtering processes on the form

$$C_i(t) = I(t > V_i),$$

where V_i are random variables for $i = 1, ..., n$. The requirement for independent filtering in this case reads

$$C_i(t)\lambda_i^*(t) = P_O(dN_i(t) = 1|\mathcal{F}_t^i).$$

Owing to the repeated conditioning argument, this condition will be true if the observed filtration contains the relevant information about $\lambda_i^*(t)$ from the truncation time and up to time t.

Example 3.1.8 (Left-truncated survival data)

Recall that $N^*(t) = (N_1^*(t), ..., N_n^*(t))$ is adapted to the filtration $(\mathcal{F}_t^*)$ and where we in the failure time data setting can define $N^*(t)$ from i.i.d. failure times $T_1^*, ..., T_n^*$ such that $N_i^*(t) = I(T_i^* \leq t)$. The basic model is that N^* has $(\mathcal{F}_t^*)$-compensator Λ^* with respect to a probability measure P where

$$\Lambda^*(t, \theta) = \int_0^t \lambda_i^*(s, \theta)\, ds$$

with θ being some parameter. In addition to the survival times we are also given i.i.d. truncation times $V_1, ..., V_n$ such that $T_i^* > V_i$. The most important difference from the right-censoring case is that events are seen *conditional* on the truncation event.

We start by noting that the observed counting processes can be written as

$$N_i(t) = \int_0^t C_i(s)\, dN_i^*(s),$$

where $C_i(t) = I(t \geq V_i)$.

Independent filtering is somewhat more complicated in this setting because the relevant probability measure is conditional on the event $A = \cap_{i=1,...,n}(T_i^* > V_i)$. To check for independent filtering we therefore have to validate that

$$C_i(t)P(t \leq T_i^* < t + dt\,|\,\mathcal{F}_{t-}^*) = P_O(t \leq T_i^* < t + dt\,|\,\mathcal{F}_{t-}), \qquad (3.12)$$

or that

$$C_i(t)P(t \leq T_i^* < t + dt\,|\,T_i^* \geq t) = P(t \leq T_i^* < t + dt\,|\,T_i^* \geq t, T_i^* \geq V_i, V_i). \qquad (3.13)$$

Condition (3.13) simply states that being included in the study after time V_i should contain no information about the intensity at any point in time where the subject is at risk.

There is an equivalent condition in the case of general counting process data, but it is important to point out that the conditioning should include all relevant information from the past of the observed counting processes in addition to the truncation variable for the left-truncation to lead to independent filtering. Therefore one would typically need to condition on the behavior of the process prior to it being included in the study, and this would often constitute a practical problem.

In the case of i.i.d. survival data that we consider here, however, things simplify because the only relevant information about the past is contained in the fact that the subject is at risk, and the independent filtering condition (Definition 3.1.1) is fulfilled even though an unconditional probability measure is used when the at risk indicator is defined as

$$Y_i(t) = C_i(t)Y_i^*(t) = I(T_i \geq t, t \geq V_i).$$

Using the observed intensity for inference it is seen that the individuals are at risk from their (individual) truncation time and onwards. This is referred to as *delayed entry* . □

Right-censoring and left-truncation will often be combined in survival studies. This corresponds to a filtering process on the form $C_i(t) = I(V_i \leq t \leq U_i)$ and where the intensity is observed subject to the information contained in $\mathcal{F}_{V_i}^{i*}$.

Example 3.1.9 (Left-censoring and current status data)

Left-censoring occurs when observation of the primary outcome (e.g. time to failure) is prevented by some lower limit V_i for the ith unit, see Figure 3.1. The filtering processes in this situation are also given by $C_i(t) = I(t > V_i)$, $i = 1, \ldots, n$. Left-censoring is frequently encountered in bioassays due to inherent limit of detection of the response of interest; see, for example, Lynn (2001) for an example of left-censored plasma HIV RNA data. If the filtering induced by the left-censoring is independent and the basic model is an Aalen multiplicative model, then the observed ith intensity is $Y_i(t)\alpha_i^\theta(t)$ with $Y_i(t) = I(V_i < t \leq T_i^*)$, and inference based on the observed intensity will be valid, but clearly not efficient as the left-censored units are not used at all in the analysis. If the left-censored units are not used in the analysis, then one should use the left-truncated version of the complete observations induced by the observed at risk indicators; otherwise one introduces a length-bias as higher observations are selected for analysis (by excluding the low ones). Usually, for such data, more traditional parametric likelihood based analyses are applied using all available information.

62   3. Estimation for filtered counting process data

An observation scheme more often encountered in survival analysis is the so-called *current status data*. Such data arise when the only knowledge about the failure time is whether the failure occurs before or after a (random) monitoring time. For instance, in carcinogenicity experiments, where one is interested in time to tumor onset, one only knows at the time where the animal is sacrificed whether or not tumor is present. Current status data are examined in Exercises 3.10 and 6.9. □

One aspect of interest in AIDS studies is the time from infection (HIV) to outbreak of clinical AIDS. When following prospectively a cohort of infected individuals, the problem arises that the time at first infection of the individuals is unknown as they were all infected prior to the start of follow-up. This is a so-called prevalent cohort (Brookmeyer & Gail, 1987), and here it is not possible to apply the delayed entry technique since the time origin is unknown.

3.2 Likelihood constructions

Consider a counting process N^* adapted to a filtration $(\mathcal{F}_t^*)$ leading to the intensity $\lambda^*(t)$. Denote the ith jump time of $N^*(t)$ by τ_i^* and let τ_i^* be infinity if $N(t)$ does not make i jumps. For convenience we let $\tau_0^* = 0$. The compensator $\Lambda^*(t) = \int_0^t \lambda^*(s)\, ds$ makes $M^* = N^* - \Lambda^*$ into a (local square integrable) martingale. We think of the intensity as being on a parametric form such that $\lambda^*(t) = \lambda^*(t, \theta)$, but do not make the notation explicit.

The likelihood function for a counting process observed up to time t is given as

$$L(\theta, t) = \left\{ \prod_{\tau_i^* \leq t} \lambda^*(\tau_i^*) \right\} \exp\left(-\int_0^t \lambda^*(s)\, ds \right)$$

$$= \left\{ \prod_{\tau_i^* \leq t} \exp\left(-\int_{\tau_{i-1}^*}^{\tau_i^*} \lambda^*(s)\, ds\right) \lambda^*(\tau_i^*) \right\} \exp\left(-\int_{\tau_{N^*(t)}^*}^{t} \lambda^*(s)\, ds \right). \quad (3.14)$$

Equation (3.14) gives the intuition behind the likelihood function; each term contributes the probability of experiencing no events between $[\tau_{i-1}^*, \tau_i^*[$ and then experiencing an event at time τ_i^* all conditional on the past of the process, and with the last term specifying the probability of experiencing no events from the last jump time to the end of the observation period conditional on the past of the counting process. The likelihood function is proportional to

$$L(\theta, t) = \left\{ \prod_{\tau_i^* \leq t} d\Lambda^*(\tau_i^*) \right\} \exp\left(-\int_0^t d\Lambda^*(s) \right)$$

$$= \prod_{s \leq t} \{d\Lambda^*(s)\}^{\Delta N^*(s)} \exp\left(-\int_0^t d\Lambda^*(s) \right), \quad (3.15)$$

where $\Delta N^*(t) = N^*(t) - N^*(t-)$. We shall see later that (3.15) is a convenient form of the likelihood to work with.

For a multivariate counting process $N^* = (N_1^*, \ldots, N_k^*)$ with intensity process $\lambda^* = (\lambda_1^*, \ldots, \lambda_k^*)$, the likelihood function reads

$$L(\theta, t) = \prod_h \prod_{s \leq t} \{\lambda_h^*(s)\}^{\Delta N_h^*(s)} \exp\left(-\int_0^t \lambda_\cdot^*(s)\, ds \right),$$

where $\lambda_\cdot^*(s) = \sum_h \lambda_h^*(s)$. The log-likelihood function up to time t for a multivariate counting process can be written elegantly as

$$l(\theta, t) = \log(L(\theta, t))$$
$$= \sum_h \left[\int_0^t \log(\lambda_h^*(s))\, dN_h^*(s) - \int_0^t \lambda_h^*(s)\, ds \right],$$

thus implying that the score process has the form (assuming that the derivative may be taken under the integral sign)

$$U(\theta, t) = \frac{\partial}{\partial \theta} l(\theta, t)$$
$$= \sum_h \left[\int_0^t \frac{\partial}{\partial \theta} \log(\lambda_h^*(s))\, dN_h^*(s) - \int_0^t \frac{\partial}{\partial \theta} \lambda_h^*(s)\, ds \right].$$

The score evaluated in the true parameter value, θ_0, can then under weak regularity conditions be written as

$$U(\theta_0, t) = \sum_h \int_0^t \frac{\partial}{\partial \theta} \log(\lambda_h^*(s))\, dM_h^*(s),$$

thus being a martingale if $\frac{\partial}{\partial \theta} \log(\lambda_h^*(t))$, $h = 1, \ldots, k$, are locally bounded and predictable. In the above display,

$$M_h^*(s) = N_h^*(s) - \int_0^s \lambda_h^*(u, \theta_0)\, du.$$

Given i.i.d. observations of counting processes $N_i^*(t)$, $i = 1, \ldots, n$, the maximum likelihood estimate $\hat{\theta}$ is computed by solving

$$U_n(\theta, t) = \sum_{i=1}^n \int \frac{\partial}{\partial \theta} \log(\lambda_i^*(s))\, dN_i^*(s) - \int \frac{\partial}{\partial \theta} \lambda_i^*(s)\, ds = 0.$$

Under regularity conditions, $n^{1/2}(\hat{\theta} - \theta_0)$ is asymptotically normal with variance

$$\mathcal{I}^{-1}(\theta_0, t), \tag{3.16}$$

where the j, k-element of the information matrix $\mathcal{I}$ is given as the mean of the second derivative of minus the log-likelihood evaluated at the true θ_0, that is the j, k-element is

$$\mathcal{I}_{j,k}(\theta, t) = E(-\frac{\partial^2}{\partial \theta_j \partial \theta_k} l_n(\theta, t)),$$

evaluated at θ_0. The information matrix may be estimated consistently by the observed information $I(\hat{\theta}, t)$ with elements

$$I_{j,k}(\theta, t) = -n^{-1} \sum_{i=1}^{n} \int_0^t \frac{\partial^2}{\partial \theta_j \partial \theta_k} \log(\lambda_i^*(s)) \, dN_i^*(s) + \int_0^t \frac{\partial^2}{\partial \theta_j \partial \theta_k} \lambda_i^*(s) \, ds,$$

evaluated in $\hat{\theta}$, or by the optional variation process with elements

$$[U_n(\theta, \cdot)](t) = \sum_{i=1}^{n} \int_0^t (\frac{\partial}{\partial \theta} \log(\lambda_i^*(s)))^{\otimes 2} \, dN_i^*(s)$$

also evaluated in $\hat{\theta}$. Recall that for a $p \times 1$ vector a, $a^{\otimes 2} = aa^T$. Additional details can be found in Borgan (1984).

As mentioned in the previous subsection one usually only observes an incomplete version of the underlying counting process N^* due to filtering with the prime example being right-censoring. If the filtering is independent (see Definition 3.1.1), then it is still possible to apply likelihood techniques for inference using expression (3.15) with λ^* replaced by $\lambda = C\lambda^*$:

$$L(\theta, t) = \prod_{\tau_i \leq t} \{\lambda(\tau_i)\} \exp(-\int_0^t \lambda(s) ds) \tag{3.17}$$

corresponding to that we observe N, and where the τ_i's denote the jump times of the observed counting process. The observed information will often, however, be larger than that generated by the filtered counting process and, in that case, the expression (3.17) is referred to as a *partial likelihood*. For example, in the case of right-censored failure times, the full likelihood also contains terms adhering to the censoring variables, and (3.17) will in that case only be the part corresponding to the right-censored failure times (Exercise 3.6). If the partial likelihood is equivalent to the full likelihood, meaning that the omitted part does not depend on the parameters of interest, then the filtering is said to be *noninformative*. If we also have information on covariates, then the considered likelihood function is conditional on the covariates.

The following example develops the partial likelihood for right-censored survival data.

3.2 Likelihood constructions 65

Example 3.2.1 (Partial likelihood for right-censored survival data)

Consider a survival time T^*, a right-censoring variable U and let $\Delta = I(T \leq U)$ be the censoring indicator and define $T = T^* \wedge U$. Denote the hazard function of the survival time by $\alpha(t)$. If the filtering induced by the right-censoring is independent, then the partial likelihood (3.17) of the filtered counting process is

$$L(\theta, \infty) = \alpha(T)^\Delta \exp(-\int_0^T \alpha(s)ds).$$

□

The following example considers left-truncated survival data.

Example 3.2.2 (Partial likelihood for left-truncated survival data)

Consider a survival time T^* with hazard function $\alpha(t)$ and a left-truncation variable V, such that we only observe T^* conditionally on $T^* > V$. In the case of independent filtering the partial likelihood related to the survival time conditional on being observed is given as (ignoring the dt-term)

$$P(T^* \in [t, t+dt]|T^* > V) = \frac{\alpha(t)\exp(-\int_0^t \alpha(s)ds)}{\exp(-\int_0^V \alpha(s)ds)}$$

$$= \alpha(t)\exp(-\int_V^t \alpha(s)ds),$$

which is equivalent to the expression (3.17) for the filtered counting process.

□

Almost all survival data will be right-censored so left-truncation is typically not present alone. The partial likelihood in the case of right-censored and left-truncated survival data is considered in the next example.

Example 3.2.3 (Left-truncated and right-censored survival data)

Consider a survival time T^* with hazard function $\alpha(t)$, a left-truncation variable V, and a right-censoring variable U. We observe $T = T^* \wedge U$ and the censoring indicator $\Delta = I(T^* \leq U)$ conditionally on $T^* > V$.

If this filtering induced by the censoring and truncation is independent, then the partial likelihood of the filtered counting process is

$$\alpha(T)^\Delta \exp(-\int_V^T \alpha(s)ds).$$

□

66   3. Estimation for filtered counting process data

Example 3.2.4 (Exponential distribution)

If the survival time T^* has constant hazard λ, then T^* is *exponential distributed* with mean $1/\lambda$. Assume we observe in the time interval $[0, \tau]$ and that we have independent right-censoring by $U = U^* \wedge \tau$ with U^* a positive random variable. The observed counting process $N(t) = \int_0^t Y(s) dN^*(s)$ then has intensity $Y(t)\lambda$, where $Y(t) = I(t \leq U \wedge T^*)$ and $N^*(t) = I(T^* \leq t)$. The score function is

$$U(\lambda) = \int_0^\tau \frac{1}{\lambda} dN(t) - \int_0^\tau Y(t) dt = \frac{\Delta}{\lambda} - T,$$

where $T = T^* \wedge U$ and $\Delta = I(T = T^*)$, and

$$I(\lambda) = \frac{\Delta}{\lambda^2}.$$

With n i.i.d. observations from this model, the maximum likelihood estimator of λ is therefore

$$\hat{\lambda} = \frac{\Delta_\cdot}{T_\cdot},$$

which is the ratio of number of events (occurrences) $\Delta_\cdot = \sum_{i=1}^n \Delta_i$ and the total at risk time (exposure) $T_\cdot = \sum_{i=1}^n T_i$. The standard error is estimated consistently by

$$\frac{(\Delta_\cdot)^{1/2}}{T_\cdot}.$$

□

The following example deals with the case where the intensity is piecewise constant. It thus generalizes the results of the previous example and gives important intuition about intensity estimation.

Example 3.2.5 (Piecewise constant intensities)

Consider a filtered counting process $N(t)$ adapted to a filtration $(\mathcal{F}_t)$ leading to the intensity $\lambda(t)$. Let $a_0 = 0, a_1, ..., a_L = \tau$ be an increasing sequence of numbers such that the sets $A_l = [a_{l-1}, a_l]$, $l = 1, .., L$ partition the interval $[0, \tau]$. We assume that the intensity is piecewise constant and is defined by

$$\lambda(t) = Y(t) \sum_{l=1}^L \lambda_l I(t \in A_l),$$

where $Y(t)$ is an at risk indicator, and we now wish to estimate the positive parameters λ_l, $l = 1, .., L$. For left-truncated (with truncation time V) and right-censored (with censoring time U) survival data with survival time T^* the at risk indicator equals $Y(t) = I(V \leq t \leq U) I(T^* \geq t)$.

3.2 Likelihood constructions

We assume that n i.i.d. counting processes are observed over the observation period $[0, \tau]$, and denote the ordered jump-times of the ith counting process by τ_{ij}, $j = 1, ..., N_i(\tau)$. Let $\theta = (\lambda_1, ..., \lambda_L)$. The likelihood function is

$$L(\theta, \tau) = \prod_i \{ \prod_{\tau_{ij} \leq \tau} \lambda(\tau_{ij}) \} \exp(-\int_0^\tau \lambda_i(s) ds)$$

$$= \prod_{l=1}^L \lambda_l^{O_l} \exp(-\lambda_l E_l),$$

where

$$O_l = \sum_i \int_{a_{l-1}}^{a_l} dN_i(s) = \sum_{i,j} I(\tau_{ij} \in [a_{l-1}, a_l]),$$

$$E_l = \sum_i \int_{a_{l-1}}^{a_l} Y_i(s) ds.$$

In the above display, O_l is the number of events (occurrences) and E_l is the total at risk time (exposure) in the interval $[a_{l-1}, a_l]$. The log-likelihood and the lth component of the score function equals

$$l(\theta, \tau) = \sum_{l=1}^L \{ O_l \log(\lambda_l) - \lambda_l E_l \},$$

$$U_l(\theta, \tau) = O_l \frac{1}{\lambda_l} - E_l,$$

respectively. The maximum likelihood estimate is thus

$$\hat{\lambda}_l = \frac{O_l}{E_l},$$

which is the occurrence/exposure rate for the lth interval. The derivative of the score equals

$$\text{diag}(-\frac{O_l}{\lambda_l^2})$$

and the inverse of the observed information can thus be estimated by

$$\text{diag}(\frac{\hat{\lambda}_l^2}{O_l}) = \text{diag}(\frac{O_l}{E_l^2}).$$

The asymptotic variance of $n^{1/2}(\hat{\lambda}_l - \lambda_l)$ is therefore estimated by O_l / E_l^2. Note that $\hat{\lambda}_1, ..., \hat{\lambda}_L$ are asymptotically independent.

It is standard procedure to consider the log-transform of the rates as a means of improving the normal approximation to the small sample distribution of the estimates. With $\mu_l = \log(\lambda_l)$,

$$n^{1/2}(\hat{\mu}_l - \mu_l)$$

68   3. Estimation for filtered counting process data

is asymptotically normal with zero-mean and a variance that is estimated consistently by
$$\frac{1}{O_l}$$
using here for example the delta-method, see Section 2.5. □

Example 3.2.6 (Weibull distribution)

Consider the setup from Example 3.2.4, but so that T^* follows a *Weibull distribution* yielding the hazard function
$$\alpha^*(t) = \lambda\gamma(\lambda t)^{\gamma-1}$$
with $\lambda, \gamma > 0$. The exponential distribution is obtained by taking $\gamma = 1$. The score equations (based on one observation) for the two parameters are
$$\frac{\gamma}{\lambda}(\Delta - (\lambda T)^\gamma) = 0; \quad \Delta(\frac{1}{\gamma} + \log(\lambda T)) - (\lambda T)^\gamma \log(\lambda T) = 0.$$
that needs to be solved iteratively. Note that
$$\int_0^t \alpha^*(s)\, ds = (\lambda t)^\gamma$$
so that the log-cumulative hazard function is linear in $\log(t)$. If a (p-dimensional) covariate, X, is present, one may use the Weibull regression model that has hazard function
$$\lambda\gamma(\lambda t)^{\gamma-1} \exp(X^T \beta), \tag{3.18}$$
where the β denotes the regression parameters. An individual with the zero covariate thus has the baseline-hazard function on the Weibull form. The hazard (3.18) may be written as a so-called proportional hazards model
$$\lambda_0(t) \exp(X^T \beta),$$
where $\lambda_0(t)$ is an arbitrary unspecified baseline hazard. For proportional hazards, the covariates act multiplicatively on the baseline hazard. Proportional hazards models are described in much detail in Chapter 6. Another type of model is the accelerated failure time model, where the hazard has the form
$$\lambda_0(\exp(X^T \phi)t) \exp(X^T \phi)$$
using ϕ to denote the regression parameters. For this model the covariates act multiplicatively on time so that their effect is to accelerate or decelerate time to failure relative to $\lambda_0(t)$. We return to this model in Chapter 8. By writing (3.18) as
$$\lambda^\gamma \gamma \left(\exp\{X^T(\beta/\gamma)\}t\right)^{\gamma-1} \exp\{X^T(\beta/\gamma)\},$$

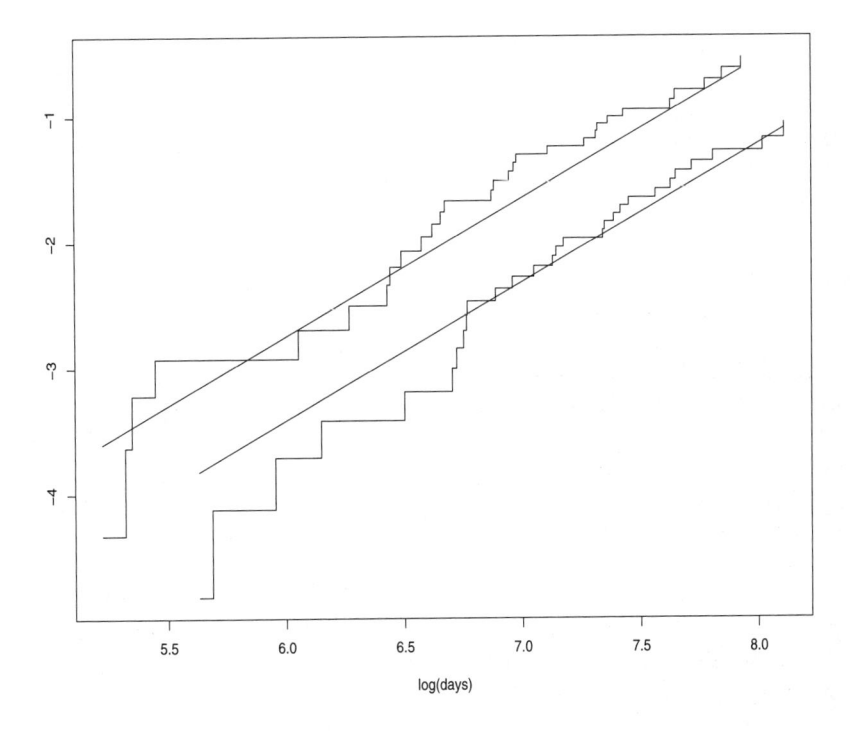

FIGURE 3.2: Melanoma data. Straight line estimates of log Nelson-Aalen curves for males and females based on Weibull regression model.

the Weibull model is also an accelerated failure time model with $\phi = \beta/\gamma$, see also Exercise 3.7.

Let us fit the Weibull regression model to the melanoma data using sex as explanatory variable. This may be done in R using the function survreg.

```
> fit.Wei<-survreg(Surv(days,status==1)~sex,data=melanoma)
> fit.Wei
Call:
survreg(formula = Surv(days, status == 1) ~ sex)

Coefficients:
(Intercept)          sex
  9.1156248   -0.6103966

Scale= 0.9116392

Loglik(model)= -564   Loglik(intercept only)= -567.2
        Chisq= 6.29 on 1 degrees of freedom, p= 0.012
n= 205
```

The estimates reported by R are those estimating the parameters in (3.24) (Exercise 3.7) so $\hat\beta = 0.6104/0.9116$, $\hat\gamma = 1/0.9116$, and $\hat\lambda = \exp(-9.1156)$. Figure 3.2 displays the log of the Nelson-Aalen estimators (computed for each sex) and plotted against log time. The straight line estimates are obtained using the above estimates from the Weibull regression. It seems that the Weibull regression model gives a reasonable fit to the melanoma data when we only include sex as explanatory variable □

3.3 Estimating equations

In some cases, it turns out that the likelihood score equations may be hard to use if not impossible. Therefore, rather than basing estimation on the likelihood, one may instead establish various estimating equations based on the observed counting processes. Let $N_i(t)$ be a (possible filtered) counting process adapted to a filtration $\mathcal{F}_t^i$ leading to the intensity $\lambda_i(t)$, $i = 1,\ldots,n$, such that the counting processes are independent and identically distributed. As in the previous sections we think of the intensity as being on a parametric form such that $\lambda_i(t) = \lambda_i(t,\theta)$.

To estimate θ one may compare the counting process $N_i(t)$ with its compensator $\Lambda_i(t) = \int_0^t \lambda_i(s,\theta)\,ds$ keeping in mind that the difference between the two is a (local square integrable) martingale with zero-mean. Formally one may consider the estimating equation

$$U(\theta,t) = \sum_{i=1}^n \int_0^t W_i(s,\theta) D_i(s,\theta)(dN_i(s) - \lambda_i(s)\,ds) = 0, \qquad (3.19)$$

where

$$D_i(t,\theta) = \frac{\partial}{\partial \theta}\lambda_i(t,\theta)$$

and $W_i(t,\theta)$ is some weight function. Because of the martingale property, this estimating equation will have mean zero when evaluated in the true parameter, θ_0. Note also that the estimating equation having zero-mean only requires that $W_i(t,\theta)$ and $D_i(t,\theta)$ are predictable and locally bounded processes.

The estimating equation (3.19) looks a lot like the score function that was equal to

$$\sum_{i=1}^n \int_0^t \frac{\partial}{\partial \theta}\log(\lambda_i(s))\,(dN_i(s) - \lambda_i(s)\,ds),$$

and the two are equivalent when $W_i(t,\theta) = 1/\lambda_i(t,\theta)$.

Under regularity conditions it follows that the solution to $U(\theta,t) = 0$, $\tilde\theta$, is asymptotically normal such that $n^{1/2}(\tilde\theta - \theta_0)$ converges in distribution towards a multivariate normal distribution with zero-mean and variance given by

$$I^{-1}(t,\theta_0)V(t,\theta_0)I^{-1}(t,\theta_0), \quad (3.20)$$

where

$$I(t,\theta_0) = E(-\int_0^t W_i(s,\theta_0)D_i^{\otimes 2}(s,\theta_0)ds) \quad (3.21)$$

is the mean of $-\partial U(\theta,t)/\partial\theta$ evaluated in θ_0 and

$$V(t,\theta_0) = E(\int_0^t W_i^2(s,\theta_0)D_i^{\otimes 2}(s,\theta_0)\lambda_i(s)\,ds) \quad (3.22)$$

is the variance of $U(\theta_0,t)$. Note that the formula simplifies when $W_i(t) = 1/\lambda_i(t)$ (the maximum likelihood case) where $I(t,\theta_0)$ and $V(t,\theta_0)$ are equal.

The above quantities defining the variance may be estimated by plugging in the estimated θ and using the i.i.d. structure. The mean of the derivative of the estimating equation is estimated consistently by the observed information

$$\hat{I}(\tilde{\theta}) = -n^{-1}\sum_{i=1}^n \int_0^t W_i(s,\tilde{\theta})D_i^{\otimes 2}(s,\tilde{\theta})\,ds.$$

The variance of the score can be estimated consistently by the observed second moment

$$\sum_{i=1}^n \int_0^t W_i^2(s,\tilde{\theta})D_i^{\otimes 2}(s,\tilde{\theta})\lambda_i(s,\tilde{\theta})\,ds,$$

or by the optional variation process with elements

$$\sum_{i=1}^n \int_0^t W_i^2(s,\tilde{\theta})D_i^{\otimes 2}(s,\tilde{\theta})\,dN_i(s),$$

or by a robust estimator

$$\sum_{i=1}^n \{\int_0^t W_i(s,\tilde{\theta})D_i(s,\tilde{\theta})(dN_i(s) - \lambda_i(s,\tilde{\theta}))\,ds\}^{\otimes 2}.$$

The structure of these estimating equations are very useful and used for essentially all models considered in Chapters 5, 6 and 7 on regression models for survival data. None of these models are purely parametric but luckily it turns out that the estimating equations can be extended to deal with both nonparametric and semiparametric models. A general treatment of estimation and inference in semiparametric models is given by Bickel et al. (1993).

3. Estimation for filtered counting process data

We here consider the basic principles in developing a score function that may be used for semiparametric intensity models and focus on the particular situation where the nonparametric terms are unspecified functions of time. To give a simple exposition we focus on the situation where the intensity is additive. Based on this special case we develop some important heuristics that lead to useful efficient score equations for all models considered in this monograph.

Consider the additive hazard model suggested by Aalen (1980), where

$$\lambda_i(t) = Y_i(t) X_i^T(t) \beta(t), \tag{3.23}$$

where $X_i(t) = (X_{i1}(t), ..., X_{ip}(t))$ is a p-dimensional predictable covariate, $Y_i(t)$ is the at risk indicator, and $\beta(t) = (\beta_1(t), ..., \beta_p(t))^T$ is a p-dimensional regression coefficient function of locally integrable functions. We deal with this in detail in Chapter 5. To estimate the infinite-dimensional parameters of this model, one considers all parametric sub-models of the form $\beta(t) = \beta_0(t) + \eta b(t)$, where η is one-dimensional parameter and b is a given p-vector of functions, and look for an estimator that makes all scores with respect to η equal to 0, see Sasieni (1992b) and Greenwood & Wefelmeyer (1990). The estimating equation then reads

$$U(\eta, t) = \sum_{i=1}^{n} \int_0^t W_i(s, \eta) D_i(s, \eta) (dN_i(s) - \lambda_i(s) \, ds),$$

where

$$D_i(t, \eta) = Y_i(t) X_i^T(t) b(t)$$

and where we ignore the precise choice of $W_i(t, \eta)$ for now and set it to 1. As noted earlier $W_i(t, \eta) = 1/\lambda_i(t)$ makes the estimates equivalent to the maximum-likelihood estimates. Then the score equation reads

$$U(\eta, t) = \sum_{i=1}^{n} \int_0^t Y_i(s) X_i^T(s) b(s) (dN_i(s) - Y_i(s) X_i^T(s) \beta(s) ds)$$

and should equal zero for all choices of $b(t)$ (within a class of suitably regular functions). For the estimating function to equal zero for all choices of $b(t)$ it follows that the increments must equal zero, that is

$$\sum_{i=1}^{n} Y_i(t) X_i^T(t) (dN_i(t) - Y_i(t) X_i^T(t) \beta(t) dt) = 0.$$

With $B(t) = \int_0^t \beta(s) ds$, we solve the score equation to obtain

$$d\hat{B}(t) = (\sum_{i=1}^{n} Y_i(t) X_i^T(t) X_i(t))^{-1} \sum_{i=1}^{n} Y_i(t) X_i^T(t) dN_i(t),$$

or

$$\hat{B}(t) = \int_0^t (\sum_{i=1}^n Y_i(s)X_i^T(s)X_i(s))^{-1} \sum_{i=1}^n Y_i(s)X_i^T(s)dN_i(s).$$

It is relatively straightforward to develop the large sample properties of this estimator, see Section 5.1.

3.4 Exercises

3.1 (Continuation of Example 3.1.4)

(a) Show that the independent censoring condition of ABGK (3.5) reduces to (3.8) in the case of right-censored survival data as described in the example.

(b) Assume that T^* and U are conditionally independent given an explanatory variable X, and that the distribution of T^* and U depends on X. Show that the right-censoring induced by U is independent.

(c) Assume that T^* and U are conditionally independent given X, but that we never observe X. So $N^*(t)$ has intensity $\lambda^*(t)$ with respect to $\mathcal{F}_t^* = \mathcal{F}_t^{N^*}$. Is the filtering of $N^*(t)$ generated by U independent?

3.2 Let $\tilde{T}_1, \ldots, \tilde{T}_n$ be i.i.d. finite lifetimes with hazard function $\alpha(t)$. Assume that $\tilde{T}_i$ is right-censored at time U_i, where

$$U_1 = \infty, \quad U_i = U_{i-1} \wedge \tilde{T}_{i-1}, i \geq 2.$$

We thus observe $T_i = \tilde{T}_i \wedge U_i$ and $\Delta_i = I(\tilde{T}_i \leq U_i), i = 1, \ldots, n$.

(a) Show that this censoring is independent.

Let $\tilde{T}_{(1)} = \tilde{T}_1 \wedge \cdots \wedge \tilde{T}_n$.

(b) Compute the Nelson-Aalen estimator $\hat{A}(t)$ for estimation of $A(t) = \int_0^t \alpha(s)\,ds$ on the set where $\tilde{T}_{(1)} = \tilde{T}_1$.

(c) Show that $\tilde{T}_n$ is observed if and only if $\tilde{T}_n = \tilde{T}_{(1)}$.

(d) Can the situation arise where all $\tilde{T}_1, \ldots, \tilde{T}_n$ are observed?

(e) Show that $T_1 \wedge \cdots T_n = \tilde{T}_{(1)}$ and that $\hat{A}(t)$ always jumps at $\tilde{T}_{(1)}$.

(f) Compute the jump size of $\hat{A}(t)$ at $\tilde{T}_{(1)}$.

3.3 (Progressive type II censoring) Let T^* be a lifetime and X a covariate vector such that the hazard of T^*, conditional on X, is $\alpha(t; X)$. Let $(T_1^*, X_1), \ldots, (T_n^*, X_n)$ be n independent copies of (T^*, X) and let $r_1, \ldots, r_m$ be some given integers such that $r_1 + \cdots r_m + m = n$. We consider the lifetimes $T_1^*, \ldots, T_n^*$ as the failure times of n units. The progressively type II censored sample is obtained in the following way. Let $T_{(1)}$ denote the first failure time. At time $T_{(1)}$ we remove (censor) at random r_1 units. We denote the second observed failure time by $T_{(2)}$, and at that point in time we remove at random r_2 surviving units. This process continues until, at the time $T_{(m)}$ of the mth observed failure the remaining surviving units are removed. Let I_i denote the set of numbers of the units censored at time $T_{(i)}$ and the number of the unit failing at time $T_{(i)}$, $i = 1, \ldots, m$.

(a) Argue that the observed filtration is

$$\mathcal{F}_t = \sigma\{(T_{(i)}, I_i) : i \leq m \text{ and } T_{(i)} \leq t\}, \quad t \geq 0.$$

Let $T_i = T_{(k)}$ if $i \in I_k$ and put $\Delta_i = 1$ if T_i is an observed failure time, and $\Delta_i = 0$ otherwise. Let $N_i(t) = I(T_i \leq t, \Delta_i = 1)$, $i = 1, \ldots, n$.

(b) Show that $N_i(t)$ has intensity

$$\lambda_i(t; X) = I(t \leq T_i)\alpha(t; X)$$

with respect to $\mathcal{F}_t$, that is, the censoring is independent.

3.4 (Failure intensity depending on censoring value) Let T^* be a failure time and put $N^*(t) = I(T^* \leq t)$. Suppose that the filtering of $N^*(t)$ is induced by $C(t) = I(t \leq U)$, where U is a positive stochastic variable with density f. As usual we let $T = T^* \wedge U$ denote the observed waiting time. Assume that

$$E(dN^*(t) \mid \mathcal{G}_{t-}^*) = I(t \leq T^*)(C(t)\alpha_1(t)dt + D(t)h(U)\alpha_2(t)dt),$$

where $\mathcal{G}_t^*$ is defined by (3.4), $\alpha_1(t)$ and $\alpha_2(t)$ are to deterministic functions $D(t) = 1 - C(t)$, and h is some function.

(a) Compute the intensity of N^* with respect to $\mathcal{F}_t^*$. Is the censoring independent according to the ABGK definition?

(b) Compute the intensity of N with respect to $\mathcal{F}_t$. Is the censoring independent according to Definition 3.1.1?

(c) Is the classification of the considered censoring depending on which definition that is used?

3.5 (Left-truncated survival time) Let the survival time T^* be left-truncated by the random V and consider the setup described in Example 3.1.2.

(a) Show that this filtering is independent if the conditional density (assumed to exist) of (T^*, V) given $T^* > V$ may be written as $f(t^*)g(v)$ for $t^* > v$.

76   3. Estimation for filtered counting process data

Assume from now on that T^* and V are independent or that the condition in (a) holds.

(b) Let $\mathcal{F}_t = \sigma(I(V \leq s), I(V < T \leq s) : s \leq t)$. Show that $N(t)$ has compensator $\Lambda(t)$ with respect to $\mathcal{F}_t$ when computed under $P_{\mathcal{O}}$.

(c) Let
$$\mathcal{F}_t = \sigma(V, I(V < T \leq s), I(T > V) : V \leq s \leq V + t).$$
Show that $N(t)$ has compensator $\Lambda(t)$ with respect to $\mathcal{F}_t$ when computed under P or $P_{\mathcal{O}}$.

3.6 (Right-censoring: full likelihood function) Let (T_i, Δ_i), $i = 1, \ldots, n$, be independent replicates of (T, Δ) described in Example 3.1.4, and assume the distribution of U is absolute continuous with hazard function $\mu(t)$. Define
$$N(t) = \sum_{i=1}^n I(T_i \leq t, \Delta_i = 1) \quad \text{and} \quad Y(t) = \sum_{i=1}^n I(t \leq T_i).$$

(a) Show that the likelihood function based on observing (T_i, Δ_i), $i = 1, \ldots, n$, can be written as
$$\prod_i \left\{ \alpha^\theta(T_i)^{\Delta_i} e^{-\int_0^{T_i} \alpha^\theta(t) \, dt} \right\} \prod_i \left\{ \mu(T_i)^{1-\Delta_i} e^{-\int_0^{T_i} \mu(t) \, dt} \right\}.$$

(b) Show that the expression in (a) is proportional to the partial likelihood (3.17) defined from N.

(c) Assume that $\mu(t) = \beta \alpha^\theta(t)$ (Koziol-Green model). Show that the censoring is now informative, but that the estimator, $\hat{\theta}$, obtained by maximizing the partial likelihood defined from N is still consistent. Derive its asymptotical distribution.

(d) Show, under the assumption of (c), that Δ is ancillary for θ.

3.7 (Weibull regression model) Let T^* have hazard given by (3.18).

(a) With $Y = \log(T^*)$, show that
$$Y = \alpha + \tilde{\beta}^T X + \sigma W, \tag{3.24}$$
where $\alpha = -\log(\lambda)$, $\sigma = \gamma^{-1}$, $\tilde{\beta} = -\sigma \beta$, and W has the extreme value distribution:
$$P(W > w) = \exp(-\exp(w)).$$

(b) Based on the Weibull regression fit, estimate the survivor function $P(T^* > t)$ for the melanoma data for males and females, and give the associated 95% pointwise confidence intervals.

(c) Make the plots of the estimated survivor functions and their confidence intervals.

3.8 (Gompertz distribution) Let T^* be a survival time with hazard function
$$\lambda(t) = \mu \nu^t \tag{3.25}$$
with $\mu, \nu > 0$. This distribution is called the Gompertz distribution. For $\nu < 1$, the hazard is decreasing with t and it does not integrate to ∞, that is, there is positive probability of not experiences the event under study.

(a) If Y has a log Weibull distribution truncated at zero, then show that Y has a Gompertz distribution.

(b) Derive the score equations for (μ, ν) based on n i.i.d. right-censored (independent censoring variables) survival times that follow the Gompertz distribution, and give a consistent estimate of the asymptotic variance of the maximum likelihood estimator.

(c) Fit the Gompertz distribution to the melanoma data considering only the females.

The hazard function (3.25) may be extended to
$$\lambda(t) = \lambda + \mu \nu^t;$$
the associated distribution is called the Gompertz-Makeham distribution.

(d) Fit now the Gompertz-Makeham distribution to the melanoma data still considering only the females. Is there an improved fit?

3.9 (Missing covariates) Assume that X_1 and X_2 are two covariates that take the values $\{0, 1\}$ and have joint distribution given by $P(X_1 = 0|X_2 = 0) = 2/3$, $P(X_1 = 0|X_2 = 1) = 1/3$ and $P(X_2 = 1) = 1/2$. Let $\lambda(t)$ be a locally integrable non-negative function, and assume that the survival time T given X_1 and X_2 has hazard function
$$\lambda(t) \exp(0.1 X_1 + 0.3 X_2).$$

(a) Assume that only X_1 is observed. What is the hazard function of T given X_1? Similarly for X_2.

3. Estimation for filtered counting process data

(b) Assume that $\lambda(t) = \lambda$ and that i.i.d. survival data are obtained from the above generic model. Find the maximum likelihood estimator of λ and specify its asymptotic distribution.

(c) Assume now that a right-censoring variable C is also present and that C given X_1 has hazard function $\lambda \exp(0.1 X_1)$. Assuming that only X_1 is observed at time 0 specify how one should estimate the parameter of the survival model.

(d) As in (c) but now assume that only X_2 is observed.

3.10 (Current status data with constant hazards) Let T^* denote a failure time with hazard function

$$\alpha(t) = \theta,$$

where θ is an unknown parameter. Let C denote a random monitoring time independent of T^* and with hazard function $\mu(t)$. The observed data consist of $(C, \Delta = I(C \leq T^*))$. Such data are called current status data since at the monitoring time C it is only known whether or not the event of interest (with waiting time T^*) has occurred.

(a) Derive the intensity functions of the counting processes

$$N_1(t) = \Delta I(C \leq t), \quad N_2(t) = (1 - \Delta) I(C \leq t)$$

[hint: Use the heuristic formula for the intensity given in Exercise 2.7].

Let (C_i, Δ_i), $i = 1, \ldots, n$, be n independent replicates of $(C, \Delta = I(C \leq T))$.

(b) Derive the likelihood function L_t for estimation of θ when we observe over the interval $[0, t]$.

Let $U_t(\theta)$ denote the score function. Let further $N_{j\cdot}(t) = \sum_i N_{ji}(t)$, where $N_{ji}(t)$ is the ith realization of the above generic $N_j(t)$, $j = 1, 2$, corresponding to observing the ith subject.

(c) Show that

$$U_t(\theta) = \int_0^t \frac{s e^{-\theta s}}{1 - e^{-\theta s}} dN_{2\cdot}(s) - \int_0^t s N_{1\cdot}(s),$$

and that this is a martingale (considered as a process in t).

(d) Compute the predictable variation process $\langle U_t(\theta) \rangle$.

(e) Derive under suitable conditions the asymptotic distribution of the maximum likelihood estimator $\hat{\theta}$ of θ, and give a consistent estimator of the asymptotic variance.

4
Nonparametric procedures for survival data

In this chapter we give a brief outline of the most important fully non-parametric tools for the analysis of survival data. The non-parametric techniques have established themselves as important tools of survival analysis due to their simplicity and the fact that their properties are well studied and understood.

4.1 The Kaplan-Meier estimator

When studying the lifetimes of a population, one often has data that are incomplete, typically in form of a right-censored versions of the survival times. It turns out that even though one does not fully observe the survival times, one can still estimate the distribution of the survival times as well as the cumulative hazard function.

We here describe the Nelson-Aalen and Kaplan-Meier estimator in the situation of right-censored survival data. Let T^* be a survival time with survival distribution $S(t) = P(T^* > t)$ and hazard function $\alpha(t)$ and let C be a right-censoring time that leads to independent censoring. We thus observe $T = T^* \wedge C$ and the censoring indicator $\Delta = I(T^* \leq C)$. Denote the n independent observation form this generic model by $(T_i, \Delta_i), i = 1, \ldots, n$.

In the one-sample case it is often of interest to estimate the *survivor function*

$$S(t) = P(T_i^* > t),$$

82   4. Nonparametric procedures for survival data

or the cumulative hazard function

$$A(t) = \int_0^t \alpha(s)ds,$$

which both may be viewed as infinite dimensional parameters when nothing is assumed about the distribution of the survival time (except that a hazard function exists). Note that $S(t) = \exp(-A(t)) = \prod_{s \leq t}(1 - dA(s))$, see Andersen et al. (1993) p. 256, and these two quantities therefore contain the same information on different scales.

Without censoring one might compute the mean and standard deviation to characterize the survival (possibly log-transformed), but with censoring present one aims at estimating the entire survival distribution. In that case it will typically be difficult to summarize the results by computing means and standard deviations, but various percentiles can often be estimated from the data.

Put $N_i(t) = I(T_i \leq t, \Delta_i = 1)$, $Y_i(t) = I(t \leq T_i)$, and

$$N(t) = \sum_{i=1}^n N_i(t), \quad Y(t) = \sum_{i=1}^n Y_i(t), \quad M(t) = N(t) - \int_0^t Y(s)\alpha(s)\,ds,$$

where the latter is a local square integrable martingale.

The *Nelson-Aalen estimator* (Aalen, 1975, 1978b; Nelson, 1969, 1972) is an estimator of the cumulative hazard function A

$$\hat{A}(t) = \int_0^t \frac{J(s)}{Y(s)} dN(s), \tag{4.1}$$

where $J(s) = I(Y(s) > 0)$ and with the convention that $0/0 = 0$. The Nelson-Aalen estimator is an unbiased estimator of (the stochastic)

$$A^*(t) = \int_0^t J(s)dA(s),$$

and it follows directly that

$$\hat{n}^{1/2}(A(t) - A^*(t)) = n^{1/2} \int_0^t \frac{J(s)}{Y(s)} dM(s)$$

is a local square integrable martingale. It turns out, under regularity conditions, that $n^{1/2}(\hat{A} - A)$ converges in distribution towards a Gaussian martingale on $[0, \tau[$. The variance of $n^{1/2}(\hat{A} - A)$ is estimated consistently by the optional variation estimator

$$n \int_0^t \frac{J(s)}{Y^2(s)} dN(s),$$

see Example 2.3.3 for additional details.

4.1 The Kaplan-Meier estimator

The *Kaplan-Meier estimator* (Kaplan & Meier, 1958) of S is

$$\hat{S}(t) = \prod_{s \leq t} \left(1 - \Delta \hat{A}(s)\right) = \prod_{s \leq t} \left(1 - \frac{\Delta N(s)}{Y(s)}\right), \qquad (4.2)$$

where $\hat{A}(t)$ denotes the Nelson-Aalen estimator. The estimator can be interpreted as a product of successive conditional probabilities. Let $\tau_1, \ldots, \tau_{N(t)}$ be the jump times of N in $[0, t]$. The factor

$$\left(1 - \frac{1}{Y(\tau_k)}\right)$$

may be interpreted as the conditional probability of surviving the interval $(\tau_k, \tau_{k+1}]$ given surviving $[0, \tau_k]$. Also, since

$$S(t) = 1 - \int_0^t S(s-)dA(s),$$

a natural estimator is one that solves this equation with A replaced by the Nelson-Aalen estimator. The solution to this equation is exactly the Kaplan-Meier estimator. Finally, the Kaplan-Meier estimator may also be derived as a nonparametric maximum likelihood estimator, see Johansen (1978).

The asymptotic properties of the Kaplan-Meier estimator may be inferred very elegantly from the properties of the Nelson-Aalen estimator by use of product integration (Andersen et al., 1993). A more traditional approach is based on the following relation

$$\frac{\hat{S}(t)}{S^*(t)} - 1 = -\int_0^t \frac{\hat{S}(s-)J(s)}{S^*(s)Y(s)} dM(s) \qquad (4.3)$$

for $t \in [0, \tau)$, where $S^*(t) = \exp(-A^*(t))$ with $A^*(t) = \int_0^t J(s)\alpha(s)\,ds$. Equation (4.3) may be established by noting that both sides of (4.3) are right-continuous in t, zero for $t = 0$ and that they have the same increments (Jacobsen, 1982). Based on (4.3) one may then show, under appropriate conditions, that $\hat{S}$ is uniformly consistent on compact intervals and, for each $t \in [0, \tau)$, that $n^{1/2}(\hat{S} - S)$ converges in distribution towards $-S \cdot U$ on $D[0, t]$, where U is a Gaussian martingale. The variance of $\hat{S}(t)$ is estimated consistently by

$$\tilde{\Sigma}(t) = \hat{S}(t)^2 \int_0^t Y^{-2}(s)dN(s),$$

which is naturally arrived at by calculating the quadratic variation of the martingale term on the right-hand side of (4.3). An alternative consistent estimator of the variance is

$$\hat{\Sigma}(t) = \hat{S}(t)^2 \int_0^t \{Y(s)(Y(s) - N(s))\}^{-1} dN(s),$$

which is the so-called *Greenwood's formula* (Greenwood, 1926), see also Exercise 4.4. It seems from the literature that $\hat{\Sigma}(t)$ should be preferred to $\tilde{\Sigma}(t)$ in practice, see Andersen et al. (1993) and Therneau & Grambsch (2000).

The asymptotic results may be used to construct pointwise confidence intervals as well as confidence bands. The standard $100(1-\alpha)\%$ pointwise confidence interval is

$$\left[\hat{S}(t) - c_{\alpha/2}\hat{\Sigma}(t)^{1/2}, \hat{S}(t) + c_{\alpha/2}\hat{\Sigma}(t)^{1/2}\right],$$

where $c_{\alpha/2}$ is the $(1-\alpha/2)$-quantile of the standard normal distribution. In practice, however, it is better to use various transformations to improve the approximation to the asymptotic distribution. The default in R is the log-transform that gives the $100(1-\alpha)\%$ pointwise confidence interval

$$\left[\hat{S}(t)\exp\{-c_{\alpha/2}\frac{\hat{\Sigma}(t)^{1/2}}{\hat{S}(t)}\}, \hat{S}(t)\exp\{c_{\alpha/2}\frac{\hat{\Sigma}(t)^{1/2}}{\hat{S}(t)}\}\right]. \quad (4.4)$$

In some situations it may be preferable to use other transformations such as cloglog or logit that transforms $]0, 1[$ to $\mathbb{R}$.

The Kaplan-Meier curve may be used to estimate quantiles of the underlying lifetime distribution, and the lower and upper confidence interval curves (4.4) can be used to construct confidence intervals, see Exercise 4.2.

Example 4.1.1 (Melanoma data.)

The data concern survival with malignant melanoma (cancer of the skin) and was collected by K. T. Drzewiecki and reproduced in Andersen et al. (1993). In the period 1962-77, 205 patients had their tumor removed and were followed until the end of 1977. The time variable is time since operation and the number of deaths in the considered period was 57. The Kaplan-Meier estimator for this data sample may be obtained in R by use of the function survfit.

```
> library(survival); library(timereg)
> data(melanoma)
> attach(melanoma)
> fit.all<-survfit(Surv(days,status==1))
```

The Kaplan-Meier curve along with 95% confidence limits is obtained by

```
> plot(fit.all)
```

resulting in Figure 4.1. The censored observations are marked on the curve but can be omitted by

```
> plot(fit.all,mark.time=F)
```

Kaplan-Meier curves for groups of subjects are obtained by

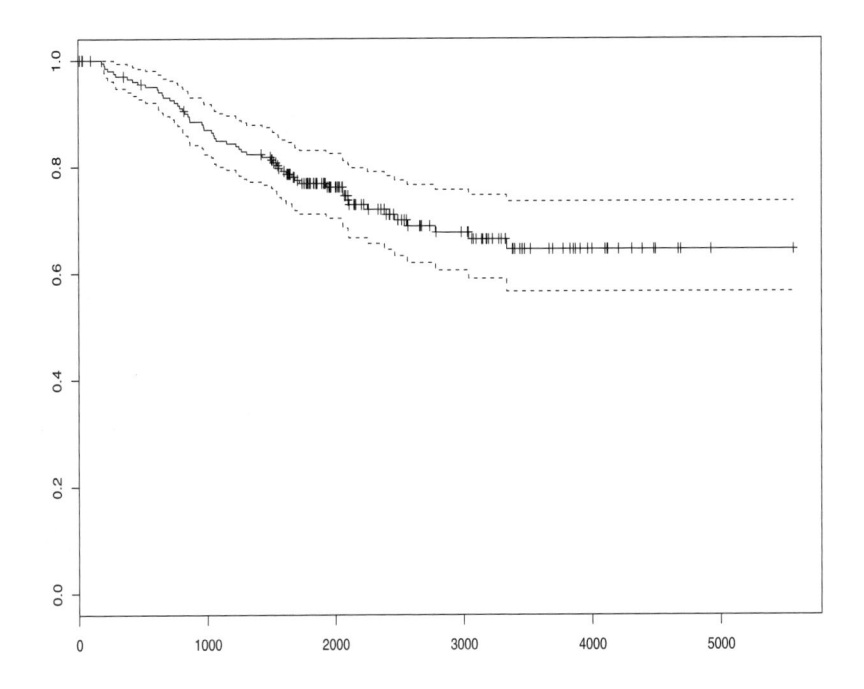

FIGURE 4.1: Melanoma data. Kaplan-Meier curve along with 95% pointwise confidence limits.

```
> fit.sex<-survfit(Surv(days,status==1)~sex)
> plot(fit.sex,mark.time=F)
```

which results in Figure 4.2 showing the curves for males and females. □

One may use the Kaplan-Meier estimator with associated 95% pointwise confidence interval to estimate specific quantiles of the underlying survival distribution. The Kaplan-Meier estimator $\hat{S}(t)$ with associated 95% pointwise confidence interval for the melanoma data is depicted in Figure 4.3. Let $\hat{S}_L(t)$ and $\hat{S}_U(t)$ denote the curves corresponding to the lower and upper limit of the confidence interval. As an illustration consider the 80% quantile, $t_{0.8}$, of $S(t)$ for the melanoma data. This quantile can be estimated by

$$\hat{t}_{0.8} = \inf_t \{t \geq 0 : \hat{S}(t) \leq 0.8\} \tag{4.5}$$

with associated 95% confidence interval

$$[\inf_t \{t \geq 0 : \hat{S}_L(t) \leq 0.8\}, \inf_t \{t \geq 0 : \hat{S}_U(t) \leq 0.8\}] \tag{4.6}$$

as illustrated on Figure 4.3.

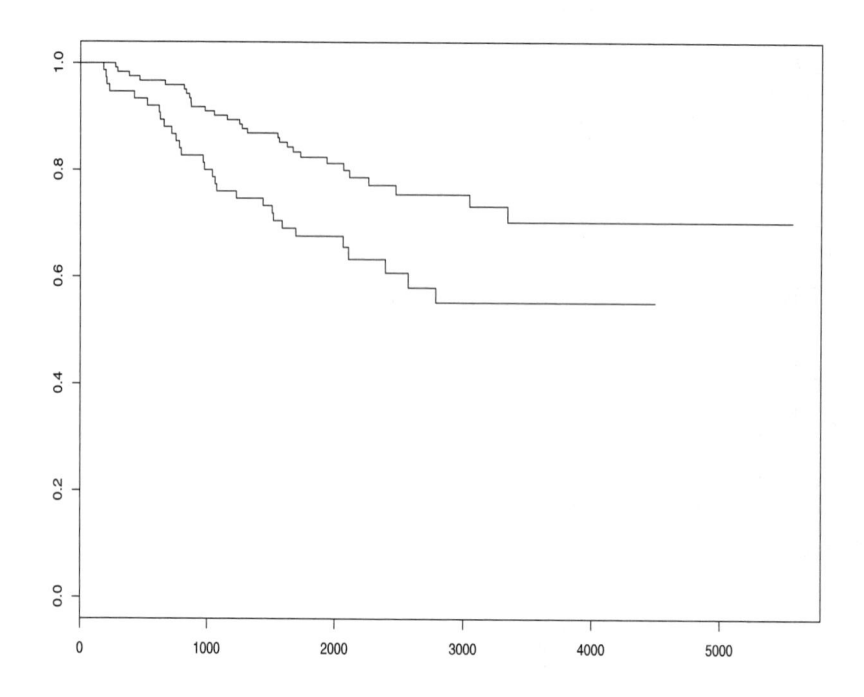

FIGURE 4.2: Melanoma data. Kaplan-Meier curves for males (lower curve) and females (upper curve).

4.2 Hypothesis testing

4.2.1 Comparisons of groups of survival data

Suppose we have a categorical explanatory variable (or several), giving rise to a grouping of the subjects into K groups. The objective is to investigate the effect of this variable on the survival, that is, to compare survival between groups. This may be done nonparametrically, for example by use of the so-called log-rank test, which is one of the tests described below.

The nonparametric tests may be derived very elegantly from the counting process setup as follows. The hazard function for a subject in the kth group, $k = 1\ldots, K$, is denoted $\alpha_k(t)$, and we want to construct tests for the hypothesis

$$H_0 : \alpha_1 = \ldots = \alpha_K.$$

To do this we assume that independent survival data from the K groups are available such that N_{ik} for $i = 1, \ldots, n_k$ represent independent survival data (possibly filtered by independent filtering) with intensity given by

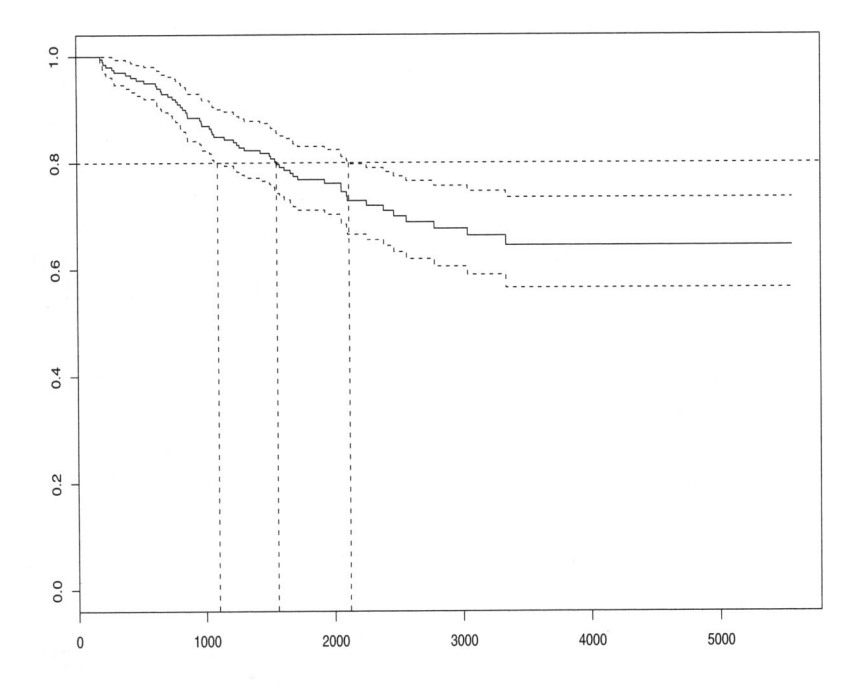

FIGURE 4.3: Melanoma data. Kaplan-Meier estimator with 95% pointwise confidence interval. Estimate of the 80% quantile with 95% confidence interval.

$Y_{ik}\alpha_k$ with at risk indicators Y_{ik}. The total group of patients $n = \sum_k n_k$ are assumed independent.

Within each group one can then estimate the cumulative hazard function, and a test may now be constructed by comparing the group specific Nelson-Aalen estimators to the Nelson-Aalen estimator computed under H_0 using all groups. To be specific, the kth group specific Nelson-Aalen estimator is

$$\hat{A}_k(t) = \int_0^t \frac{1}{Y_k(s)} dN_k(s), \qquad (4.7)$$

where

$$Y_k(t) = \sum_{i=1}^{n_k} Y_{ik}(t), \quad N_k(t) = \sum_{i=1}^{n_k} N_{ik}(t),$$

denote the number of subjects at risk at time t in group k, and the sum of the individual counting processes within group k, respectively. The Nelson-Aalen estimator, under the null, of $A(t) = \int_0^t \alpha(s)\,ds$, where α denotes the

88   4. Nonparametric procedures for survival data

common hazard function, is

$$\hat{A}(t) = \int_0^t \frac{1}{Y.(s)} dN.(s),$$

where $Y.(t) = \sum_k Y_k(t)$, $N.(t) = \sum_k N_k(t)$. Let

$$\tilde{A}_k(t) = \int_0^t J_k(s) d\hat{A}(s),$$

where $J_k(t) = I(Y_k(t) > 0)$. The key to derive the test statistics is that

$$\hat{A}_k(t) - \tilde{A}_k(t) = \left(\int_0^t \frac{J_k(s)}{Y_k(s)} Y_k(s)\alpha(s) \, ds - \int_0^t \frac{J_k(s)}{Y.(s)} Y.(s)\alpha(s) \, ds \right)$$
$$+ \left(\int_0^t \frac{J_k(s)}{Y_k(s)} dM_k(s) - \int_0^t \frac{J_k(s)}{Y.(s)} dM.(s) \right)$$
$$= \sum_{j=1}^K \int_0^t J_k(s) \left(\frac{\delta_{jk}}{Y_k(s)} - \frac{1}{Y.(s)} \right) dM_j(s)$$

is a (local) square integrable martingale under the hypothesis, and therefore should fluctuate around zero if the hypothesis is true. In the above display, δ_{jk} means $I(j = k)$. Let

$$R_k = R_k(\tau) = \int_0^\tau w_k(t) d(\hat{A}_k - \tilde{A}_k)(t),$$

where $w_k(t)$ is some (predictable) weight function to reflect specific aspects of the data. We here restrict attention to the case

$$w_k(t) = Y_k(t) w(t),$$

where $w(t)$ is a predictable weight function. With this choice of weight function we find that

$$R_k = \int_0^\tau w(t) [dN_k(t) - \frac{Y_k(t)}{Y.(t)} dN.(t)].$$

Note the constraint

$$\sum_{k=1}^K R_k = 0,$$

which is also satisfied on the incremental level: $\sum_k dR_k(t) = 0$.

With $R = (R_1, \ldots, R_{K-1})^T$ then $n^{1/2} R$ is [under some mild regularity conditions, see Andersen et al. (1993)] asymptotically normally distributed around zero with some covariance matrix Σ with elements Σ_{kl} being the limit in probability of

$$n \left\langle \int_0^\cdot w_k(t)d(\hat{A}_k - \tilde{A}_k)(t), \int_0^\cdot w_l(t)d(\hat{A}_l - \tilde{A}_l)(t) \right\rangle (\tau)$$

$$= n \int_0^\tau w_k(t) w_l(t) J_k(t) J_l(t) \frac{1}{Y_k(t) Y_\cdot(t)} \left(\delta_{kl} - \frac{Y_k(t)}{Y_\cdot(t)} \right) Y_\cdot(t) \alpha(t)\, dt,$$

which may be estimated consistently by

$$\hat{\Sigma}_{kl} = n \int_0^\tau w_k(t) w_l(t) J_k(t) J_l(t) \frac{1}{Y_k(t) Y_\cdot(t)} \left(\delta_{kl} - \frac{Y_k(t)}{Y_\cdot(t)} \right) dN_\cdot(t). \quad (4.8)$$

If the hypothesis is true, then

$$Q = nR^T \hat{\Sigma}^{-1} R \quad (4.9)$$

is asymptotically χ^2-distributed with $K - 1$ degrees of freedom. The R_K is not included in the above construction of the test since $\hat{\Sigma}$ would then be singular.

One may now construct various tests by choosing different weight functions. The *log-rank test* is obtained by choosing $w_k(t) = Y_k(t) I(Y_\cdot(t) > 0)$. For this particular choice of weight function we may write the R_k's as

$$R_k = O_k - E_k,$$

where $O_k = N_k(\tau)$ is the observed number of failures in group k and

$$E_k = \int_0^\tau Y_k(t) d\hat{A}(t)$$

is referred to as the expected number of failures under the hypothesis. This is a little imprecise since E_k is stochastic (and can hence not be an expected number) but the terminology is used since, under the hypothesis, $E(R_k) = 0$, and therefore $E(E_k) = E(O_k)$.

Example 4.2.1 (Melanoma data.)

We illustrate the nonparametric tests by use of the melanoma dataset. We here focus on the covariate: sex of the patient (coded 0 for female and 1 for male). The log-rank test for testing the hypothesis of no difference of the two groups with respect to survival may be obtained in R by use of the function `survdiff`.

```
> library(survival)
> library(timereg)
> data(melanoma)
```

90   4. Nonparametric procedures for survival data

```
> attach(melanoma)
> survdiff(Surv(days,status==1)~sex)
Call:
survdiff(formula = Surv(days, status == 1) ~ sex)

        N Observed Expected (O-E)^2/E (O-E)^2/V
sex=0 126       28     37.1     2.25      6.47
sex=1  79       29     19.9     4.21      6.47

 Chisq= 6.5  on 1 degrees of freedom, p= 0.011
```

We see that too many males die than expected if the hypothesis of no difference should be true, and the hypothesis is rejected with a p-value of 0.011. The survdiff function actually implements the S-ρ family of Harrington & Fleming (1982) (see (4.10) below) with the default of $\rho = 0$ giving the log-rank test. The Peto & Peto modification of the Gehan-Wilcoxon test is obtained by putting $\rho = 1$.

```
> survdiff(Surv(days,status==1)~sex,rho=1)
Call:
survdiff(formula = Surv(days, status == 1) ~ sex, rho = 1)

        N Observed Expected (O-E)^2/E (O-E)^2/V
sex=0 126     23.4     31.6     2.14      7.09
sex=1  79     25.2     17.0     3.98      7.09

 Chisq= 7.1  on 1 degrees of freedom, p= 0.00776
```

□

The log-rank test is the most powerful test against the alternative of proportional hazards meaning that the hazard functions at any given time of an individual in one group is proportional to the hazard function at that time to the hazard function of an individual in the other group(s). This alternative is equivalent to the Cox model assumption, which we return to in detail in Chapter 6. Actually, the log-rank test may be derived as a model based (score)-test under the assumption of proportional hazards, see Exercise 6.1.

Other tests may be better to detect other alternatives. Harrington & Fleming (1982) introduced a class of tests by letting

$$w_k(t) = Y_k(t)\hat{S}(t-)^\rho I(Y_\cdot(t) > 0), \qquad (4.10)$$

where $\hat{S}(t)$ is the Kaplan-Meier estimator, see Section 4.1, computed under the hypothesis and ρ is a fixed number between zero and one. Taking $\rho = 0$ gives the log-rank test and $\rho = 1$ gives the so-called Peto & Peto modification of the Gehan-Wilcoxon test. This class of tests is implemented in R, see the above example.

4.2 Hypothesis testing   91

The log-rank test and the entire family of S-ρ tests are well suited for detecting differences that are consistent over the considered time-range, and will be efficient against particular alternatives. Sometimes, however one would like an omnibus test that will detect any type of departure from the null hypothesis of equal intensities across the groupings.

In the two-sample case the Kolmogorov-Smirnov test may also be used. We briefly outline how it may be implemented, and how it differs from the log-rank test. We consider the two sample-situation, and thus wish to investigate the hypothesis

$$H_0 : \alpha_1 = \alpha_2.$$

The log-rank test consider the asymptotic distribution of

$$\int_0^\tau J_1(s) J_2(s) \left(\frac{Y_2(s)}{Y_\cdot(s)} dN_1(s) - \frac{Y_1(s)}{Y_\cdot(s)} dN_2(s) \right),$$

where $J(s) = \max(J_1(s), J_2(s))$. If one, however, wishes to compare the two intensities without using any prior knowledge on where to look for differences, it seems natural to compare the two Nelson-Aalen estimates

$$\Delta(t) = \int_0^t J_1(s) J_2(s) \left(\frac{1}{Y_1(s)} dN_1(s) - \frac{1}{Y_2(s)} dN_2(s) \right).$$

To obtain the log-rank test one should weight these differences with $\tilde{w}(t) = Y_1(s) Y_2(s) / Y_\cdot(t)$. An omnibus test may be constructed by considering a statistic like

$$\sup_{t \in [0,\tau]} \frac{|\Delta(t)|}{\sigma(t)}$$

where $\sigma^2(t)$ is an estimator of the variance of $\Delta(t)$. Another omnibus test could be constructed by inspecting the uniform Hall-Wellner band, see Chapter 5.

Example 4.2.2 (A Kolmogorov-Smirnov Two Sample Test.)

As in the previous example we consider the melanoma dataset, and wish to test if there is a significant difference in survival depending on sex.

The Kolmogorov-Smirnov test outlined above can be computed by using the additive hazard regression function aalen() that we describe in further detail in Chapter 5. The syntax for computing the Kolmogorov-Smirnov test-statistic and plotting the Nelson-Aalen estimates is as follows.

```
> data(melanoma)
> fit<-aalen(Surv(days/365,status==1) ~ 1 + factor(sex),
+ melanoma)
Nonparametric Additive Risk Model
Simulations start N= 1000
```

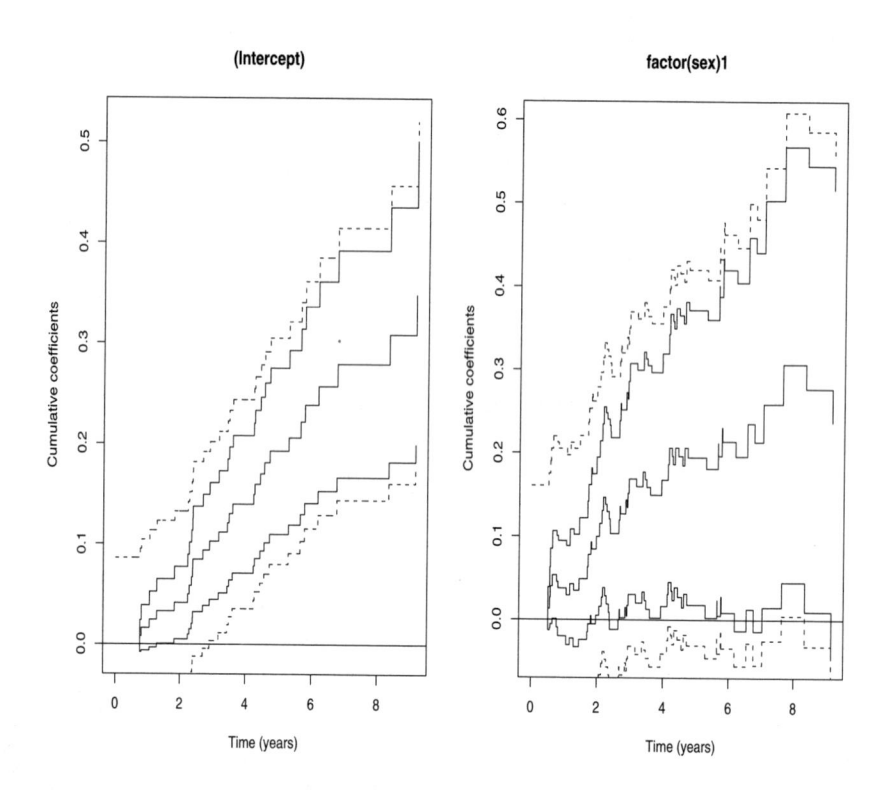

92   4. Nonparametric procedures for survival data

FIGURE 4.4: Nelson-Aalen estimates with 95% confidence intervals (full lines), and 95% Hall-Wellner confidence bands (broken lines). Intercept gives the estimate for females, and factor(sex)1 gives the difference in the estimates for males and females.

```
> summary(fit)
Additive Aalen Model

Test for nonparametric terms

Test for non-significant effects
             sup| hat B(t)/SD(t) | p-value H_0: B(t)=0
(Intercept)                 4.87                  0.00
factor(sex)1                2.67                  0.07
Test for time invariant effects
             sup| B(t) - (t/tau)B(tau)|  p-value H_0: B(t)=b t
(Intercept)                 0.0416                         0.741
factor(sex)1                0.1090                         0.422

             int (B(t)-(t/tau)B(tau))^2dt  p-value H_0: B(t)=b t
(Intercept)                 0.00245                        0.841
factor(sex)1                0.03280                        0.249
```

```
> plot(fit,xlab="Time (years)",hw.ci=2)
```

The Kolmogorov-Smirnov test results in a p-value of 0.07, and a non-significant difference at the 5 % level.

Figure 4.4 shows the Nelson-Aalen estimate for females (the intercept in the model) and the difference between the Nelson-Aalen estimates for males and females (the effect of sex). Note, that the difference between the two Nelson-Aalen estimates is essentially a straight line with positive slope, thus indicating that the hazard function for males is consistently higher than that for females. The full lines give the estimate with 95% pointwise confidence intervals, and the broken lines give the 95% Hall-Wellner confidence band. The confidence band suggest that the difference is borderline significant, with zero just escaping the confidence region around time 8. Thus giving a different conclusion than the Kolmogorov-Smirnov test.

The difference between the Nelson-Aalen estimates suggests that males have an excess hazard that is constant over time. Looking a bit ahead, formal tests for this are given in the output as "Tests for time invariant effects" thus resulting in p-values of either 0.42 or 0.25, depending on which of the two test-statistics that are applied. □

4.2.2 Stratified tests

Above we saw how various nonparametric tests could be applied to compare the survival of some K groups of subjects. Often it is an explanatory variable that gives rise to the groups being compared and we are then investigating the effect of this explanatory variable on the survival. It is often of interest to *control for other potentially important factors* when comparing differences across the primary variable. This may also be done in a nonparametric fashion and is termed a stratified analyses.

Suppose we have L strata, which may be formed from the other factor(s) that we want to control for. The hazard function for a subject in the kth group, $k = 1\ldots,K$, in the lth stratum, $l = 1\ldots,L$, is denoted $\alpha_{kl}(t)$, and we want to construct tests for the hypothesis

$$\mathrm{H}_0 : \alpha_{1l} = \ldots = \alpha_{Kl} \qquad (4.11)$$

for all $l = 1\ldots,L$. This is done by comparing the group specific Nelson-Aalen estimators in each stratum to the Nelson-Aalen estimator computed under H_0. Let

$$R_{kl} = \int_0^\tau w_{kl}(t) d(\hat{A}_{kl} - \tilde{A}_{kl})(t),$$

where $w_{kl}(t)$ is a weight function, and

$$\hat{A}_{kl}(t) = \int_0^t \frac{1}{Y_{kl}(s)} dN_{kl}(s), \quad \tilde{A}_{kl}(t) = \int_0^t \frac{J_{kl}(s)}{Y_{\cdot l}(s)} dN_{\cdot l}(s),$$

with $J_{kl}(t) = I(Y_{kl}(t) > 0)$, $Y_{\cdot l}(t) = \sum_k Y_{kl}(t)$, $N_{\cdot l}(t) = \sum_k N_{kl}(t)$, and with $Y_{kl}(t)$ and $N_{kl}(t)$ being the number at risk at time t in group k in stratum l, and the sum of the counting processes of group k and stratum l, respectively.

Put $R_l = (R_{1l}, \ldots, R_{K-1,l})^T$ and let $\hat{\Sigma}_l$ denote the estimate of the variance of R_l. A test of H_0 for l fixed, that is, within the lth stratum could be carried out using

$$R_l^T \hat{\Sigma}_l^{-1} R_l,$$

which is asymptotically χ^2-distributed with $K-1$ degrees of freedom under the hypothesis of equal hazard functions in the lth stratum. We want, however, to combine the information across strata. This may of course be done in several ways, but it is common practice to base the test on the sum of the R_l's. Hence, let $R = \sum_l R_l$ and $\hat{\Sigma} = \sum_l \hat{\Sigma}_l$. A class of (stratified) test statistics of (4.11) is then given by

$$R^T \hat{\Sigma} R, \qquad (4.12)$$

which is also asymptotically χ^2-distributed with $K-1$ degrees of freedom under the hypothesis and given some mild regularity conditions, see Andersen et al. (1993). The *stratified log-rank test* is obtained by taking $w_{kl}(t) = Y_{kl}(t) I(Y_{\cdot l}(t) > 0)$.

Example 4.2.3 (Melanoma data. Continuation of Example 4.2.1.)

We saw in Example 4.2.1 that there seemed to be a significant different survival between males and females in the melanoma dataset. Let us investigate this more closely. The variable ulc indicates (0 for absent, and 1 for present) whether the tumor was ulcerated, and it is well known that this is an important factor. It may hence be a good idea to control for this variable before comparing the survival of the two sexes. The commands

```
> fit.sex.ulc<-survfit(Surv(days,status==1)~sex+ulc)
> plot(fit.sex.ulc)
```

give the Kaplan-Meier plots for the four combinations of sex and ulceration shown in Figure 4.5. There still seems to be a difference between the survival of the two sexes. A formal test of this is given for example by the stratified log-rank test, which may be obtained as follows.

```
> survdiff(Surv(days,status==1)~sex+strata(ulc))
Call:
survdiff(formula = Surv(days, status == 1) ~ sex + strata(ulc))

        N Observed Expected (O-E)^2/E (O-E)^2/V
sex=0 126       28     34.7      1.28      3.31
sex=1  79       29     22.3      1.99      3.31

 Chisq= 3.3  on 1 degrees of freedom, p= 0.0687
```

[Figure: Kaplan-Meier curves plot]

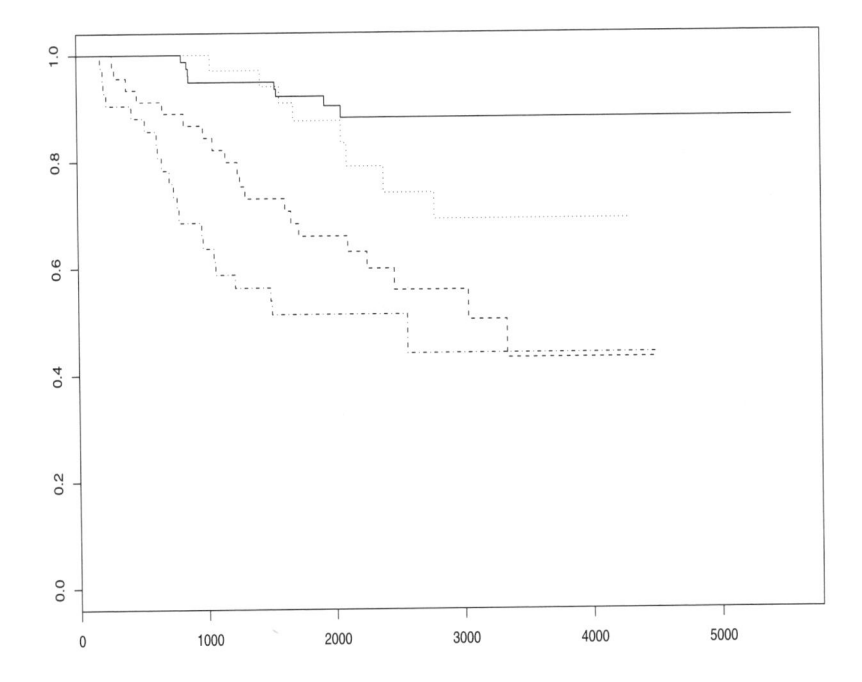

FIGURE 4.5: Melanoma data. Kaplan-Meier curves for female and males without ulceration (full curve and dotted curve), and for females and males with ulceration (broken curve and broken-dotted curve).

We see that the evidence of a difference is not as convincing now where we have controlled for ulceration, the test statistic now being 3.3 compared with 6.5 obtained in the analysis where we did not stratify. □

By taking the sum of the R_l's as in the above test statistic it is obvious that this test will only have good power against alternatives where the deviations from the hypothesis go in the same direction in all strata, see Exercise 4.7 for a test that avoids this.

4.3 Exercises

4.1 (Smoothing of the Nelson-Aalen estimator) Consider the multivariate counting process $N = (N_1, \ldots N_n)^T$, where $N_i(t)$ has intensity $\lambda_i(t) =$

96   4. Nonparametric procedures for survival data

$Y_i(t)\alpha(t)$. The Nelson-Aalen estimator of $A(t) = \int_0^t \alpha(s)\, ds$ is

$$\hat{A}(t) = \int_0^t \frac{1}{Y.(s)} dN.(s),$$

where $N.(t) = \sum_{i=1}^n N_i(t)$, $Y.(t) = \sum_{i=1}^n Y_i(t)$.

We shall now consider estimation of $\alpha(t)$ by kernel smoothing of $\hat{A}(t)$. Let $K(t)$ be a kernel function that is a bounded function vanishing outside $[-1, 1]$, and let b_n denote the bandwidth that is a positive parameter. The kernel estimator of $\alpha(t)$ is

$$\hat{\alpha}(t) = b_n^{-1} \int K(\frac{t-s}{b_n}) d\hat{A}(s).$$

This estimator was proposed and studied by Ramlau-Hansen (1983a,b).

(a) Find the compensator of $\hat{\alpha}(t)$ and compute $E\hat{\alpha}(t)$.

(b) Let $0 < t_1 < t_2 < t$. Assume that K is of bounded variation and that α is continuous on $[0, t]$. Let $b_n \to 0$ and assume that

$$\inf_{s \in [0,t]} b_n^2 Y.(s) \xrightarrow{P} \infty$$

as $n \to \infty$. Show that

$$\sup_{s \in [t_1, t_2]} |\hat{\alpha}(s) - \alpha(s)| \xrightarrow{P} 0.$$

(c) Let α be continuous at t and let y be a function, positive and continuous at t, so that

$$\sup_{s \in [t-\epsilon, t+\epsilon]} |n^{-1} Y.(s) - y(s)| \xrightarrow{P} 0,$$

for an $\epsilon > 0$. Show, as $n \to \infty$, $b_n \to 0$, and $nb_n \to \infty$, that

$$n^{1/2} b_n^{1/2} (\hat{\alpha}(t) - \tilde{\alpha}(t)) \xrightarrow{D} N(0, \tau^2(t)),$$

where

$$\tilde{\alpha}(t) = b_n^{-1} \int K(\frac{t-s}{b_n}) dA(s), \quad \tau^2(t) = \frac{\alpha(t)}{y(t)} \int_{-1}^1 K^2(s)\, ds.$$

We shall now assume that α is twice continuously differentiable on $[t_1 - c, t_2 + c]$ for $t_1 < t_2$, $c > 0$, and that

$$\int_{-1}^1 K(t)\, dt = 1, \quad \int_{-1}^1 tK(t)\, dt = 0, \quad k_2 = \int_{-1}^1 t^2 K(t)\, dt > 0.$$

(d) Show that the bias of the estimator is

$$E\hat{\alpha}(t) - \alpha(t) = \frac{1}{2}b_n^2 \alpha''(t) k_2 + o(b_n^2) + o(n^{-1}),$$

$t \in [t_1 - c, t_2 + c]$.

We shall now consider the problem of picking an optimal bandwidth. As criteria we use the mean integrated squared error

$$\text{MISE}(\hat{\alpha}) = E \int_{t_1}^{t_2} (\hat{\alpha}(t) - \alpha(t))^2 \, dt.$$

Modulo a lower order term one may decompose $\text{MISE}(\hat{\alpha})$ as

$$\text{MISE}(\hat{\alpha}) = \int_{t_1}^{t_2} (\tilde{\alpha}(t) - \alpha(t))^2 \, dt + \int_{t_1}^{t_2} E[(\hat{\alpha}(t) - \tilde{\alpha}(t))^2] \, dt,$$

which may be interpreted as the sum of a *squared bias* term and *variance* term.

(e) Show under appropriate conditions that

$$\int_{t_1}^{t_2} (\tilde{\alpha}(t) - \alpha(t))^2 \, dt = \frac{1}{4} b_n^4 k_2^2 \int_{t_1}^{t_2} \alpha''(t)^2 \, dt + o(b_n^4)$$

and

$$\int_{t_1}^{t_2} E[(\hat{\alpha}(t) - \tilde{\alpha}(t))^2] \, dt = (nb_n)^{-1} \int_{-1}^{1} K(t)^2 \, dt \int_{t_1}^{t_2} \frac{\alpha(t)}{y(t)} \, dt + o((nb_n)^{-1}),$$

where $y(t)$ is the limit in probability of $n^{-1} Y.(t)$.

It follows that the bias and the variance terms are balanced for $(nb_n)^{-1} \sim b_n^4$, which implies an optimal choice of bandwidth is equal to $b_n \sim n^{-1/5}$.

(f) Minimize (ignoring lower order terms) the expression of $\text{MISE}(\hat{\alpha})$ with respect to b_n to obtain the optimal bandwidth

$$b_{n,\text{opt}} = k_2^{-2/5} \left(\int_{-1}^{1} K(t)^2 \, dt \int_{t_1}^{t_2} \frac{\alpha(t)}{y(t)} \, dt \right)^{1/5} \left(\int_{t_1}^{t_2} \alpha''(t)^2 \, dt \right)^{-1/5} n^{-1/5}.$$

One may aim at estimating $b_{n,\text{opt}}$ using a twice differentiable kernel function to estimate the term

$$\int_{t_1}^{t_2} \alpha''(t)^2 \, dt.$$

The term

$$\int_{t_1}^{t_2} \frac{\alpha(t)}{y(t)} \, dt$$

is easily estimated by

$$\int_{t_1}^{t_2} \frac{1}{n^{-1} Y.(t)} \, d\hat{A}(t).$$

98   4. Nonparametric procedures for survival data

(g) Another way of estimating MISE goes as follows. Verify that

$$\text{MISE} = \text{E}\int_{t_1}^{t_2} \hat{a}(t)^2 \, dt - 2\text{E}\int_{t_1}^{t_2} \hat{a}(t)\alpha(t) \, dt + \int_{t_1}^{t_2} \alpha(t)^2 \, dt,$$

where the latter term does not depend on the bandwidth and thus can be ignored. The first term is easy to estimate from $\hat{a}(t)$. Show that the second term is estimated approximately unbiased by the cross-validation estimate

$$-2\sum_{j\neq k} b_n^{-1} K\left(\frac{T_j - T_k}{b_n}\right) \frac{1}{Y_\bullet(T_j)} \frac{1}{Y_\bullet(T_k)},$$

where the sum is taken over j, k so that $j \neq k$ and $t_1 \leq T_j \leq t_2$ denotes the jump times in the specified interval.

(h) Compute $\hat{a}(t)$ for the females and males of the Melanoma dataset using the Epanechnikov kernel

$$K(x) = 0.75(1 - x^2)I(-1 \leq x \leq 1).$$

Consider only the time-interval from 1 to 6 years.

4.2 (Estimation of quantiles)

(a) Show that the estimator (4.5) is consistent and derive the asymptotic distribution of $n^{1/2}(\hat{t}_{0.8} - t_{0.8})$ (use the delta-theorem).

(b) Show that (4.6) is an asymptotic 95% confidence interval for $t_{0.8}$.

4.3 (Kaplan-Meier as NPMLE)   Consider n i.i.d. survival times T_i with right-censoring times C_i such that we observe $X_i = T_i \wedge C_i$ and $\delta_i = I(T_i \leq C_i)$, for simplicity we let the survival times be ordered such that $X_1, ..., X_d$ are the d ordered death times, the remaining censored survival times are denoted $X_{d+1}, ..., X_n$. We assume that the underlying survival time has continuous survival function $G_T(\cdot)$, with $G_T(0) = 1$.

Let $\mathcal{D}$ be the set of functions that have jumps at the observed death times and that can be identified with a vector of probability masses $p = (p_1, ..., p_d)$ that are located at the ordered death times (such that $\sum p_i \leq 1, p_j \geq 0$). The survival function related to the probability masses are given

$$G(t) = 1 - \sum_{i=1}^{d} I(X_i \leq t) p_i.$$

Denote $G(X_i) = P(U > X_i) = G_i$.

The nonparametric maximum likelihood estimator for the survivor function $G \in \mathcal{D}$ is given as

$$L(G, X_1, ..., X_n, \delta_1, ..., \delta_n) = \prod_{i=1}^{d} p_i \prod_{i=d+1}^{n} G(X_i).$$

(a) Show that L is maximized for the product-limit estimator.

(b) Show that the maximizer of the above likelihood cannot be made larger by including monotonic decreasing survivor functions.

(c) Rather than maximizing the likelihood directly one may apply the EM-algorithm. Assume that full data consist of all survival times being fully observed, and work out the E and M step of the EM algorithm.

(d) Returning to (a) reparameterize the problem by considering the discrete hazard rather than p_i such that

$$\lambda_i = \frac{p_i}{G_{i-1}}$$

and maximize the likelihood.

(e) Write down the EM-algorithm for the hazard parameterization.

4.4 (Greenwood's formula) Consider the counting processes: N_i, $i = 1, \ldots, n$, so that $N_i(t)$ has compensator

$$\Lambda_i(t) = \int_0^t Y_i(s) dA(s),$$

where A may have jumps. The Nelson-Aalen estimator of $A(t)$ is

$$\hat{A}(t) = \int_0^t \frac{1}{Y(s)} dN(s),$$

where $N(t) = \sum_{i=1}^n N_i(t)$, $Y(t) = \sum_{i=1}^n Y_i(t)$. Put $A^*(t) = \int J(s) dA(s)$, where $J(t) = I(Y(t) > 0)$.

(a) Show that

$$\langle \hat{A} - A^* \rangle(t) = \int_0^t \frac{J(s)}{Y(s)} (1 - \Delta A(s)) dA(s) \quad (4.13)$$

4. Nonparametric procedures for survival data

where ΔA denotes the jumps of A, see Exercise 2.13, and that (4.13) is estimated consistently by

$$\int_0^t J(s)(Y(s) - \Delta N(s))\frac{1}{Y(s)^3}dN(s),$$

which gives an alternative estimator of the variance of the Nelson-Aalen estimator.

Let $S(t) = \exp(-A(t))$, $S^*(t) = \exp(-A^*(t))$, and

$$\hat{S}(t) = \prod_{s \leq t}\left(1 - \frac{\Delta N(s)}{Y(s)}\right).$$

denotes the Kaplan-Meier estimator of $S(t)$.

(b) Use (4.3) to show that

$$\left\langle \frac{\hat{S}}{S^*} - 1 \right\rangle(t) = \int_0^t \left(\frac{\hat{S}(s-)}{S^*(s)}\right)^2 \frac{J(s)}{Y(s)}(1 - \Delta A(s))dA(s),$$

and use this, and the fact that

$$\hat{S}(t) = \left(1 - \frac{\Delta N(t)}{Y(t)}\right)\hat{S}(t-),$$

to arrive at the Greenwood estimator of the variance of the Kaplan-Meier estimator.

4.5 (K-sample test) The test-statistic given in (4.9) could be denoted by Q_K to stress that it is constructed based on $R_1, \ldots R_{K-1}$ hence not using R_K. Now make the same construction leaving out R_j and denote the corresponding test statistic Q_j, $j = 1, \ldots, K - 1$.

(a) Show that $Q_1 = \cdots = Q_K$.

4.6 (Hypothesis testing) Consider the set-up in Section 4.2.1.

(a) Compute the optional variation process for $(R_1, \ldots, R_{K-1})$ and compare with the variance estimator given by $\hat{\Sigma}$ given by (4.8).

(b) Verify that for the log-rank $R_k = O_k - E_k$, where $O_k = N_k(\tau)$ and that $E(E_k) = E(O_k)$.

(c) We focused only on the special weight-function $w_k(t) = Y_k(t)w(t)$, where w is a weight function. Consider now the general case where w_k are arbitrary weight-functions and derive the asymptotic distribution of $(R_1, \ldots, R_K)$ that need not be singular.

(d) Consider the PBC data in R (survival-package) and compute the log-rank and the Kolmogorov-Smirnov test to evaluate the effect of edema on survival. Also, make Kaplan-Meier plots and estimate the cumulative hazard function for the two groups.

4.7 By taking sum of the R_l's in the test statistic (4.12) it is obvious that this test will only have good power against alternatives where deviations from the hypothesis go in the same direction in all strata. A test that does not require this is one based on for example the absolute values $|R_l|$, $l = 1, \ldots, L$, and such a test statistic could be

$$\left(\sum_{l=1}^{L} |R_l|\right)^T \left(\sum_{l=1}^{L} \hat{\Sigma}_l\right)^{-1} \left(\sum_{l=1}^{L} |R_l|\right). \tag{4.14}$$

(a) Do the stratified log-rank test for testing effect of x2 based on the following dataset, where time holds the right-censored waiting times and status is the indicator of whether time is a true event (status equal to one).

```
n<-400
x1<-rbinom(n,1,0.5)
x2<-rbinom(n,1,0.5)
hazard<-1+0*x1-0.2*x2+0.4*x1*x2
time.star<-rexp(n,1/hazard)
Cen<-rexp(n,0.25)
time<-apply(cbind(time.star,Cen),1,'min')
status<-as.numeric(time.star<=Cen)
```

(b) Perform the test (4.14) on the same dataset. Here you need to simulate the asymptotic distribution of the test statistic.

5
Additive Hazards Models

The additive hazards model, or the additive Aalen model, was introduced by Aalen (1980). It is a very flexible nonparametric model, which has estimators on explicit form. The model is simple to implement and its properties are well understood. It seems, however, to be somewhat overlooked in practice, probably due to the fact that the model only contains nonparametric terms, and that the handling of these terms for inferential purposes is not fully developed.

The additive Aalen model assumes that the intensity for the counting process $N(t)$ conditionally on a p-dimensional covariate,
$$X(t) = (X_1(t), ..., X_p(t))^T$$
is of the form
$$\begin{aligned}\lambda(t) &= Y(t)X^T(t)\beta(t) \\ &= Y(t)(X_1(t)\beta_1(t) + ... + X_p(t)\beta_p(t)),\end{aligned} \tag{5.1}$$

where $\beta(t) = (\beta_1(t), ..., \beta_p(t))^T$ is a p-dimensional regression coefficient. In principle $Y(t)$ may be any locally bounded predictable process but we think of it as the at risk indicator. The theory that follows may likewise be developed in a general counting process setup, but we think of it in a survival analysis setting, that is, $Y(t)$ is the at risk indicator and $X^T(t)\beta(t)$ is a conditional hazard function. We see from (5.1) that the effect of the covariates may thus change with time as the regression coefficient is allowed to depend on time. The additive Aalen model is very flexible and can be seen as a first order Taylor series expansion of a general intensity around the zero covariate: for a general hazard function $\alpha(t, X(t))$ depending on $X(t)$ we have

$$\alpha(t, X(t)) = \alpha(t, 0) + X^T(t)\alpha'(t, X^*(t))$$

for $X^*(t)$ on the line segment between 0 and $X(t)$.

It turns out that the cumulative regression coefficient

$$B(t) = \int_0^t \beta(s)ds$$

is easy to estimate and that the estimator converges at the usual $n^{1/2}$-rate. We will aim at this parameter instead of the regression coefficient itself.

The full flexibility of the additive Aalen model being completely nonparametric is sometimes superfluous, and this can make it more difficult than really necessary to report findings for a data set. Also when data are limited one can only hope to extract major contours of the data. Some regression coefficients may for example be approximately constant with time. In practice it will indeed often be of interest to test if a treatment effect is time-varying or constant with time. A very useful sub-model of the additive hazards model (5.1) is the semiparametric additive hazards model, suggested by McKeague & Sasieni (1994) and denoted as the additive semiparametric risk model. It assumes that the intensity is on the form

$$\lambda(t) = Y(t)(X^T(t)\beta(t) + Z^T(t)\gamma), \tag{5.2}$$

where $(X(t), Z(t))$ is a $(p+q)$-dimensional covariate, $Y(t)$ is the at risk indicator, $\beta(t)$ is a p-dimensional time-varying regression coefficient and γ a q-dimensional time-invariant coefficient. Hence the effect of some of the covariates may change with time while the effect of others is assumed to be constant. This model also leads to estimators on explicit form, which are easy to compute.

The semiparametric additive hazards model is needed to investigate if the time-varying regression coefficients of the semiparametric model (5.2) are in fact significantly varying with time. To perform a test of the hypothesis $H_0 : \beta_p(t) \equiv \gamma_{q+1}$, one needs to compare the two semiparametric models

$$\lambda(t) = Y(t)(X^T(t)\beta(t) + Z^T(t)\gamma)$$

and

$$\tilde{\lambda}(t) = Y(t)(X_1(t)\beta_1(t) + ... + X_{p-1}(t)\beta_{p-1}(t) + X_p(t)\gamma_{q+1} + Z^T(t)\gamma).$$

The following example illustrates how the methodology developed later in this chapter may be used in practice. Details concerning the estimators and inferential procedures follow. We apply the aalen-function (timereg) that can fit the models (5.1) and (5.2).

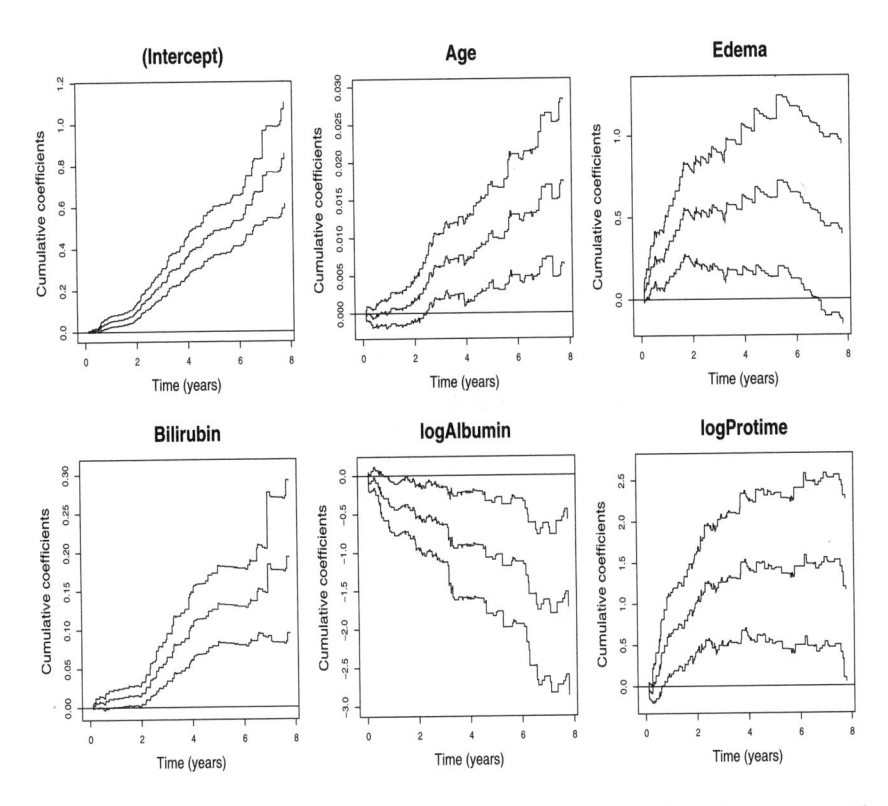

FIGURE 5.1: PBC-data. Estimated cumulative regression functions with 95% pointwise confidence intervals based on Aalen's additive model.

Example 5.0.1 (PBC-data, continuation of Example 1.1.1)

We wish to examine the predictive effect on survival of the covariates: age (years), albumin (g/dl), bilirubin (mg/dl), edema (present/not present), and prothrombin time (seconds). We consider the additive hazards model framework and start by fitting Aalen's additive hazards model where all components of the model have nonparametric time-varying effects. We fit the model with age, edema, bilirubin, log(albumin) and log(protime) using the `timereg` library. All covariates are centered around their averages in the version of the PBC data that we use.

```
> library(survival)
> library(timereg)
> fit<-aalen(Surv(time/365,status)~Age+Edema+Bilirubin+
+ logAlbumin+logProtime,pbc,max.time=8)
Nonparametric Additive Risk Model
Simulations start N= 1000
> summary(fit)
Additive Aalen Model
```

106   5. Additive Hazards Models

```
Test for nonparametric terms

Test for non-significant effects
            sup| hat B(t)/SD(t) |  p-value H_0: B(t)=0
(Intercept)          8.85                  0.000
Age                  3.35                  0.022
Edema                3.89                  0.002
Bilirubin            5.64                  0.000
logAlbumin           3.77                  0.008
logProtime           3.12                  0.029
Test for time invariant effects
            sup| B(t) - (t/tau)B(tau)|  p-value H_0: B(t)=b t
(Intercept)          0.13000                    0.139
Age                  0.00297                    0.829
Edema                0.47000                    0.005
Bilirubin            0.03430                    0.369
logAlbumin           0.29200                    0.883
logProtime           0.96200                    0.002

            int (B(t)-(t/tau)B(tau))^2dt  p-value H_0: B(t)=b t
(Intercept)          5.72e-02                   0.037
Age                  1.86e-05                   0.665
Edema                8.73e-01                   0.000
Bilirubin            1.85e-03                   0.420
logAlbumin           7.92e-02                   0.963
logProtime           3.10e+00                   0.001

> plot(fit,xlab="Time (years)");
```

The output contains a number of summary statistics. First we see, using a supremum test, that all covariate effects are significant. Figure 5.1 depicts the estimated cumulative regression coefficients with 95% pointwise confidence intervals. It appears from these that the effect of at least age and log(albumin) is constant with time as the estimated cumulatives are approximately straight lines. Below, this is studied further.

We now start to simplify the model by a number of successive tests with the purpose of reducing the number of nonparametric components. First, we note that the log(albumin) does not seem to have a time-varying effect (p=0.88, using the supremum test), which, as mentioned above, is consistent with the cumulative estimate being approximately a straight line in Figure 5.1. Fitting the model with the effect of log(albumin) being constant (output not shown) we find that the effect of age is also constant (p=0.86). The model where both log(albumin) and age have constant effects shows that the effect of bilirubin also can be described as being constant (p=0.56). The reduced semiparametric model is then fitted resulting in the below output.

```
> fit.semi<-aalen( Surv(time/365,status)~const(Age)+Edema+
+ const(Bilirubin)+const(logAlbumin)+logProtime,pbc,
+ max.time=8)
Semiparametric Additive Risk Model
Simulations start N= 1000
> summary(fit.semi)
Additive Aalen Model

Test for nonparametric terms

Test for non-significant effects
            sup| hat B(t)/SD(t) | p-value H_0: B(t)=0
(Intercept)              21.80                  0.000
Edema                     3.28                  0.011
logProtime                2.80                  0.057
Test for time invariant effects
            sup| B(t) - (t/tau)B(tau)| p-value H_0: B(t)=b t
(Intercept)              0.101                  0.001
Edema                    0.439                  0.000
logProtime               0.937                  0.001

            int (B(t)-(t/tau)B(tau))^2dt p-value H_0: B(t)=b t
(Intercept)              0.0419                 0.001
Edema                    0.7890                 0.000
logProtime               2.5200                 0.002

Parametric terms :
                    Coef.       SE  Robust SE     z    P-val
const(Age)         0.00201  0.000579   0.00060  3.47  5.16e-04
const(Bilirubin)   0.02070  0.003870   0.00328  5.34  9.24e-08
const(logAlbumin) -0.22800  0.069200   0.06170 -3.29  9.89e-04

> plot(fit.semi,score=T,xlab="Time (years)",ylab="Test Process")
```

The fit of the semiparametric model shows that edema and log(protime) have effects that are significantly time-varying (p<0.001 and p=0.001, using the supremum test-statistic). The impact of the remaining covariates is characterized by their constant effects. Increasing age by one year, for example, leads to an estimated increased intensity of 0.002 (0.00058). □

5.1 Additive hazards models

We now give the estimators associated with the Aalen additive model and describe their asymptotic properties. The model was originally suggested by Aalen (1980) and further studied in Aalen (1989, 1993). Asymptotic properties were given by McKeague (1988) and Huffer & McKeague (1991).

The model states that the intensity for the counting process $N(t)$, $t \in [0, \tau]$, $\tau < \infty$, of a subject with a p-dimensional predictable bounded covariate, $X(t) = (X_1(t), ..., X_p(t))^T$, and at risk indicator, $Y(t)$, is of the form

$$\lambda(t) = Y(t) X^T(t) \beta(t), \tag{5.3}$$

where $\beta(t) = (\beta_1(t), ..., \beta_p(t))^T$ is a p-dimensional locally integrable regression coefficient ($\int_0^t |\beta_j(s)| ds < \infty$ for $j = 1, ..., p$). One may relax the assumption about the covariates being bounded to only require that they are locally bounded, but as this seems to of very little importance in practice it will not be pursued here.

It turns out that it is very easy to estimate the cumulative regression coefficients

$$B(t) = \int_0^t \beta(s) ds$$

of the additive Aalen model. Let

$$(N_i(t), Y_i(t), X_i(t)), \quad i = 1, \ldots, n,$$

be independent replicates of the above model, that is, the intensity $\lambda_i(t)$ for the ith counting process $N_i(t)$ is on the form (5.3). Define

$$N(t) = (N_1(t), ..., N_n(t))^T, \quad \lambda(t) = (\lambda_1(t), ..., \lambda_n(t))^T,$$

the n-dimensional counting process of all subjects and its intensity. We also organize the covariates into a design matrix of dimension $n \times p$:

$$X(t) = (Y_1(t) X_1(t), ..., Y_n(t) X_n(t))^T.$$

Further denote the n-dimensional cumulative intensities as $\Lambda(t) = \int_0^t \lambda(s) ds$ such that $M(t) = N(t) - \Lambda(t)$ is a n-dimensional martingale. We thus have that

$$\begin{aligned} dN(t) &= \lambda(t) dt + dM(t) \\ &= X(t) \beta(t) dt + dM(t), \end{aligned} \tag{5.4}$$

and since the increments of the martingale are uncorrelated and have zero mean, this equation suggests that the increments of $\beta(t) dt$, which we write suggestively as $dB(t)$, can be estimated by simple multiple linear regression techniques. To solve the multiple linear regression problem define the generalized inverse of $X(t)$ as the $p \times n$ matrix

$$X^-(t) = (X^T(t) W(t) X(t))^{-1} X^T(t) W(t), \tag{5.5}$$

where W(t) is a predictable $n \times n$ diagonal weight matrix. We make the convention that $X^-(t)$ is zero when the inverse does not exist, and let $J(t)$ be one when the inverse exists and zero otherwise. The generalized inverse satisfies the relation

$$X^-(t)X(t) = J(t)I_p,$$

where I_p is the $p \times p$ identity matrix. Equation (5.4) leads to the estimator

$$d\hat{B}(t) = X^-(t)dN(t),$$

which can be written in integral form as

$$\hat{B}(t) = \int_0^t X^-(s)dN(s). \tag{5.6}$$

Note, that

$$\hat{B}(t) = \int_0^t J(s)dB(s) + \int_0^t X^-(s)dM(s),$$

which implies that, if the rank of $X(t)$ is full for all t (asymptotically at least), then $\hat{B}(t)$ is essentially an unbiased estimator of $B(t)$, since the mean of the martingale $\int_0^t X^-(s)dM(s)$ is zero. But more can be said since, given some regularity conditions, the root-n difference between the estimator and true cumulative regression function converges in distribution to a Gaussian martingale, see the below Theorem 5.1.1.

Define for $j, k, l = 1 \ldots p$, $t \in [0, \tau]$,

$$R_{2jk}(t) = \sum_{i=1}^n Y_i(t)W_i(t)X_{ij}(t)X_{ik}(t),$$

$$R_{3jkl}(t) = \sum_{i=1}^n Y_i(t)W_i^2(t)X_{ij}(t)X_{ik}(t)X_{il}(t).$$

The matrix $R_2(t) = X^T(t)W(t)X(t)$ has elements $R_{2jk}(t)$, $j, k = 1 \ldots p$. The regularity conditions needed are formulated below.

Condition 5.1

(a) $\sup_{t \in [0,\tau]} E(Y_i(t)W_i^2(t)X_{ij}(t)X_{ik}(t)X_{il}(t)) < \infty$ for all $j, k, l = 1, .., p$;

(b) $r_2(t) = E(Y_i(t)W_i(t)X_i^{\otimes 2}(t))$ is non-singular for all $t \in [0, \tau]$.

□

Given that Condition 5.1 is fulfilled we have the following results, which follow using functional forms of the strong law of large numbers (Andersen & Gill, 1982).

110   5. Additive Hazards Models

Lemma 5.1.1 *If Condition 5.1 holds, then there exist continuous functions $r_{2jk}(t)$ and $r_{3jkl}(t)$ such that as $n \to \infty$*

$$\sup_{t \in [0,\tau]} |n^{-1} R_{2jk}(t) - r_{2jk}(t)| \xrightarrow{P} 0,$$

$$\sup_{t \in [0,\tau]} |n^{-1} R_{3jkl}(t) - r_{3jkl}(t)| \xrightarrow{P} 0,$$

for $j, k, l = 1 \ldots p$.

We can now give the asymptotic result concerning the estimator of the cumulative regression coefficients.

Theorem 5.1.1 *If Condition 5.1 holds, then, as $n \to \infty$,*

$$n^{1/2}(\hat{B} - B) \xrightarrow{D} U \tag{5.7}$$

on $D[0,\tau]^p$, where U is a Gaussian martingale with covariance function

$$\Phi(t) = \int_0^t \phi(s) ds \tag{5.8}$$

with

$$\phi(t) = r_2^{-1}(t) E\left[Y_i(t) W_i^2(t) X_i^{\otimes 2}(t) X_i^T(t) \beta(t)\right] r_2^{-1}(t). \tag{5.9}$$

PROOF. The key to the proof is the following decomposition

$$n^{1/2}(\hat{B}(t) - B(t)) = \tilde{M}(t) + Z_1(t) + Z_2(t),$$

where

$$\tilde{M}(t) = n^{-1/2} \int_0^t J(s)(r_2(s))^{-1} X^T(s) W(s) dM(s),$$

$$Z_1(t) = n^{-1/2} \int_0^t J(s) \left\{(n^{-1} R_2(s))^{-1} - r_2^{-1}(s))\right\} X^T(s) W(s) dM(s),$$

$$Z_2(t) = n^{1/2} \int_0^t (J(s) - 1) \beta(s) \, ds.$$

We want to show, as $n \to \infty$, that $Z_1(t)$ and $Z_2(t)$ converge uniformly to zero in probability and that $\tilde{M}(t)$ converges in distribution to a Gaussian martingale with the postulated covariance function. The latter is established using the martingale central limit theorem, see Theorem 2.5.1. We deal with these three terms separately below.

Since $(1 - J(t)) \leq 1 - J$ with $J = I(n^{-1} R_2(t)$ invertible for all $t \in [0,\tau])$ we have

$$\sup_t |Z_2(t)| \leq n^{1/2} I(K_n) \int_0^\tau |\beta(t)| \, dt, \tag{5.10}$$

where
$$K_n = (\exists t : n^{-1}R_2(t) \text{ is singular}) \subseteq (\sup_t ||n^{-1}R_2(t) - r_2(t)|| \geq \epsilon) = L_n$$

for some $\epsilon > 0$. The right-hand side of (5.10) therefore converges to zero in probability since $\beta(t)$ is assumed locally integrable, $P(L_n) \to 0$, and $n^{1/2} I(K_n) \xrightarrow{P} 0$ when $I(K_n) \xrightarrow{P} 0$.

The jth component of $Z_1(t)$ is a square integrable martingale and may be written as
$$Z_{1j}(t) = n^{-1/2} \sum_{i=1}^{n} \int_0^t J(s) V_{ji}(s) dM_i(s),$$

where
$$V_{ji}(t) = \sum_{l=1}^{p} \left\{ (n^{-1} R_2(t))^{-1} - r_2^{-1}(t) \right\}_{jl} Y_i(t) X_{il}(t) W_i(t).$$

Using the inequality of Cauchy-Schwarz we get
$$\langle Z_{1j} \rangle (\tau) = n^{-1} \sum_{i=1}^{n} \int_0^\tau J(t) V_{ji}^2(t) \lambda_i(t) \, dt \leq \int_0^\tau G_j(t) \, dt,$$

where
$$G_j(t) = \sum_{k,l=1}^{p} J \left\{ (n^{-1} R_2)^{-1} - r_2^{-1} \right\}_{jl}^2 \times \left(n^{-1} \sum_{i=1}^{n} Y_i X_{il}^2 X_{ik} W_i^2 \right) \beta_k,$$

and where we have suppressed dependency on time in the expression on the right-hand side of the latter equality. Since inversion of a matrix is a continuous operation we have for all t that $G_j(t) \xrightarrow{P} 0$ as $n \to \infty$. Since the random functions in $G_j(t)$ converges in probability towards continuous functions, we also have that
$$\int_0^\tau G_j(t) \, dt \xrightarrow{P} 0$$

as $n \to \infty$ using Gill's lemma (2.27). It then follows, as $n \to \infty$, that
$$\sup_t |Z_{1j}(t)| \xrightarrow{P} 0$$

by use of Lenglart's inequality (2.25).

The process $\tilde{M}(t)$ is local square integrable martingale with predictable variation process
$$\langle \tilde{M} \rangle (t) = n^{-1} \int_0^t J(s) r_2^{-1}(s) \left(\sum_{i=1}^{n} Y_i(s) W_i(s)^2 X_i(s)^{\otimes 2} X_i^T(s) \beta(s) \right) r_2^{-1}(s) \, ds$$

that converges in probability to $\Phi(t)$ uniformly in t as $n \xrightarrow{P} \infty$ using similar arguments as above. The process containing all the jumps larger in absolute value than ϵ of the jth component of $\tilde{M}_j(t)$ is
$$\tilde{M}_{j\epsilon}(t) = \sum_{i=1}^{n} \int_0^t n^{-1/2} \tilde{V}_{ji}(s) I(|n^{-1/2} \tilde{V}_{ji}(s)| > \epsilon) dM_i(s),$$

112   5. Additive Hazards Models

where
$$\tilde{V}_{ji}(t) = \sum_{l=1}^{p} (r_2(t))_{jl}^{-1} Y_i(t) W_i(t) X_{il}(t).$$

Since
$$|n^{-1/2}\tilde{V}_{ji}(t)| \leq p \cdot \sup_{t,j,l} |(r_2(t))_{jl}^{-1}| n^{-1/2} \sup_{t,i,l} |Y_i(t)W_i(t)X_{il}(t)| \equiv H \xrightarrow{P} 0,$$

as $n \to \infty$, we have
$$\langle \tilde{M}_{j\epsilon}\rangle(t) \leq n^{-1} \sum_{i=1}^{n} \int_0^t \tilde{V}_{ji}^2(s)\lambda_i(s)\, ds I(H > \epsilon) \xrightarrow{P} 0$$

as $n \to \infty$, which completes the proof. □

The cumulative regression coefficients, $B(t)$, are, as we have just seen, easy to estimate nonparametrically and with the uniform asymptotic description given in Theorem 5.1.1 they furthermore provide an excellent basis for doing inference. In Section 5.2 we give a detailed description of how this theorem may be used for testing hypothesis such as $H_0 : \beta_j(t) \equiv 0$, that one of the components is non-significant, or $H_0 : \beta_j(t) \equiv \gamma$, that one of the components is constant with time.

The variance of the estimator (5.6) is easily estimated. Since, under Condition 5.1,

$$n^{1/2}(\hat{B}(t) - B(t)) = n^{1/2} \int_0^t X^-(s) dM(s) + o_p(1), \quad (5.11)$$

and a uniformly consistent estimator of the variance function is therefore given by optional variation process of the martingale in the latter display:

$$\hat{\Phi}(t) = n \int_0^t X^-(s) \text{diag}(dN(s))(X^-(s))^T, \quad (5.12)$$

or by the empirical version of the asymptotic variance (5.8),

$$\tilde{\Phi}(t) = n \int_0^t R_2^{-1}(s) X^T(s) W(s) \text{diag}(X_i^T(s) d\hat{B}(s)) W(s) X(s) R_2^{-1}(s). \quad (5.13)$$

That the latter estimator of the variance is uniformly consistent follows using Lenglart's inequality (2.25). The optional variation process (5.12) estimator is slightly simpler to implement than (5.13) and is the one implemented in the aalen-function. In Section 5.6 we give yet another variance estimator, which is also simple to compute and in addition possesses some robustness properties.

A pointwise $(1-\alpha)$ confidence interval for $B(t)$ can be constructed as

$$\hat{B}_j(t) \pm n^{-1/2} c_{\alpha/2} \cdot \hat{\Phi}_{jj}^{1/2}(t),$$

Edema

[Figure: Cumulative coefficients vs Time (years), showing estimated cumulative regression function with 95% pointwise confidence intervals]

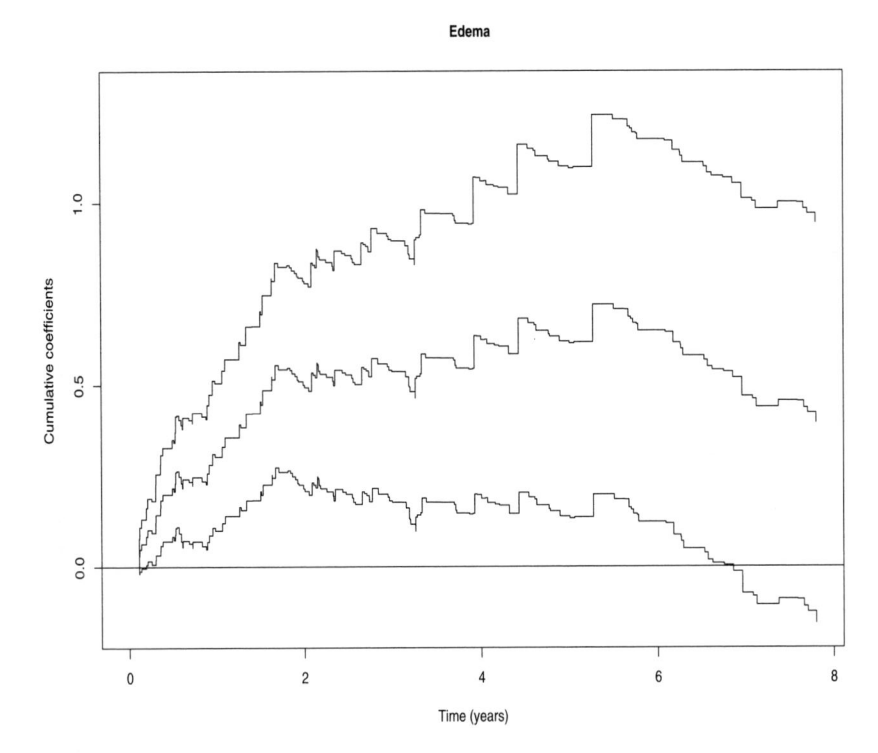

FIGURE 5.2: PBC-data. Estimated cumulative regression function along with 95% pointwise confidence intervals based on the optional variation standard errors.

where $\hat{\Phi}_{jj}(t)$ is the jth diagonal element of $\hat{\Phi}(t)$ and $c_{\alpha/2}$ is the $(1 - \alpha/2)$-quantile of the standard normal distribution. In the next section we show how to construct confidence bands, and how to perform inference about the regression coefficients.

Example 5.1.1 (PBC-data)

Reconsider the PBC data from Example 5.0.1. The estimated cumulative effect of edema is depicted in Figure 5.2. The optional variation standard errors are used to give the shown 95%-pointwise confidence intervals.

```
> plot(fit,xlab="Time (years)",specific.comps=3)
```

These intervals are useful for doing inference at fixed (and preplanned) time-points. They are not well suited for inferential purposes about the shape of the entire curve, however. A simple test for significance of edema could for example be based on the cumulative estimate at time 8, and then

114   5. Additive Hazards Models

the effect edema is deemed non-significant. If we, on the other hand, test the effect at time 2, then we conclude that it has a significant effect. This is obviously due to the changing behavior of the effect of edema with an initial excess risk that vanishes around time 2 to just before time 6 and then in the final part of the interval suggests a negative excess risk corresponding to a protective effect. We shall address these questions in more detail later. □

We motivated the estimator $\hat{B}(t)$ by the least squares arguments, which goes back to the original paper Aalen (1980), but it turns out that the estimator can also be thought of as an approximate maximum likelihood estimator. The (partial) log-likelihood function can be written as

$$\sum_{i=1}^{n} \left\{ \int \log(\lambda_i(t)) dN_i(t) - \int \lambda_i(t) dt \right\}$$
$$= \sum_{i=1}^{n} \left\{ \int \log(Y_i(t) X_i^T(t) \beta(t)) dN_i(t) - \int Y_i(t) X_i^T(t) \beta(t) dt \right\}.$$

Taking derivative with respect to $\beta(t)$ (heuristically) leads to the score equation

$$X^T(t) \text{diag}(Y_i(t)/\lambda_i(t))(dN(t) - X(t) dB(t)) = 0.$$

Solving with respect to $dB(t)$ while assuming that $\lambda_i(t)$ is known leads to

$$d\tilde{B}(t) = (X^T(t) W(t) X(t))^{-1} X^T(t) W(t) dN(t),$$

with $W(t) = \text{diag}(Y_i(t)/\lambda_i(t))$. This equation can be written on integral form as

$$\tilde{B}(t) = \int_0^t (X^T(s) W(s) X(s))^{-1} X^T(s) W(s) dN(s). \qquad (5.14)$$

A formal derivation of the score for the infinite dimensional parameter $\beta(t)$ was carried out by Greenwood & Wefelmeyer (1991) and Sasieni (1992b), see also the description at the end of Chapter 3.

The estimator (5.14) is not a real estimator since it depends on the unknown parameter $\beta(t)$. One solution is to plug in estimates based on the unweighted estimator:

(i) First, obtain initial estimates, $\hat{\beta}(t)$, of $\beta(t)$ by smoothing (5.6) with $W(t) = I$, see (5.15) below.

(ii) Secondly, use the weighted least squares estimator with weights $\hat{W}(t) = \text{diag}(Y_i(t)/\hat{\lambda}_i(t))$, where $\hat{\lambda}_i(t) = Y_i(t) X_i^T(t) \hat{\beta}(t)$.

Huffer & McKeague (1991) and McKeague (1988) showed that with a uniformly consistent estimator of $\beta(t)$ the asymptotic properties stated in Theorem 5.1.1 are still valid, and that the properties of the estimator are equivalent to those for known weights. This is true even for non-predictable estimates of the subject specific intensities, but then many technical problems are encountered, and it is therefore often assumed that a predictable smoothing based estimator of $\beta(t)$ is used.

To estimate the optimal weights $\lambda_i(t)$ smoothing techniques must be applied. A simple estimator of $\beta(t)$ is

$$\hat{\beta}(t) = \int_0^\tau \frac{1}{b} K(\frac{t-u}{b}) d\hat{B}(u) \qquad (5.15)$$

where $b \in]0, \infty[$ and K is a bounded kernel function with compact support $[-1, 1]$ satisfying that $\int K(u)du = 1$ and $\int uK(u)du = 0$, see Exercise 4.1 for more details on kernel smoothing. An often applied kernel function is the Epanechikov kernel

$$K(x) = \frac{3}{4}(1 - x^2)I(-1 \le x \le 1).$$

Standard considerations can be applied to decide on the degree of smoothing, see e.g. Simonoff (1996) and references therein. The simple kernel estimator (5.15) can be improved by an estimator that avoids edge problems, such as for example the local linear estimator, see Fan & Gijbels (1996).

Greenwood & Wefelmeyer (1991) and Sasieni (1992b) showed that the estimator with weight matrix $W(t) = \text{diag}(Y_i(t)/X_i^T(t)\beta(t))$ is efficient, and since the estimator with consistently estimated weights has the same asymptotic properties this estimator is efficient as well. It is important to realize, however, that the result about efficiency is an asymptotic result. It is our experience that in practice the unweighted estimator, $W(t) = I$, does as well as the maximum likelihood estimator. This is also supported by simulations in (Huffer & McKeague, 1991) showing that the efficiently weighted estimator does not improve on the unweighted least squares estimator unless one has a very large dataset. Obviously, one appealing property of the unweighted estimator is that one does not need to bother about choosing some smoothing parameter. The smoothing needed in the maximum likelihood estimator can in fact be quite a nuisance to carry out in practice. One problem often encountered is that some of the estimated intensities, $\hat{\lambda}_i(t)$, may become negative or very close to zero. The former is unacceptable and the latter may result in an unreliable estimator of $B(t)$. Such problems are hard to tackle in a satisfying way and are often dealt with in an ad hoc manner.

5.2 Inference for additive hazards models

In this section we present some approaches for conducting inference in the additive hazards model. The material here may be viewed as a special case of the later Section 5.4 on inference for the semiparametric additive hazards model, but since all formulas are considerably simpler for the additive hazards model this section will provide a good introduction to some of the main ideas without the notation getting to heavy.

Various hypotheses about the regression coefficients may be of interest and it is often possible to construct a sensible test-statistic based on the estimated cumulative regression coefficients to investigate a given hypothesis. Although one at first sight might find it unappealing to work with the cumulative regression coefficients rather than the regression coefficients directly, the cumulative coefficients are much better suited for inferential purposes. The uniform asymptotic description of order $n^{1/2}$ leads to a simpler theory than is possible for procedures based directly on $\hat{\beta}(t)$. One problem with inferential procedures based on $\hat{\beta}(t)$ is that the asymptotic distribution of $\hat{\beta}(t)$ will have a bias part and variance part. Although a uniform confidence band can be constructed for $\hat{\beta}(t)$, along the lines of for example Fan & Zhang (2000b), one drawback is that $\hat{\beta}(t)$ converges at a slower rate than $\hat{B}(t)$.

In the following we consider the two hypotheses

$$H_{01} : \beta_p(t) \equiv 0,$$
$$H_{02} : \beta_p(t) \equiv \gamma,$$

where we, without loss of generality, formulate the hypothesis for the pth regression coefficient function. Both these hypotheses are about the functional behavior of the regression coefficient function and the stated equalities are for the entire considered time range $[0, \tau]$. Obviously, these hypotheses may also be of relevance for multiple regression coefficients simultaneously and even though we only cover the one-dimensional case, all the procedures can be generalized to a multivariate setting.

The hypotheses above can be translated directly into hypotheses about the cumulative regression coefficients:

$$H_{01} : B_p(t) \equiv 0$$
$$H_{02} : B_p(t) \equiv \gamma t.$$

The hypothesis H_{01} differs from H_{02} since the null hypothesis H_{02} involve semiparametric models. The null of H_{02} is exactly the semiparametric risk model, which we describe in detail in Section 5.3. When evaluating H_{02} in this section, however, we will do so without fitting the model under the null, that is by considering only the properties of the process $\hat{B}_p(t)$.

We start by considering the hypothesis H_{01}, which, as already indicated, can be evaluated by the Hall-Wellner confidence band given in (5.16) below.

5.2 Inference for additive hazards models

Alternatively, one may consider a maximal deviation test statistic such as

$$\tilde{T}_{1S} = \sup_{t \in [0,\tau]} |\hat{B}_p(t)|$$

or modified versions of it that take the variability of $\hat{B}_p(t)$ into account; we illustrate this in Example 5.2.1. If $B_p(t)$ is expected to be monotone, then one may simply use $\hat{B}_p(\tau)$ to test the null hypothesis, but this test statistic will obviously have low power if $B_p(\tau) = 0$ but so that H_{01} is not true. On the other hand the test statistic, $\tilde{T}_{1S}$, will have low power if $\beta_p(t)$ differs only substantially from 0 towards the end of the time period $[0, \tau]$, and then a test statistic like

$$\sup_{s,t \in [0,\tau]} |\hat{B}_p(s) - \hat{B}_p(t)|$$

should be better at detecting departures of $\beta_p(t)$ from the null hypothesis.

The latter test statistic and $\tilde{T}_{1S}$ are easy to compute but approximate quantiles are more difficult to obtain. Under the additive Aalen model and Condition 5.1 we established that $U^{(n)} = n^{1/2}(\hat{B} - B)$ converges in distribution towards a Gaussian martingale U with variance function $\Phi(t)$. Since the mappings that map $(U^{(n)}(t) : t \in [0,\tau])$ into the suggested test statistics are continuous (see Exercise 5.7), it follows that the test statistic $n^{1/2}\tilde{T}_{1S}$, e.g., has a limiting distribution that is equivalent to $\sup_{t \in [0,\tau]} |U_p(t)|$, where U_p denotes the pth component of U, and we can therefore obtain approximate asymptotic quantiles by using the asymptotic distribution U with an estimate of the variance function $\hat{\Phi}(t)$. This distribution must then be simulated based on $\hat{\Phi}(t)$. Alternatively, one can transform the process to obtain a known limit distribution. The Hall-Wellner band is based on the fact that for the Gaussian martingale, $U_p(t)$, with covariance function $\Phi_{pp}(t)$,

$$U_p(t) \frac{\Phi_{pp}(\tau)^{1/2}}{\Phi_{pp}(\tau) + \Phi_{pp}(t)}$$

has the same distribution as

$$B^0 \left(\frac{\Phi_{pp}(t)}{\Phi_{pp}(\tau) + \Phi_{pp}(t)} \right)$$

where B^0 is the Brownian bridge. This leads to the Hall-Wellner band

$$\hat{B}_p(t) \pm n^{-1/2} d_\alpha \cdot \hat{\Phi}_{pp}(\tau)^{1/2} \left(1 + \frac{\hat{\Phi}_{pp}(t)}{\hat{\Phi}_{pp}(\tau)} \right), \quad t \in [0,\tau], \quad (5.16)$$

where $\hat{\Phi}_{pp}$ is the pth diagonal element of $\hat{\Phi}$ and d_α is the the upper α-quantile of $\sup_{t \in [0,1/2]} |B^0(t)|$.

The confidence band may be used for testing hypotheses such as H$_{01}$ by observing whether or not the zero function is contained within the band. Note, however, that the hypothesis that the regression coefficient is time invariant, H$_{02}$, cannot be evaluated by looking at the band, because the uncertainty of not knowing γ is not reflected.

Before we move on to discuss how to test the hypothesis H$_{02}$, we first present a general resampling approach, which can be used to evaluate the variability of various test statistics. Considering the martingale term in (5.11) and using the i.i.d. structure we may write it as

$$n^{-1/2} \sum_{i=1}^{n} \epsilon_i(t), \qquad (5.17)$$

where

$$\epsilon_i(t) = \int_0^t (n^{-1} X(s)^T X(s))^{-1} X_i(s) dM_i(s), \qquad (5.18)$$

and

$$M_i(t) = N_i(t) - \int_0^t Y_i(s) X_i(s)^T dB(s).$$

For simplicity we have used the un-weighted version of the estimator. When n is large, (5.17) is essentially equivalent to a sum of the independent and identically distributed martingales

$$\tilde{\epsilon}_i(t) = \int_0^t \left[E(Y_i(s) X_i^{\otimes 2}(s)) \right]^{-1} X_i(s) dM_i(s). \qquad (5.19)$$

The variance of $n^{1/2}(\hat{B}(t) - B(t))$ may therefore be estimated consistently by

$$\hat{\Psi}(t) = n^{-1} \sum_{i=1}^{n} \hat{\epsilon}_i^{\otimes 2}(t),$$

where

$$\hat{\epsilon}_i(t) = \int_0^t (n^{-1} X^T(s) X(s))^{-1} X_i(s) d\hat{M}_i(s), \qquad (5.20)$$

with

$$\hat{M}_i(t) = N_i(t) - \int_0^t Y_i(s) X_i(s)^T d\hat{B}(s).$$

The above representation of $n^{1/2}(\hat{B}(t) - B(t))$ as a sum of i.i.d. terms may also be used to simulate its limit distribution.

Theorem 5.2.1 *Let $G_1, ..., G_n$ be independent and standard normally distributed. Under Condition 5.1 and with the additional assumption that*

5.2 Inference for additive hazards models

$Y_i(t)X_i(t)$ are uniformly bounded with bounded variation, it follows that $n^{1/2}(\hat{B}(t) - B(t))$ has the same limit distribution as

$$\Delta_1(t) = n^{-1/2} \sum_{i=1}^{n} \hat{\epsilon}_i(t) G_i$$

conditional on the data $(N_i(\cdot), Y_i(\cdot), X_i(\cdot))\ i = 1, \ldots, n$. Further, $\hat{\Psi}(t)$ is a consistent estimator of the asymptotic variance of $n^{1/2}(\hat{B}(t) - B(t))$.

PROOF. We start by showing that the i.i.d. representation leads to the same asymptotic distribution. The process $n^{1/2}(\hat{B}(t) - B(t))$ is asymptotically equivalent to

$$n^{-1/2} \sum_{i=1}^{n} \epsilon_i(t)$$

where only an $o_p(1)$ term due to lack of invertibility has been removed, see Theorem 5.1.1, and where ϵ_i was defined in (5.18). We now show that the i.i.d. representation has the same asymptotic distribution by showing that

$$n^{-1/2} \sum_{i=1}^{n} (\tilde{\epsilon}_i(t) - \epsilon_i(t)) = o_p(1)$$

where $\tilde{\epsilon}_i$ is defined in (5.19) and $o_p(1)$ is uniformly in $t \in [0, \tau]$. This difference is equivalent to

$$n^{-1/2} \sum_{i=1}^{n} \int_0^t \delta(s) X_i(s) dM_i(s) = \int_0^t \delta(s) d\tilde{M}(s)$$

with

$$\delta(t) = [E(Y_i(t) X_i^{\otimes 2}(t))]^{-1} - n(X^T X)^{-1}(t)$$

and with

$$\tilde{M}(t) = n^{-1/2} \sum_{i=1}^{n} \int_0^t X_i(s) dM_i(s).$$

It is a consequence of the central limit theorem for random processes that $\tilde{M}$ converges in distribution towards a zero mean continuous Gaussian process, or by the martingale central limit theorem due to its uniformly bounded second moments. That the random process converges in the non-martingale case can be shown by using the central limit theorem for all finite dimensional distributions and establishing tightness. It follows by the assumptions that δ is bounded in variation and that it converges uniformly to zero in probability, therefore applying the Lemma by Spiekerman & Lin (1998) given in Chapter 2 it follows that $\int_0^t \delta d\tilde{M}$ converges uniformly to zero. For more on this detail see also Lin et al. (2000). Note, that the key-assumptions are the convergence to zero in probability of the bounded variation process δ and the convergence in distribution of $\tilde{M}$. A consequence is that the asymptotic variance of $n^{1/2}(\hat{B} - B)$ is given by $E(\tilde{\epsilon}_i^{\otimes 2})$. Note also that the asymptotic covariance function of $n^{1/2}(\hat{B} - B)$ is $E(\tilde{\epsilon}_i(s)\tilde{\epsilon}_i^T(t))$.

We now consider $\Delta_1(t)$ conditional on the data and proceed as Lin et al. (2000) where additional details can be found. First, its conditional mean is 0 and its variance equals $\hat{\Psi}(t)$. It therfore suffices to show that $\hat{\Psi}(s,t)$ converges to $\Psi(s,t)$ almost surely (that the finite dimensional distributions converge), and that $\Delta_1(t)$ is tight.

We know that

$$\tilde{\Psi}(s,t) = n^{-1} \sum_{i=1}^{n} \tilde{\epsilon}_i(s)\tilde{\epsilon}_i^T(t),$$

converges to $\Psi(s,t)$ uniformly when the second moments are uniformly bounded because of the central limit theorem. We consider the one dimensional case for notational simplicity and show that $\hat{\Psi}(t)$ converges to $\Psi(t)$

$$n^{-1} \sum_{i=1}^{n} \{(\hat{\epsilon}_i - \epsilon_i) + (\epsilon_i - \tilde{\epsilon})\}^2 (t) \qquad (5.21)$$

converges uniformly to zero. Then it follows that

$$\tilde{\Psi}(t) - \hat{\Psi}(t)$$

converges uniformly to zero since

$$\hat{\Psi}(t) = \tilde{\Psi}(t) + n^{-1} \sum_{i=1}^{n} \{(\hat{\epsilon}_i - \tilde{\epsilon}_i)\}^2 (t) + 2n^{-1} \sum_{i=1}^{n} \tilde{\epsilon}_i(t) \{(\hat{\epsilon}_i - \tilde{\epsilon}_i)\} (t)$$

by use of Cauchy-Schwarz on the last term and (5.21). This follows by showing that

$$n^{-1} \sum_{i=1}^{n} (\hat{\epsilon}_i - \epsilon_i)^2 (t)$$

and

$$n^{-1} \sum_{i=1}^{n} (\epsilon_i - \tilde{\epsilon}_i)^2 (t)$$

both converges uniformly to zero almost surely for almost all sequences of the data.

An alternative proof using modern empirical process theory is to use the conditional multiplier central limit theorem (see van der Vaart & Wellner (1996), Theorem 2.9.6) to see that

$$n^{-1/2} \sum_{i=1}^{n} \tilde{\epsilon}_i(t) G_i \qquad (5.22)$$

has the same asymptotic distribution as $n^{1/2}(\hat{B} - B)$ both conditional and unconditional on the data. Then the result follows after showing that Δ_1 (with the estimated residuals) has the same asymptotic distribution as (5.22) for almost all sequences of the data.

□

Edema

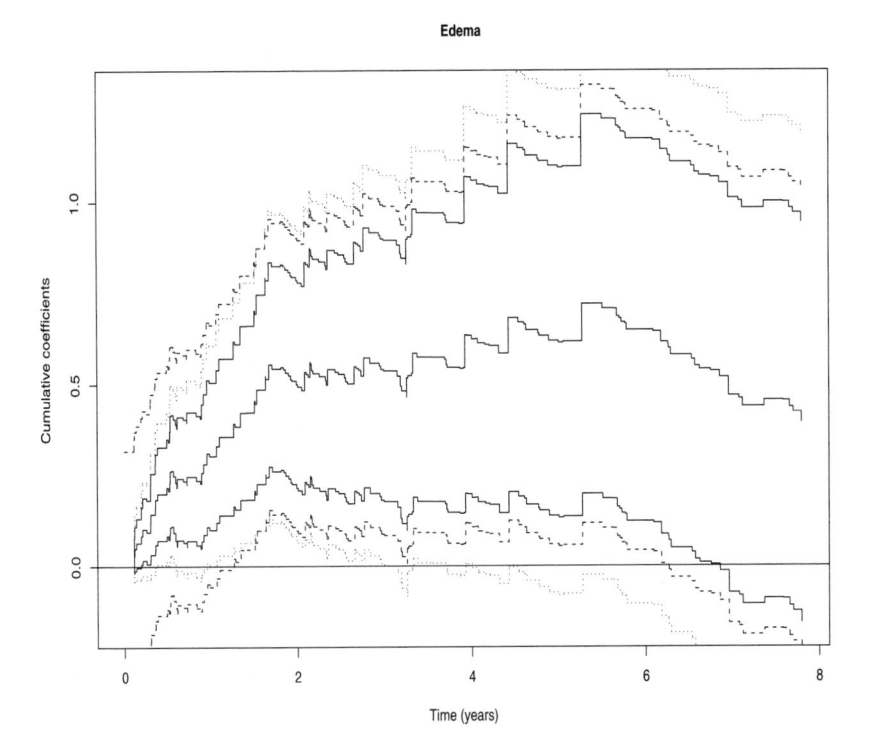

FIGURE 5.3: PBC-data. Estimated cumulative regression functions with 95% confidence intervals (solid lines). Hall-Wellner bands (broken lines) and simulation based bands (dotted lines).

This resampling approach for the additive Aalen model was suggested in Scheike (2002).

A uniform confidence band and a test for $H_{01} : B_p(t) \equiv 0$ may now be constructed based on replicates of $\Delta_1(t)$ by repeatedly generating normal variates $\{G_i^{(k)}\}_{i=1,\ldots,n}$ while holding the observed data fixed. Using the test statistic $\tilde{T}_{1S}$, one can approximate its distribution by sampling of $\Delta_1(t)$, $t \in [0, \tau]$, using the empirical distribution of

$$\sup_{t \in [0,\tau]} |\Delta_{1k,p}(t)|$$

where $\Delta_{1k,p}(t)$ denotes the kth resample of the pth component. Alternatively, a variance weighted test statistic is

$$T_{1S} = F_{1S}(n^{1/2}(\hat{B}_p(t) - B_p(t)), \hat{\Psi}_{pp}(t))$$
$$= \sup_{t \in [0,\tau]} |\frac{n^{1/2} \hat{B}_p(t)}{\hat{\Psi}_{pp}^{1/2}(t)}|$$

122   5. Additive Hazards Models

where $\hat{\Psi}_{pp}(t)$ is the pth diagonal element of $\hat{\Psi}(t)$, and now $F_{1S}(\Delta_1(t), \hat{\Psi}_{pp}(t))$ will have the same asymptotic distribution as T_{1S}.

Example 5.2.1 (PBC-data. Example 5.0.1 continued)

The estimate of the cumulative regression coefficients related to edema is depicted in Figure 5.3 along with 95% confidence bands. The Hall-Wellner band is shown with broken lines and the band based on T_{1S} (obtained by the above resampling technique) is shown with dotted lines. The pointwise confidence intervals are given for comparison (solid lines). The two types of bands are obtained as follows:

```
> plot(fit,xlab="Time (years)",hw.ci=2,sim.ci=3,specific.comps=3)
```

Note that the shape of the two confidence bands differ considerably. The Hall-Wellner band being wide initially and narrower later in contrast to the simulation based band. Both bands show that the effect of edema is significant having the zero-function outside the bands. The p-value associated with the resampling based approach is the one reported in the output shown in Example 5.0.1. □

To test $H_{02} : \beta_p(t) \equiv \gamma$, we consider the following simple test statistics

$$T_{2S} = F_{2S}(n^{1/2}(\hat{B}_p - B_p)) = n^{1/2} \sup_{t \in [0,\tau]} |\hat{B}_p(t) - \hat{B}_p(\tau)\frac{t}{\tau}|,$$

and

$$T_{2I} = n \int_0^\tau (\hat{B}_p(t) - \hat{B}_p(\tau)\frac{t}{\tau})^2 dt,$$

the idea being that $\hat{B}_p(\tau)/\tau$ is an estimate of the underlying constant under the null hypothesis. The basic test process in this context is

$$n^{1/2}(\hat{B}_p(t) - \hat{B}_p(\tau)\frac{t}{\tau})$$

for $t \in [0, \tau]$, that under the null should have the same asymptotic distribution as the resampled processes

$$\Delta_1(t) - \Delta_1(\tau)\frac{t}{\tau}.$$

By fitting the model under the null hypothesis, as is done in Section 5.4, one could also use

$$n^{1/2} \sup_{t \in [0,\tau]} |\hat{B}_p(t) - \hat{\gamma}t|,$$

or
$$n \int_0^\tau (\hat{B}_p(t) - \hat{\gamma} t)^2 dt.$$

We here consider only the test statistics, T_{2S} and T_{2I}, which only involves $\hat{B}_p(t)$.

One potential drawback of the above test statistics is that they depend on the considered time-interval and a test for constant effect over $[0, \tau]$ may be accepted even though one finds that the null hypothesis is rejected on a smaller time-interval $[0, \tau_1]$ with $\tau_1 < \tau$.

The test statistic T_{2S}, for example, has an asymptotic distribution that can be derived directly as a consequence of the asymptotic distribution of $n^{1/2}(\hat{B} - B)$ in Theorem 5.1.1. The quantiles of this distribution are, however, difficult to obtain, and must be simulated based on one of the estimators of the variance function such as $\hat{\Phi}$, $\tilde{\Phi}$ or $\hat{\Psi}$. This may be circumvented using the Khamaladze transformation of the test statistic yielding an asymptotic distribution with quantiles that can be found in standard tables. Further details are given in the below note.

The resampling approach motivated by Theorem 5.2.1 is conceptually simpler to carry out as the asymptotic distribution of $F_{2S}(n^{1/2}(\hat{B}_p - B_p))$ according to the theorem can be approximated by $F_{2S}(\Delta_1)$.

Note. Khmaladzes transformation.
Suppose we are interested in testing the hypothesis $H_{02} : \beta_p(t) = \gamma$. Assume that the hypothesis is true and define
$$\hat{V}_p(t) = n^{1/2}(\hat{B}_p(t) - \hat{B}_p(\tau)\frac{t}{\tau})$$
$$= n^{1/2}\left(\hat{B}_p(t) - B_p(t)\right) - n^{1/2}\left(\hat{B}_p(\tau) - B_p(\tau)\right)\frac{t}{\tau}.$$

By Theorem 5.1.1 it follows that $\hat{V}_p(t)$ converges in distribution towards a Gaussian process $V_p(t)$ that may be decomposed as
$$V_p(t) = U_p(t) - U_p(\tau)\frac{t}{\tau},$$

where U_p is a Gaussian martingale as described in Theorem 5.1.1. The process V_p is not a martingale, however, but it may transformed to one using the so-called Khmaladzes transformation, see Appendix A for more details. The martingale property of V_p is destroyed by the second component on the right-hand side of the latter display. The idea of Khmaladzes transformation is to project the process into the orthogonal space spanned by that component hence removing it. In this situation it reads (Appendix A)

$$V_p^*(t) = V_p(t) - \int_0^t d\Phi_{pp}(s)\phi_p^{-1}(s)\left\{\int_s^\tau \phi_p^{-1}(u)d\Phi_{pp}(u)\phi_p^{-1}(u)\right\}^{-1}$$
$$\times \int_s^\tau \phi_p^{-1}(u)dV_p(u),$$

where $\Phi_p(t)$ is the variance of $U_p(t)$ and $\phi_p(t)$ is the pth component of $\phi(t)$ given in (5.9). An empirical version is

$$\hat{V}_p^*(t,\tau) = \hat{V}_p(t) - \int_0^t d\hat{\Phi}_{pp}(s)\hat{\phi}_p^{-1}(s)\left\{\int_s^\tau \hat{\phi}_p^{-1}(u)d\hat{\Phi}_{pp}(u)\hat{\phi}_p^{-1}(u)\right\}^{-1}$$
$$\times \int_s^\tau \hat{\phi}_p^{-1}(u)d\hat{V}_p(u), \qquad (5.23)$$

where $\hat{\Phi}(t)$ is the optional variation estimator, and $\hat{\phi}(t)$ is obtained by inserting empirical quantities in the expression of $\phi(t)$, see (5.9). To do this, one needs to estimate $\beta(t)$ for example by smoothing of $\hat{B}(t)$. The basic message is now that the limit distribution of $\hat{V}_p^*(t,\tau)$ is the same as $U_p(t)$. Some technical difficulties arise, however, when trying to show convergence on the whole of $[0,\tau]$. What may be shown easily is that $\hat{V}_p^*(t,\tau_2)$ converges weakly in $D([0,\tau_1])$, $\tau_1 < \tau_2 < \tau$, to the Gaussian martingale $U_p(t)$. Based on this result one may then construct various tests such as the Kolmogorov-Smirnov test and the Cramér-von Mises test.

The Kolmogorov-Smirnov test rejects at level α if

$$\sup_{t \leq \tau_1} \left|\hat{V}_p^*(t,\tau_2)/(n\hat{\Phi}_{pp})^{1/2}\right| \geq f_\alpha, \qquad (5.24)$$

where f_α is the $(1-\alpha)$-quantile in the distribution of $\sup_{0\leq x\leq 1}|B(x)|$ with B the standard Brownian motion and $\hat{\Phi}_{pp} = \hat{\Phi}_{pp}(\tau_1)$. Specific values of f_α are $f_{0.01} = 2.81$, $f_{0.05} = 2.24$ and $f_{0.1} = 1.96$ (Schumacher, 1984).

The Cramér-von Mises test rejects at level α if

$$\int_0^{\tau_1}\left(\frac{\hat{V}_p^*(t,\tau_2)/(n\hat{\Phi}_{pp})^{1/2}}{1+\hat{\Gamma}(t)}\right)^2 d\left(\frac{\hat{\Gamma}(t)}{1+\hat{\Gamma}(t)}\right) \geq e_\alpha \qquad (5.25)$$

where e_α is the $(1-\alpha)$-quantile in the distribution of $\int_0^{1/2} B^0(u)^2\,du$ with B^0 the standard Brownian bridge and $\hat{\Gamma}(t) = \hat{\Phi}_{pp}(t)/\hat{\Phi}_{pp}$. Specific values of e_α were given in Chapter 2.

Example 5.2.2 (PBC data. Example 5.0.1 continued)

Considering the estimates depicted in Figure 5.1 it is not clear based on the pointwise confidence intervals shown there which of the components that have time-varying effects. The uniform bands depicted in Figure 5.3 are also inappropriate to test for constant effects because the bands do not reflect the uncertainty of the estimate of the constant effect such as T_{2S} and T_{2I} that we consider in the following. The table of statistics and p-values for testing for time invariant effects obtained in Example 5.0.1 are

```
Test for time invariant effects
           sup| B(t) - (t/tau)B(tau)| p-value H_0: B(t)=b t
(Intercept)                   0.13000                 0.139
```

5.2 Inference for additive hazards models

Edema

logAlbumin

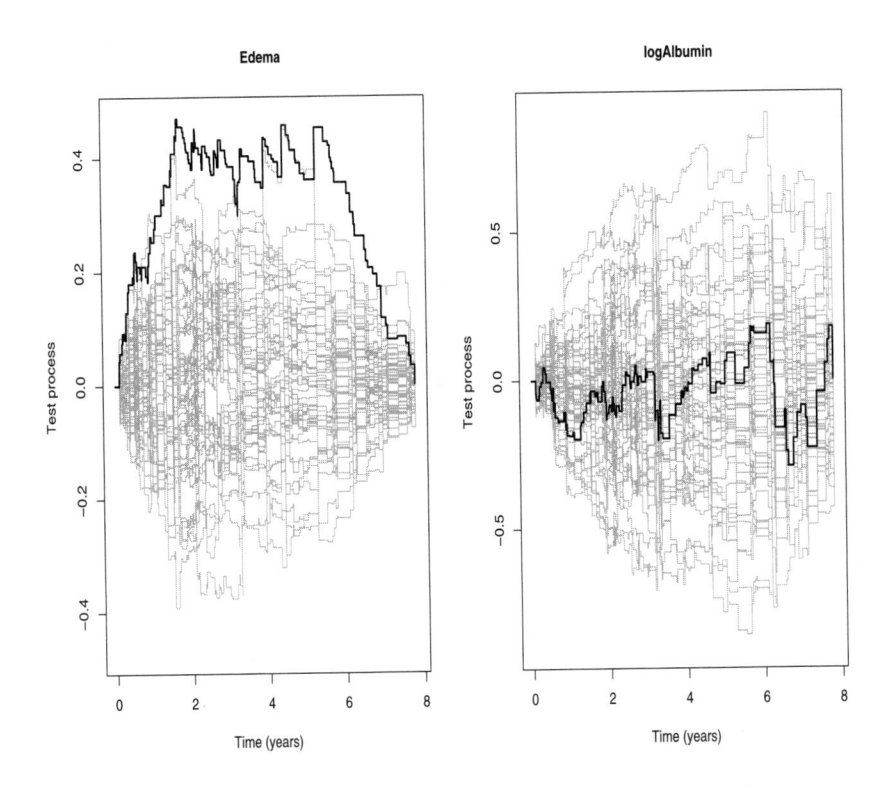

FIGURE 5.4: Test processes for testing constant effects with 50 simulated processes under the null. Processes shown for edema and log(albumin).

```
            Age          0.00297              0.829
            Edema        0.47000              0.005
            Bilirubin    0.03430              0.369
            logAlbumin   0.29200              0.883
            logProtime   0.96200              0.002

                int (B(t)-(t/tau)B(tau))^2dt p-value H_0: B(t)=b t
(Intercept)         5.72e-02                     0.037
Age                 1.86e-05                     0.665
Edema               8.73e-01                     0.000
Bilirubin           1.85e-03                     0.420
logAlbumin          7.92e-02                     0.963
logProtime          3.10e+00                     0.001

  Call:
  aalen(Surv(time/365, status) ~ Age + Edema + Bilirubin + logAlbumin +
      logProtime, pbc, max.time = 8)
```

Both T_{2S} and T_{2I} lead to very similar p-values, and it is seen that the intercept, edema and log(protime) do have effects that vary with time. We plot the processes used for computing the test-statistics T_{2S} and T_{2I} with 50 random realizations under the null of constant effects for edema and log(albumin) (Figure 5.4).

```
> plot(fit,xlab="Time (years)",ylab="Test process",score=T,
+ specific.comps=3)
> plot(fit,xlab="Time (years)",ylab="Test process",score=T,
+ specific.comps=5)
```

The two plots of the test-statistic processes indicate that edema has a time-varying effect, and that log(albumin) has a performance consistent with the null of time-invariant effect. As seen above the simulation based p-values were 0.005 for edema and 0.88 for log(albumin) thus clearly rejecting the hypothesis of constant effect of edema. □

5.3 Semiparametric additive hazards models

The additive Aalen model (5.3) is very flexible with all regression coefficients being time-varying. In many practical settings, however, it is of interest to investigate if the risk associated with some of the covariates is constant with time, that is, if some of the regression coefficients do not depend on time. This is of practical relevance in a number of settings when there is a desire to look more closely at the time-dynamics of covariates effects, such as for example treatment effects in medical studies. Also, when data is limited it is sometimes necessary, as well as sensible, to limit the degrees of freedom of the considered model to avoid too much variance, thus making a variance-bias trade-off to get more precise information.

McKeague & Sasieni (1994) considered the semiparametric additive intensity model

$$\lambda_i(t) = Y_i(t)\{X_i^T(t)\beta(t) + Z_i^T(t)\gamma\}, \qquad (5.26)$$

where $Y_i(t)$ is the at risk indicator, $X_i(t)$ and $Z_i(t)$ are predictable locally bounded covariate vectors of dimensions p and q, respectively, $\beta(t)$ is a p-dimensional locally integrable function and γ is a q-dimensional regression vector. Lin & Ying (1994) considered the special case of this model where $p = 1$ and

$$\lambda_i(t) = Y_i(t)\{\beta(t) + Z_i^T(t)\gamma\}, \qquad (5.27)$$

which parallels the proportional hazards model of Cox (1972), see Section 6.1. The added generality of the general semiparametric risk model (5.26) by McKeague & Sasieni (1994) is, however, at no extra cost in terms of added complexity in estimation. From a practical point of view it is preferable with a more elaborate model that can describe time-dynamics of covariate effects when needed, rather than forcing all covariate effects to have constant effects. Much of the literature on semiparametric additive hazards models, that we also term semiparametric additive hazards models, have focused on the simple version (5.27) of the model apparently being unaware of the important parallel development for the general version (5.26) of the model. McKeague & Sasieni (1994) derived explicit formulas for approximate maximum likelihood estimators of the cumulative $B(t) = \int_0^t \beta(s)\,ds$ and γ for model (5.26). The estimators may be motivated by least squares reasoning or as solutions to approximate score equations similarly to what was done for the general additive Aalen model in the previous section.

As for the additive Aalen model we organize the design vectors into matrices
$$X(t) = (Y_1(t)X_1(t), ..., Y_n(t)X_n(t))^T$$
and
$$Z(t) = (Y_1(t)Z_1(t), ..., Y_n(t)Z_n(t))^T.$$

The martingale decomposition of the counting process is
$$\begin{aligned} dN(t) &= \lambda(t)dt + dM(t) \\ &= X(t)dB(t) + Z(t)\gamma dt + dM(t), \end{aligned} \quad (5.28)$$

which suggests, since the martingale increments are uncorrelated with zero-mean, that $dB(t)$ and γ can be estimated from the least squares equations
$$X^T(t)W(t)(dN(t) - \lambda(t)dt) = 0, \quad (5.29)$$
$$\int Z^T(t)W(t)(dN(t) - \lambda(t)dt) = 0, \quad (5.30)$$

where $W(t)$ is a diagonal weight matrix. These equations can be solved successively as follows. Solving (5.29) for fixed γ gives
$$d\hat{B}(t) = X^-(t)\{dN(t) - Z(t)\gamma dt\}. \quad (5.31)$$

Plugging this solution into (5.30) and solving for γ as well as integrating we get
$$\hat{\gamma} = \left\{\int_0^\tau Z^T(t)H(t)Z(t)dt\right\}^{-1}\int_0^\tau Z^T(t)H(t)dN(t), \quad (5.32)$$

where
$$H(t) = W(t)(I - X(t)X^-(t)),$$

and with the convention that $H(t)$ is zero when the matrix inverse does not exist. The matrix $X^-(t)$ is the generalized inverse of $X(t)$ defined in (5.5).

128   5. Additive Hazards Models

Note that the matrix $H(t)$ projects onto the orthogonal space spanned by the columns of $X(t)$. By using (5.31) with $\hat{\gamma}$ inserted in place of γ we get the following estimator of $B(t)$:

$$\hat{B}(t) = \int_0^t X^-(s)(dN(s) - Z(s)\hat{\gamma}ds). \tag{5.33}$$

The asymptotic properties of the estimators $\hat{B}(t)$ and $\hat{\gamma}$ are given in the below theorem. Before giving the results we need some regularity conditions.

Condition 5.2   With $\tilde{X}_i = (X_i, Z_i)$ and $l = p + q$

(a) $\sup_{t \in [0,\tau]} E(W_i(t) Y_i(t) \tilde{X}_{ij}(t) \tilde{X}_{ik}(t) \tilde{X}_{im}(t)) < \infty$ for all $j, k, m = 1, .., l$;

(b) $r_2(t) = E(Y_i(t) W_i(t) (\tilde{X}_i)^{\otimes 2}(t))$ is non-singular for all $t \in [0, \tau]$.

$\square$

Theorem 5.3.1 *If Condition 5.2 holds, then, as $n \to \infty$,*

$$n^{1/2}(\hat{\gamma} - \gamma) \xrightarrow{D} V, \tag{5.34}$$

where V is a zero-mean normal with variance Σ, and

$$n^{1/2}(\hat{B} - B)(t) \xrightarrow{D} U(t) \quad \text{as } n \to \infty \tag{5.35}$$

in $D[0,\tau]^p$, where $U(t)$ is a zero-mean Gaussian process with variance $\Phi(t)$.

PROOF.   The key to the proof is the following decomposition:

$$n^{1/2}(\hat{\gamma} - \gamma) = \left\{ n^{-1} \int_0^\tau Z^T H Z dt \right\}^{-1} n^{-1/2} \int_0^\tau Z^T H dM + o_p(1) \tag{5.36}$$

where the $o_p(1)$ term is due to the possible non-invertibility of the involved matrices. This term is handled in the same way as in Theorem 5.1.1. To show that $n^{1/2}(\hat{\gamma} - \gamma)$ is asymptotically normal with the suggested covariance matrix, it therefore suffices to use the martingale central limit theorem and to show that the matrix $n^{-1} \int_0^\tau Z^T H Z dt$ converges in probability, the latter being a simple consequence of the i.i.d. assumption and Condition 5.2.

Similarly, it follows that

$$n^{1/2}(\hat{B}(t) - B(t)) = n^{1/2} \int_0^t X^- dM - \int_0^t X^- Z ds \, n^{1/2}(\hat{\gamma} - \gamma) + o_p(1). \tag{5.37}$$

5.3 Semiparametric additive hazards models

The second term that arises from the asymptotic distribution of $n^{1/2}(\hat\gamma-\gamma)$ can be written as a martingale using the above (5.36). It is a simple consequence of the i.i.d. assumption and Condition 5.2 that $\int_0^t X^- Z ds$ converges uniformly in probability towards a deterministic matrix function, that we may denote by $p(t)$. We can use the martingale central limit theorem to deal with the martingale $(n^{1/2}\int_0^t X^- dM, n^{-1/2}\int_0^t Z^T H dM)$. It is now a simple application of the continuous mapping theorem to get the asymptotic distribution of $n^{1/2}(\hat B - B)$. If the weights $W_i(t) = Y_i(t)/\lambda_i(t)$, $i=1,\ldots,n$, are used, then

$$\langle n^{-1/2}\int_0^\cdot Z^T H dM, n^{1/2}\int_0^\cdot X^- dM\rangle(t) = 0$$

so in that case the covariance between the two leading terms in the above (5.37) is equal to zero. □

Note that the asymptotic distribution of $n^{1/2}(\hat B - B)$ is not a Gaussian martingale due to the term $\hat\gamma$ in (5.33). This has consequences for the construction of confidence bands. The asymptotic variance of the estimators (5.32) and (5.33) are easily derived from martingale decompositions of the estimators. First note that

$$n^{1/2}(\hat\gamma - \gamma) = C_1^{-1} M_1(\tau) + o_p(1), \qquad (5.38)$$

where

$$C_1 = n^{-1}\int_0^\tau Z^T(t) H(t) Z(t) dt, \quad M_1(t) = n^{-1/2}\int_0^t Z^T(s) H(s) dM(s). \qquad (5.39)$$

Similarly, it follows that

$$\begin{aligned} n^{1/2}(\hat B(t) - B(t)) &= n^{1/2}\int_0^t X^-(s) dM(s) \\ &\quad - \int_0^t X^-(s) Z(s) ds\, n^{1/2}(\hat\gamma - \gamma) + o_p(1) \\ &= M_2(t) - P(t) C_1^{-1} M_1(\tau) + o_p(1), \end{aligned}$$

where

$$P(t) = \int_0^t X^-(s) Z(s) ds, \quad M_2(t) = n^{1/2}\int_0^t X^-(s) dM(s). \qquad (5.40)$$

The variances in Theorem 5.3.1 are estimated consistently, under the assumptions of the theorem for example by the optional variation processes. There exist theoretical expressions for the variances similarly to the expression for Aalen's additive model (5.8) but since the expressions are of little practical use we omit them. The optional variation estimators for Σ and Φ have the form

$$\hat{\Sigma} = C_1^{-1}[M_1](\tau)C_1^{-1}, \tag{5.41}$$

$$\hat{\Phi}(t) = [M_2](t) + P(t)C_1^{-1}[M_1](\tau)C_1^{-1}P^T(t)$$
$$- [M_2, M_1](t)C_1^{-1}P^T(t) - P(t)C_1^{-1}[M_1, M_2](t). \tag{5.42}$$

The optional variation processes and optional covariation processes are computed as

$$[M_1](t) = n^{-1}\int_0^t Z^T(s)H(s)\text{diag}(dN(s))H(s)Z(s),$$

$$[M_2](t) = n\int_0^t X^-(s)\text{diag}(dN(s))X^-(s),$$

$$[M_1, M_2](t) = \int_0^t Z^T(s)H(s)\text{diag}(dN(s))(X^-(s))^T.$$

The predictable variation estimator is obtained by replacing $\text{diag}(dN(t))$ by $\text{diag}(X_i^T(t)d\hat{B}(t) + Z_i^T(t)\hat{\gamma}dt)$ in the above expressions. This expression is more difficult to compute because it involves Lebesgue integration, and the optional variation estimator is therefore preferred in practice.

Example 5.3.1 (PBC-data.)

In Example 5.0.1 we considered the semiparametric additive hazards model with log(albumin), age and bilirubin having constant effects. The estimates and their standard errors were

```
Parametric terms :
                    Coef.      SE Robust SE     z    P-val
const(Age)       0.00201 0.000579   0.00060  3.47 5.16e-04
const(Bilirubin) 0.02070 0.003870   0.00328  5.34 9.24e-08
const(logAlbumin) -0.22800 0.069200  0.06170 -3.29 9.89e-04

  Call:
aalen(Surv(time/365, status) ~ const(Age) + Edema +
    const(Bilirubin) + const(logAlbumin) + logProtime, pbc,
    max.time = 8)
```

This gives a simple summary of these effects, while the model still allows the needed complexity for the remaining two effects that are shown in Figure 5.5 together with the estimated cumulative baseline. The shown 95% pointwise confidence intervals (full lines) are based on the optional variation formula just given, and the 95% confidence bands (broken lines) are based on a resampling technique described in Section 5.6. The plots are obtained by

5.3 Semiparametric additive hazards models

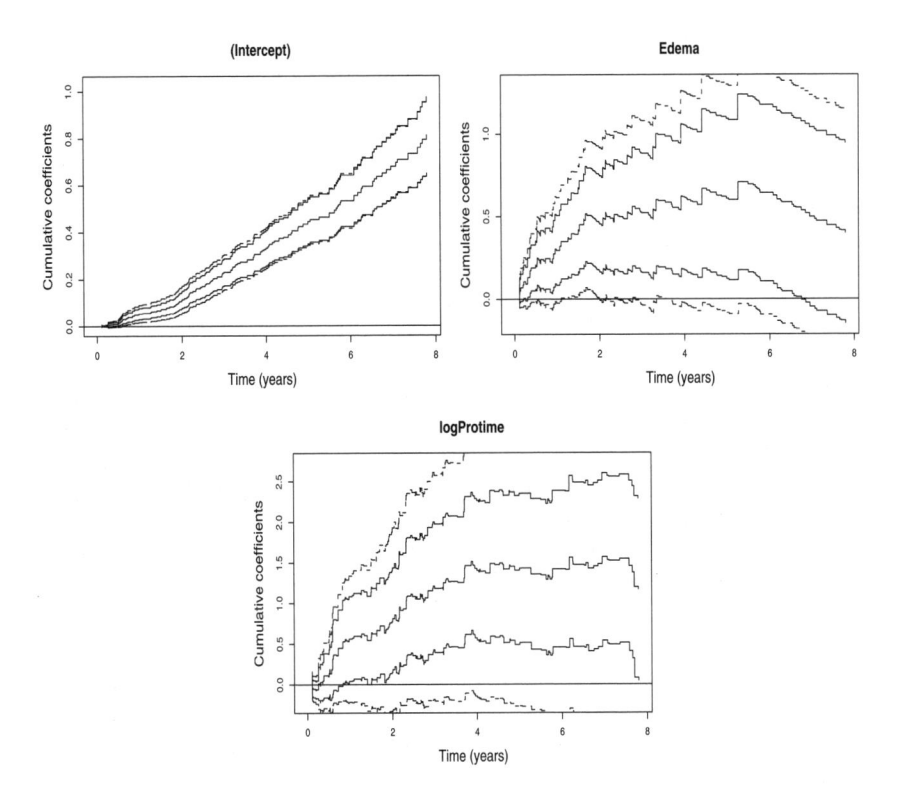

FIGURE 5.5: PBC-data. Estimated cumulative regression coefficients in the semiparametric additive hazards model with 95% pointwise confidence intervals (solid lines) and 95% confidence band (broken lines).

```
> plot(fit.semi,sim.ci=2,xlab="Time (years)")
```

Compare with the appropriate plots given in Figure 5.1 and note that both the estimates and the standard errors are almost equivalent. Given that the straight line approximations fit so well one might have expected a gain in efficiency for the nonparametric components, but these appear to be estimated just as well in the full model with all components being nonparametric for this particular dataset, see also Exercise 5.8. □

We motivated the estimator by least squares arguments similarly to what was done for the Aalen additive model in Section 5.1, but the original work by McKeague & Sasieni (1994) derived the estimator as an approximate maximum likelihood estimator. The log-likelihood function of the

132   5. Additive Hazards Models

i.i.d. counting processes can be written as

$$\sum_{i=1}^{n}(\int \log(X_i^T(t)\beta(t) + Z_i^T(t)\gamma)dN_i(t) - \int Y_i(t)(X_i^T(t)\beta(t) + Z_i^T(t)\gamma)dt).$$

Taking derivatives with respect to $\beta(t)$ and γ leads to the score equations

$$X(t)\operatorname{diag}(Y_i(t)/\lambda_i(t))(dN(t) - X(t)dB(t) - Z(t)\gamma dt) = 0,$$

$$\int Z(t)\operatorname{diag}(Y_i(t)/\lambda_i(t))(dN(t) - X(t)dB(t) - Z(t)\gamma dt) = 0.$$

These are on the same form as the least squares score equations (5.29) and (5.30) if the $\lambda_i(t)$'s in the above displays are assumed known. McKeague & Sasieni (1994) showed that with these weights and even with consistent estimates of the weights these estimators are asymptotically efficient. Efficient estimates can thus be constructed by a two-step procedure similarly to what was done for the simple additive hazards model. For practical use we recommend, however, using the unweighted estimators, that is, to take $W(t) = I$ in the expressions (5.32) and (5.33).

The estimator of γ was derived by integrating the score equation (5.30) before solving it. An alternative estimator $\tilde{\gamma}$ may be constructed by solving for the increments γdt and then cumulate these increments. This alternative estimator has certain robustness properties as shown in the following examples. The alternative estimator is

$$\tilde{\gamma} = \frac{1}{\tau}\int_0^\tau \{Z^T(t)H(t)Z(t)\}^{-1} Z^T(t)H(t)dN(t), \qquad (5.43)$$

and then an alternative estimator of $B(t)$ is given by

$$\tilde{B}(t) = \int_0^t X^-(s)(dN(s) - Z(s)\tilde{\gamma}ds). \qquad (5.44)$$

These estimators have the same asymptotic properties as $\hat{\gamma}$ and $\hat{B}(t)$ and are thus also efficient, see Exercise 5.12, when efficiently weighted. The matrix inverse in (5.43) may make $\tilde{\gamma}$ numerically more unstable than $\hat{\gamma}$, but there are also some advantages of the alternative estimators as illustrated in the following two examples.

Example 5.3.2 (The alternative semiparametric estimator)

One advantage of the alternative estimator is that it results in something sensible even if it is not specified correctly which of the effects that are time-varying. To realize this consider the additive hazards model on Aalen form, where

$$\lambda_i(t) = X_i^T(t)\alpha(t) + Z_i^T(t)\beta(t).$$

5.3 Semiparametric additive hazards models

Then one can estimate the cumulatives of α and β by the least-squares Aalen estimator (5.6). The estimator for the $B(t) = \int_0^t \beta(s)ds$ component of the model can be written as

$$\hat{B}(t) = \int_0^t \{Z^T(s)H(s)Z(s)\}^{-1} Z^T(s)H(s)dN(s)$$

with $H = (I - XX^-)$, see Exercise 5.12. Therefore $\tilde{\gamma}$, that is $\tau^{-1}\hat{B}(\tau)$, makes sense even if $\beta(t)$ is not constant over the considered time interval. □

A similar point to the one just made in the previous example can be formulated as a robustness property in the case of a misspecification of which of the effects that are time-varying.

Example 5.3.3 (Misspecified additive models)

In models with time-varying effects, such as the semiparametric additive hazards model, the primary interest may be on one covariate while it is still important to correct for another. We here consider two covariates and wish to investigate what consequences it has if the model is misspecified in terms of which of the covariates that has time-varying effect. Assume that the true hazard is on the form

$$\tilde{\lambda}(t) = Z(t)\beta_0(t) + X(t)\gamma_0.$$

We assume that the nonparametric effect $\beta_0(t)$ is non-constant. We shall now take a closer look at the consequences of working with the incorrectly specified model

$$\lambda(t) = X(t)\beta(t) + Z(t)\gamma.$$

We start by estimating the parameters of the misspecified model, by using the usual un-weighted estimates of γ and B, (5.32) and (5.33), respectively,

$$\hat{\gamma} = C_1^{-1} \int_0^\tau Z^T(t)H(t)dN(t),$$

$$\hat{B}(t) = \int_0^t X^-(s)(dN(s) - Z(s)\hat{\gamma}ds),$$

where $H(t) = (I - X(t)X^-(t))$. The martingale decomposition under the true model gives

$$\hat{\gamma} = n^{-1/2} C_1^{-1} M_1(\tau) + n^{-1} C_1^{-1} \int_0^\tau Z^T(t)H(t)Z(t)\beta_0(t)dt,$$

$$\hat{B}(t) = M_3(t,\tau) + \gamma_0 t$$
$$+ \int_0^t X^-(s)Z(s)\beta_0(s)ds - n^{-1}P(t)C_1^{-1}\int_0^\tau Z^T(s)H(s)Z(s)\beta_0(s)ds,$$

where
$$M_3(t,\tau) = \int_0^t X^-(s)dM(s) + n^{-1/2}P(t)C_1^{-1}M_1(\tau).$$

We see that $\hat{\gamma}$, apart from the martingale term, is a weighted average of $\beta_0(t)$, so, when $\beta_0(t)$ is non-constant with time, $\hat{\gamma}$ is not an unbiased (or even consistent) estimator of $\int_0^\tau \beta_0(t)dt$. The nonparametric estimate $\hat{B}(t)$ will not be a consistent estimator of $\gamma_0 t$ unless

$$\int_0^t X^-(s)Z(s)\beta_0(s)ds = n^{-1}P(t)C_1^{-1}\int_0^t Z^T(s)H(s)Z(s)\beta_0(s)ds,$$

and this will typically not be the case when $\beta_0(t)$ is non-constant. Note, however, that if $X^-(t)Z(t)$ are small for all $t \in [0,\tau]$, indicating that $X(t)$ and $Z(t)$ are almost uncorrelated for all t then the two integrals will both be close to zero. Also, if $\beta_0(t)$ does not vary to much then the two expressions will be close to each other.

If we instead use the alternative estimator (5.43) of γ, we get that

$$\tilde{\gamma} = \tau^{-1}\int_0^\tau \{Z^T(t)H(t)Z(t)\}^{-1}Z^T(t)H(t)dM(t) + \tau^{-1}\int_0^\tau \beta_0(t)dt$$

$$\tilde{B}(t) = \gamma_0 t + n^{-1/2}M_2(t)$$
$$- \tau^{-1}P(t)\int_0^\tau \{Z^T(t)H(t)Z(t)\}^{-1}Z^T(t)H(t)dM(t)$$
$$+ \int_0^t X^-(s)Z(s)\beta_0(s)ds - P(t)\tau^{-1}\int_0^t \beta_0(s)ds.$$

Therefore $\tilde{\gamma}$ is an unbiased (assuming that the involved inverses exist) estimator of $\tau^{-1}\int_0^\tau \beta_0(t)dt$ even though the applied model is misspecified. The nonparametric estimate $\tilde{B}(t)$ will still not be a consistent estimator of $\gamma_0 t$ unless

$$\int_0^t X^-(s)Z(s)\beta_0(s)ds = P(t)\tau^{-1}\int_0^t \beta_0(s)ds.$$

If $X^-(t)Z(t)$ is small for all $t \in [0,\tau]$, or if $\beta_0(t)$ does not vary too much, then the two expressions in the later display will be close to each other.

Consider the simple case with time-fixed covariates $X_i(t) = Y_i(t)X_i$ and $Z_i(t) = Y_i(t)Z_i$ with the at risk indicator $Y_i(t)$ absorbed into the design. Even if X_i and Z_i are independent, then $X_i(t)$ and $Z_i(t)$ will be correlated (if $\gamma \neq 0$ and $\beta \neq 0$) for those subjects at risk at a particular point in time. This is due to the correlation induced by the subjects being at risk.

We conclude that it is important to carefully investigate if each of the effects of the covariates are time-varying before reducing to the semiparametric model. A simple strategy is to start with the flexible model that allows all effects to be time-varying and then investigate if some of the effects are well described by constants and then successively simplifying the model as appropriate. □

5.4 Inference for the semiparametric hazards model

The semiparametric additive hazards model is easy to fit when it has been decided if covariate effects are time-varying or constant with time. In Section 5.2 we showed how to test if a covariate effect was significant and to test if a covariate had a time-invariant effect using the full Aalen additive model as starting point. The test for time-invariance was limited to considering just one covariate, and even though we could have constructed a multidimensional version of the test, it is often natural and preferable with successive test for time-varying effects that is testing one component at a time using the reduced model as the starting point for the next analysis and test. In this section we show how to perform such successive test for deciding if effects are time invariant or not. This question is of great practical importance in many settings as already illustrated in the introductory Example 5.0.1.

Within the semiparametric model

$$\lambda_i(t) = Y_i(t)\{X_i^T(t)\beta(t) + Z_i^T(t)\gamma\}$$

we shall focus on the two hypothesis

H_{01} : $\beta_p(t) \equiv 0$ or equivalently $B_p(t) \equiv 0$;

H_{02} : $\beta_p(t) \equiv \gamma_{q+1}$ or equivalently $B_p(t) \equiv \gamma_{q+1} t$;

where we, without loss of generality, consider only the last nonparametric component of the model. Note, however, that the effect of the Z-covariates is now constant in contrast to what was assumed in Section 5.2.

Considering H_{01} we may apply Theorem 5.3.1 directly to obtain a confidence band for $B_p(t)$. The asymptotic distribution of $n^{1/2}(\hat{B}_p(t) - B_p(t))$ is a Gaussian process, but is does not have independent increments, and therefore the standard Hall-Wellner band can not be applied directly. One could apply the Khmaladze transformation to obtain a well described limit distribution. We use, however, a resampling approach that is easier to implement in practice (Scheike, 2002).

The resampling approach is based on the following decomposition into i.i.d. residuals. First, note that

$$n^{1/2}(\hat{\gamma} - \gamma) = C_1^{-1} n^{-1/2} \sum_{i=1}^n \epsilon_{2i} + o_p(1),$$

where C_1 was given in (5.39) and

$$\epsilon_{2i} = \int_0^\tau \{Z_i(t) - (Z(t)^T X(t))(X(t)^T X(t))^{-1} X_i(t)\} dM_i(t),$$

136   5. Additive Hazards Models

using the un-weighted version of $\hat{\gamma}$. The basic martingales (residuals) are given by

$$M_i(t) = N_i(t) - \int_0^t Y_i(s)(X_i^T(s)dB(s) + Z_i^T(s)\gamma ds).$$

The sum of the residuals is asymptotically equivalent to a sum of i.i.d. terms

$$\tilde{\epsilon}_{2i} = \int_0^T \left\{ Z_i(t) - E(Y_i(t)Z_i(t)X_i^T(t))E(Y_i(t)X_i(t)X_i^T(t))^{-1}X_i(t) \right\} dM_i(t),$$

where we use that the limit of for example $n^{-1}Z^T(t)X(t)$ is given by $E(Y_i(t)Z_i(t)X_i^T(t))$.

This implies for example that the variance of $n^{1/2}(\hat{\gamma}-\gamma)$ can be estimated consistently by

$$C_1^{-1}(n^{-1}\sum_{i=1}^n \hat{\epsilon}_{2i}^{\otimes 2})C_1^{-1}, \qquad (5.45)$$

where $\hat{\epsilon}_{2i}$ is estimated using

$$\hat{M}_i(t) = N_i(t) - \int_0^t Y_i(s)(X_i^T(s)d\hat{B}(s) + Z_i^T(s)\hat{\gamma}ds)$$

in the expression for ϵ_{2i}. Further, and more interestingly, we can also make an i.i.d. decomposition of the nonparametric estimator. Note that

$$n^{1/2}(\hat{B}(t) - B(t)) = n^{-1/2}\sum_{i=1}^n \epsilon_{3i}(t) + o_p(1),$$

where

$$\epsilon_{3i}(t) = \epsilon_{4i}(t) - P(t)C_1^{-1}\epsilon_{2i},$$

$$\epsilon_{4i}(t) = \int_0^t \left(n^{-1}X^T(s)X(s) \right)^{-1} X_i(s)dM_i(s),$$

with C_1 and $P(t)$ defined in (5.39) and (5.40), respectively. The asymptotically equivalent i.i.d. decomposition is obtained by a modification similarly to what was applied to go from ϵ_{2i} to $\tilde{\epsilon}_{2i}$. This suggests that the variance of $n^{1/2}(\hat{B}(t) - B(t))$ can be estimated by the robust variance estimator

$$\hat{\Psi}(t) = n^{-1}\sum_{i=1}^n \hat{\epsilon}_{3i}^{\otimes 2}(t), \qquad (5.46)$$

again substituting $\hat{M}_i$ in the expressions for ϵ_{3i} and ϵ_{4i}. In Section 5.6 we discuss which robustness properties the estimator $\hat{\Psi}(t)$ possesses. The following theorem justifies the resampling approach utilized later in this section.

5.4 Inference for the semiparametric hazards model

Theorem 5.4.1 *Under the conditions of Theorem 5.3.1 and with $G_1, ..., G_n$ independent standard normals, it follows that*

$$\Delta_2 = C_1^{-1} n^{-1/2} \sum_{i=1}^{n} \hat{\epsilon}_{2i} G_i,$$

$$\Delta_3(\cdot) = n^{-1/2} \sum_{i=1}^{n} \hat{\epsilon}_{3i}(\cdot) G_i,$$

has the same asymptotic distribution as $n^{1/2}(\hat{\gamma} - \gamma, \hat{B} - B)$. Further, (5.45) and (5.46) are consistent estimators of the variance of $n^{1/2}(\hat{\gamma} - \gamma)$ and $n^{1/2}(\hat{B} - B)$, respectively.

PROOF. Follows along the lines of the equivalent theorem for the additive Aalen model, Theorem 5.2.1. □

Example 5.4.1 (PBC-data.)

Consider the semiparametric model, as in Example 5.0.1, where age, bilirubin and log(albumin) have constant effect. The remaining two covariates, edema and log(protime), have time-varying effect. In Figure 5.6 we depict 95% confidence intervals for the cumulative coefficients based on the robust standard errors (broken lines) and those based on the optional variation process (solid lines). For this dataset the two types of confidence intervals are almost equivalent.

```
> for (i in 1:3) {
+ plot(fit.semi,xlab="Time (years)",specific.comps=i,
+ robust=2,pointwise.ci=0)
+ plot(fit.semi,xlab="Time (years)",specific.comps=i,
  pointwise.ci=1,add.to.plot=T) }
```

□

The resampling theorem may be used to construct a confidence band for the pth component of B. We use the following simple functional

$$T_{1S} = F_{1S}(n^{1/2}(\hat{B}_p - B_p), \hat{\Psi}_{pp}) = \sup_{t \in [0,\tau]} |\frac{n^{1/2} \hat{B}_p(t)}{\hat{\Psi}_{pp}(t)}|,$$

where $\hat{\Psi}_{pp}(t)$ is the pth diagonal element of $\hat{\Psi}(t)$. To approximate the quantiles one may make simulations based on the limiting distribution of $n^{1/2}(\hat{B}_p(t) - B_p(t))$ or by using the above resampling theorem that implies that $F_{1S}(\Delta_3, \hat{\Psi}_{pp})$ has the same asymptotic distribution as T_{1S}.

138   5. Additive Hazards Models

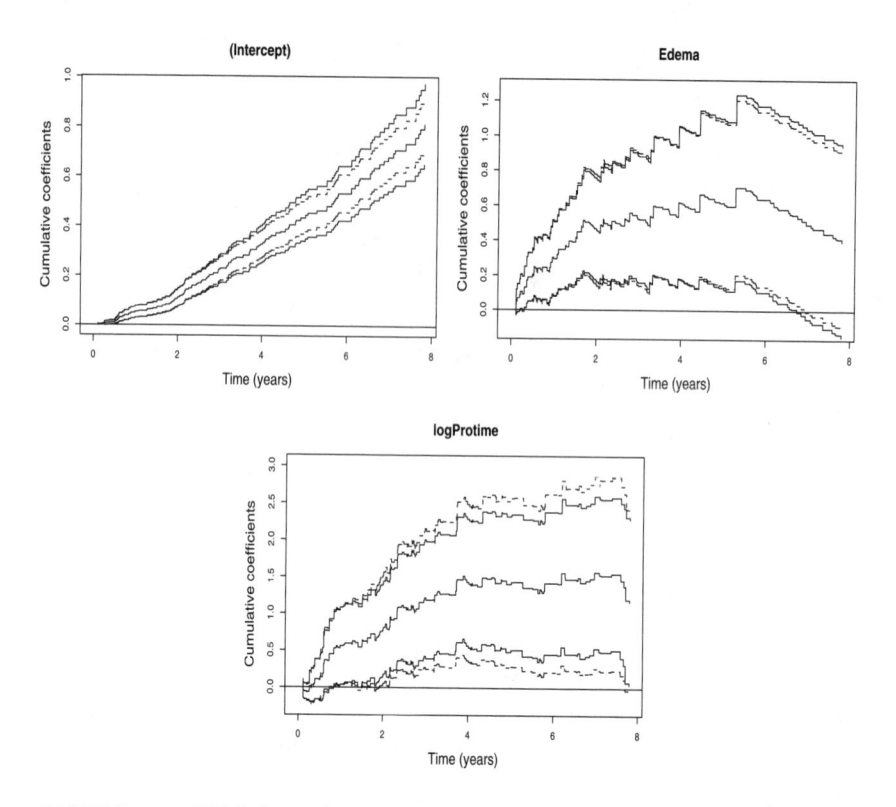

FIGURE 5.6: PBC-data. Estimated cumulative regression coefficients in semiparametric additive hazards model with 95% confidence intervals based on robust (broken lines) and optional variation (solid lines) variance estimates.

The key point of this section is to construct a formal procedure for testing the hypothesis

$$H_{02} : \beta_p(t) \equiv \gamma_{q+1}.$$

A simple test, based on $\hat{B}_p$ only, is to compute

$$T_{2S} = F_{2S}(n^{1/2}(\hat{B}_p - B_p)) = n^{1/2} \sup_{t \in [0,\tau]} |\hat{B}_p(t) - \hat{B}_p(\tau)\frac{t}{\tau}|.$$

The asymptotic properties of this test statistic may be simulated as a direct consequence of Theorem 5.4.1, by computing $F_{2S}(\Delta_3)$. An alternative to this test statistic is

$$T_{2I} = F_{2I}(n^{1/2}(\hat{B}_p - B_p)) = n \int_0^\tau (\hat{B}_p(t) - \hat{B}_p(\tau)\frac{t}{\tau})^2 dt,$$

5.4 Inference for the semiparametric hazards model

that under the null equals $F_{2I}(n^{1/2}(\hat{B}_p - B_p))$. The test-process associated with these two test statistics is

$$\hat{B}_p(t) - \hat{B}_p(\tau)\frac{t}{\tau},$$

which will carry much information about the type of deviation from the null hypothesis.

A more complicated test statistic is based on both $\hat{B}_p(\cdot)$ and $\hat{\gamma}_{q+1}$, where $\hat{B}_p(\cdot)$ is obtained in the full model and $\hat{\gamma}_{q+1}$ is computed under the null-hypothesis, see Martinussen & Scheike (1999) and Scheike (2002) for similar ideas in a regression set-up. To distinguish the design under the model with freely varying $\beta_p(t)$ and under the semiparametric null, we let the designs under the null be denoted $\tilde{X}(t)$ and $\tilde{Z}(t)$, and use a similar notation for other quantities defined under the null.

Two functionals to test the null are

$$n^{1/2} \sup_{t \in [0,\tau]} |\hat{B}_p(t) - \hat{\gamma}_{q+1}t|$$

and

$$n \int_0^\tau (\hat{B}_p(t) - \hat{\gamma}_{q+1}t)^2 dt.$$

One may also consider test statistics where the variance is taken into account. To approximate the quantiles of these test statistics make an i.i.d. representation and note that $n^{1/2}(\hat{B}_p(t) - \hat{\gamma}_{q+1}t)$ is asymptotically equivalent to a Gaussian process that can be approximated by

$$n^{-1/2} \sum_{i=1}^n \epsilon_{5i}(t),$$

where

$$\epsilon_{5i}(t) = \epsilon_{4i}(t) - t\tilde{P}(t)\tilde{C}_1^{-1}\tilde{\epsilon}_{2i},$$

and where the last term is computed under the null. Further, similarly to Theorem 5.3.1, it can be shown that the asymptotic distribution of $n^{1/2}(\hat{B}_p(t) - \hat{\gamma}_{q+1}t)$ (and $n^{-1/2}\sum_i \epsilon_{5i}(t)$) is the same as the asymptotic distribution of

$$\Delta_4(t) = n^{-1/2} \sum_{i=1}^n \hat{\epsilon}_{5i}(t) G_i,$$

where $G_1, ..., G_n$ are independent standard normals. Therefore the quantiles of the two test-statistics may be obtained from random samples of $\Delta_4(\cdot)$.

The suggested test statistics are easy to modify in the current framework. For example the test statistic

$$n^{1/2} \sup_{s,t \in [0,\tau]} |(\hat{B}_p(t) - \hat{B}_p(s)) - \hat{\gamma}_{q+1}(t-s)|$$

may be better to detect local departures from the null around s.

5. Additive Hazards Models

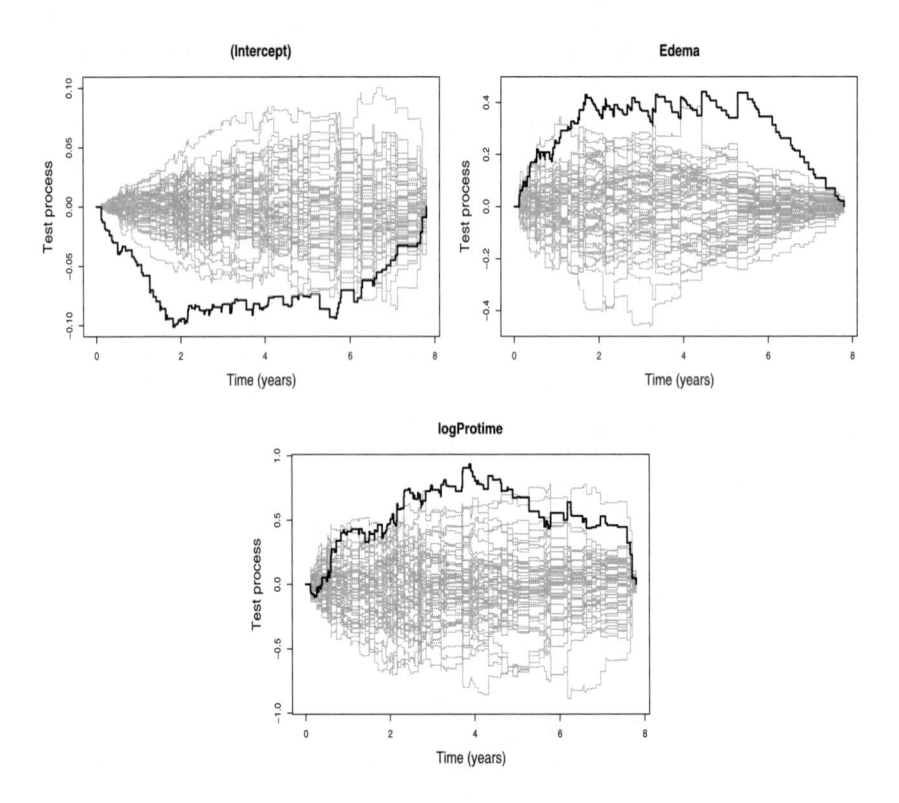

FIGURE 5.7: Test processes for time-varying effects with 50 random processes under the null.

Example 5.4.2 (PBC-data.)

This example illustrates the use of the test statistics T_{2S} and T_{2I}. Consider the semiparametric model, as in Example 5.0.1, where log(albumin), age and bilirubin have constant parametric effects. The computed test statistics are given in the below output with p-values being approximated based on 1000 replications.

```
> fit.semi<-aalen( Surv(time/365,status)~const(Age)+Edema+
+ const(Bilirubin)+const(logAlbumin)+logProtime,pbc,
+ max.time=8)
Semiparametric Additive Risk Model
Simulations start N= 1000
> summary(fit.semi)
Additive Aalen Model

Test for nonparametric terms

Test for non-significant effects
```

5.4 Inference for the semiparametric hazards model 141

```
                  sup| hat B(t)/SD(t) | p-value H_0: B(t)=0
(Intercept)                21.80                      0.000
Edema                       3.28                      0.011
logProtime                  2.80                      0.057
Test for time invariant effects
                  sup| B(t) - (t/tau)B(tau)|  p-value H_0: B(t)=b t
(Intercept)                     0.101                      0.001
Edema                           0.439                      0.000
logProtime                      0.937                      0.001

                  int (B(t)-(t/tau)B(tau))^2dt  p-value H_0: B(t)=b t
(Intercept)                    0.0419                       0.001
Edema                          0.7890                       0.000
logProtime                     2.5200                       0.002


Parametric terms :
                       Coef.        SE Robust SE      z     P-val
const(Age)         0.00201 0.000579    0.00060    3.47  5.16e-04
const(Bilirubin)   0.02070 0.003870    0.00328    5.34  9.24e-08
const(logAlbumin) -0.22800 0.069200    0.06170   -3.29  9.89e-04

> plot(fit.semi,score=T,xlab="Time (years)",ylab="Test Process")
```

The observed test-processes may be used to learn where the departure from the null is present. Figure 5.7 shows the underlying process along with 50 resampled processes. The behavior of the observed test-process for edema indicates, just as the estimate of the effect of edema, that the effect of edema is much higher initially. Note, that the figures are consistent with the computed supremum test-statistic.

Sometimes the observed test-process will deviate from the behavior under the null without it being reflected in the test-statistics considered here. The supremum test-statistic will tend to be large at places with large variation, and sometimes one should rather look for departures between the observed test-process and the null at places with small variation. One way of remedying this is to use a modified version of the test-statistics that takes the variance into account. These are computed using the option `weighted.test=1` as shown below.

```
> fit.semi.w<-aalen( Surv(time/365,status)~const(Age)+Edema+
+ const(Bilirubin)+const(logAlbumin)+logProtime,pbc,
+ max.time=8,weighted.test=2)
Semiparametric Additive Risk Model
Simulations start N= 1000
> summary(fit.semi.w)
Additive Aalen Model

Test for nonparametric terms
```

142   5. Additive Hazards Models

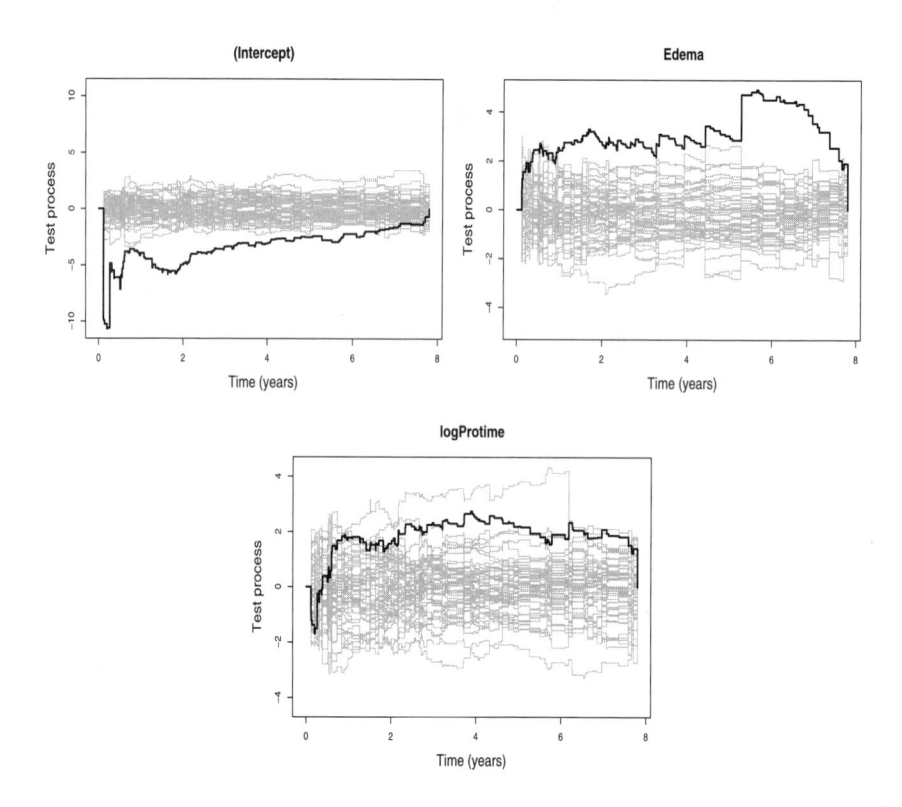

FIGURE 5.8: Weighted test-processes for time-varying effects with 50 random processes under the null.

```
Test for non-significant effects
            sup| hat B(t)/SD(t) |  p-value H_0: B(t)=0
(Intercept)              21.80                  0.000
Edema                     3.28                  0.015
logProtime                2.80                  0.044
Test for time invariant effects
            sup| B(t) - (t/tau)B(tau)|  p-value H_0: B(t)=b t
(Intercept)              13.30                  0.000
Edema                     5.21                  0.000
logProtime                3.42                  0.006

            int (B(t)-(t/tau)B(tau))^2dt p-value H_0: B(t)=b t
(Intercept)              396                    0.000
Edema                    115                    0.000
logProtime                57                    0.002

Parametric terms :
                Coef.      SE  Robust SE     z    P-val
const(Age)    0.00201 0.000579   0.00060  3.47 5.16e-04
```

```
const(Bilirubin)      0.02070 0.003870    0.00328  5.34 9.24e-08
const(logAlbumin)    -0.22800 0.069200    0.06170 -3.29 9.89e-04

> plot(fit.semi.w,score=T,xlab="Time (years)",ylab="Test process");
```

The weighted version of the observed test-processes are shown in Figure 5.8. They result have a behavior quite similar to the unweighted case for this dataset as is evident from comparing Figure 5.7 and Figure 5.8. The weighted test-statistics shows a somewhat erratic behavior at the start and end of the time-interval. This is due to the fact that the test-statistic that is almost zero is divided with a standard error that is also almost zero. This can be remedied by not considering the edge area's, in the above example `weighted.test=2` thus ignoring the first and last two jump times edge points. Note, however, that the weighted supremum test-statistic may lead to different conclusions, because the different summary statistics reflect different types of departures from the null. □

Example 5.4.3 (Time-varying U-shaped risk function)

In this example we consider another type of hypothesis:

$$H_{03}: \beta_p(t) \equiv \theta \beta_{p-1}(t);$$

supposing that the ratio between two of the regression functions is constant. This is of interest to investigate if one encounters a so-called U-shaped relationship between mortality and certain risk factors such as body mass index (BMI, weight in kilograms divided by square of height in meters) with low and high BMI being unfavorable. It then becomes an issue whether the nadir, which is the value of the covariate associated with the lowest risk, remains stable by advancing time during which the risk factor may change at the individual level.

The Aalen model is well suited to investigate such questions since the influence of each covariate in the model can vary separately with time thus allowing a possible nadir (related to a given covariate) to vary with time. To be specific: If $X_{ip}(t)$ is set to $X_{ip-1}^2(t)$, the nadir of the quadratic relationship between the covariate $X_{ip-1}(t)$ and the intensity $\lambda_i(t, X_i(t))$ is

$$-\frac{\beta_{p-1}(t)}{2\beta_p(t)},$$

and since we are interested in investigating a possible time-dependency of such a nadir, the null-hypothesis $H_{03}: \beta_p(t) \equiv \gamma \beta_{p-1}(t)$. is of interest. Below we address estimation of γ and testing of the hypothesis of constant nadir, see Martinussen & Sørensen (1998) for further details. The following notation will be used: for a $(p \times l)$-matrix A, A_i denotes the $(1 \times l)$-matrix consisting of the ith row in A, $\tilde{A}_i$ denotes the $(i \times l)$-matrix consisting of

144   5. Additive Hazards Models

the first i rows in A, and $\tilde{A}_{ij}$ denotes the $(1 \times j)$-matrix consisting of the first j elements in the ith row of A. Solving the parametric score equation (differentiate the log-likelihood function with respect to γ) yields

$$\gamma = \left(\int_0^\tau \tilde{Y}_p(t)^T W(t)\tilde{Y}_p(t)\, dB_{p-1}(t)\right)^{-1}$$
$$\times \left(\int_0^\tau \tilde{Y}_p(t)^T W(t)\, dN(t) - \int_0^\tau \tilde{Y}_p(t)^T W(t)\tilde{Y}_{p-1}(t)d\tilde{B}_{p-1}(t)\right). \tag{5.47}$$

Here,

$$\tilde{Y}_p(t) = (Y_{1p}(t),\ldots,Y_{np})^T, \quad \tilde{Y}_{p-1}(t) = (\tilde{Y}_{1p-1}^T(t),\ldots,\tilde{Y}_{np-1}^T(t))^T,$$
$$\tilde{B}_{p-1}(t) = \int_0^t \tilde{\beta}_{p-1}\, ds, \quad \text{and} \quad W(t) = \beta_{p-1}(t)\mathrm{diag}(1/\lambda_i(t)).$$

The expression given by (5.47) cannot be used as an estimate of γ since it depends on the unknown regression functions. However, replacing the weight matrix $W(t)$ by the identity matrix I_n, $B_{p-1}(t)$ and $\tilde{B}_{p-1}(t)$ by the estimates under the unconstraint Aalen additive model leads to the following unweighted least squares estimator

$$\hat{\gamma} = \left(\int_0^\tau \tilde{Y}_p(t)^T \tilde{Y}_p(t)\, d\hat{B}_{p-1}(t)\right)^{-1} \int_0^\tau J(t)\tilde{Y}_p(t)^T H(t)\, dN(t), \tag{5.48}$$

where $H(t) = (I_n - \tilde{Y}_{p-1}(t)(Y^-(t))\tilde{}_{p-1})$. To test the null-hypothesis one may consider the maximal deviation test statistic:

$$T_S = \sup_{t \in [0,\tau]} \left|\hat{B}_p(t) - \hat{\gamma}\hat{B}_{p-1}(t)\right|.$$

Under the null-hypothesis we have that

$$n^{1/2}(\hat{B}_p(t) - \hat{\gamma}\hat{B}_{p-1}(t)) = n^{1/2}(\hat{B}_p(t) - \gamma\hat{B}_{p-1}(t)) - \hat{B}_{p-1}(t)n^{1/2}(\hat{\gamma} - \gamma)$$
$$= \tilde{M}_1(t) - \hat{B}_{p-1}(t)\left(n^{-1}\int_0^\tau \tilde{Y}_p^T \tilde{Y}_p\, d\hat{B}_{p-1}\right)^{-1}\tilde{M}_2(\tau),$$

where

$$\tilde{M}_1(t) = n^{1/2}\int_0^t \gamma^* Y^-\, dM,$$

$$\tilde{M}_2(t) = n^{-1/2}\int_0^t \tilde{Y}_p^T H(I_n - \gamma\tilde{Y}_p(Y^-)_{p-1})\, dM$$

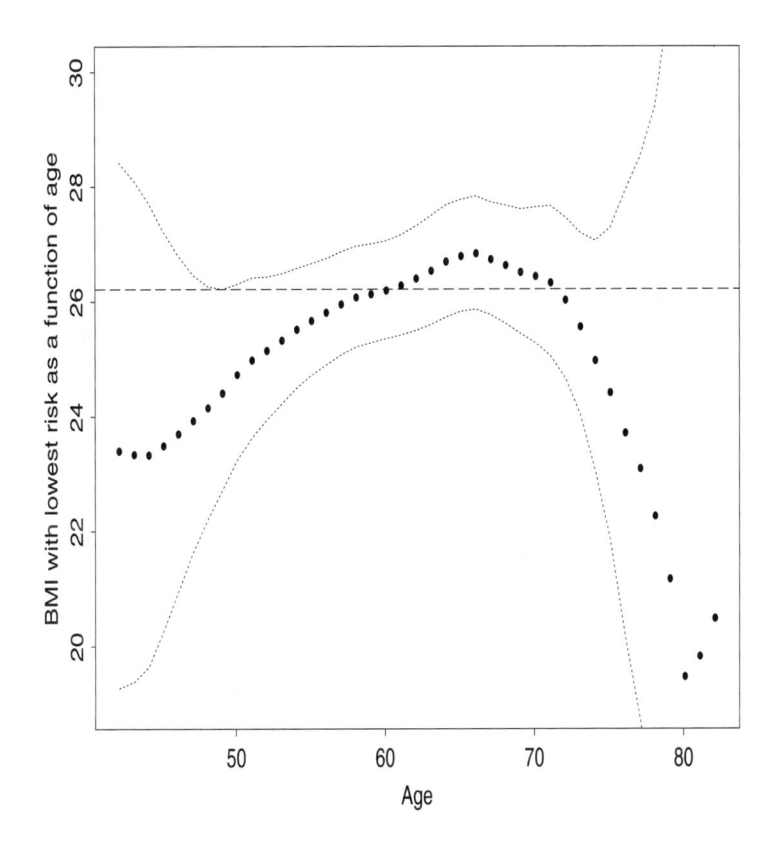

FIGURE 5.9: Time-dependent nadir of risk with 95% pointwise confidence limits. The straight line estimate is given by $\hat{\gamma}$. Adapted from Martinussen & Sørensen (1998).

with $M(t) = (M_1(t), \ldots, M_n(t))^T$, $M_i(t) = N_i(t) - \int_0^t \lambda_i \, ds$ the basic martingales, and γ^* the $(1 \times p)$-vector $(0, \ldots, 0, -\gamma, 1)$

In Martinussen & Sørensen (1998) this method was applied to data from the Copenhagen City Heart Study. The dataset that were analyzed consisted of 8443 women. The time scale is age and failures beyond age 85 were excluded, that is, $\tau = 85$. The following covariates are considered: $X_{i1}=1$, $X_{i2}=$ex-smoker (1 if yes, 0 otherwise), $X_{i3}=$smoker (1 if yes, 0 otherwise), $X_{i4} = \log(\text{BMI}) - \text{constant}$ and $X_{i5} = X_{i4}^2$ the quadratic term defining the U-shape of interest. The applied model is thus

$$\lambda_i(t, X_i(t)) = Y_i(t)\{\beta_1(t) + \beta_2(t)X_{i2}(t) + \beta_3(t)X_{i3}(t) \\ + \beta_4(t)X_{i4}(t) + \beta_5(t)X_{i4}^2(t)\}.$$

The estimated cumulative regression functions were smoothed using the Epanechnikov kernel with bandwidth 15 years to get estimates of the regression functions. In Figure 5.9 we have used these estimates to obtain a plot of the evolution of the nadir related to BMI (recall that the nadir at time t is $-\beta_4(t)/2\beta_5(t)$). The included pointwise confidence limits are based on the confidence limits for the regression functions. Since the estimates of the regression functions are biased, see Exercise 4.1, these limits should be interpreted with some caution.

From Figure 5.9, it seems that the nadir could be constant within the interval where the estimate is well determined. Using (5.48), a time-invariant nadir is estimated to a body mass index at 26.2 kg/m², which seems acceptable judging from Figure 5.9. The distribution of the teststatistic T_S were simulated and it was found that the null-hypothesis is acceptable with a p-value of 0.24. It therefore seems reasonable to conclude that an age-independent nadir is in agreement with the data, and is estimated to be 26.2 kg/m². □

5.5 Estimating the survival function

We now show how to estimate subject specific survival using the semiparametric additive survival model. Note, that the Aalen additive hazards model is a special case of this taking $q = 0$ in the semiparametric model. Assume that a subject with covariates X_0 and Z_0, that do not depend on time, have additive hazard function

$$\lambda_0(t) = X_0^T \beta(t) + Z_0^T \gamma.$$

The survival probability is given as

$$S_0(t) = S_0(B, \gamma, t) = \exp(-X_0^T B(t) - Z_0^T t\gamma)$$

that obviously can be estimated by

$$\hat{S}_0(t) = S_0(\hat{B}, \hat{\gamma}, t) = \exp(-X_0^T \hat{B}(t) - Z_0^T t\hat{\gamma}).$$

It is a consequence of Theorem 5.3.1 and the functional delta method that the continuous functional $n^{1/2}(\hat{S}_0 - S_0)$ has an asymptotic distribution that is easy to derive (see Exercise 5.13). It can be shown, under Condition 5.2, that $n^{1/2}(\hat{S}_0 - S_0)$ converges towards a zero-mean Gaussian process U with variance function Q on $[0, \tau]$ (see Exercise 5.13). A Taylor series expansion yields (up to $o_p(1)$) that

$$n^{1/2}(S_0(\hat{B}, \hat{\gamma}, t) - S_0(B, \gamma, t)) = \\ - S_0(B, \gamma, t) \left\{ X_0^T n^{1/2}(\hat{B}(t) - B(t)) + t Z_0^T n^{1/2}(\hat{\gamma} - \gamma) \right\}. \quad (5.49)$$

5.5 Estimating the survival function

The last expression on the right hand side of (5.49) can be written as

$$X_0^T\{M_2(t) - P(t)C_1^{-1}M_1(\tau)\} + tZ_0^T C_1^{-1} M_1(\tau),$$

see (5.39) and (5.40). Based on this martingale decomposition we may give a optional variation process estimator of its variance, see Exercise 5.13, which we here denote by $\hat{\Upsilon}(t)$ without deriving an explicit formula. The variance function Q can then be estimated consistently by

$$\tilde{Q}(t) = \hat{S}_0^2(t)\hat{\Upsilon}(t).$$

This will lead to pointwise $(1-\alpha)$-confidence intervals of the form

$$\hat{S}_0(t) \pm n^{-1/2} c_{\alpha/2} \tilde{Q}^{1/2}(t).$$

where $c_{\alpha/2}$ is the $(1-\alpha/2)$-quantile of the standard normal distribution. The above method to construct confidence intervals is in principle straightforward. Below, however, we outline a resampling approach that is simpler to implement and also will lead to a confidence band.

With the notation from Section 5.4 we derived in Theorem 5.4.1 that $n^{1/2}(\hat{\gamma} - \gamma)$ and $n^{1/2}(\hat{B} - B)$ are asymptotically equivalent to

$$\Delta_2 = n^{-1/2} \sum_{i=1}^n \hat{\epsilon}_{2,i} G_i,$$

$$\Delta_3(t) = n^{-1/2} \sum_{i=1}^n \hat{\epsilon}_{3,i}(t) G_i,$$

where $G_1, \ldots, G_n$ are independent and standard normally distributed. Therefore, applying the functional delta method to these asymptotically equivalent resampling processes will lead to an equivalent limit distribution, which may be used to construct a confidence band. We now make an i.i.d. representation of the term

$$X_0^T n^{1/2}(\hat{B} - B)(t) + tZ_0^T n^{1/2}(\hat{\gamma} - \gamma)$$

from (5.49). Define

$$\epsilon_{5,i}(t) = X_0^T \epsilon_{3,i}(t) + tZ_0^T \epsilon_{2,i}.$$

It follows that that $n^{1/2}(\hat{S}_0 - S_0)(t)$ has the same asymptotic distribution as

$$\Delta_S(t) = -S_0(t) n^{-1/2} \sum_{i=1}^n \hat{\epsilon}_{5,i}(t) G_i. \qquad (5.50)$$

It also follows that

$$\hat{Q}(t) = \hat{S}_0^2(t) n^{-1} \sum_{i=1}^n \hat{\epsilon}_{5,i}^2(t),$$

148   5. Additive Hazards Models

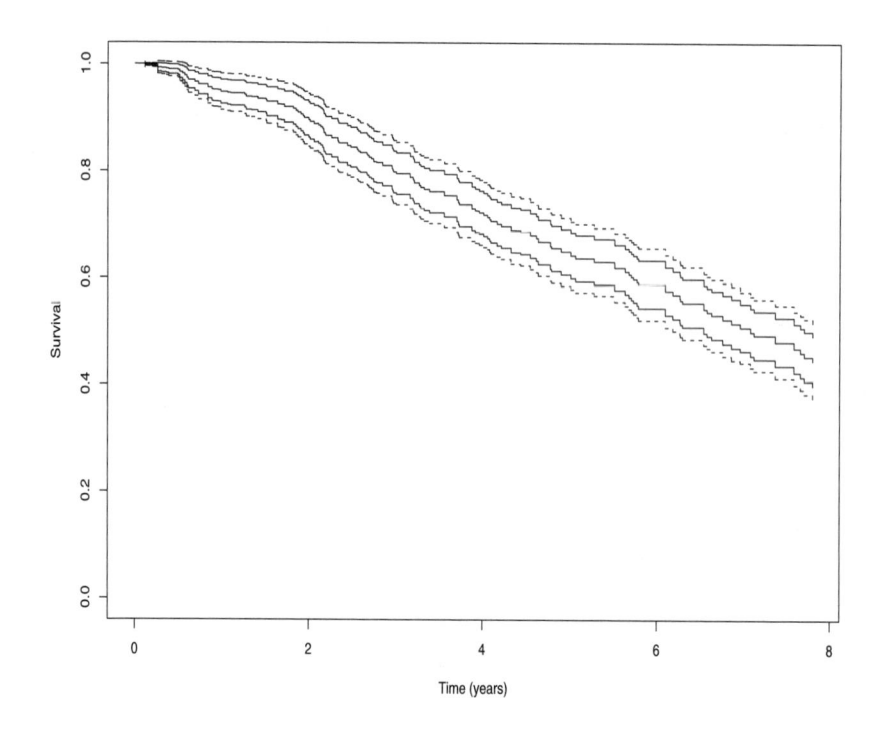

FIGURE 5.10: PBC-data. Survival prediction with 95% pointwise confidence intervals (solid lines) and 95% confidence band (broken lines).

is a consistent estimator of the variance of $n^{1/2}(\hat{S}_0 - S_0)$, and an approximate $(1-\alpha)$-confidence band is on the form

$$\hat{S}_0(t) \pm C_\alpha n^{-1/2} \hat{Q}^{1/2}(t),$$

where C_α is the $(1-\alpha)$-quantile of

$$\sup_{t \in [0,\tau]} |\frac{\Delta_S^k(t)}{\hat{Q}^{1/2}(t)}|$$

with $\Delta_S^k(t)$ the kth resampled process, $k = 1, \ldots, K$.

Example 5.5.1 (Survival prediction for PBC-data)

Consider the PBC-data using the semiparametric additive hazards model with edema and log(protime) having timevarying effect and with age, bilirubin, and log(albumin) having constant effect.

We first fit the model to get the i.i.d. representation, and then compute the approximate constant to construct a 95% confidence band based on resampling.

```
> fit<-aalen(Surv(time/365,status)~const(Age)+Edema
+ +const(Bilirubin)+const(logAlbumin)+logProtime,max.time=8,
+ pbc,resample.iid=1)
Semiparametric Additive Risk Model
Simulations start N= 1000
> # fit$B.iid and fit$gamma.iid contains i.i.d. representation
> x0<-c(1,0,0); z0<-c(0,0,0);
> delta<-matrix(0,144,418);
> for (i in 1:418) {delta[,i]<-x0 %*% t(fit$B.iid[[i]])+
+ fit$cum[,1]*sum(z0*fit$gamma.iid[i,]);}
> S0<-S0.add<-exp(- x0 %*% t(fit$cum[,-1]))
> se<-apply(delta^2,1,sum)^.5
> ### pointwise confidence intervals
> plot(fit$cum[,1],S0,type="s",ylim=c(0,1),xlab="Time (years)",
+ ylab="Survival")
> lines(fit$cum[,1],S0-1.96*S0*se,type="s");
> lines(fit$cum[,1],S0+1.96*S0*se,type="s")
> ### uniform confidence bands
> mpt<-c()
> for (i in 1:418) {
+ g<-rnorm(418); pt<-abs(delta %*% g)/se;  mpt<-c(mpt,max(pt[-1])); }
> Cband<-percen(mpt,0.95);
> lines(fit$cum[,1],S0-Cband*S0*se,lty=2,type="s");
> lines(fit$cum[,1],S0+Cband*S0*se,lty=2,type="s")
```

The 95% uniform band shown in Figure 5.10 is as expected wider than the 95% pointwise confidence interval. The estimated survival function is for a subject without presence of edema and with average values for all the other covariates. □

5.6 Additive rate models

The additive Aalen model (5.3) or the semiparametric version (5.26) of it are models for the intensity of the observed counting processes. The intensity gives the instantaneous risk of an event given the history. Considering the Aalen model, as we set it up, as an example, the intensity is equivalent to

$$\lambda(t)dt = E[dN(t)|\sigma(N(s), X(s), Y(s), \ s \in [0, t[)],$$

with $dN(t) = N((t+dt)-) - N(t-)$. The intensity *should* therefore reflect the dependence on the past of $N(t)$, $Y(t)$ and $X(t)$. If, for example, the

150   5. Additive Hazards Models

covariate process exhibit a path that indicates a particularly high risk, this should be reflected in the expression for the intensity. In applications it may be a difficult task to understand the subject matter well enough to correctly specify the intensity, although it may be possible to construct a sufficiently good approximation. The consequences of working with the intensity are reflected in the formulas for the variances of the suggested estimators. If the intensity is misspecified, these variance estimates will be biased. This section describes a framework for remedying this problem by constructing models for the rate of the counting process instead. The rate function at time t given the at risk indicator and selected covariates of interest, $X(t)$, is assumed to be on the Aalen additive form

$$E(\lambda(t)|Y(t), X(t)) = Y(t)X(t)^T \beta(t), \qquad (5.51)$$

where the important distinction is that the p-dimensional $X(t)$ does not necessarily reflect the entire history but is only known to give an unbiased linear prediction of the rate in the sense of (5.51). The model may be stated in alternative fashion as giving the instantaneous probability of an event given the at risk indicator and the selected covariates, such that

$$E(dN(t)|Y(t), X(t)) = Y(t)X(t)^T \beta(t)dt.$$

Note that the model may be used for both survival and recurrent events data. It is important to stress that the traditional analysis, which is based on the assumption that the specified model is the intensity, rely on stronger assumptions than the rate model.

The semiparametric version of the rate function is

$$E(\lambda(t)|Y(t), X(t), Z(t)) = Y(t)(X(t)^T \beta(t) + Z(t)^T \gamma). \qquad (5.52)$$

The key message of this section is that the usual estimators given in Sections 5.1 and 5.3 are valid also in the rate context, but that the martingale based standard error estimates, for example the optional variation estimators, may be biased and therefore should be applied with caution. The inferential procedures based on the resampling approach, however, continues to be valid. Note, that in the case of survival data with fixed covarites the rate and the intensity will be the same. In Scheike (2002) a simulation study indicated that the martingale standard errors typically perform quite well even when the considered model is in fact a rate model. Since the robust standard errors are just as easy to compute, however, we recommend them for general use.

We summarize the results for the semiparametric rate model (5.52) in the following two theorems.

Theorem 5.6.1 *If Condition 5.2 holds and the rate model is on the semiparametric risk form (5.52), then, as $n \to \infty$,*

$$n^{1/2}(\hat{\gamma} - \gamma) \xrightarrow{\mathcal{D}} V, \qquad (5.53)$$

where V is a zero-mean normal with variance Σ, and

$$n^{1/2}(\hat{B}-B)(t) \xrightarrow{D} U(t) \tag{5.54}$$

in $D[0,\tau]^p$, where $U(t)$ is a zero-mean Gaussian process with variance Ψ. Further, $\hat{\Psi}(t)$ given in (5.46) is a uniformly consistent estimator of $\Psi(t)$.

Just as in the intensity case we can approximate the asymptotic distributions in the above theorem by resampling of the residuals and we can estimate the variance of the estimators consistently by the squared residual estimators.

Theorem 5.6.2 *Under the conditions of Theorem 5.6.1 and with $G_1, ..., G_n$ independent standard normals, it follows that*

$$\Delta_2 = n^{-1/2} \sum_{i=1}^{n} \hat{\epsilon}_{2i} G_i,$$

$$\Delta_3(\cdot) = n^{-1/2} \sum_{i=1}^{n} \hat{\epsilon}_{3i}(\cdot) G_i,$$

distributed, has the same limit distribution as $n^{1/2}(\hat{\gamma}-\gamma, \hat{B}-B)$. Further, (5.45) and (5.46) are consistent estimators of the variance of $n^{1/2}(\hat{\gamma}-\gamma)$ and $n^{1/2}(\hat{B}-B)$, respectively.

Note that the terms

$$M_i(t) = N_i(t) - \int_0^t Y_i(s)(X_i^T(s)dB(s) + Z_i^T(s)\gamma ds), \quad i=1,\ldots,n,$$

are no longer martingales but that

$$\hat{M}_i(t) = N_i(t) - \int_0^t Y_i(s)(X_i^T(s)d\hat{B}(s) + Z_i^T(s)\hat{\gamma} ds), \quad i=1,\ldots,n,$$

used in the above variance estimators still make sense in the rate context.

5.7 Goodness-of-fit procedures

Although the additive Aalen model is very flexible, it is still important to check that the model provides an adequate fit to the data. The true model may for instance not be additive, the effect of some covariates may not be linear on the scale where they are included and various interactions may have been overlooked. We consider only how to access the goodness-of-fit of the additive Aalen hazards model because the semiparametric additive hazards model is considered a submodel of this model. To evaluate the fit of the model we consider various martingale residuals and then check if their behavior is consistent with what should be expected under the model.

We start by considering the underlying martingale residuals
$$M(t) = (M_1(t), ..., M_n(t))^T$$
with
$$M_i(t) = N_i(t) - \int_0^t Y_i(s) X_i(s)^T dB(s).$$
The martingale residuals are estimated by
$$\hat{M}(t) = N(t) - \int_0^t X(s) d\hat{B}(s)$$
$$= N(t) - \int_0^t X(s) X^-(s) dN(s) = \int_0^t G(s) dN(s),$$
where $G(t) = I - X(t)X^-(t)$ and considering only the time-range where the design has full rank. Under the additive Aalen model the residual vector is an exact martingale
$$\hat{M}(t) = \int_0^t G(s) dM(s),$$
because $G(t)X(t) = 0$. The particular structure of the residuals implies that
$$X^T(t) d\hat{M}(t) = X^T(t) G(t) dM(t) = 0.$$
In the case with covariates that are constant with time, thus leading to $X(t) = \text{diag}(Y_i(t))X(0)$, it follows that
$$X^T(0) d\hat{M}(t) = X^T(0) G(t) dM(t) = X^T(t) G(t) dM(t) = 0.$$
One special implication of this (for models with an intercept term) is that
$$\sum_{i=1}^n Y_i(t) d\hat{M}_i(t) = 0,$$
that is, the estimated martingale increments are zero when summed over the subjects at risk.

To validate the model fit one possibility is to sum the residuals depending on the level of the covariates (Aalen, 1993). Define therefore an $n \times m$ matrix,
$$K(t) = (K_1^T(t), \ldots, K_n^T(t))^T,$$
possibly depending on time. A K-cumulative residual process is then defined as
$$M_K(t) = \int_0^t K^T(s) d\hat{M}(s) = \int_0^t K^T(s) G(s) dM(s).$$

5.7 Goodness-of-fit procedures

A typical choice of K is to let it be a factor with levels defined by the quartiles of the considered covariates, as we do in the below Example 5.7.1. The variance of $M_K(t)$ can be estimated by the optional variation process

$$[M_K](t) = \int_0^t K^T(s)G(s)\mathrm{diag}(dN(s))G(s)K(s).$$

We give an alternative robust variance estimator in (5.55) below.

Plotting the observed cumulative residual process $M_K(t)$ with 95% pointwise confidence intervals or 95% Hall-Wellner confidence band will give an indication of whether or not the observed residuals are consistent with the model. When a large number of residuals are computed it is convenient with a p-value to help summarize how serious a departure from the null that is seen. We therefore suggest to compute the test-statistics $\sup |M_K(t)|$, and approximate its distribution under the model by resampling. Resampling can also be used to construct confidence bands, the key is to establish an i.i.d. representation of the cumulative residual process. To do this simply note that

$$M_K(t) = \sum_{i=1}^n \int_0^t \left(K_i(s)^T - K(s)^T X(s)(X(s)^T X(s))^{-1} X_i(s) \right) dM_i(s),$$

The asymptotic distribution of $M_K(t)$ is equivalent to the asymptotic distribution of

$$\sum_{i=1}^n G_i \int_0^t \left(K_i(s)^T - K(s)^T X(s)(X(s)^T X(s))^{-1} X_i(s) \right) d\hat{M}_i(s)$$

where $G_1, ..., G_n$ are independent standard normals.

To estimate the variance of $M_K(t)$ a simple estimator based on the i.i.d. decomposition is given by

$$\sum_{i=1}^n \left[\int_0^t \left(K_i^T(s) - K(s)^T X(s)(X(s)^T X(s))^{-1} X_i(s) \right) d\hat{M}_i(s) \right]^{\otimes 2}. \quad (5.55)$$

It may be shown that the resampling approximation has the same asymptotic limit as $n^{-1/2} M_K(t)$ and that the variance estimator is consistent.

One may also consider the following test statistics to evaluate the performance of the cumulative residuals:

$$\sup_{t \in [0,\tau]} |M_{K,j}(t)|, \qquad \int_0^\tau (M_{K,j}(t))^2 dt,$$

for $j = 1, ..., m$, where $M_{K,j}$ denotes the jth component of the vector M_K.

Example 5.7.1 (PBC-data)

We consider the additive hazards model with the covariates edema, bilirubin, log(protime), age and log(albumin). To evaluate the fit we transformed

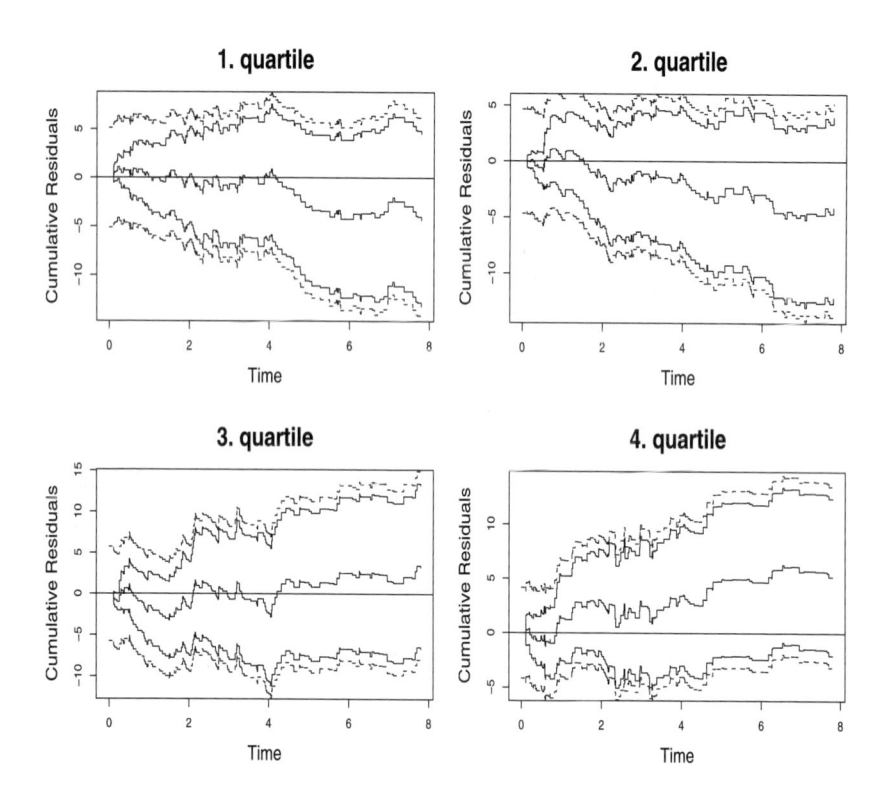

FIGURE 5.11: Observed cumulative residuals for quartiles of bilirubin with 95% confidence intervals (solid lines) and 95% Hall-Wellner confidence bands (broken lines).

all continuous covariates into factors with 4 levels defined by the quartiles, and computed the cumulative martingale residuals. We only show the result for bilirubin. The covariate log(albumin) indicated some minor problems with the fit, and we quantify this further in the below Example 5.7.2. All other covariates did not give any indication of a poor fit.

```
> fit<-aalen(Surv(time/365,status)~Age+Edema+Bilirubin+
+ logAlbumin+logProtime,max.time=8,pbc,residuals=1,n.sim=0)
Nonparametric Additive Risk Model
> X<-model.matrix(~-1+cut(Bilirubin,quantile(Bilirubin),
+ include.lowest=T),pbc)
> colnames(X)<-c("1. quartile","2. quartile","3. quartile","4. quartile")
> resids<-cum.residuals(fit,pbc,X,n.sim=1000)
Cumulative martingale residuals for Right censored survival times
> plot(resids,hw.ci=2)
> summary(resids)
Test for cumulative MG-residuals
```

5.7 Goodness-of-fit procedures

Grouped Residuals consistent with model

	sup| hat B(t) |	p-value H_0: B(t)=0
1. quartile	4.334	0.582
2. quartile	5.175	0.365
3. quartile	3.471	0.873
4. quartile	6.273	0.172

	int (B(t))^2 dt	p-value H_0: B(t)=0
1. quartile	40.070	0.544
2. quartile	58.986	0.392
3. quartile	21.707	0.826
4. quartile	111.898	0.182

The cumulative residuals with confidence intervals and bands, Figure 5.11, clearly indicate that the fit is acceptable for all levels of bilirubin.

For the PBC data example it is well established that when fitting a Cox model one should use log-bilirubin to get an acceptable fit of the proportional model. This is in contrast to the conclusion for the additive model, and to show that the use of log-bilirubin leads to a poor fit for the additive hazards model we computed the cumulative residuals for this model for the quartiles of bilirubin.

```
> nfit<-aalen(Surv(time/365,status)~Age+Edema+logBilirubin
+ +logAlbumin+logProtime,max.time=8,pbc,residuals=1,n.sim=0)
Nonparametric Additive Risk Model
> X<-model.matrix(~-1+cut(Bilirubin,quantile(Bilirubin),
+ include.lowest=T),pbc)
> colnames(X)<-c("1. quartile","2. quartile","3. quartile",
+ "4. quartile");
> resids<-cum.residuals(nfit,pbc,X,n.sim=1000)
Cumulative martingale residuals for Right censored survival times
> plot(resids,score=1)
> summary(resids)
Test for cumulative MG-residuals
```

Grouped Residuals consistent with model

	sup| hat B(t) |	p-value H_0: B(t)=0
1. quartile	13.045	0.002
2. quartile	9.980	0.050
3. quartile	13.888	0.022
4. quartile	8.885	0.007

	int (B(t))^2 dt	p-value H_0: B(t)=0
1. quartile	666.869	0.002
2. quartile	268.896	0.063
3. quartile	659.609	0.032

156   5. Additive Hazards Models

1. quartile
2. quartile
3. quartile
4. quartile

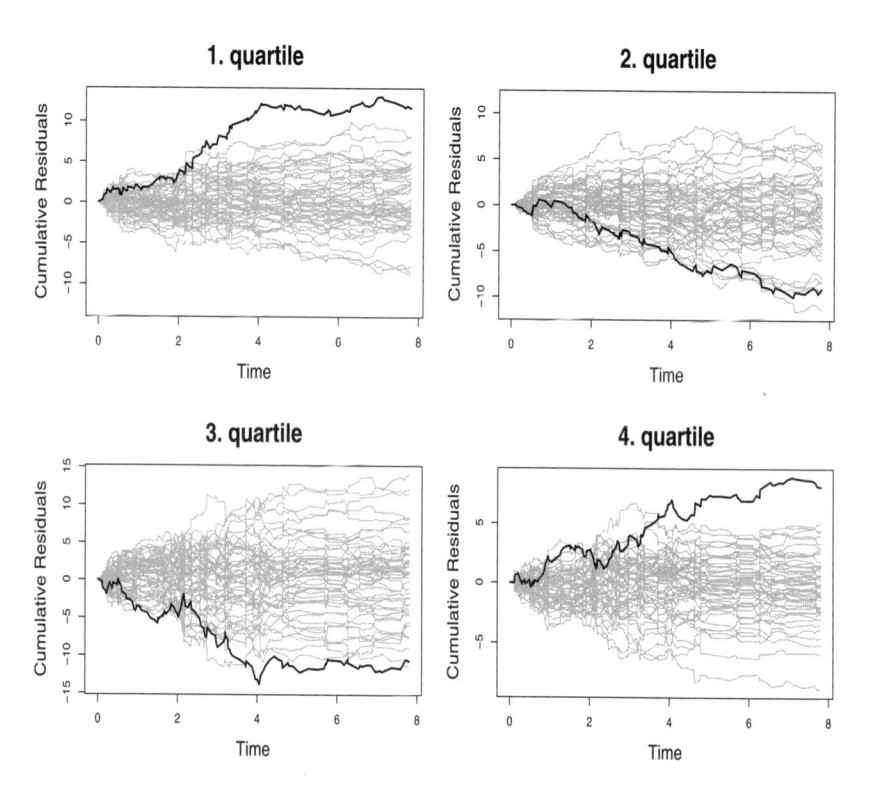

FIGURE 5.12: PBC-data. Observed cumulative residuals for quartiles of bilirubin and 50 random realizations under the model using log(bilirubin) in the model.

    4. quartile   255.224   0.014

Figure 5.12 shows the cumulative test processes with 50 random simulations under the null, which is summarized into p-values in the output. All quartiles indicating that there are severe problems with the fit. This suggests that the effect of bilirubin is not additive when it is log-transformed. □

These K-cumulative residual plots are useful, but it is somewhat inconvenient that one needs to group the continuous covariates. An alternative procedure similar in spirit but avoiding this grouping was suggested by Lin et al. (1993) in the context of the Cox model, see Section 6.2. We adopt it here in the case of the additive Aalen model.

Considering the first continuous covariate of the model we show how one can construct a cumulative residual process that will carry information about the fit of the model as a function of the level of the covariate. We start by considering a cumulative residual process

$$M_c(t,z) = \int_0^t K_z^T(s) d\hat{M}(s) = \int_0^t K_z^T(s) G(s) dM(s).$$

where $K_z(t)$ is an $1 \times n$ matrix with elements $I(X_{i1}(t) \le z)$ for $i = 1, \ldots, n$ focusing here on the fit with regard to the first covariate X_1. Integrating over the entire time span we get a process only in z:

$$M_c(z) = \int_0^T K_z^T(t) d\hat{M}(t) = \int_0^T K_z^T(t) G(t) dM(t). \tag{5.56}$$

This process has a decomposition similarly to M_K developed above, and resampling may thus be used to validate the fit of the model. One may also consider the process as a function of both z, t, and a resampling scheme to approximate its asymptotic distribution is also possible in this case. A different version, but very similar in spirit, was given by McKeague & Utikal (1990a) and McKeague & Utikal (1990b) who considered double cumulative processes as a general mean for doing goodness-of-fit for structured models.

Example 5.7.2 (PBC-data, Example 5.7.1 continued)

We again consider the additive risk model with the covariates edema, bilirubin, log(protime), age and log(albumin). The following commands compute the cumulative residuals (5.56) versus the covariates (with more than two levels).

```
> resids<-cum.residuals(fit,pbc,cum.resid=1)
Cumulative martingale residuals for Right censored survival times
Simulations start N= 500
> plot(resids,score=2);
> summary(resids)
Test for cumulative MG-residuals

Residual versus covariates consistent with model

            sup| hat B(t) |  p-value H_0: B(t)=0
Age                 5.730              0.796
Bilirubin          10.250              0.170
logAlbumin          7.838              0.356
logProtime          4.603              0.890
```

The output suggests that all covariates lead to a performance that is consistent with the model. Figure 5.13 shows the cumulative residuals with 50 resampled processes under the model. Age, log(bilirubin) and log(protime) show observed cumulative processes that behave as they should under the

158   5. Additive Hazards Models

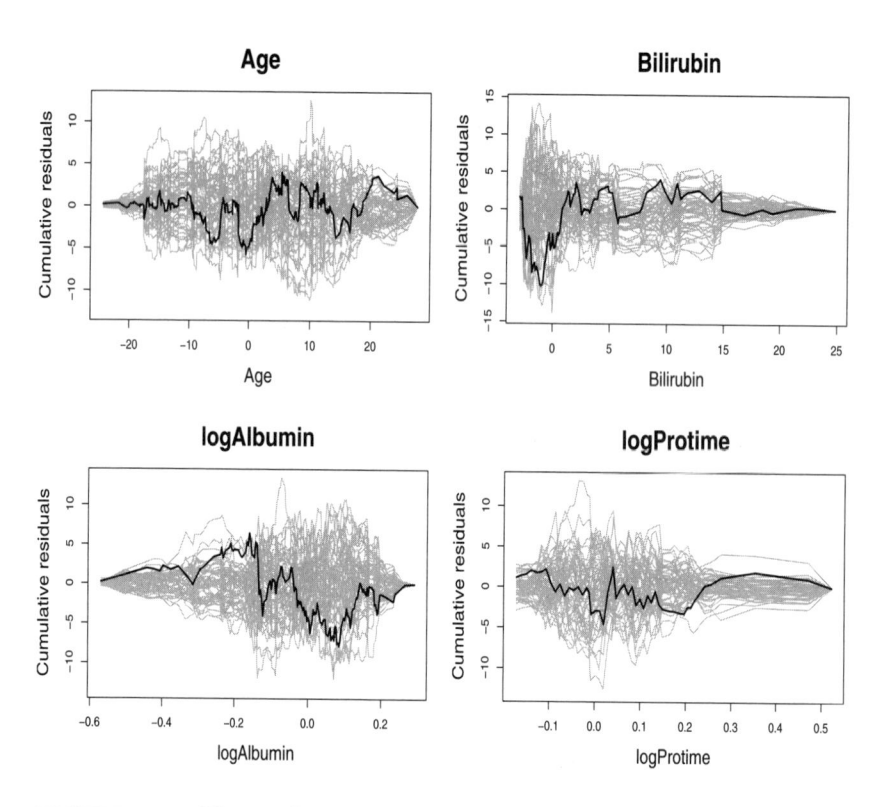

FIGURE 5.13: Observed cumulative residuals versus continuous covariates and 50 random realizations under the model.

null, but log(albumin) shows a performance that is not completely consistent with the performance expected under the model. Note that the deviation from the null is not dramatic and that the supremum test-statistic is insignificant.

We finally show the similar plots for an additive hazards model with log-bilirubin.

```
> resids<-cum.residuals(nfit,pbc,cum.resid=1)
Cumulative martingale residuals for Right censored survival times
Simulations start N= 500
> plot(resids,score=2);
> summary(resids)
Test for cumulative MG-residuals

Residual versus covariates consistent with model

              sup| hat B(t) |  p-value H_0: B(t)=0
Age                  5.154                   0.914
logBilirubin        12.588                   0.004
```

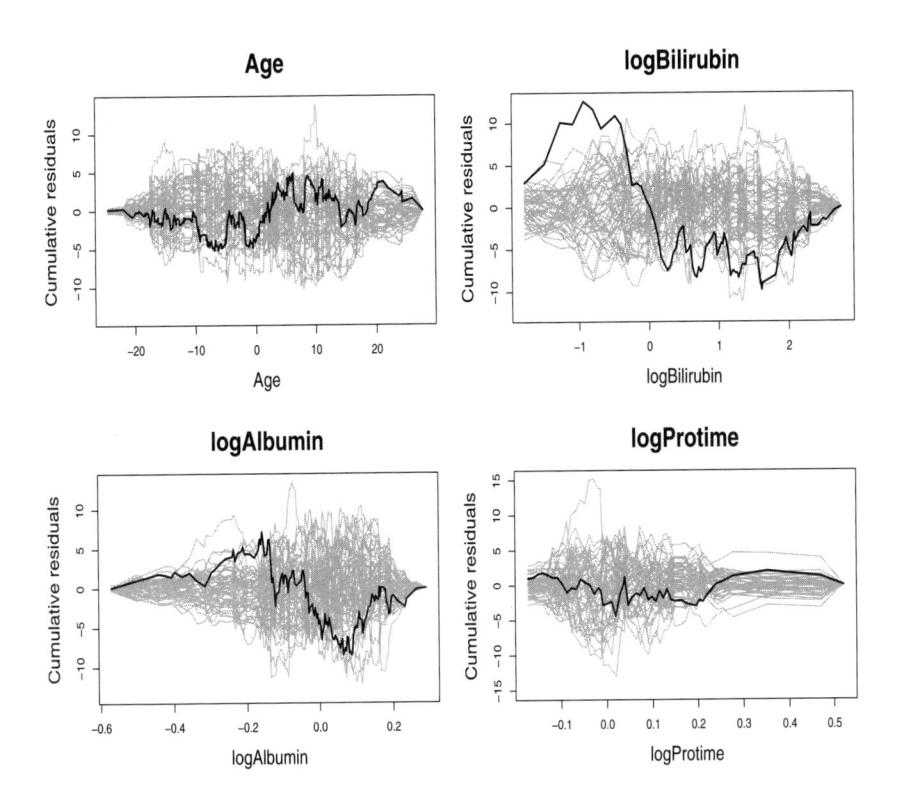

FIGURE 5.14: Observed cumulative residuals versus continuous covariates and 50 random realizations under the model.

```
logAlbumin          8.485           0.248
logProtime          4.387           0.936
```

The output and Figure 5.14 clearly show that there are problems with the fit of the model indicated by the extreme behavior of the residuals cumulated versus log(bilirubin). □

5.8 Example

In this section we show a worked example of how to use the semiparametric additive hazards model to predict the survival of patients with myocardial infarction based on the TRACE data (Jensen et al., 1997).

Example 5.8.1 (TRACE Data)

The TRACE study group, see Jensen et al. (1997), studied the prognos-

160   5. Additive Hazards Models

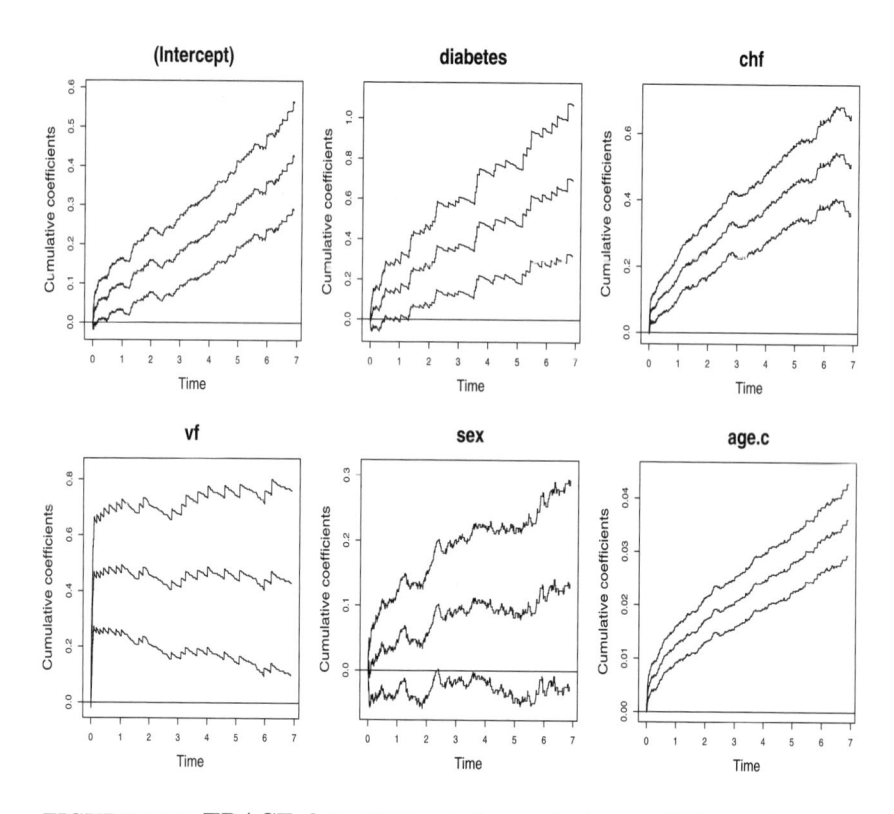

FIGURE 5.15: TRACE-data. Estimated cumulative coefficients along with 95% confidence intervals

tic importance of various risk factors on mortality for approximately 6600 patients with myocardial infarction. The TRACE data included in the `timereg` package is a random sample of 1877 of these patients. In this example we consider 1000 of these patients and this is the tTRACE data set used below.

The risk factors that we consider are age, sex (male=1), clinical heart failure (CHF) (present=1), ventricular fibrillation (VF) (present=1), and diabetes (present=1). Some risk factors were expected to have strongly timevarying effects, in particular, ventricular fibrillation. The effect of diabetes was also expected to decay with time. The considered time scale was time since prognosis, and the total number of deaths in an 7 year period after prognosis was 958, and of these, 115 took place within the two first months. We start by fitting an additive hazards regression model with age centered around its mean

```
> age.c<-tTRACE$age-mean(tTRACE$age)
> fit.trace<-aalen(Surv(time,status==9)~diabetes+chf+vf+sex+age.c,
+ tTRACE,max.time=7,residuals=1)
```

5.8 Example

```
Nonparametric Additive Risk Model
Simulations start N= 1000
> plot(fit.trace)
> summary(fit.trace)
Additive Aalen Model

Test for nonparametric terms

Test for non-significant effects
            sup| hat B(t)/SD(t) |  p-value H_0: B(t)=0
(Intercept)         6.15                    0.000
diabetes            4.09                    0.000
chf                 7.72                    0.000
vf                  4.79                    0.000
sex                 2.11                    0.427
age.c              11.10                    0.000
Test for time invariant effects
            sup| B(t) - (t/tau)B(tau)|  p-value H_0: B(t)=b t
(Intercept)         0.05040                 0.598
diabetes            0.14300                 0.483
chf                 0.13000                 0.003
vf                  0.46200                 0.000
sex                 0.05530                 0.703
age.c               0.00742                 0.001

            int (B(t)-(t/tau)B(tau))^2dt  p-value H_0: B(t)=b t
(Intercept)         0.003520                0.613
diabetes            0.023600                0.598
chf                 0.049400                0.003
vf                  0.499000                0.000
sex                 0.003500                0.749
age.c               0.000142                0.001
```

Figure 5.15 and the output clearly show that VF has a strongly time-varying effect. The effect of VF is highly predictive initially (the first 3 months approximately) and then its predictive effect disappears. Thus, if this serious condition is survived, then the prognosis is similar to other subjects without the prognosis. It seems also that the effect of age and CHF varies with time whereas the effect of diabetes and sex result in a constant increase in the hazard. One may therefore consider a model with the effects of these latter two covariates being summarized by constant excess risk parameters.

Before considering the semiparametric submodels we do some goodness-of-fit analysis of the model and here for illustration purposes focus on how age should be included in the model. We therefore make the cumulative residual plot versus age.

162   5. Additive Hazards Models

age.c

I(exp(age.c/10))

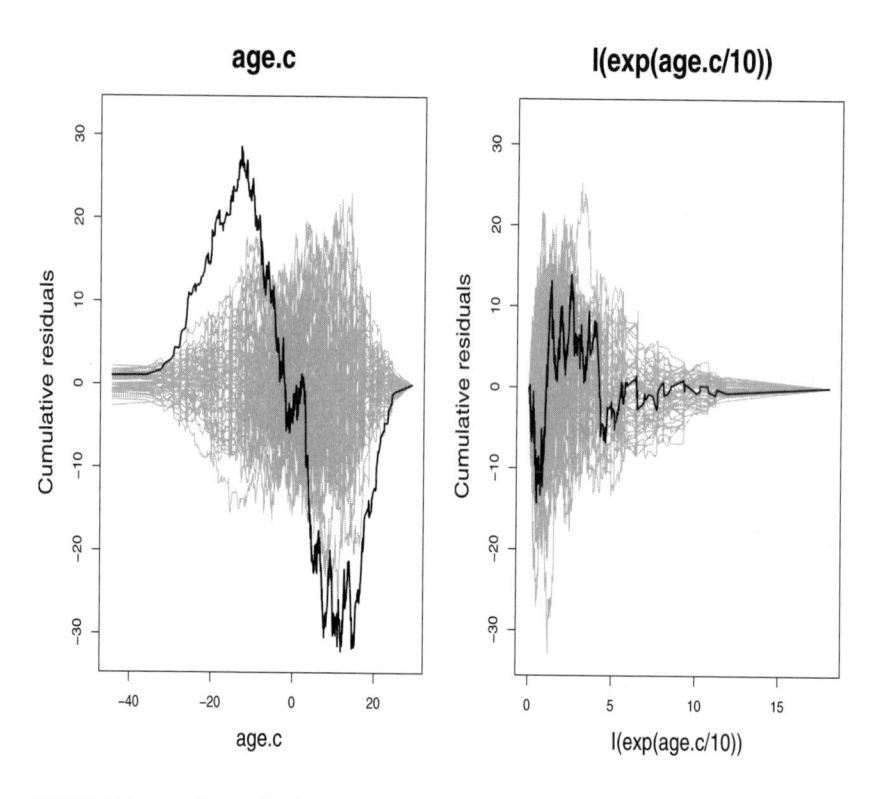

FIGURE 5.16: Cumulative residuals versus age with 50 random realizations under the model for age (left panel) and exp(age.c/10) (right panel).

This reveals that the effect of age is not well-described by the model; the corresponding cumulative residual plot is given in Figure 5.16 left panel. When age enters the model on exponential scale (exp(age.c/10), (cumulative residual plot is shown in Figure 5.16 right panel), the Aalen model with all covariates having time-varying effects seems to give an adequate fit to the data. One can then go on testing successively whether the effect of the covariates can be described as being constant with time. This is acceptable for the covariates diabetes, sex and exp(age.c/10). The results from this model is reported below.

```
> age.c<-tTRACE$age-mean(tTRACE$age)
> fit.trace.semi<-aalen(Surv(time,status==9)~const(diabetes)+chf
+ +vf+const(sex)+const(I(exp(age.c/10))),tTRACE,
+ max.time=7,resample.iid=1)
Semiparametric Additive Risk Model
Simulations start N= 1000
> summary(fit.trace.semi)
Additive Aalen Model
```

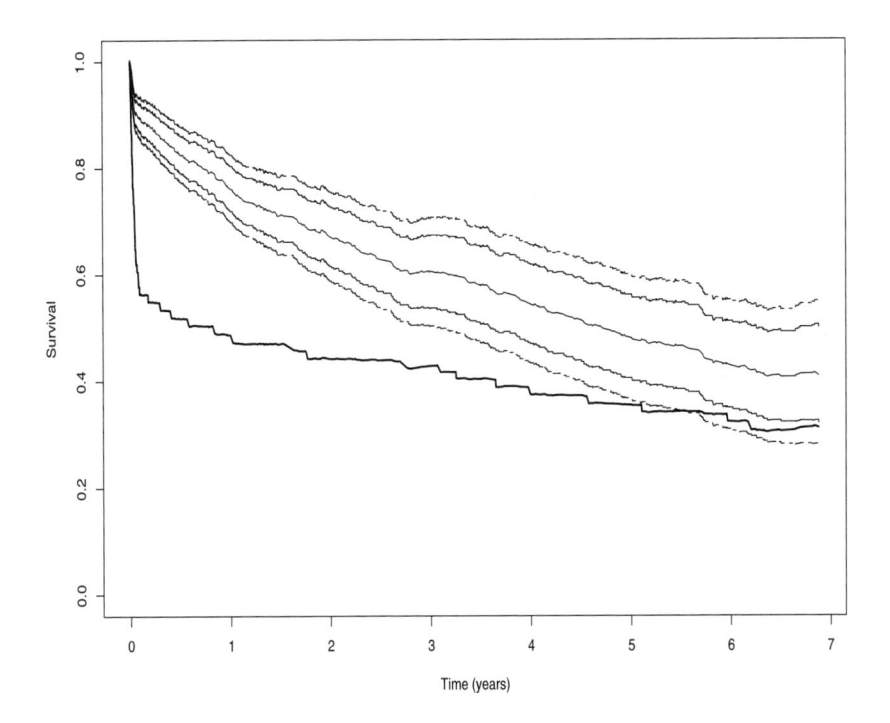

FIGURE 5.17: Survival function estimates for two females without diabetes with VF (thick solid line) and without VF (thin lines). Subject without VF condition is shown with 95% confidence intervals (solid lines) and with 95% confidence band (broken lines).

```
Test for nonparametric terms

Test for non-significant effects
            sup| hat B(t)/SD(t) |  p-value H_0: B(t)=0
(Intercept)          5.30                  0.000
chf                  5.78                  0.000
vf                   4.60                  0.001
Test for time invariant effects
            sup| B(t) - (t/tau)B(tau)|  p-value H_0: B(t)=b t
(Intercept)          0.032                 0.195
chf                  0.155                 0.000
vf                   0.447                 0.000

            int (B(t)-(t/tau)B(tau))^2dt  p-value H_0: B(t)=b t
(Intercept)          0.00237               0.132
chf                  0.07580               0.000
```

164   5. Additive Hazards Models

```
vf                              0.46300              0.000
```

```
Parametric terms :
                         Coef.      SE   Robust SE     z      P-val
const(diabetes)         0.1200   0.02970   0.04140   4.02   5.82e-05
const(sex)              0.0301   0.01270   0.01880   2.36   1.81e-02
const(I(exp(age.c/10))) 0.0619   0.00744   0.00995   8.32   0.00e+00
```

Finally, we compute estimates of the survival function for two females with the chf conditions, with average age, without diabetes and with (solid thick line) and without the vf condition (solid thin line), respectively. These survival function estimates are depicted in Figure 5.17 where it is seen that VF is indeed a serious condition with a marked impact on survival. The R output shows how to compute the survival estimates and make the uniform confidence band.

```
> age.c<-tTRACE$age-mean(tTRACE$age);
> fit<-aalen(Surv(time,status==9)~const(I(exp(age.c/10)))+vf+chf
+ +const(sex)+const(diabetes),tTRACE,max.time=7,n.sim=0,resample.iid=1)
Semiparametric Additive Risk Model
> # fit$B.iid and fit$gamma.iid contains i.i.d. representation
> x0<-c(0,0,1); z0<-c(1,0,0);
> delta<-matrix(0,length(fit$cum[,1]),500);
> for (i in 1:500) {delta[,i]<-x0%*%t(fit$B.iid[[i]])+
+ fit$cum[,1]*sum(z0*fit$gamma.iid[i,]);}
> S0<-exp(- x0 %*% t(fit$cum[,-1])- fit$cum[,1]*sum(z0*fit$gamma))
> se<-apply(delta^2,1,sum)^.5
> ### pointwise confidence intervals
> plot(fit$cum[,1],S0,type="l",ylim=c(0,1),xlab="Time (years)",
+ ylab="Survival")
> lines(fit$cum[,1],S0-1.96*S0*se,type="s")
> lines(fit$cum[,1],S0+1.96*S0*se,type="s")
> x0.VF<-c(1,1,1);
> S0.VF<-exp(- x0.VF %*% t(fit$cum[,-1])- fit$cum[,1]*sum(z0*fit$gamma))
> lines(fit$cum[,1],S0.VF,lwd=2)
> ### uniform confidence band
> mpt<-c()
> for (i in 1:500) {
+ g<-rnorm(500); pt<-abs(delta %*% g)/c(se);mpt<-c(mpt,max(pt[-1])); }
> Cband<-percen(mpt,0.95);
> lines(fit$cum[,1],S0-Cband*S0*se,lty=2,type="s");
> lines(fit$cum[,1],S0+Cband*S0*se,lty=2,type="s")
```

□

5.9 Exercises

5.1 (Aalen, 1989) Let $N(t) = I(T \leq t)$ have intensity according to Aalen's additive model:

$$\lambda^{(p)}(t) = Y(t)(\alpha_0(t) + \alpha_1(t)X_1 + \cdots + \alpha_p(t)X_p),$$

where $X_1, \ldots, X_p$ denote time-invariant covariates.

(a) Assume that X_p is independent of the other covariates. Show that the intensity of N with respect to the filtration spanned by N and the covariates $X_1, \ldots, X_{p-1}$ is

$$\lambda^{(p-1)}(t) = Y(t)(\alpha_0(t) - f'_p(A_p(t))\alpha_p(t) + \alpha_1(t)X_1 + \cdots + \alpha_{p-1}(t)X_{p-1}),$$

where f_p denotes the logarithm of the Laplace transform of X_p (assumed to exist), $A_p(t) = \int_0^t \alpha_p(s)\,ds$ and $Y(t) = I(t \leq T)$.

(b) Assume now that $(X_1, \ldots, X_p)$ have a multivariate normal distribution. Show that $\lambda^{(p-1)}(t)$ is still an additive intensity.

Consider now the situation where we only condition on one covariate, Z, and assume that the intensity is $\lambda(t) = Y(t)(\alpha_0(t) + \alpha(t)Z)$. The covariate Z is, however, not observed as we only observe $X = Z + e$ (error in covariate).

(c) Assume that Z and e are independent and normally distributed with mean μ and 0, and variances σ_Z^2 and σ_e^2, respectively. Show that the conditional intensity given X is

$$Y(t)(\alpha_0(t) + (1-\rho)\alpha(t)(\mu - \sigma_Z^2 A(t)) + \rho\alpha(t)X),$$

where $A(t) = \int_0^t \alpha(s)\,ds$ and $\rho = \sigma_Z^2/(\sigma_Z^2 + \sigma_e^2)$.

5.2 In this exercise, we shall consider the estimator in Aalen's additive model when $p = 1$, that is we consider the model

$$\lambda_i(t) = \beta_1(t)Y_i(t).$$

(a) For this model, write out the matrix $X(t)$, and compute $X^-(t)$ taking $W(t) = I$.

(b) Compute the (unweighted) estimator for $B_1(t) = \int_0^t \beta_1(s)\,ds$. Does it hold generally that this estimator, $\hat{B}_1(t)$, is always the same as the Nelson-Aalen estimator?

166   5. Additive Hazards Models

(c) Determine
$$X^-(t) = (X(t)^T W(t) X(t))^{-1} X(t)^T W(t),$$
where $W_i(t) = I(Y_i(t) > 0)/\lambda_i(t)$. Comment on the estimator $\hat{B}_1(t)$ that is obtained now. Note by the way that $W_i(t)$ is set to $W_i(t) = Y_i(t)/\lambda_i(t)$ in Chapter 5, which is the same as above in the case where $Y_i(t)$ is an at risk indicator.

5.3 (Melanoma-data) In this exercise, we wish to apply the additive Aalen model to the melanoma data. We consider the effect of sex, ulceration and log(thickness).

(a) Consider first only the covariate sex using the Aalen additive model with unweighted generalized inverse of $X(t)$. The covariate sex (X_i) is coded as 1 if the ith individual is a male and 0 otherwise. Show that the estimators obtained in this situation, $\hat{B}_1(t)$ and $\hat{B}_1(t) + \hat{B}_2(t)$, are the Nelson-Aalen estimators for the female and male groups, respectively. Now fit the Aalen additive model in this situation using the aalen-function. What is the conclusion regarding the effect of sex based on this analyis?

(b) Include now also the covariates ulceration and log(thickness) into the analysis. Specify the Aalen additive model in this situation, and fit it to the data.

(c) Simplify the model as appropriate focusing first on time-varying effects of the covariates. Specify a final model. Has your conclusion regarding the effect of sex changed?

5.4 (Melanoma data. Excess and relative mortality) In this exercise we shall compare the mortality of the melanoma patients to the population mortality. The population mortality $\mu_i(t)$ (taking into account age and sex) obtained from life tables published by the Danish Central Bureau of Statistics (Table A.2 in Andersen et al. (1993), p. 714). The melanoma data and the associated population mortality are given in the dataset mela.pop in the timereg-package. Let $\alpha_i(t)$ be the hazard rate t years after operation for the ith patient. The models for relative mortality
$$\alpha_i(t) = \alpha(t)\mu_i(t) \qquad (5.57)$$
and for excess mortality
$$\alpha_i(t) = \gamma(t) + \mu_i(t) \qquad (5.58)$$

with $\mu_i(t)$ the population mortality are both contained in the model

$$\alpha_i(t) = \gamma(t) + \alpha(t)\mu_i(t), \qquad (5.59)$$

as noted by Andersen & Væth (1989).

(a) Argue that the model (5.59) is an example of Aalen's additive hazards model.

(b) The Table A.2 in Andersen et al. (1993) gives, as described above, the population mortality $\mu_i(t)$ taking into account age and sex. Think about how the data set mela.pop is prepared so that the model (5.59) can be fitted using the aalen-function from timereg using the id-option. Explain the first 10 lines in the data set mela.pop.

(c) Use the model (5.59) to investigate (using the data in mela.pop) whether the models (5.57) and (5.58) provide a sufficient description to the melanoma data [simplify first to an appropriate semiparametric version of the additive Aalen model].

(d) Formulate and investigate the hypothesis that the mortality for the melanoma patients are identical to the general Danish population.

5.5 (Aalen, 1993) Consider n i.i.d.

$$(N_i(t), Y_i(t), X_i)$$

with $X_i = (X_{i1}, \ldots, X_{ip})$ so that $N_i(t)$ has intensity

$$\lambda_i(t) = Y_i(t)(\beta_0(t) + \beta_1(t)X_{i1} + \cdots + \beta_p(t)X_{ip}).$$

(a) Show that the vector of martingale residuals processes

$$M_{\text{res}}(t) = N(t) - \int_0^t X(s)d\hat{B}(s),$$

where $X(t)$ is the design matrix and $\hat{B}(t)$ denotes the usual least squares estimator of $B(t) = \int_0^t \beta(s)\,ds$, is a (vector) martingale.

(b) Show that

$$X(0)^T M_{\text{res}}(\tau) = 0,$$

meaning that there are no linear trends in the martingale residuals with respect to the covariates.

5. Additive Hazards Models

5.6 (Tests in Aalen's additive hazards model)   Consider n i.i.d.
$$(N_i(t), Y_i(t), X_i)$$
with $X_i = (X_{i1}, \ldots, X_{ip})$ so that $N_i(t)$ has intensity
$$\lambda_i(t) = Y_i(t)(\beta_0(t) + \beta_1(t)X_{i1} + \cdots + \beta_p(t)X_{ip}),$$
that is, Aalen's additive intensity model is assumed.

(a) Show that the unweighted least squares estimator of $B(t)$ may be written as
$$\hat{B}(t) = \int (X_Y(t)^T G(t) X_Y(t))^{-1} X_Y(t)^T G(t) dN(t),$$
where $X_Y(t)$ is the $n \times p$-matrix with ith row $Y_i(t)(X_{i1}, \ldots, X_{ip})$, and $G(t) = I - 1(t)1^-(t)$ with $1(t) = (Y_1(t), \ldots, Y_n(t))^T$ assuming in these expressions that the inverses exist.

Tests of the hypothesis
$$H_0 : \beta_j(t) = 0 \quad \text{for all } t$$
and for $j \in J \subseteq \{1, \ldots, p\}$ with $|J| = q(\leq p)$ may be based on
$$Z_j(t) = \int_0^t L_j(s) d\hat{B}_j(s),$$
where $L_j(t)$ denotes a (predictable) weight process. One choice of weight function is to take $L_j(t)$ equal to the reciprocal of the $(j+1)$th diagonal element of $(X(t)^T X(t))^{-1}$, where $X(t)$ denotes the usual design matrix of the Aalen model.

(b) Derive, under H_0, the asymptotic distribution of
$$T(t) = Z(t)^T \hat{\Sigma}(t)^{-1} Z(t),$$
where $Z(t) = (Z_1, \ldots Z_p(t))^T$,
$$\hat{\Sigma}(t) = \int_0^t \text{diag}(L(s)) d[\hat{B}](s) \text{diag}(L(s))$$
with $\text{diag}(L(t))$ the diagonal matrix with jth diagonal element equal to $L_j(t)$.

Consider now the situation where we have three treatments and want to judge their effects on survival. We then have $p = 2$ and the covariates are indicator variables of two of the three treatments. A somewhat unpleasant property is that the value of the above test depends on which group is taken as the baseline if the applied weight functions vary with groups.

(c) Show by a direct calculation that the value of the test statistic $T(t)$ depends on which group is taken as the baseline group in the case where the weight functions vary with groups (as for example the weight function described above).

We finally consider the situation where one wishes to test that a factor leads to constant excess risk for all groups.

(d) Make precise suggestions for what hypotheses that may be of interest.

(e) Suggest a test-statistic that can evaluate the hypotheses, and think about alternative parameterizations and the consequences thereof.

5.7 (Tests for H_{01} and H_{02}) Consider n i.i.d. $(N_i(t), Y_i(t), X_i)$ with $X_i = (X_{i1}, \ldots, X_{ip})$ so that $N_i(t)$ has intensity

$$\lambda_i(t) = Y_i(t)(\beta_0(t) + \beta_1(t)X_{i1} + \cdots + \beta_p(t)X_{ip}),$$

that is, Aalen's additive intensity model is assumed. Let $\hat{B}$ denote the Aalen estimator of the cumulative regression functions for the Aalen additive intensity model.

(a) Consider the two test statistics for H_{01}:

$$\sup_{t \in [0,\tau]} |\hat{B}(t)| \quad \sup_{s,t \in [0,\tau]} |\hat{B}(s) - \hat{B}(t)|.$$

Derive the asymptotic distribution of the two test-statistics under H_{01} (use the continuous mapping theorem).

(b) Answer the same question for two test statistics for H_{02}:

$$\sup_{t \in [0,\tau]} |\hat{B}(t) - \hat{B}(\tau)/\tau| \quad \sup_{s,t \in [0,\tau]} |(\hat{B}(s) - \hat{B}(t)) - (s-t)\hat{B}(\tau)/\tau|.$$

5.8 (An alternative estimator for the semiparametric model) Consider n i.i.d. $(N_i(t), Y_i(t), X_i, Z_i)$ so that $N_i(t)$ has intensity

$$\lambda_i(t) = X_i^T(t)\beta(t) + Z_i^T(t)\gamma,$$

on the semiparametric risk form. One may consider the joint covariate vector $\tilde{X}_i = (X_i, Z_i)$ and fit the larger model

$$\lambda_i(t) = Y_i(t)\tilde{X}_i^T(t)\alpha(t).$$

Then $A(t) = \int_0^t \alpha(s)ds$ may be estimated by $\hat{A}$ the Aalen estimator of the cumulative regression functions. We denote the coefficients related to X by A_1 and the coefficients related to Z by A_2, such that $A = (A_1, A_2)$, and $\hat{A} = (\hat{A}_1, \hat{A}_2)$.

(a) To estimate γ of the semiparametric model one may use

$$\tilde{\gamma}_w = \int_0^\tau w(t) d\hat{A}_2(s),$$

where $w(t)$ denote a weight matrix. Derive the asymptotic distribution of $\tilde{\gamma}$, and find the optimal weights.

(b) Show that $\tilde{\gamma}_w$ for the right choice of w may be efficient.

(c) Which estimator would you expect to be superior. Do a small simulation study that compares the performance of the unweighted $\hat{\gamma}$ (5.32) and the un-weighted γ_w.

5.9 (K-cumulative residual processes) Consider n i.i.d. $(N_i(t), Y_i(t), X_i)$ so that $N_i(t)$ has intensity

$$\lambda_i(t) = X_i^T(t)\beta(t).$$

Define, a $n \times m$-matrix, $K(t)$. The K-cumulative residual process is then defined as

$$M_K(t) = \int_0^t K^T(s) d\hat{M}(s) = \int_0^t K^T(s) G(s) dM(s).$$

(a) Derive the asymptotic distribution of M_K and provide a consistent estimator of its variance under Condition 5.1.

(b) Show that the resampling version given in Section 5.7 has the same asymptotic distribution as M_K and that the (5.55) is a consistent estimator of its variance.

5.10 (Constant additive regression effects (Lin & Ying, 1994)) Consider the multivariate counting process $N = (N_1, \ldots N_n)^T$ so that $N_i(t)$ has intensity

$$\lambda_i(t) = Y_i(t)(\alpha_0(t) + \beta^T Z_i)$$

where the covariates Z_i, $i = 1, \ldots, n$ (p-vectors) are contained in the given filtration, $Y_i(t)$ is the usual at risk indicator, $\alpha_0(t)$ is locally integrable baseline intensity and β denotes a p-vector of regression parameters. Let $M_i(t) = N_i(t) - \Lambda_i(t)$, $i = 1, \ldots, n$, where $\Lambda_i(t) = \int_0^t \lambda_i(s)\,ds$. Define also $N.(t) = \sum_{i=1}^n N_i(t)$, $Y.(t) = \sum_{i=1}^n Y_i(t)$, og $A_0(t) = \int_0^t \alpha_0(s)\,ds$. The processes are observed in the interval $[0, \tau]$ with $\tau < \infty$.

(a) Suppose first that β is known. Explain why a natural estimator of $A_0(t)$ is

$$\hat{A}_0(t,\beta) = \int_0^t \frac{1}{Y_.(s)} dN_.(s) - \sum_{i=1}^n \int_0^t \frac{Y_i(s)}{Y_.(s)} \beta^T Z_i(s)\, ds, \quad (5.60)$$

where $Y_i(t)/Y_.(t)$ is defined as 0 if $Y_.(t) = 0$.

By mimicking the Cox-partial score function the following estimating function for estimation of β is obtained:

$$U(\beta) = \sum_{i=1}^n \int_0^\tau Z_i(t)\, (dN_i(t) - Y_i(t)\, d\hat{A}_0(t,\beta) - Y_i(t)\beta^T Z_i(t)\, dt),$$

in the case where β again is supposed unknown.

(b) Show that the above estimating function can be written

$$U(\beta) = \sum_{i=1}^n \int_0^\tau (Z_i(t) - \overline{Z}(t))(dN_i(t) - Y_i(t)\beta^T Z_i(t)\, dt),$$

where

$$\overline{Z}(t) = \sum_{i=1}^n Y_i(t) Z_i(t) \Big/ \sum_{i=1}^n Y_i(t).$$

(c) The value of β that satisfies $U(\beta) = 0$ is denoted $\hat{\beta}$. Show that

$$\hat{\beta} = \Big(\sum_{i=1}^n \int_0^\tau Y_i(t)(Z_i(t) - \overline{Z}(t))^{\otimes 2}\, dt\Big)^{-1} \Big(\sum_{i=1}^n \int_0^\tau (Z_i(t) - \overline{Z}(t))\, dN_i(t)\Big), \quad (5.61)$$

when $\sum_{i=1}^n \int_0^\tau Y_i(t)(Z_i(t) - \overline{Z}(t))^{\otimes 2}\, dt$ is assumed to be regular.

(d) Show that $U(\beta)$ can be written as $U(\beta) = \tilde{M}(\tau)$, where

$$\tilde{M}(t) = \sum_{i=1}^n \int_0^t (Z_i(s) - \overline{Z}(s))\, dM_i(s),$$

and that $\tilde{M}(t)$ is a (local) square integrable martingale and find its predictable variation process.

(e) Show, under suitable conditions, that $n^{-\frac{1}{2}} U(\beta)$ converges in distribution towards a p-dimensional normal distribution for $n \to \infty$, and identify the mean and variance. Show that the variance is estimated consistently by

$$B = \frac{1}{n} \sum_{i=1}^n \int_0^\tau (Z_i(t) - \overline{Z}(t))^{\otimes 2}\, dN_i(t).$$

172   5. Additive Hazards Models

(f) Show that

$$n^{1/2}(\hat{\beta} - \beta) = \Big(\frac{1}{n}\sum_{i=1}^n \int_0^\tau Y_i(t)(Z_i(t) - \overline{Z}(t))^{\otimes 2}\, dt\Big)^{-1}\big(n^{-\frac{1}{2}}U(\beta)\big),$$

and, under suitable conditions, that this stochastic variable converges in distribution towards a p-dimensional normal for $n \to \infty$. Identify the mean and variance of the limit distribution, and show that the variance is estimated consistently by $A^{-1}BA^{-1}$, where

$$A = \frac{1}{n}\sum_{i=1}^n \int_0^\tau Y_i(t)(Z_i(t) - \overline{Z}(t))^{\otimes 2}\, dt.$$

The above estimator (5.61) corresponds to (5.32) with $W(t) = I$.

5.11 (Additive hazard breakpoint model, Chen et al. (2002)) Let T be a failure time, U the latent treatment effectiveness lag time, and $Z = (W^T, R^T)^T$ a p-vector of covariates. Assume that the conditional hazard function for the failure time T given Z and U is

$$\lambda(t\,|\,Z, U) = \lambda_0(t) + \gamma^T R + I(U \le t)\beta^T W,$$

where $\theta = (\beta^T, \gamma^T)^T$ is a p-vector of regression parameters and $\lambda_0(t)$ is an unknown baseline hazard function. The above hazard function is $\lambda_0(t) + \gamma^T R$ before U and $\lambda_0(t) + \gamma^T R + \beta^T W$ after, and β therefore characterizes the full effect of W (treatment) after the individual (unobserved) lag time.

(a) Show that the observed hazard function has the form

$$\lambda(t\,|\,Z) = \lambda_0(t) + \gamma^T R + \beta^T W H(t),$$

so the additive hazard structure is preserved. In the above display

$$H(t) = \frac{\int_0^t \exp\left(-\beta^T W(t-u)\right) dG(u)}{\int_0^t \exp\left(-\beta^T W(t-u)\right) dG(u) + 1 - G(u)}$$

with G denoting the distribution function of U.

Suppose G is known.

(b) Derive estimating equations for estimation of (γ, β).

5.12 (Semiparametric model)

(a) Work out expressions for the theoretical values of the variance for (5.32) and (5.33).

(b) Construct an estimator of the covariance between (5.32) and (5.33), and show it is consistent.

(c) Derive the asymptotic distribution of the alternative estimators for the semiparametric model given by (5.43) and (5.44).

(d) Validate that the estimator $\hat{B}(t)$ from Example 5.3.2 is equivalent to the least squares estimator for the model
$$\lambda_i(t) = (X_i(t), Z_i(t))^T (\alpha(t), \eta(t)).$$

5.13 (Estimating the survival function) Assume that we observe n i.i.d. subjects in the time period from $[0, \tau]$ that are assumed to originate as outcomes from the semiparametric risk model. We start by computing the usual un-weighted estimates $\hat{B}$ and $\hat{\gamma}$. Consider a subject with covariates X_0 and Z_0 that for simplicity do not depend on time.

(a) Show that the mapping
$$S_0(B, \gamma, t) = \exp(-X_0^T B(t) - t Z_0^T \gamma)$$
is a continuously differentiable mapping and that the functional delta method can be applied to derive the asymptotic distribution of S_0.

(b) Show that the resampling scheme is on the form given in equation (5.50) leads to the same asymptotic distribution and the squared residual process is a consistent estimator of the variance of S_0.

(c) Give an explicit formulae for the optional variation based estimator of the variance of $\hat{S}_0 - S_0$.

6
Multiplicative hazards models

In the previous chapter we studied hazards models where the effect of covariates were modeled on an additive scale. In some cases it may be more appropriate with models where the effect of covariates are modeled on a multiplicative scale. The multiplicative hazards models encompass the famous proportional hazards model, or the Cox model as it is also called. The Cox model was introduced by Cox (1972) in the context of survival data, and Andersen & Gill (1982) extended it to the counting process framework and gave elegant martingale proofs for the asymptotic properties of the associated estimators, which we return to later in this chapter. Others that have contributed to establishing asymptotic results for the model are Tsiatis (1981) and Næs (1982).

The Cox model assumes that the intensity is of the form

$$\lambda(t) = Y(t)\lambda_0(t)\exp(X^T(t)\beta) \qquad (6.1)$$

where $X(t) = (X_1(t), ..., X_p(t))$ is a p-dimensional bounded predictable covariate vector and $Y(t)$ is the at risk indicator. In principle $Y(t)$ may be any locally bounded predictable process but we think of it as the at risk indicator. The parameters of the model are the p-dimensional regression parameter β and the nonparametric baseline intensity function $\lambda_0(t)$ that is assumed to be locally integrable: $\int_0^\tau \lambda_0(t)\,dt < \infty$ with τ denoting the timepoint where the study is stopped. The intensity $\lambda(t)$ for an individual with covariate vector equal to zero is $\lambda_0(t)$, which explains why it is called the baseline intensity. It is important to realize that no structure is imposed on $\lambda_0(t)$, which gives the model a great deal of flexibility. In a survival study

176   6. Multiplicative hazards models

it means that no assumption is made on the distribution of the lifetimes of the baseline population (those with zero covariate values).

A key assumption in (6.1) is that the relative risks are constant with time. Consider for a moment the special case where $p = 1$ and X_1 is time-invariant, for example a treatment indicator. The *relative risk* is the ratio

$$\frac{\lambda(t, X_1 + 1)}{\lambda(t, X_1)} = \exp(\beta_1), \tag{6.2}$$

which is seen not to depend on time because only the baseline intensity reflects dependence on time. If there is more than one covariate in the model, we get the same type of result if we compare two individuals with the same covariate vector except that they differ on X_1 (with the value 1) as above.

Example 6.0.1 (PBC-data. Continuation of Example 1.1.1)

Let us consider the PBC data again and use the Cox model with the covariates identified in Fleming & Harrington (1991) as being important: age, edema, log(bilirubin), log(albumin) and log(protime). The Cox model is easily fitted in R using the function coxph:

```
> fit.pbc<-coxph(Surv(time/365,status)~Age+Edema+logBilirubin
+ +logAlbumin+logProtime,pbc);
> fit.pbc
Call:
coxph(formula = Surv(time/365, status) ~ Age + Edema +
    logBilirubin + logAlbumin + logProtime, data = pbc)


              coef  exp(coef) se(coef)       z       p
Age         0.0383     1.0390  0.00768    4.98 6.2e-07
Edema       0.6599     1.9345  0.20588    3.21 1.4e-03
logBilirubin 0.8971    2.4525  0.08269   10.85 0.0e+00
logAlbumin  -2.4574    0.0857  0.65733   -3.74 1.9e-04
logProtime   2.3489   10.4736  0.77408    3.03 2.4e-03

Likelihood ratio test=234  on 5 df, p=0  n= 418
```

The estimated regression coefficients (the $\hat{\beta}$'s) are given in the first column of the output from coxph and the estimated relative risks in the second column. The covariate edema is binary with the value 1 for an individual with presence of edema (swelling). Thus, comparing two individuals that have the same covariate values except on edema gives an estimated effect of edema (controlled for the other covariates) in terms of the relative risk that is estimated to 1.979. So, keeping the value of the other covariates fixed, presence of edema almost doubles the risk (relying for the moment on the assumption that the Cox model gives a satisfactory fit to the data). This result is significant according to the associated p-value (we return to how this value is computed in a moment). Similar interpretation can be given for the other covariates. Age is given in months, so increasing age by one month gives an estimated relative risk of 1.037 (still keeping everything else fixed), and so on. □

The assumption that the relative risks are constant with time may be reasonable in some settings but fails in others. The Cox model may thus not reflect all important aspects of the data and may even give misleading summaries. It is therefore important to have good diagnostic tools to check the adequacy of the model in specific applications; we return to goodness-of fit tools later in this chapter. The fit of the model, however, is typically not examined that carefully in practice. The PBC data are one example of data that are not well described by the Cox model in its simplest form because of the strongly time-varying effect of some of the covariates, see Example 6.0.2 below.

A natural extension of the Cox model to accommodate time-varying covariate effects is

$$\lambda(t) = Y(t)\lambda_0(t)\exp(X^T(t)\beta(t)), \tag{6.3}$$

where $\beta(t) = (\beta_1(t), ..., \beta_p(t))$ is a p-dimensional time-varying regression coefficient that satisfies certain smoothness conditions. This model has been studied by a number of authors, e.g., Zucker & Karr (1990), Murphy & Sen (1991), Grambsch & Therneau (1994), and more recently by Pons (2000), Martinussen et al. (2002), Cai & Sun (2003) and Winnett & Sasieni (2003).

The extended version (6.3) of the Cox model is very flexible and can be derived as a first order Taylor series expansion of the log of a general conditional intensity given covariates. The flexibility of model (6.3) may in some situations not be needed for all covariates, however. Therefore we also consider the important semiparametric version of the model:

$$\lambda(t) = Y(t)\lambda_0(t)\exp(X^T(t)\beta(t) + Z^T(t)\gamma), \tag{6.4}$$

where $(X(t), Z(t))$ is a $(p+q)$-dimensional covariate and the parameters of the model are the nonparametric p-dimensional $\beta(t)$ and the q-dimensional regression parameter γ. This model was studied in Martinussen et al. (2002) and Scheike & Martinussen (2004). The semiparametric model (6.4) is as easy to fit as (6.3) and has the ability to summarize covariate effects as much as the data or subject matter suggests. For small to medium sized data the fully nonparametric version of the extended Cox model (6.3) with all covariate effects being time-varying may further be difficult to fit, and the semiparametric model can then give a more reasonable compromise between model complexity and size of the data.

Further, as we also described for the additive hazards model in Chapter 5, the semiparametric model is crucial when inferential procedures are developed. We shall consider procedures for testing if covariate effects in the semiparametric model are time-varying or time invariant, such as the hypothesis

$$H_0 : \beta_p(t) = \gamma_{q+1}.$$

Investigating this hypothesis amounts to comparing the fit of the two semiparametric models

$$\lambda(t) = Y(t)\lambda_0(t) \exp(X^T(t)\beta(t) + Z^T(t)\gamma)$$

and

$$\tilde{\lambda}(t) = Y(t)\lambda_0(t) \exp(X_1(t)\beta_1(t)+...+X_{p-1}(t)\beta_{p-1}(t)+X_p(t)\gamma_{q+1}+Z^T(t)\gamma).$$

It turns out, as for the additive hazards model, that the cumulative regression function

$$B(t) = \int_0^t \beta(s)\, ds$$

is easy to estimate and well suited for inference. With such inferential procedures to compare the above two semiparametric models we can do successive testing of time-varying effects. For a given dataset we may start with the model where all effects are allowed to be time-varying. Using that model we may then investigate for each of the covariates whether their effects could be time-invariant. If this is acceptable for at least one of them, we go on with the reduced model where this covariate has time-invariant effect while the others are still allowed to have time-varying effects. Using the simplified model, the question about time-invariance is then investigated again for the remaining variables with possible time-varying effects, and so on until further simplification of the model is unacceptable. We illustrate this procedure using the PBC data in the following example using the timecox-function that can be used for fitting the models (6.3) and (6.4).

Example 6.0.2 (PBC data)

Consider the PBC data. We restrict attention to the first 8 years days of the study. The reader might compare with Example 5.0.1 where we considered the Aalen additive hazards model for these data. We consider the covariates: age, edema, log(albumin), log(bilirubin) and log(protime). First we fit the flexible model with all covariates having nonparametric time-varying effects.

```
> fit<-timecox(Surv(time/365,status)~Age+Edema+logBilirubin
+ +logAlbumin+logProtime,pbc,max.time=8);
Nonparametric Multiplicative Hazard Model
Simulations start N= 1000
> plot(fit,ylab="Cumulative coefficients",xlab="Time (years)");
> summary(fit)
```

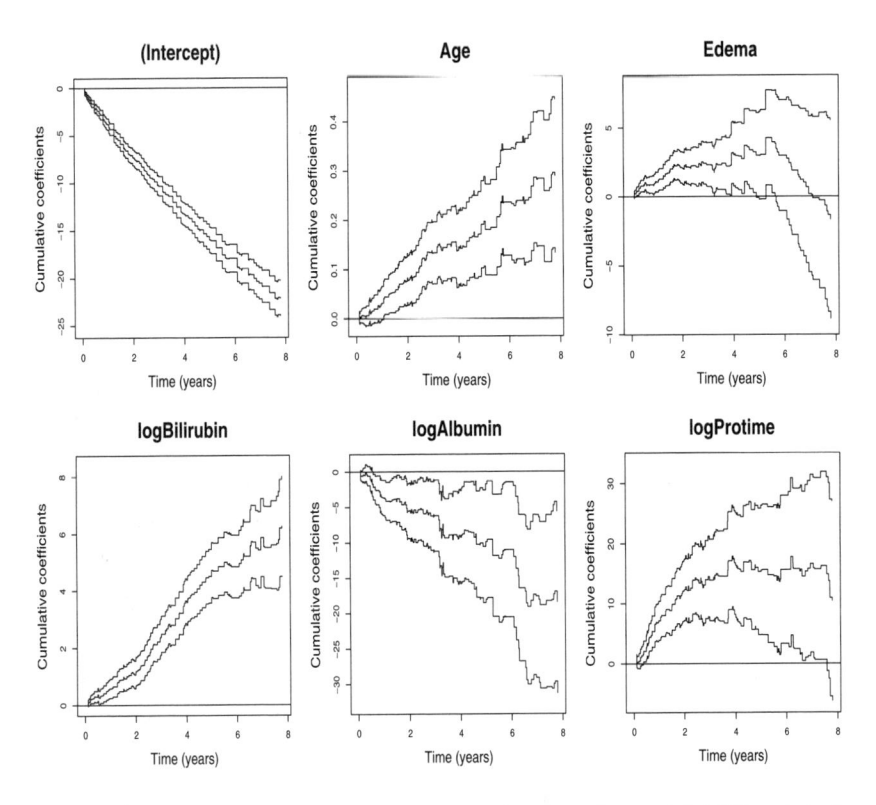

FIGURE 6.1: Estimated cumulative regression functions with 95% pointwise confidence intervals.

```
Multiplicative Hazard Model

Test for nonparametric terms

Test for non-significant effects
            sup| hat B(t)/SD(t) | p-value H_0: B(t)=0
(Intercept)           43.40                0.000
Age                    4.52                0.000
Edema                  4.32                0.001
logBilirubin          10.40                0.000
logAlbumin             5.15                0.000
logProtime             6.24                0.000
Test for time invariant effects
            sup| B(t) - (t/tau)B(tau)| p-value H_0: B(t)=b t
(Intercept)           2.0700               0.000
Age                   0.0353               0.940
Edema                 5.4000               0.000
logBilirubin          0.7170               0.559
logAlbumin            3.4200               0.851
```

180   6. Multiplicative hazards models

```
logProtime                          12.7000                       0.004
```

	int (B(t)-(t/tau)B(tau))^2dt	p-value H_0: B(t)=b t
(Intercept)	1.79e+01	0.000
Age	1.29e-03	0.976
Edema	7.41e+01	0.000
logBilirubin	9.16e-01	0.478
logAlbumin	1.12e+01	0.943
logProtime	5.28e+02	0.000

The output contains information about the nonparametric effects and Figure 6.1 displays the estimated cumulative regression coefficients with 95% pointwise confidence intervals. Later in this chapter we return to how these are actually computed.

The cumulative estimates with the pointwise confidence intervals clearly indicate that all effects are significant, and this is also reflected by the supremum test for significant effects in the output. The p-value for the significance of edema, for example, is p=0.001.

The tests for time-invariant effects shows that some of the effects are well described by constant effects. Two tests are computed and we here focus on the supremum test and return later to a discussion of the integrated squared difference test. The supremum test for time invariant effects shows that age (p=0.940), and log(albumin) (p=0.851) are well described by constant multiplicative effects. We therefore consider the model where log(albumin) has constant effect (output not shown) and for this model it is found that age (p=0.98) and log(bilirubin) (p=0.29) have a constant effect. Now considering the model with age and log(albumin) having constant effects and testing for constant effect of log(bilirubin) gives the p-value of 0.303. We therefore fit the model where age, log(albumin) and log(bilirubin) have constant effects while the other effects are allowed to be time-varying.

```
> fit.semi<-timecox(Surv(time/365,status)~const(Age)+Edema
+ +const(logBilirubin)+const(logAlbumin)+logProtime,
+ pbc,max.time=8)
Semiparametric Multiplicative Risk Model
Simulations start N= 1000
> summary(fit.semi)
Multiplicative Hazard Model

Test for nonparametric terms

Test for non-significant effects
             sup| hat B(t)/SD(t) |  p-value H_0: B(t)=0
(Intercept)                32.10                      0
Edema                       4.58                      0
logProtime                  5.50                      0
Test for time invariant effects
```

```
                sup| B(t) - (t/tau)B(tau)|  p-value H_0: B(t)=b t
(Intercept)                       2.08                     0.000
Edema                             5.09                     0.000
logProtime                       12.40                     0.006

                int (B(t)-(t/tau)B(tau))^2dt  p-value H_0: B(t)=b t
(Intercept)                      19.4                      0.000
Edema                            72.8                      0.000
logProtime                      508.0                      0.001

Parametric terms :
                         Coef.       SE    Robust SE     z    P-val
const(Age)              0.0377   0.00931    0.00921    4.05  5.2e-05
const(logBilirubin)     0.8210   0.09840    0.08200    8.34  0.0e+00
const(logAlbumin)      -2.4500   0.67300    0.60600   -3.64  2.7e-04
```

The fit of the semiparametric model, which has been validated by successive testing, shows that edema and log(protime) have effects that are significantly time-varying (p<0.001 and p=0.006) and that the effects are significant (p<0.001 and p<0.001).

The constant log-relative risk of age, log(bilirubin) and log(albumin) are estimated to (with estimated se's in parenthesis) 0.038 (0.009), 0.821 (0.098) and -2.450 (0.673), respectively. Note that these effects fits well with the slopes of the cumulative coefficients in Figure 6.1. Compare also with the output from the Cox regression analysis given in Example 6.0.1. □

6.1 The Cox model

The Cox regression model is by far the most used regression model for counting process data, and has been studied in an enormous number of papers. It assumes that the intensity is of the form

$$\lambda(t) = Y(t)\lambda_0(t)\exp(X^T(t)\beta), \qquad (6.5)$$

where $X(t) = (X_1(t), ..., X_p(t))$ is a p-dimensional bounded predictable covariate and $Y(t)$ is an at risk indicator. The parameters of the model are the p-dimensional regression parameter β and the nonparametric locally integrable baseline hazard function $\lambda_0(t)$. A key assumption is as mentioned earlier that the relative risks are constant with time, see (6.2).

In the following we show how to estimate the log-relative risk parameter β and the cumulative baseline hazard function $\Lambda_0(t) = \int_0^t \lambda_0(s)ds$, and describe the asymptotic properties of these estimators based on i.i.d. replicates from the Cox model. Assume thus that n independent copies

182   6. Multiplicative hazards models

$(N_i(t), Y_i(t), X_i(t))$, $i = 1, \ldots, n$, are being observed in some time interval $[0, \tau]$, $\tau < \infty$, and that each $N_i(t)$ has intensity on the Cox form (6.5).

The regression parameter β is estimated as the maximizer to Cox's partial likelihood function (Cox, 1972, 1975)

$$L(\beta) = \prod_t \prod_i \left(\frac{\exp\left(X_i^T(t)\beta\right)}{S_0(t, \beta)} \right)^{\Delta N_i(t)}, \qquad (6.6)$$

where

$$S_0(t, \beta) = \sum_{i=1}^n Y_i(t) \exp(X_i^T(t)\beta).$$

Define the first and second order partial derivative of $S_0(t, \beta)$ with respect to β:

$$S_1(t, \beta) = \sum_{i=1}^n Y_i(t) \exp(X_i^T(t)\beta) X_i(t),$$

$$S_2(t, \beta) = \sum_{i=1}^n Y_i(t) \exp(X_i^T(t)\beta) X_i(t)^{\otimes 2}.$$

The estimator $\hat{\beta}$ is thus found as the solution to the score equation $U(\hat{\beta}) = 0$, where

$$U(\beta) = \sum_{i=1}^n \int_0^\tau (X_i(t) - E(t, \beta)) dN_i(t) \qquad (6.7)$$

with

$$E(t, \beta) = \frac{S_1(t, \beta)}{S_0(t, \beta)}.$$

There are several ways of arriving at (6.6) and (6.7) as natural estimation functions, some of which we describe below.

An appealing interpretation of (6.6) is that it can be seen as profile likelihood function where the cumulative baseline hazard function has been profiled out. If the value of β is fixed then a natural estimator of $\Lambda_0(t)$ is the Nelson-Aalen type estimator

$$\hat{\Lambda}_0(t, \beta) = \int_0^t \frac{1}{S_0(s, \beta)} dN_\cdot(s), \qquad (6.8)$$

where $N_\cdot(t) = \sum_i N_i(t)$. The estimator (6.8) can be interpreted as the maximizer, for fixed value of β, of the likelihood function

$$\prod_t \prod_i \left((d\Lambda_0(t) \exp(X_i(t)\beta))^{\Delta N_i(t)} \right) \exp\left(-\int_0^\tau S_0(t, \beta) d\Lambda_0(t) \right) \qquad (6.9)$$

with respect to the jumps $\Delta \Lambda_0(t)$. Replacing $d\Lambda_0(t)$ in (6.9) with $d\hat{\Lambda}_0(t, \beta)$ gives Cox's partial likelihood function (6.6).

6.1 The Cox model

The score function (6.7), which is the derivative of $\log L(\beta)$ with respect to β, may also be obtained from a least squares principle. Let

$$N(t) = (N_1(t), .., N_n(t))^T$$

denote the multivariate counting process with intensity

$$\lambda(t) = (\lambda_1(t), ..., \lambda_n(t))^T,$$

and organize the covariates into a design matrix of dimension $n \times p$:

$$X(t) = (Y_1(t)X_1(t), ..., Y_n(t)X_n(t))^T.$$

Further denote the n-dimensional cumulative intensities as $\Lambda(t) = \int_0^t \lambda(s)ds$ such that $M(t) = N(t) - \Lambda(t)$ is a n-dimensional (local square integrable) martingale. The martingale decomposition of $dN(t)$ then reads

$$dN(t) = \lambda(t)dt + dM(t) = \text{diag}(\exp(X_i^T(t)\beta))Y(t)d\Lambda_0(t) + dM(t), \quad (6.10)$$

where

$$Y(t) = (Y_1(t), ..., Y_n(t))^T$$

is the at-risk vector. Since the increments of the martingale are uncorrelated and have mean 0, equation (6.10) suggests that estimation of $\lambda_0(t)dt$ and β can be done by considering the least squares score equations

$$\int X^T \text{diag}(\lambda_i) W_1 \{dN - \text{diag}(\exp(X_i^T\beta))Y d\Lambda_0\} = 0, \quad (6.11)$$

$$Y^T \text{diag}(\exp(X_i^T\beta)) W_2 \{dN - \text{diag}(\exp(X_i^T\beta))Y d\Lambda_0\} = 0, \quad (6.12)$$

where $W_1(t)$ and $W_2(t)$ are diagonal weight matrices, and where we have suppressed the dependency on time in the display. It may be shown that the optimal choice of $W_1(t)$ and $W_2(t)$ is $\text{diag}(Y_i(t)/\lambda_i(t))$. The least squares score equations (6.11) and (6.12) can be solved successively as follows. Solving (6.12) for fixed β gives

$$\tilde{\Lambda}_0(t) = \int_0^t Y^-(s)dN(s), \quad (6.13)$$

where $Y^-(t)$ is the generalized inverse

$$Y^-(t) = (Y^T(t)\text{diag}(\exp(X_i^T(t)\beta))Y(t))^{-1}Y^T(t)$$

of $Y(t)$. Observe that (6.13) is equal to (6.8). We make the convention that $Y^-(t)$ is 0 when the inverse does not exist. Inserting this solution into (6.11) and solving for β gives

$$\int X^T(t)(dN(t) - \text{diag}(\exp(X_i^T(t)\beta))Y(t)Y^-(t)dN(t)) = 0, \quad (6.14)$$

6. Multiplicative hazards models

which is nothing but $U(\beta) = 0$.

Given $\hat{\beta}$, as the solution to $U(\beta) = 0$, we estimate $\Lambda_0(t)$ from (6.8) by the Breslow estimator

$$\hat{\Lambda}_0(t) = \hat{\Lambda}_0(t, \hat{\beta}) = \int_0^t \frac{1}{S_0(s, \hat{\beta})} dN.(s). \tag{6.15}$$

Before we describe the asymptotic properties of these estimators we need some conditions taken from Andersen & Gill (1982). Let minus the derivative of the score with respect to β be denoted by $I(\beta) = I(\tau, \beta)$, where

$$I(t, \beta) = \sum_{i=1}^n \int_0^t \left(\frac{S_2(s, \beta)}{S_0(s, \beta)} - E(s, \beta)^{\otimes 2} \right) dN_i(s)$$

$$= \int_0^t V(s, \beta) dN.(s) \tag{6.16}$$

with

$$V(t, \beta) = \frac{S_2(t, \beta)}{S_0(t, \beta)} - E(t, \beta)^{\otimes 2}. \tag{6.17}$$

We use the notation β_0 to denote true value of β defining the Cox model (6.5).

Condition 6.1 There exists a neighborhood $\mathcal{B}$ of β_0 so that

(a) $E\left[\sup_{t \in [0,\tau], \beta \in \mathcal{B}} Y_i(t) |X_{ij}(t) X_{ik}(t)| \exp(X_i^T(t)\beta)\right] < \infty$ for all $j, k = 1, ..., p$;

(b) $P(Y_i(t) = 1 \text{ for all } t \in [0, \tau]) > 0$;

(c) The limit in probability of $n^{-1} \int_0^\tau V(t, \beta_0) S_0(t, \beta_0) d\Lambda_0(t)$ is positive definite and is denoted Σ.

□

These conditions are sufficient to show that $\hat{\beta}$ is a consistent estimator, see Andersen & Gill (1982) and Andersen et al. (1993). The asymptotic properties of $\hat{\beta}$ needed to do inference about β_0 is given in the below theorem.

Theorem 6.1.1 If Condition 6.1 holds, then, as $n \to \infty$,

$$n^{-1/2} U(\beta_0) \xrightarrow{\mathcal{D}} N(0, \Sigma),$$

$$n^{1/2}(\hat{\beta} - \beta_0) \xrightarrow{\mathcal{D}} N(0, \Sigma^{-1}),$$

and Σ is estimated consistently by $n^{-1} I(\hat{\beta})$.

6.1 The Cox model

PROOF. The key to the proof is that the score evaluated in the true point β_0 is a (local square integrable) martingale (evaluated in τ):

$$U(\beta_0) = \sum_{i=1}^{n} \int_0^{\tau} (X_i(t) - E(t, \beta_0)) dM_i(t) \qquad (6.18)$$

since the compensator of $U(\beta_0)$ given by (6.7) is

$$\sum_{i=1}^{n} \int_0^{\tau} (X_i(t) - \frac{S_1(t, \beta_0)}{S_0(t, \beta_0)}) Y_i(t) \exp(X_i^T(t)) d\Lambda_0(t) = 0.$$

The predictable variation process of $n^{-1/2} U(\beta_0)$ is

$$\langle n^{-1/2} U(\beta_0) \rangle = n^{-1} \sum_{i=1}^{n} \int_0^{\tau} (X_i(t) - E(t, \beta_0))^{\otimes 2} Y_i(t) \exp(X_i^T(t) \beta_0) d\Lambda_0(t)$$

$$= n^{-1} \int_0^{\tau} V(t, \beta_0) S_0(t, \beta_0) d\Lambda_0(t) \xrightarrow{P} \Sigma.$$

The Lindeberg condition of the martingale CLT may also be seen to be fulfilled so it follows that $U(\beta_0)$ converges in distribution to a normal variate with zero-mean and variance Σ. Furthermore, $n^{-1} \langle U(\beta_0) \rangle$ is the compensator of $n^{-1} I(\beta_0)$ so, by Lenglart's inequality, it follows that the difference between these two converges to zero in probability. Also, $n^{-1} I(\hat{\beta}) - n^{-1} I(\beta_0)$ converges to zero in probability and $n^{-1} I(\hat{\beta})$ is thus a consistent estimator of Σ.

A Taylor series expansion of the score gives

$$n^{1/2} (\hat{\beta} - \beta_0) = (n^{-1} I(\beta^*))^{-1} n^{-1/2} U(\beta_0),$$

where β^* is on the line segment between β_0 and $\hat{\beta}$. Consistency of $\hat{\beta}$ and the results above give that $n^{1/2}(\hat{\beta} - \beta_0)$ converges to the postulated normal distribution. □

By Theorem 6.1.1 it follows directly that the *Wald test statistic*

$$(\hat{\beta} - \beta_0)^T I(\hat{\beta})(\hat{\beta} - \beta_0)$$

for test of the hypothesis $H_0 : \beta = \beta_0$ is asymptotically χ^2 with p degrees of freedom. It also holds true, using standard arguments from asymptotic theory, that the *likelihood ratio statistic*

$$-2 \log \left(\frac{L(\beta_0)}{L(\hat{\beta})} \right)$$

and the *score test statistic*

$$U(\beta_0)^T I(\beta_0)^{-1} U(\beta_0)$$

both are asymptotically χ^2 with p degrees of freedom under the null.

186   6. Multiplicative hazards models

Note. The above test statistics can be used to investigate $H_0 : \beta = \beta_0$ that is called a simple hypothesis. In practice one is rarely interested in testing all parameters equal to a fixed value, but rather testing some of the parameters equal to a fixed value leaving the remaining parameters unrestricted. The above test statistics can easily be accommodated to such a situation, which is a special case of so-called differentiable hypotheses. This is summarized below and may be shown using arguments from standard asymptotic theory for maximum likelihood estimation.

Let ϕ be a mapping from an open subset of $\mathbb{R}^q$, $q < p$, into the domain of β so that ϕ is three times continuous differentiable and the $p \times q$-matrix $D_\gamma \phi(\gamma)$ has full rank q. Write $\phi(\hat{\gamma})$ as $\hat{\phi}$. Under the (differentiable) hypothesis

$$H_0 : \beta = \phi(\gamma)$$

one may show that the likelihood ratio test statistic

$$-2 \log \left(\frac{L(\hat{\phi})}{L(\hat{\beta})} \right),$$

the Wald test statistic

$$(\hat{\beta} - \hat{\phi})^T I(\hat{\phi})(\hat{\beta} - \hat{\phi}),$$

and the score test statistic

$$U(\hat{\phi}) I(\hat{\phi})^{-1} U(\hat{\phi})$$

are asymptotically equivalent and asymptotically χ^2-distributed with $p - q$ degrees of freedom.

Example 6.1.1 (Continuation of Example 6.0.1)

Consider again the output from the Cox regression analysis in Example 6.0.1:

```
> fit.pbc<-coxph(Surv(time/365,status)~Age+Edema+logBilirubin
+logAlbumin+logProtime,pbc);
> fit.pbc
                coef exp(coef) se(coef)       z       p
Age           0.0362    1.037   0.00806    4.49 7.0e-06
Edema         0.6828    1.979   0.21483    3.18 1.5e-03
logBilirubin  0.8643    2.373   0.08493   10.18 0.0e+00
logAlbumin   -2.4641    0.085   0.67562   -3.65 2.7e-04
logProtime    2.6637   14.349   0.85476    3.12 1.8e-03

Likelihood ratio test=215  on 5 df, p=0  n= 418
```

The test made for effect of the individual covariates is the Wald-test (z^2 is the Wald test statistic). The likelihood ratio test for testing overall effect of the covariates is also given. Compare with Example 6.0.2 to find that the effect of the covariates that were well described there as having constant effects are almost equivalent to those of the standard Cox regression analysis shown above. The linear approximations based on the above estimated coefficients to the cumulative coefficients curves associated with edema and log(protime), given in Figure 6.1, are seen to be poor, however. The effect of these two covariates on survival, based on the above Cox-regression analysis, is therefore hard to interpret. □

Using martingale calculus again, one may also derive the asymptotic behavior of the Breslow-estimator. This is summarized in the following theorem.

Theorem 6.1.2 *If Condition 6.1 holds, then, as $n \to \infty$,*

$$n^{1/2}(\hat{\Lambda}_0(t,\hat{\beta}) - \Lambda_0(t)) \xrightarrow{D} U(t)$$

where $U(t)$ is a Gaussian process with zero-mean and covariance function $\Phi(t)$ that is estimated consistently by

$$n\left(\int_0^t S_0(s,\hat{\beta})^{-2} dN.(s) + \int_0^t E(s,\hat{\beta})^T d\hat{\Lambda}_0(s,\hat{\beta})(n^{-1}I(\hat{\beta}))^{-1} \int_0^t E(s,\hat{\beta}) d\hat{\Lambda}_0(s,\hat{\beta})\right).$$

PROOF. A detailed proof can be found in Andersen et al. (1993) but the following sketch makes it clear how the proof proceeds. Define $J(t) = I(S_0(t,\hat{\beta}) > 0)$. Since

$$\hat{\Lambda}_0(t,\hat{\beta}) = \int_0^t \frac{J(s)}{S_0(s,\hat{\beta})} dN.(s)$$

$$= \int_0^t \frac{J(s)}{S_0(s,\hat{\beta})} S_0(s,\beta_0) d\Lambda_0(s) + \int_0^t \frac{J(s)}{S_0(s,\hat{\beta})} dM.(s)$$

and

$$S_0(t,\hat{\beta}) - S_0(t,\beta_0) = S_1(t,\beta^*)^T(\hat{\beta} - \beta_0)$$

with β^* on the line segment between β_0 and $\hat{\beta}$, one obtains

$$n^{1/2}(\hat{\Lambda}_0(t,\hat{\beta}) - \Lambda_0(t)) = -\int_0^t J(s)E(s,\beta_0)^T d\Lambda_0(s) n^{1/2}(\hat{\beta} - \beta_0)$$

$$+ n^{-1/2} \int_0^t \frac{J(s)}{n^{-1}S_0(s,\beta_0)} dM.(s) + \epsilon(t), \quad (6.19)$$

where $\epsilon(t)$ converges to zero in probability uniformly in t. Also

$$n^{1/2}(\hat{\beta} - \beta_0) = (n^{-1}I(\beta_0))^{-1} n^{-1/2} U(\beta_0) + \tilde{\epsilon} = (n^{-1}I(\beta_0))^{-1} n^{-1/2} \tilde{M}(\tau) + \tilde{\epsilon},$$

188   6. Multiplicative hazards models

where $\tilde{\epsilon} \xrightarrow{P} 0$, and

$$\tilde{M}(t) = \sum_{i=1}^{n} \int_0^t (X_i(s) - E(s, \beta_0))dM_i(s).$$

Finally note that

$$\langle \tilde{M}, \int_0^\cdot \frac{J(s)}{S_0(s,\beta_0)} dM_\cdot(s) \rangle (t)$$
$$= \sum_{i=1}^{n} \int_0^t J(s) \frac{(X_i(s) - E(s,\beta_0))}{S_0(s,\beta_0)} Y_i(s) \exp(X_i(s)^T \beta) d\Lambda_0(s) = 0$$

so that the covariance between the two leading terms on the right hand side of (6.19) is zero. □

It is clear from (6.19) that the limit distribution of $n^{1/2}(\hat{\Lambda}_0(t, \hat{\beta}) - \Lambda_0(t))$ cannot be a Gaussian martingale due to the term $(\hat{\beta} - \beta_0)$ destroying the independent increments requirement. The estimator of the variance function may be used to construct pointwise confidence intervals but not to construct confidence bands as for example the Hall-Wellner band. Such a band may, however, be constructed using an i.i.d. decomposition of $n^{1/2}(\hat{\Lambda}_0(t, \hat{\beta}) - \Lambda_0(t))$, see Chapter 7.1 for a treatment of this in a more general setting. These band and confidence intervals may be computed using the cox-aalen function, see Appendix C, as illustrated in the below example. One may also approximate the joint asymptotic distribution of

$$\left(n^{1/2}(\hat{\beta} - \beta), n^{1/2}(\hat{\Lambda}_0(\cdot, \hat{\beta}) - \Lambda_0(\cdot))\right),$$

which is of importance when we for instance want to construct confidence band accompanying survival predictions

$$\hat{S}_{X_0}(\cdot) = \exp(-\int_0^\cdot \exp(X_0(t)^T \hat{\beta}) d\hat{\Lambda}_0(t, \hat{\beta}))$$

for an individual with covariate vector X_0, see again Chapter 7.1 for a treatment of this in a more general setting.

Example 6.1.2 (Estimated cumulative baseline function for PBC-data)

Consider again the PBC-data. We want to apply the Cox model to this dataset and further to show the estimated cumulative baseline function along with 95% confidence intervals and simulation based 95% confidence band. Recall that the baseline function $\lambda_0(t)$ is the hazard function for an individual with zero covariate values. Before applying the Cox model it may therefore be sensible to center the continuous covariates around their average value to obtain a $\lambda_0(t)$ that is the hazard function for an individual with average covariate values (for the continuous variates).

6.1 The Cox model 189

(Intercept)

[Figure: plot of Cumulative baseline function vs Time (years), with step functions and confidence intervals/bands]

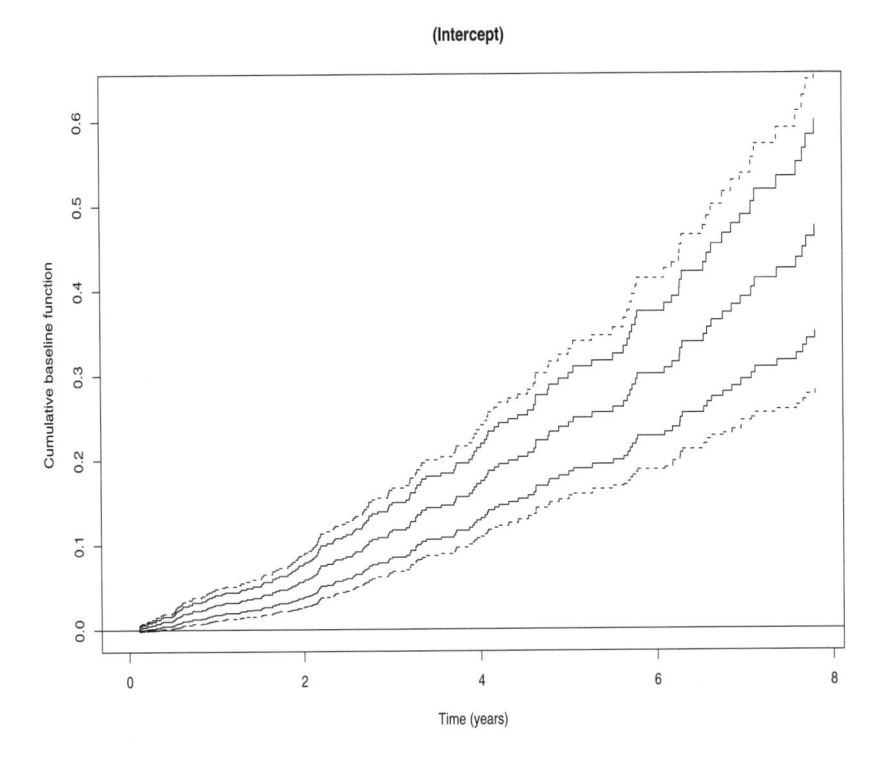

FIGURE 6.2: Estimated cumulative baseline hazard function along with 95% pointwise confidence intervals (full lines) and 95% simulation based confidence bands (broken lines)

```
> fit<-cox.aalen(Surv(time/365,status)~prop(Age)+prop(Edema)+
+ prop(logBilirubin)+prop(logAlbumin)+prop(logProtime),
+ pbc,n.sim=1000,max.time=8);
Cox-Aalen Survival Model
Simulations start N= 1000
> plot(fit,sim.ci=2,robust=0,xlab="Time (years)",
+ ylab="Cumulative baseline function")
```

The `cox.aalen` function is described in further detail later in Chapter 7.1 and can fit the Cox regression model as a special case. The shown estimated cumulative hazard function, see Figure 6.2, estimates $\Lambda_0(t) = \int_0^t \lambda_0(s)\,ds$ with $\lambda_0(t)$ the hazard function for an individual with no swelling (edema=0) and with average values for the other applied covariates. □

The asymptotic results for the estimators of the parameters of the Cox model derived above are the basis for inference. These results are asymptotic but seem to work very well also in small samples as reported in the literature where a huge amount of real datasets have been analyzed using the Cox model. Many simulation studies have also been made to investigate the performance of the estimators and their properties, and in general these results are very reassuring. The maximization of the partial likelihood function (6.6) may, however, break down in some situations. This was studied by Jacobsen (1989) who gave a necessary and sufficient condition ensuring that (6.6) attains its maximal value at a unique point $\hat{\beta}$. This is summarized in the following note.

Note. Let $t_1, \ldots, t_K$ denote the jumps of $\sum_i N_i(t)$ on $[0, \tau]$, R_j is the risk set at time t_j (includes the individual that is going to fail at t_j) and k_j is the individual that fails at t_j, $j = 1, \ldots, K$. The partial likelihood function (6.6) attains its maximal value at a unique point $\hat{\beta}$ if and only if there is no $\theta \in \mathbb{R}^p$, $\theta \neq 0$, such that for all $j, k \in R_j \setminus k_j$:

$$\sum_{l=1}^{p} \theta_l X_{kl}(t_j) \geq \sum_{l=1}^{p} \theta_l X_{k_j l}(t_j). \qquad (6.20)$$

In words, at each failure time the individual that fails must not be extreme in the risk group as described by (6.20), that is, there must be no linear combination of the p covariates such that the value of the linear combination for the failing individual exceeds or equals the value for all other at risk at that time. For the pbc-data it would be impossible to maximize the partial likelihood if the failing subject at each failure time has an extreme linear combination of the covariates used in the model. For example, at each failure time the failing subject must not have the largest value of protime among those at risk, or the sum of log(protime) and log(albumin) (using the log-transform of these covariates in the model), and so on.

As mentioned earlier the assumption that the relative risks are constant with time may not hold in practice. There are various ways of circumventing this assumption, but most of them somewhat ad hoc. Below we describe two of the most commonly applied approaches.

- If the proportional hazards assumption is questionable for a given categorical covariate, X_1, one may extend the model to the so-called *stratified Cox model*:

$$\lambda(t) = Y(t)\lambda_{0k}(t) \exp(\beta_2 X_2(t) + \cdots + \beta_p X_p(t)), \qquad (6.21)$$

when $X_1 = k$ with $k = 1, \ldots, K$ denoting the K possible values of X_1. The baseline intensity function λ_0 is thus replaced by K baseline intensity functions $\lambda_{01}, \ldots, \lambda_{0K}$, one for each strata defined by X_1. The baseline functions may reflect various nonproportional developments of the relative risks with time. If the specific covariate is continuous, this method is not really satisfying since one needs to construct the strata (more or less arbitrarily).

6.1 The Cox model 191

- A typical violation of the model in practice is time-dependent effects of the covariates. This phenomenon can actually, to a certain degree, be modeled within the Cox model by use of time-dependent covariates. Suppose for a moment that X_1 is the only covariate in the model, that it is continuous, and that it is suspected to have a time-dependent effect. Suppose further that the relative risk changes at some specific points in time as for example after one year and two years. A possible model is then the Cox model with the covariates X_1, $X_2(t) = X_1 I(1 \leq t)$ and $X_3(t) = X_1 I(2 \leq t)$. Hence

$$\beta_1 X_1 + \beta_2 X_2(t) + \beta_3 X_3(t) = \begin{cases} \beta_1 X_1 & t < 1 \\ (\beta_1 + \beta_2) X_1 & 1 \leq t < 2 \\ (\beta_1 + \beta_2 + \beta_3) X_1 & 2 \leq t \end{cases}$$

so β_2 gives the change in the interval from 1 to 2, and β_3 gives the additional change in the last interval. This approach may of course be extended to include other covariates, and may in some applications capture what is going on. The down side is that the cut points (here 1 and 2) will not be known a priori but need to be chosen in an ad hoc manner.

We now consider the situation where regression effects are estimated using Cox's maximum partial likelihood estimator but the underlying true model may not be the Cox model.

Example 6.1.3 (Misspecified proportional hazards model)

Consider the situation where some true intensity regression model holds for a particular dataset and the Cox model is fitted to the data. If the true model is not the Cox model, then what does the maximum partial likelihood estimator converge to? This was investigated by Struthers & Kalbfleisch (1986). Let $(N_1, \ldots, N_n)$ be n i.i.d. counting processes obtained from right-censored life-times. Suppose that the intensity with respect to the observed filtration is

$$Y_i(t) \alpha(t, X_i), \qquad (6.22)$$

where the covariates X_i, $i = 1, \ldots, n$, are time-invariant and contained in the given filtration and $Y_i(t)$ is the usual at risk indicator. Assume for simplicity that X_i is one-dimensional, $i = 1, \ldots, n$. Note that (6.22) needs not be of the Cox-form. Under some standard regularity conditions, Struthers & Kalbfleisch (1986) showed that Cox's maximum partial likelihood estimator $\hat{\beta}$ is a consistent estimator of β^*, where β^* is the solution to the equation $h(\beta) = 0$ with

$$h(\beta) = \int_0^\tau \left(\frac{s_1(t)}{s_0(t)} - \frac{s_1(t, \beta)}{s_0(t, \beta)} \right) s_0(t) \, dt, \qquad (6.23)$$

where $s_j(t) = E(S_j(t))$, $s_j(t, \beta) = E(S_j(t, \beta))$ with

$$S_j(t) = n^{-1} \sum_{i=1}^{n} X_i^j Y_i(t) \alpha(t, X_i), \quad S_j(t, \beta) = n^{-1} \sum_{i=1}^{n} X_i^j Y_i(t) \exp(X_i \beta),$$

$j = 0, 1$. Lin & Wei (1989) further showed that $n^{1/2}(\hat{\beta} - \beta^*)$ is asymptotically normal and gave a consistent estimator of variance-covariance matrix, see Exercise 6.7.

Note that β^* will depend on the censoring pattern due to the term $s_0(t)$ in (6.23). This led Xu & O'Quigley (2000) to consider an alternative to the Cox score equation:

$$\tilde{U}(\beta) = \sum_{i=1}^{n} \int_0^\tau W(t)(X_i - E(t, \beta)) \, dN_i(t),$$

where $W(t) = \hat{S}(t-)/\sum_i Y_i(t)$ with $\hat{S}(t-)$ the left-continuous version of the Kaplan-Meier estimator of the marginal survivor function. If the censoring is independent of the life-times and covariates, then the solution to $\tilde{U}(\beta) = 0$ will converge to a quantity $\tilde{\beta}$ that does not depend on the censoring pattern. If the true model is

$$\alpha(t, X_i) = \alpha_0(t) \exp(X_i \beta(t))$$

and the limit in probability of (6.17) evaluated in $\beta = \beta(t)$ is denoted by $v(t, \beta(t))$, then $\tilde{\beta}$ is approximately equal to

$$\frac{\int_0^\tau v(t, \beta(t)) \beta(t) \, dF(t)}{\int_0^\tau v(t, \beta(t)) \, dF(t)},$$

which may be interpreted as an weighted average of $\beta(t)$ over $[0, \tau]$. In the above display $F(t) = 1 - S(t)$. Although this approach is appealing it is usually preferable to make as few assumptions as possible about the distribution of the censoring times. Also it may seem more satisfactory to take the model with time-dependent regression coefficients as a starting point and then try to simplify the model as appropriate, see Section 6.6.

Lin (1991) also considered a weighted Cox-score function

$$U_w(\beta) = \sum_{i=1}^{n} \int_0^\tau W(t)(X_i - E(t, \beta)) \, dN_i(t),$$

where $W(t)$ is some predictable weight function. Assume that $W(t)$ converges uniformly in probability to a non-negative bounded function $w(t)$. Similarly to above one may show that the solution, $\hat{\beta}_w$, to $U_w(\beta) = 0$ converges in probability to a quantity β_w that solves the equation $h_w(\beta) = 0$ with

$$h_w(\beta) = \int_0^\tau w(t) \left(\frac{s_1(t)}{s_0(t)} - \frac{s_1(t, \beta)}{s_0(t, \beta)} \right) s_0(t) \, dt.$$

Lin (1991) then derived a test based on the asymptotic distribution of $n^{1/2}(\hat{\beta}_w - \hat{\beta})$ that is consistent against any model misspecification of the Cox model under which $h_w(\beta^*) \neq 0$, see Exercise 6.8. □

The nonparametric element, $\lambda_0(t)$, of the Cox model makes the model quite flexible and for many applications it may be a sensible model to use. In fact in applied biomedical work there seems to be just this regression model for survival data, and the biomedical researchers are so used to the model and how to interpret its parameters that they will settle for nothing else. This is somewhat unfortunate if the Cox model does not fit the data since the summaries obtained from the model can then be misleading. In any case it is pertinent to investigate whether the model gives an acceptable fit to the data (as it is for any model). This is the topic of the next section where some diagnostic tools are discussed.

6.2 Goodness-of-fit procedures for the Cox model

The Cox regression model

$$\lambda(t) = Y(t)\lambda_0(t)\exp(X^T(t)\beta)$$

can fail in various ways. The functional form of the individual covariates may be misspecified, the link function, exp, may be misspecified meaning that the relationship between the intensity function and the linear predictor $X^T(t)\beta$ may not be log-linear, and the regression coefficients may not be constant with time (the proportional hazards assumption). In practice one often encounters covariate effects, such as treatment effects, that are weakened with time.

We focus on the proportional hazards assumption that has been the study of much work. One of the simplest procedures to examine if the proportional hazards assumption is violated is to make plots of the estimated cumulative baseline hazards in the stratified model (6.21). Consider again the stratified model where the stratification is based on $X_1(t)$:

$$\lambda(t) = Y(t)\lambda_{0k}(t)\exp(\beta_2 X_2(t) + \cdots + \beta_p X_p(t)),$$

when $X_1(t) = k$ with $k = 1, \ldots, K$ denoting the K possible strata. If the Cox model is correct, then the estimated cumulative baselines $\hat{\Lambda}_{0k}(t)$ of the stratified Cox model should be approximately proportional. One usually make the plots $(t, \log(\hat{\Lambda}_{0k}(t)))$, $k = 1, \ldots, K$, noting that these curves should be approximately parallel. These plots may be quite difficult to use in practice, however, since it is unclear how large deviations from the null (parallel curves) are acceptable. An improvement to this procedure is instead to plot the differences between these curves because these can fairly easy be provided with confidence intervals as illustrated in the next example.

194   6. Multiplicative hazards models

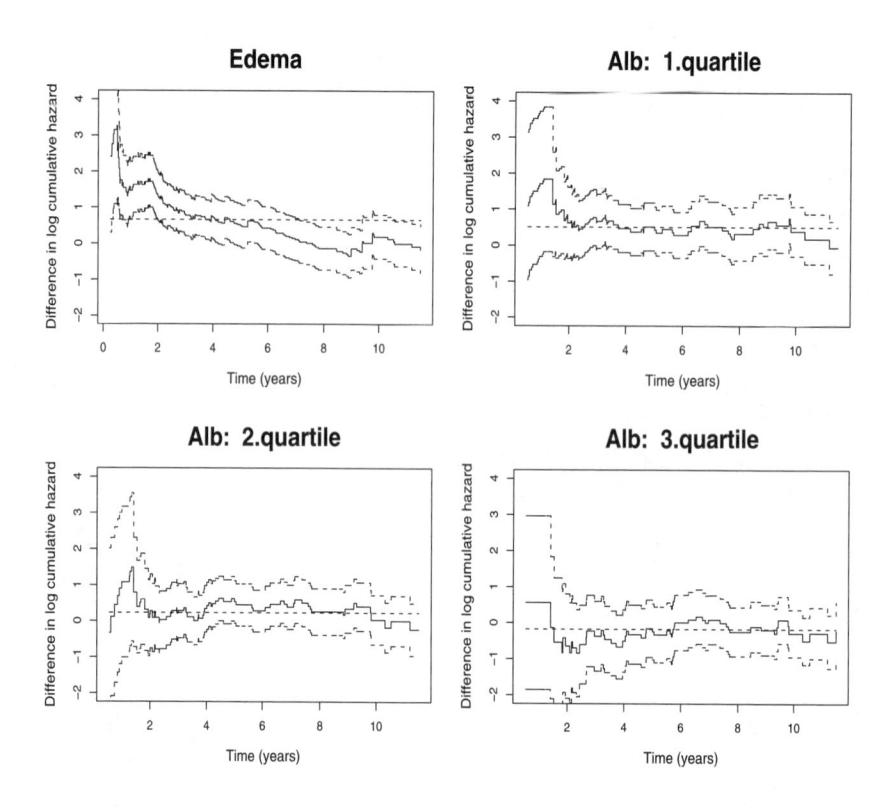

FIGURE 6.3: Estimated log-cumulative hazards difference along with 95% pointwise confidence intervals. The straight lines (dashed lines) are based on the Cox model.

Example 6.2.1 (Proportional hazards assumption for the PBC-data)

We wish to check the proportional hazards assumption for the PBC-data using the plots

$$(t, \log(\hat{\Lambda}_{0k}(t)) - \log(\hat{\Lambda}_{01}(t))), \quad k = 2, \ldots, K, \qquad (6.24)$$

based on the stratified Cox model. Under the model these curves should be approximately constant and equal to the estimated coefficients under the model. Confidence intervals may be obtained using the `cox.aalen` function and some additional calculations. We focus on the covariates edema and albumin to illustrate the technique. The latter covariate is continuous and is therefore grouped using here four groups based on the quartiles of the covariate. The `cox.aalen` function gives the estimated variance covariance-matrix for $\hat{\Lambda}_{0k}(t)$, $k = 1, \ldots, K$ as follows:

```
> fit1<-cox.aalen(Surv(time,status)~-1+prop(Age)+factor(Edema)
    +prop(logProtime)+prop(logAlbumin)+prop(logBilirubin),
```

```
covariance=1)
```

focusing here on edema and where we have centered the other covariates. One may then apply the delta-method (see Chapter 2) to obtain 95% confidence intervals for the curves (6.24) as shown in Figure 6.3 along with the straight line estimates based on the Cox model. The plot for edema indicates that the proportional hazards assumption may not hold for edema. The plots for the grouped version of albumin are also shown, and for this covariate there seems to be no indication of lacking fit of the Cox model if we include albumin as a categorical variable in the model based on the quartiles of the variate. □

Checking this property for all covariates will give some insight into whether the proportional hazards assumption is violated. Considering the performance of this procedure in the model defined by the extended Cox model with time-varying coefficients

$$\lambda(t) = Y(t)\lambda_0(t)\exp(X^T(t)\beta(t)) \tag{6.25}$$

it is apparent that the procedure will do quite well in the one-dimensional case where the stratified baselines can be used to approximate the shape of $\beta(t)$. With more than one covariate in the model, however, it is unclear how the individual plots will reflect the departure from the null. There are two other obvious drawbacks with this approach. First, if a covariate is continuous, then one needs to define some strata (more or less arbitrarily) based on the covariate values, but it is a different model that one really wishes to check, namely the one where the covariate is included as a continuous variate. Secondly, the model is checked one covariate at a time assuming that the model is okay for all the other covariates, which might obviously not be the case. If none of these plots indicate departure from the null, however, then this of course suggests that one may have some confidence in the model.

We now describe a class of tests that are often performed in practice along with the graphical procedure just discussed. We are looking for deviations from the Cox model of the type (6.25). Write, for the moment, the time-varying regression coefficients as

$$\beta_j(t) = \beta_j + \theta_j g_j(t), \tag{6.26}$$

where $g_j(t)$ is considered as known and assumed to be predictable. Examples are $g_j(t) = \log(t)$, $g_j(t) = N.(t-)$ but we return to that in a moment. The interest is in testing the hypothesis $H_0 : \theta = 0$ with $\theta = (\theta_1, \ldots, \theta_p)$. Note that, when the g_j's are known functions (predictable), then the model with coefficients (6.26) is still a Cox model and the asymptotic results developed in the previous section may be invoked to test the hypothesis H_0. It turns out indeed that the score test statistic gives many of the suggested goodness of fit tests in the literature when the g_j's are chosen appropriately as pointed out by Therneau & Grambsch (2000). If we denote the score function by $U = (U_1^T, U_2^T)^T$ (suppressing the dependency on (β, θ)), where the first component is the derivative of partial likelihood with respect to β, and the second component is the derivative with respect to θ. Similarly let $(I_{kl})_{k,l=1,2}$ denote the empirical information matrix written as a block matrix reflecting that we have two parameter vectors in play. Denote the inverse of the empirical information matrix by $(I^{kl})_{k,l=1,2}$. The score test statistic may thus be written

$$(U_1^T, U_2^T) \begin{pmatrix} I^{11} & I^{12} \\ I^{21} & I^{22} \end{pmatrix} \begin{pmatrix} U_1 \\ U_2 \end{pmatrix},$$

which reduces to

$$T(G) = U_2^T(\hat{\beta}, 0) I^{22}(\hat{\beta}, 0) U_2(\hat{\beta}, 0)$$

when evaluated in $(\hat{\beta}, 0)$, where $\hat{\beta}$ denotes the maximum partial likelihood estimator under the null and $G(t)$ is the vector of g_j's. The score test $T(G)$ is asymptotically χ^2 with p degrees of freedom under the null. Different choices of $G(t)$ lead to most of the suggested test-statistics for proportionality of the Cox regression model, see Therneau & Grambsch (2000) for more details. Instead of computing the above score test one could of course also use the likelihood ratio or the Wald test.

One typical application of this type of testing is to let $g_j(t) = \log(t)$ (Cox, 1972) for $j = 1, \ldots, p$. If this is done multivariately, and all components have departures from proportionality of this type, the test will give a good idea about the lacking fit of the Cox model. It is a standard procedure to consider the covariates one at a time, and then test for departures of $g(t)$ type (log for example), thus assuming that only θ_p, say, differs from 0 and then testing $H_0 : \theta_p = 0$. This leads to an asymptotically χ^2 with 1 degree of freedom if the null is true.

Example 6.2.2 (Continuation of Example 1.1.1)

Consider again the PBC data. To test if there is a departure from proportionality given by the log-function we fit the model

```
> cox<-coxph(Surv(time/365,status)~Age+Edema+logBilirubin
+ +logAlbumin+logProtime,data=pbc);
> time.test<- cox.zph(cox,transform="log")
> print(time.test)
                    rho     chisq         p
Age             0.00147  2.92e-04  0.986372
Edema          -0.24982  9.46e+00  0.002103
logBilirubin    0.07891  8.44e-01  0.358245
logAlbumin      0.02139  7.87e-02  0.779066
```

```
logProtime   -0.24983 6.93e+00 0.008472
GLOBAL                NA 2.35e+01 0.000266
```

The combined GLOBAL test, which is an approximation to the above $T(G)$ with the g_j's chosen as the log-function, suggests strongly that there is departure from the standard Cox form with p < 0.001. The individual covariate tests point to that it is edema and log(protime) that have departure from constant effects. These findings are in line with the results obtained from the successive type of testing done in Example 6.0.2. □

The tests against specific deviations from the Cox model using prespecified g_j-functions may give an indication of a possible lack fit of the Cox model, but it is important to realize that the individual tests associated with each covariate in the model are only valid if the Cox model is true for all the other covariates. One should therefore be cautious with these procedures. Scheike & Martinussen (2004) showed that the test for individual components can be far from the nominal level when other components do not have proportional effects. For many applications the sample size will be small and the degree of non-proportionality will not be dramatic and the individual testing of components may therefore do quite well. Another problem with this testing procedure is that one has to specify the g_j-functions so one needs to have a clear idea about the type of departure from proportionality to look for, which we believe is seldom the case in practice. Different g_j's may result in different conclusions.

Lin et al. (1993) and Wei (1984) suggested an important class of test statistics based on cumulative residuals. These test statistics can be designed to investigate different departures from the model including misspecification of the link function and the functional form of the covariates. The martingales under the Cox regression model can be written as

$$M_i(t) = N_i(t) - \int_0^t Y_i(s)\exp(X_i^T(s)\beta)\lambda_0(s)ds$$
$$= N_i(t) - \int_0^t Y_i(s)\exp(X_i^T(s)\beta)d\Lambda_0(s)$$

and these can be estimated using the estimates from the Cox model, see Section 6.1, leading to

$$\hat{M}_i(t) = N_i(t) - \int_0^t Y_i(s)\exp(X_i^T(s)\hat{\beta})d\hat{\Lambda}_0(s)$$
$$= N_i(t) - \int_0^t Y_i(s)\exp(X_i^T(s)\hat{\beta})\frac{1}{S_0(s,\hat{\beta})}dN_\cdot(s).$$

The idea is now to look at different functionals of these estimated residuals and see if they behave as they should under the model. Note for example

198   6. Multiplicative hazards models

that the score function, evaluated in the estimate $\hat{\beta}$, and seen as a function of time, can be written as

$$U(\hat{\beta}, t) = \sum_{i=1}^{n} \int_0^t X_i(s) d\hat{M}_i(s).$$

A closer analysis of the score process evaluated at $\hat{\beta}$ shows that $n^{-1/2}U(\hat{\beta}, t)$ is asymptotically equivalent to the process

$$n^{-1/2} \left(M_1(t) - I(t, \hat{\beta}) I^{-1}(\tau, \hat{\beta}) M_1(\tau) \right), \qquad (6.27)$$

where

$$M_1(t) = \sum_{i=1}^{n} M_{1i}(t) = \sum_{i=1}^{n} \int_0^t (X_i(s) - e(s, \beta_0)) dM_i(s)$$

with $e(t, \beta_0)$ the limit in probability of $E(t, \beta_0)$. The asymptotic distribution of (6.27) may be evaluated using a resampling procedure. The distribution of the process $n^{-1/2} M_1(t)$ ($t \in [0, \tau]$) is asymptotically equivalent to

$$n^{-1/2} \sum_{i=1}^{n} \int_0^t (X_i(s) - E(s, \hat{\beta})) dN_i(s) G_i$$

where $G_1, ..., G_n$ are independent standard normals. The key reasoning is that the M_i's are i.i.d. with variance $E(N_i)$ and therefore can be approximated by $G_i N_i$. Alternatively to this resampling approach one may also, as in Lin et al. (2000), establish that $n^{-1/2} M_1(t)$ is asymptotically equivalent to

$$n^{-1/2} \sum_{i=1}^{n} \int_0^t (X_i(s) - E(s, \hat{\beta})) d\hat{M}_i(s) G_i.$$

The last martingale residual resampling approach has certain desirable robustness properties, see Section 6.8. With the ability to assess the behavior of the observed score process under the null, the Cox model, one can proceed to suggest some appropriate test statistics like

$$\sup_{t \in [0, \tau]} |U_j(\hat{\beta}, t)| \quad \text{or} \qquad (6.28)$$

$$\sup_{t \in [\delta, \tau - \delta]} |\frac{U_j(\hat{\beta}, t)}{\hat{\text{var}}(U_j(\hat{\beta}, t))}|, \quad j = 1 \ldots, p, \qquad (6.29)$$

where δ is a small positive number to avoid numerical problems at the edges, and $\hat{\text{var}}(U(\hat{\beta}, t))$ is a consistent estimator of the variance of the observed score process such as

$$\sum_{i=1}^{n} \left(\hat{M}_{1i}(t) - I(t, \hat{\beta}) I^{-1}(\tau, \hat{\beta}) \hat{M}_{1i}(\tau) \right)^{\otimes 2},$$

6.2 Goodness-of-fit procedures for the Cox model

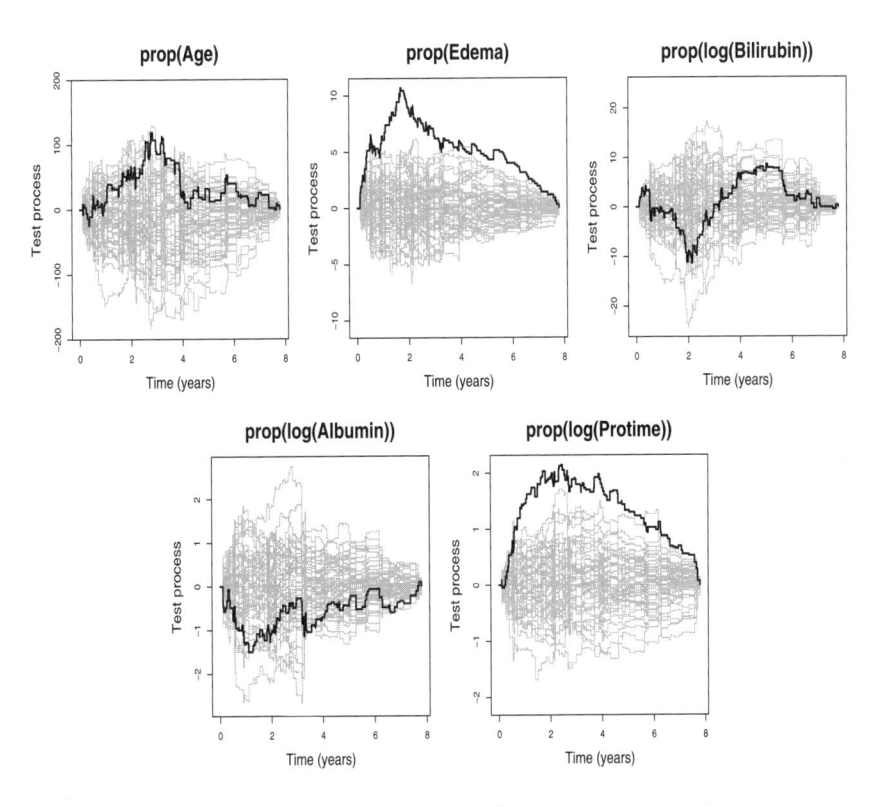

FIGURE 6.4: Score processes (unweighted) with 50 simulated processes under the model.

where
$$\hat{M}_{1i}(t) = \int_0^t (X_i(s) - E(s,\hat{\beta}))d\hat{M}_i(s).$$

Note that these test statistics are easily modified and evaluated by the resampling approach.

Example 6.2.3 (Continuation of Example 1.1.1)

The Lin, Wei, and Ying score process test for proportionality, (6.28), has the advantage that no specific functional form needs to be specified when looking for lack of fit of the model for a specific covariate. The test can be computed as follows using the cox.aalen function. The shown output is slightly edited.

```
> fit.cox<-cox.aalen(Surv(time/365,status)~prop(Age)+prop(Edema)
+ +prop(logBilirubin)+prop(logAlbumin)+prop(logProtime),
+ weighted.test=0,pbc);
Cox-Aalen Survival Model
```

200   6. Multiplicative hazards models

```
Simulations start N= 500
> summary(fit.cox)
Cox-Aalen Model

Proportional Cox terms :
                      Coef.       SE  Robust SE  D2log(L)^-1    P-val
prop(Age)            0.0383  0.00701    0.00926      0.00768  4.88e-08
prop(Edema)          0.6600  0.20000    0.24500      0.20600  9.54e-04
prop(logBilirubin)   0.8970  0.07590    0.08820      0.08270  0.00e+00
prop(logAlbumin)    -2.4600  0.67900    0.64100      0.65700  2.98e-04
prop(logProtime)     2.3500  0.64300    0.94700      0.77400  2.59e-04

Test for Proportionality
                   sup| hat U(t) |  p-value H_0
prop(Age)                 108.00          0.350
prop(Edema)                10.90          0.002
prop(logBilirubin)         12.50          0.170
prop(logAlbumin)            1.48          0.324
prop(logProtime)            2.29          0.004
```

The output differs slightly from the results from the standard coxph function because the ties are handled differently. To plot the score processes, see Figure 6.4, just do as follows.

```
> plot(fit.cox,score=T,xlab="Time (years)")
```

When the score processes are evaluated under the null using the unweighted supremum test-statistic we see that there is lacking fit of the Cox model with respect to edema and log(protime). Also for log(albumin) the model shows lacking fit towards the end of the time-period, see Figure 6.4, but this is not reflected in the unweighted supremum test statistic. We also compute the weighted version of the supremum test statistics taking the variance of score processes into account (6.29), see Figure 6.5. The following output is edited just focusing on the weighted score process.

```
> fit.cox.w<-cox.aalen(Surv(time/365,status)~prop(Age)+prop(Edema)
+ +prop(logBilirubin)+prop(logAlbumin)+prop(logProtime),
+ pbc,weighted.test=1)
Cox-Aalen Survival Model
Simulations start N= 500
> summary(fit.cox.w)
Cox-Aalen Model

Proportional Cox terms :
                Coef.       SE  Robust SE  D2log(L)^-1    P-val
prop(Age)      0.0383  0.00701    0.00926      0.00768  4.88e-08
prop(Edema)    0.6600  0.20000    0.24500      0.20600  9.54e-04
```

6.2 Goodness-of-fit procedures for the Cox model

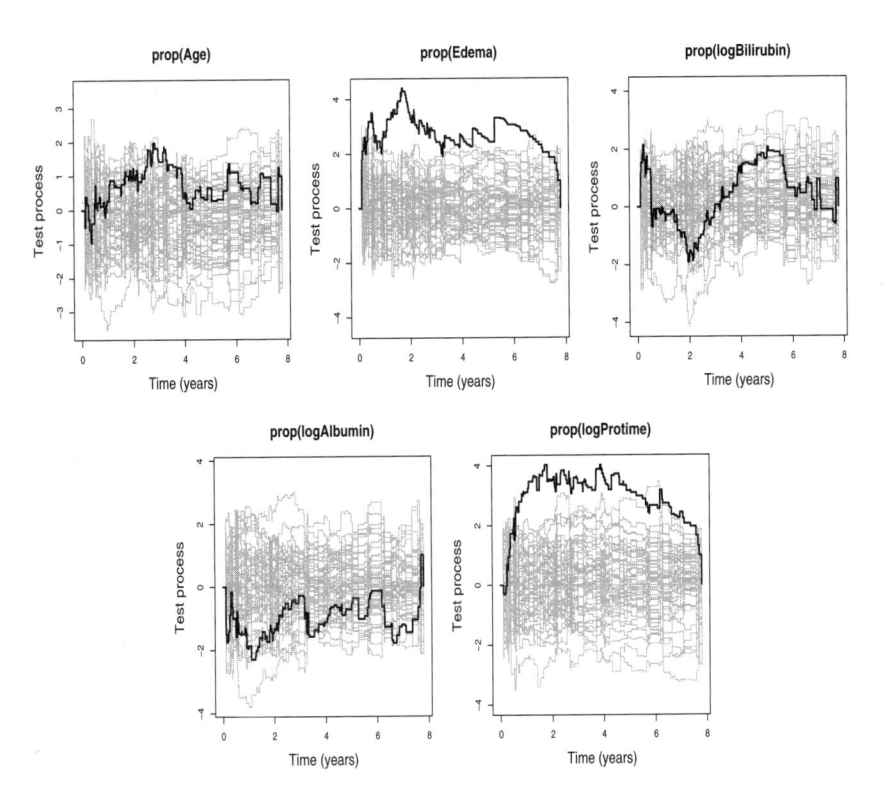

FIGURE 6.5: Score processes (weighted) with 50 simulated processes under the model.

```
prop(logBilirubin)   0.8970  0.07590   0.08820   0.08270  0.00e+00
prop(logAlbumin)    -2.4600  0.67900   0.64100   0.65700  2.98e-04
prop(logProtime)     2.3500  0.64300   0.94700   0.77400  2.59e-04

Test for Proportionality
                  sup| hat U(t) |   p-value H_0
prop(Age)                   1.82        0.732
prop(Edema)                 9.42        0.000
prop(logBilirubin)          3.08        0.060
prop(logAlbumin)            2.27        0.380
prop(logProtime)            3.94        0.002

> plot(fit.cox.w,score=T,xlab="Time (years)",ylab="Test process")
```

These tests lead in this case to similar conclusions as the unweighted test statistics. □

202   6. Multiplicative hazards models

The supremum tests outlined above are appealing in that no arbitrary grouping of (continuous) covariates or specific deviations from proportionality are needed. The tests do, however, suffer the drawback that the model is assumed to be correct with respect to all the other covariates when the proportionality assumption is investigated for a specific covariate. One may therefore overlook important features of the data as well as not being able to pin point exactly where a possible lack of proportionality is present.

Lin et al. (1993) also suggested to consider the two-dimensional cumulative residual process

$$M_c(t, z) = \int_0^t K_z^T(s) d\hat{M}(s)$$

where $K_z(t)$ is an $n \times 1$ matrix with elements $I(X_{i1}(t) \leq z)$ for $i = 1, \ldots, n$ focusing here on the first continuous covariate X_1, say. Thus cumulating residuals versus both time and the covariate values. The cumulative residual process M_c is useful to study possible misspecification of the functional form of covariates and the interaction with time. To summarize things further one may integrate over the entire time span to get a process only in z:

$$M_c(z) = \int_0^\tau K_z^T(t) d\hat{M}(t), \tag{6.30}$$

which can be plotted against z. The cumulative residual processes may also be decomposed into a sum of i.i.d. components making resampling possible to approximate their asymptotic distributions. We illustrate the use of $M_c(z)$ in the following example.

Example 6.2.4 (PBC-data: cumulative residuals)

We shall see that the cumulative residuals do reveal information about misspecification of the functional form of the covariates. To make this point for the PBC data we compare the fit of the models, where it is assumed that either bilirubin or log(bilirubin) leads to constant relative risk. First consider the model with log(bilirubin):

```
> fit<-cox.aalen(Surv(time/365,status)~prop(Age)+prop(Edema)
+ +prop(logBilirubin)+prop(logAlbumin)+prop(logProtime)
+ ,max.time=8,pbc,residuals=1,n.sim=0)
Cox-Aalen Survival Model
> resids<-cum.residuals(fit,pbc,cum.resid=1);
Cumulative martingale residuals for Right censored survival times
Simulations start N= 500
> summary(resids)
Test for cumulative MG-residuals

Residual versus covariates consistent with model
```

6.2 Goodness-of-fit procedures for the Cox model

prop(Age)

prop(logBilirubin)

prop(logAlbumin)

prop(logProtime)

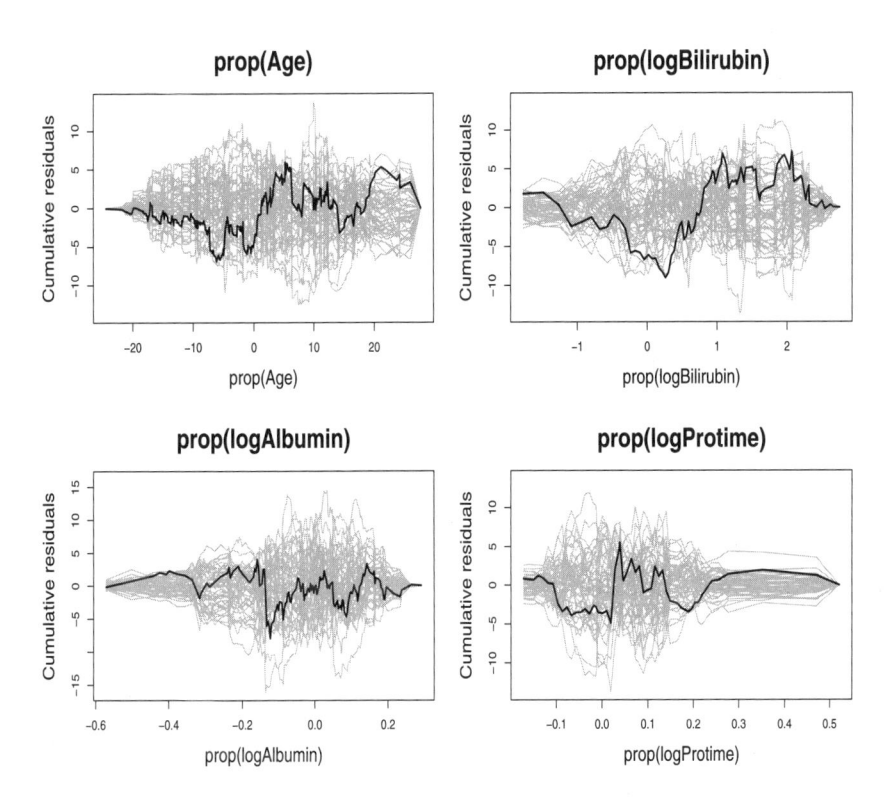

FIGURE 6.6: PBC-data. Observed cumulative residuals versus continuous covariates with 50 random realizations under the model.

```
                   sup| hat B(t) |  p-value H_0: B(t)=0
prop(Age)              6.857                  0.694
prop(logBilirubin)     9.030                  0.172
prop(logAlbumin)       7.998                  0.450
prop(logProtime)       5.525                  0.814

> plot(resids,score=2)
```

We know that there is lacking fit for the model with respect to edema and log(protime) but the summary statistics and Figure 6.6 suggest that the functional representation of the covariates seems to be sensible enough.

Consider now the model where we use bilirubin on its original scale as a covariate in the model:

```
> fit<-cox.aalen(Surv(time/365,status)~prop(Age)+prop(Edema)
+ +prop(Bilirubin)+prop(logAlbumin)+prop(logProtime),
+ max.time=8,pbc,residuals=1,n.sim=0)
```

204   6. Multiplicative hazards models

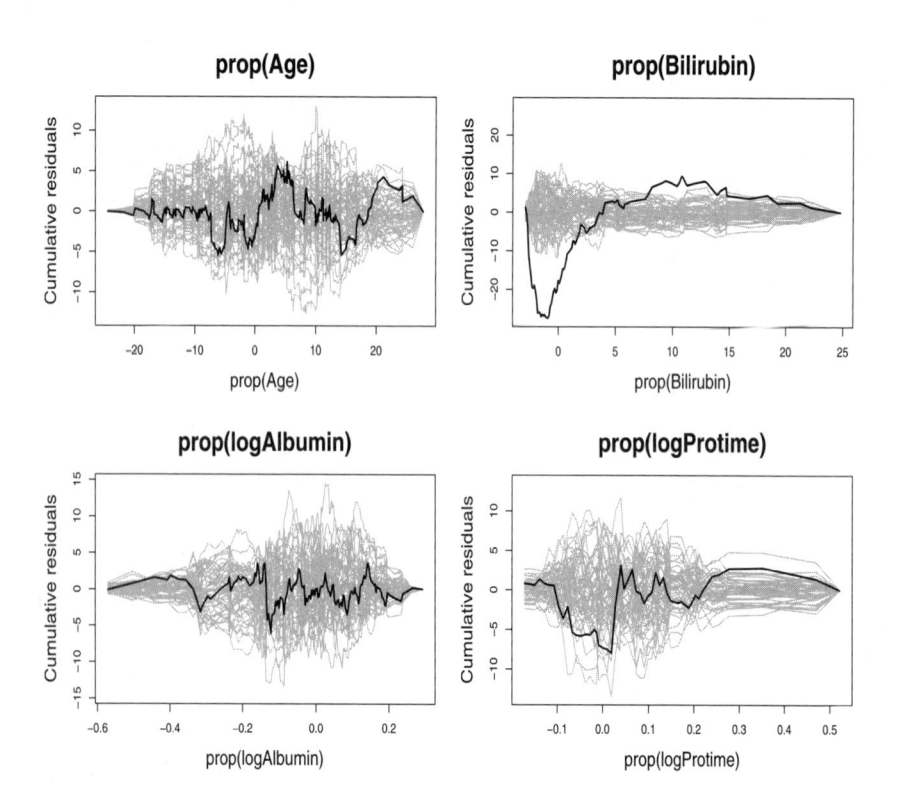

FIGURE 6.7: PBC-data. Observed cumulative residuals versus continuous covariates with 50 random realizations under the model.

```
Cox-Aalen Survival Model
> resids<-cum.residuals(fit,pbc,cum.resid=1);
Cumulative martingale residuals for Right censored survival times
Simulations start N= 500
> summary(resids)
Test for cumulative MG-residuals

Residual versus covariates consistent with model

                sup| hat B(t) |  p-value H_0: B(t)=0
prop(Age)              6.139                  0.788
prop(Bilirubin)       27.530                  0.000
prop(logAlbumin)       6.045                  0.830
prop(logProtime)       7.983                  0.356

> plot(resids,score=2)
```

The summary statistics and Figure 6.7 clearly suggest that bilirubin should not be included in the model on its original scale. □

In Section 6.6 we suggest a model based approach for successive testing of timevarying effects based on the semiparametric model (6.4).

6.3 Extended Cox model with time-varying regression effects

The Cox model is far the most used model in applications. As stressed in the two previous sections it relies on some assumptions that should be checked in each application. Taking another perspective one may extend the Cox model relaxing some of the assumptions. Ideally one can hope for inferential tools that can be used to investigate whether the more general model can be simplified, eventually perhaps to the Cox model. There are many ways to extend the Cox model. One extension that seems natural, however, is the model where the relative risk parameters are allowed to depend on time so that the effect of a treatment, say, can change with time. We study the Cox model with time-varying regression coefficients in this section and we shall see indeed (Section 6.6) that inferential tools can be developed, which allow for investigating whether the Cox model is an acceptable submodel to use in specific applications.

The Cox model with time-varying regression coefficients is a very flexible model, and it will give a good first order approximation to most hazards models. The model assumes that the intensity has the form

$$\lambda(t) = Y(t)\lambda_0(t) \exp(X^T(t)\beta(t)), \qquad (6.31)$$

where $Y(t)$ is the at risk process and $X(t)$ a p-dimensional predictable bounded covariate vector. The baseline $\lambda_0(t)$ function still gives the intensity for an individual with covariates equal to zero. The regression coefficients of the Cox model have been replaced by a vector $\beta(t)$ of time-dependent regression functions.

Most work on this model (see references in the beginning of this chapter) aims directly at estimating $\beta(t)$ utilizing smoothness assumptions. Large sample properties for these estimators have been derived but due to presence of bias in the estimation it has been difficult to develop inferential tools such as confidence bands. This problem has, however, been overcome in the recent paper by Tian et al. (2005) who used a resampling method to construct confidence bands. This procedure seems to work but one should still keep in mind that estimators of $\beta(t)$ converge at a slower rate than the usual $n^{1/2}$-rate, which inevitably will lead to less powerful inference. Murphy & Sen (1991) studied a histogram sieve estimator of $\beta(t)$ and then integrated this estimator to obtain an estimator of the cumulative time-varying effects, $B(t) = \int_0^t \beta(s)ds$. Practically, the histogram sieve estimator may be difficult to use since one needs to choose a suitable number of time segments and endpoints, see Murphy (1993) for an example. In this section, we focus also on the cumulative regression coefficients because these quantities can be estimated at the usual $n^{1/2}$-rate. Since most hypotheses about the regression coefficients, such as time-invariance, can be directly transferred to hypotheses concerning the cumulatives it is in most cases no limitation to work with the cumulatives. A further benefit, when working with the cumulatives, is that martingale calculus may be invoked to establish large sample properties of the suggested estimators. One may establish convergence over the entire time span in contrast to pointwise convergence so that for example uniform confidence bands may be easily constructed.

We shall assume that $\lambda_0(t) > 0$ and rewrite the model as

$$\lambda(t) = Y(t) \exp(X^T(t)\beta(t)), \tag{6.32}$$

where the baseline has been absorbed into the design vector. We prefer to work with this parameterization because it leads to simpler formulas, but return to a discussion of how to deal with the more standard parameterization (6.31) later in this section.

Assume that n independent copies $(N_i(t), Y_i(t), X_i(t))$, $i = 1, \ldots, n$, are being observed in some time interval $[0, \tau]$, $\tau < \infty$, and that each $N_i(t)$ has intensity (6.32). Let

$$N(t) = (N_1(t), \ldots, N_n(t))^T$$

denote the multivariate counting process with intensity

$$\lambda(t) = (\lambda_1(t), \ldots, \lambda_n(t))^T,$$

and organize the covariates into a design matrix of dimension $n \times p$:

$$X(t) = (Y_1(t)X_1(t), \ldots, Y_n(t)X_n(t))^T.$$

Further denote the n-dimensional cumulative intensity as $\Lambda(t) = \int_0^t \lambda(s)ds$ such that $M(t) = N(t) - \Lambda(t)$ is a n-dimensional (square integrable) martingale.

We base the estimation on the log-likelihood function

$$\sum_{i=1}^n \left\{ \int_0^\tau X_i(t)^T \beta(t) \, dN_i(t) - \int_0^\tau Y_i(t) \exp(X_i(t)^T \beta(t)) \, dt \right\}.$$

Taking the derivative with respect to $\beta(t)$ leads to the score equation (written on differential form)

$$X(t)^T (dN(t) - \lambda(t)dt) = 0. \tag{6.33}$$

Equation (6.33) will be the starting point for our estimation procedure although it has no solution as it is written here, because the first term

6.3 Extended Cox model with time-varying regression effects

represents a pure jump process while the second is absolutely continuous. We use it, however, to construct an iteration procedure based on an initial estimate, $\tilde{\beta}$. For this we need the second derivative of the log-likelihood function

$$-\left\{\sum_{i=1}^{n} Y_i(t) e^{X_i(t)^T \tilde{\beta}(t)} X_i(t) X_i(t)^T\right\} dt = -\tilde{A}(t)\, dt,$$

where $\tilde{A} = A_{\tilde{\beta}}$ with

$$A_\beta(t) = X^T(t) W(t) X(t)$$

and $W(t) = \text{diag}(\lambda_i(t))$. A Taylor series expansion of (6.33) gives the iteration step

$$\tilde{\beta}_{\text{new}}(t) = \tilde{\beta}(t) + \tilde{A}(t)^{-1} X(t)^T \left(dN(t) - \tilde{\lambda}(t)\, dt \right), \quad (6.34)$$

where $\tilde{\lambda}$ is λ evaluated with $\beta = \tilde{\beta}$. The iteration steps will not lead to a solution, as already pointed out, and we need to bring in some smoothness assumptions to obtain a solution. We integrate the linearized equation (6.34) to estimate the cumulative regression coefficients instead. This leads to the iteration step $\tilde{B}^{(k+1)} = g(\tilde{B}^{(k)})$ where

$$g(\tilde{B})(t) = \int_0^t \tilde{\beta}(s)\, ds + \int_0^t \tilde{A}(s)^{-1} X(s)^T dN(s)$$
$$- \int_0^t \tilde{A}(s)^{-1} X(s)^T \tilde{\lambda}(s)\, ds, \quad (6.35)$$

and introduce smoothness of the underlying regression coefficients through the estimation of $\beta(t)$. For simplicity, $\tilde{\beta}(t)$ is taken to be a simple kernel estimator of $\beta(t)$, that is,

$$\tilde{\beta}(t) = \int b^{-1} K\left(\frac{s-t}{b}\right) d\tilde{B}(s),$$

with b the bandwidth parameter and K a uniformly continuous kernel with support $[-1, 1]$ satisfying

$$\int K(s)\, ds = 1, \qquad \int s K(s)\, ds = 0.$$

The iteration scheme may be summarized as follows:

- Start with an initial $\tilde{\beta}^{(0)}(t)$;
- Use the iteration step (6.35) to obtain $\tilde{B}^{(1)}(t)$;
- Smooth $\tilde{B}^{(1)}(t)$ to obtain $\tilde{\beta}^{(1)}(t)$ and apply (6.35) again. Iterate until convergence.

The properties of the obtained estimator are described in the following theorem. The norm $\|C\|$ of a matrix C is here defined as $\max_{i,j} |C_{ij}|$. Let $A(t) = A_{\beta_0}(t)$ with $\beta_0(t)$ the true regression function.

Condition 6.2

(a) The regression function $\beta(t)$ is three times continuously differentiable;

(b) The bandwidth b is of order $n^{-\alpha}$, where $1/8 < \alpha < 1/4$;

(c) Convergence of $n^{-1}A(t)$:

$$\sup_{t \in [0,\tau]} \|n^{-1}A(t) - a(t)\| \xrightarrow{P} 0,$$

where a is non-singular with continuous components.

□

Theorem 6.3.1 *Assume Condition 6.2. Then, with a probability tending to 1 as $n \to \infty$, (6.35) has a solution $g(\hat{B}) = \hat{B}$ such that $\|\hat{B} - B\| = O_p(n^{-1/2})$. Furthermore,*

$$n^{1/2}(\hat{B} - B) \xrightarrow{D} U \quad \text{as } n \to \infty$$

in $D[0,\tau]^p$, where U is a zero-mean Gaussian martingale with variance function

$$\Phi(t) = \int_0^t a^{-1}(u)\, du. \tag{6.36}$$

PROOF. In this proof we focus on only establishing the asymptotic normality result. That (6.35) has a solution $g(\hat{B}) = \hat{B}$ such that $\|\hat{B} - B\| = O_p(n^{-1/2})$ is shown in Martinussen et al. (2002) using the fix point theorem.

We can decompose the counting process as

$$dN(t) = \lambda(t)\, dt + dM(t), \tag{6.37}$$

where M is a (local square integrable) vector martingale. By use of the martingale central limit theorem and Condition 6.2 (a), it may be seen that

$$n^{1/2} \int_0^\cdot A(s)^{-1} X(s)^T\, dM(s) \xrightarrow{D} U \quad \text{as } n \to \infty, \tag{6.38}$$

where U is a zero-mean Gaussian martingale with covariance function given by (6.36). The latter point follows since the predictable variation process of the martingale in (6.38) is

$$n \left\langle \int_0^\cdot A(s)^{-1} X(s)^T\, dM(s) \right\rangle = n \int_0^t A(s)^{-1} X(s)^T W(s) X(s) A(s)^{-1}\, ds$$

$$= \int_0^t (n^{-1} A(s))^{-1}\, ds,$$

6.3 Extended Cox model with time-varying regression effects

which converges in probability to the expression (6.36). The asymptotic distribution of $\hat{B}$ is obtained from equation (6.35) starting from $\hat{B}$. Since $g(\hat{B}) = \hat{B}$, we have

$$\hat{B}(t) - B(t) = \int_0^t \hat{A}(s)^{-1} X(s)^T \, dM(s)$$
$$+ \int_0^t \hat{A}(s)^{-1} \left\{ A^*(s) - \hat{A}(s) \right\} \left\{ \hat{\beta}(s) - \beta(s) \right\} ds$$
$$= \int_0^t \hat{A}(s)^{-1} X(s)^T \, dM(s) + O(\|\beta - \hat{\beta}\|^2),$$

where $\hat{A}(t) = A_{\hat{\beta}}(t)$, $A^*(t) = A_{\beta^*}(t)$ and with $\beta^*(t)$ on the line segment between $\hat{\beta}$ and $\beta(t)$. If

(i) $n^{1/2} \int_0^t (\hat{A}(s)^{-1} - A(s)^{-1}) X(s)^T \, dM(s) = o_p(1),$

such that $\hat{A}$ can be replaced by the predictable A, and

(ii) $n^{1/2} O(\|\beta - \hat{\beta}\|^2) = o_p(1),$

then the proof follows from (6.38).
To show (ii), it suffices to choose b such that

$$\|\hat{\beta} - \beta\| = o_p(n^{-1/4}). \tag{6.39}$$

To this end we split the error of $\hat{\beta} - \beta$ into a bias part and a random part,

$$\hat{\beta}(t) - \beta(t) = \int b^{-1} K\left(\frac{u-t}{b}\right) d(\hat{B}(u) - B(u)) + \overline{\beta}(t) - \beta(t),$$

where

$$\overline{\beta}(t) = \int b^{-1} K\left(\frac{u-t}{b}\right) dB(u)$$

denote the smoothed derivative of $B(t)$. Hence

$$\|\hat{\beta} - \beta\| \leq O(b^{-1}\|\hat{B} - B\|) + O(b^2)$$

and (6.39) is seen to be met with

$$b = n^{-\alpha}, \qquad 1/8 < \alpha < 1/4,$$

which is Condition 6.2 (b).
To show that (i) is valid, we Taylor expand the matrix function $A(t)^{-1}$. For ease of notation we consider only the one-dimensional case. Let

$$C(t) = X(t)^T \operatorname{diag}(X_{i1}(t)) W(t) X(t).$$

6. Multiplicative hazards models

We then obtain for the leading term of (i):

$$\int A(t)^{-1}C(t)b^{-1}\int K\left(\frac{u-t}{b}\right)d(\hat{B}-B)(u)A(t)^{-1}X(t)^T\,dM(t)$$
$$=\int A(t)^{-1}C(t)b^{-2}\int K_d\left(\frac{u-t}{b}\right)(\hat{B}-B)(u)\,du\,A(t)^{-1}X(t)^T\,dM(t)$$
$$=b^{-2}\int\int A(t)^{-1}C(t)K_d\left(\frac{u-t}{b}\right)A(t)^{-1}X(t)^T\,dM(t)(\hat{B}-B)(u)\,du$$
$$\leq\|\hat{B}-B\|b^{-2}\left\|\int\left|\int A(t)^{-1}C(t)A(t)^{-1}K_d\left(\frac{u-t}{b}\right)X(t)^T\,dM(t)\right|\,du\right\|,$$

where K_d is the derivative of K. Since $\hat{\beta}$ is a smoothed version of $\hat{B}$ the above change of integrals effectively smoothes the martingale rather than $\hat{B}$ and the martingale central limit theorem applies. By use of Lenglart's inequality it is seen that (i) holds, and the proof is complete. □

Winnett & Sasieni (2003) studied a related procedure that estimates $\beta(t)$ and establishes a stronger consistency than the one given by the above theorem. It also follows that with a probability tending to one that the solution is unique within a ball of radius $O(n^{-\delta})$ from B where $2\alpha < \delta < 1/2$, $1/8 < \alpha < 1/4$.

It is worth pointing out that, if a consistent starting point is given, then it suffices with one iteration step to obtain efficiency. That the estimator is in fact efficient follows by comparing the estimator's variance with the information bound for this model, see Sasieni (1992b).

Consistent estimates of the variance function $\Phi(t)$ are provided either by

$$n\int_0^t \hat{A}(s)^{-1}\,ds,$$

where $\hat{A}(t)=A_{\hat{\beta}}(t)$, or by the optional variation process

$$n\int_0^t \hat{A}(s)^{-1}X(s)^T\,\text{diag}\,(dN(s))\,X(s)\hat{A}(s)^{-1}$$

with the latter referring to the martingale decomposition

$$n^{1/2}(\hat{B}(t)-B(t))=n^{1/2}\int_0^t \hat{A}(s)^{-1}X(s)^T\,dM(s)+o_p(1).$$

Example 6.3.1 (PBC-data. Example 6.0.2 continued.)

The optional variation standard errors are used to give 95% pointwise confidence intervals in Figure 6.8 obtained by the command.

6.3 Extended Cox model with time-varying regression effects

Edema

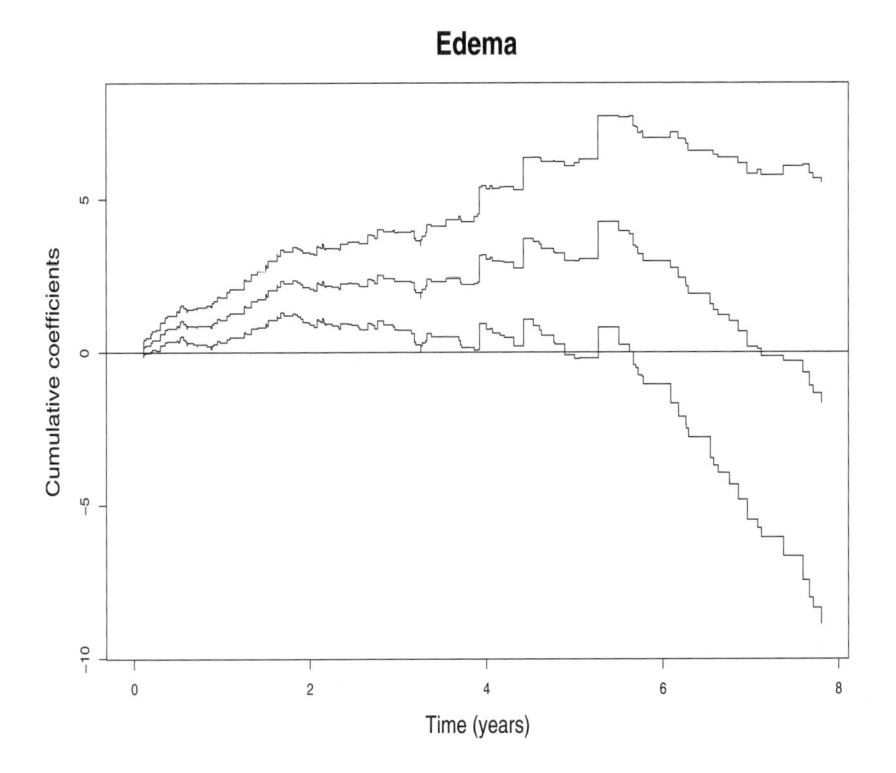

FIGURE 6.8: PBC-data. Estimated cumulative regression function with 95% pointwise confidence intervals for edema.

```
> fit<-timecox(Surv(time/365,status)~Age+Edema+logBilirubin
+ +logAlbumin+logProtime,pbc,max.time=8)
> plot(fit,xlab="Time (years)",ylab="Cumulative coefficients",
+ specific.comps=3)
```

Even though the pointwise confidence intervals are useful in evaluating the cumulative effect at specific timepoints, they are not well suited for inferential purposes about the shape of the entire curve. A simple test for significance of edema could for example be based on the cumulative estimate at time 6, and then edema is deemed non-significant. If we, on the other hand, test the effect at time 2, we conclude that it is significant. This is obviously due to the changing behavior of the effect of edema. Later we construct confidence bands. □

In the note below the asymptotic properties for the estimators within the standard parameterization (6.31) are sketched.

Note. We now give some details to indicate how similar asymptotics is obtained with the standard parameterization (6.31). Write thus the model as

$$\lambda_i(t) = \lambda_0(t) Y_i(t) \exp(X_i(t)^T \beta(t)) = \lambda_0(t)\phi_i(t), \qquad (6.40)$$

where $\phi_i(t,\beta) = Y_i(t)\exp(X_i(t)^T\beta(t))$. The score equations for $\beta(t)$ and $d\Lambda_0(t)$ are

$$X^T(t)\left(dN(t) - \mathrm{diag}(\exp(X_i^T(t)\beta(t)))Y(t)d\Lambda_0(t)\right) = 0, \qquad (6.41)$$

$$Y^T(t)\left(dN(t) - \mathrm{diag}(\exp(X_i^T(t)\beta(t)))Y(t)d\Lambda_0(t)\right) = 0, \qquad (6.42)$$

and solving these successively, as for the Cox model (see Section 6.1), we get

$$\tilde{\Lambda}_0(t) = \int_0^t \frac{1}{S_0(s,\beta(s))} dN_\bullet(s), \qquad (6.43)$$

where

$$S_0(t,\beta(t)) = \sum_{i=1}^n Y_i(t)\exp(X_i^T(t)\beta(t)).$$

With this solution inserted into (6.41) and solving for $\beta(t)$ we obtain

$$X^T(t)(dN(t) - \mathrm{diag}(\exp(X_i^T(t)\beta(t)))Y(t)(S_0(t,\beta(t))^{-1}dN_\bullet(t)) = 0. \qquad (6.44)$$

With an initial estimator $(\tilde{\Lambda}_0(t), \tilde{\beta}(t))$ and $\tilde{\phi}_i(t) = \phi_i(t,\tilde{\beta})$ we get the updating step for the cumulated parameter vector:

$$g(\tilde{B})(t) = \int_0^t \tilde{\beta}(s)ds + \int_0^t \tilde{\Gamma}(s)^{-1}\frac{1}{\tilde{\lambda}_0(s)}\{X(s) - \bar{X}(s)\}^T dN(s), \qquad (6.45)$$

where

$$\tilde{\Gamma}(t) = (X(t) - \bar{X}(t))^T \mathrm{diag}(\tilde{\phi}_i(t))(X(t) - \bar{X}(t)),$$

and $\bar{X}(t)$ is the matrix with rows

$$\sum_{i=1}^n \tilde{\phi}_i(t)X_i(t)^T / S_0(\tilde{\beta}(t), t).$$

The asymptotic variance of the estimator may be estimated consistently by

$$\int_0^\cdot \{\hat{\lambda}_0(t)\hat{\Gamma}(t)\}^{-1} dt,$$

where the quantities in the last display are those based on the final estimator (at convergence). See Scheike & Martinussen (2004) for more details on this approach.

Grambsch & Therneau (1994) considered the scaled Schoenfeld residuals (Schoenfeld, 1982) based on estimates from the Cox model to learn about the behavior of $\beta(t)$. With

$$E(t,\beta) = S_1(t,\beta)/S_0(t,\beta); \quad V(t,\beta) = \frac{S_2(t,\beta)}{S_0(t,\beta)} - \left\{\frac{S_1(t,\beta)}{S_0(t,\beta)}\right\}^{\otimes 2},$$

the scaled Schoenfeld residual is defined as

$$r_k^* = V^{-1}(t_k, \hat{\beta}) r_k(\hat{\beta}),$$

where

$$r_k(\beta) = X_{(k)}(t_k) - E(t_k, \beta)$$

with $X_{(k)}$ the covariate vector of the subject with an event at time t_k and $\hat{\beta}$ denoting the usual maximum partial likelihood estimator under the Cox model. Using a Taylor-series expansion, Grambsch & Therneau (1994) noted that direct smoothing of the scaled Schoenfeld residuals added onto $\hat{\beta}$, $r_k^* + \hat{\beta}$, gives a way of estimating $\beta(t)$. Their estimator may be seen as a one-step estimator based on the initial time-constant estimator $\hat{\beta}$, the maximum partial likelihood estimator. Since $\hat{\beta}$ is not a consistent estimator of the time-varying regression function $\beta(t)$ it is not possible to show that such a one-step procedure will give a consistent estimator. The procedure may do well in practice, however, if the regression functions do not vary too dramatically. Winnett & Sasieni (2001) considered variations of how to smooth the residuals.

6.4 Inference for the extended Cox model

Considering the general version of the extended Cox model (6.31) with time-varying regression coefficients, we shall present various approaches for making inference about the regression coefficients of the model. We have already presented some goodness of fit procedures for the standard Cox model, but now focus more specifically on how to carry out inference about the time-varying regression coefficients of the extended Cox model. Although some of the methods are related, the hypotheses considered in this section are more specific and precise as they relate to a specific model. The earlier goodness of fit procedures in reality all considered the hypothesis that all the time-varying regression coefficient are constant $H_0 : \beta(t) \equiv \beta$. In contrast to this we now wish to consider the regression coefficients individually and investigate the two hypotheses

$$H_{01} : \beta_p(t) \equiv 0;$$
$$H_{02} : \beta_p(t) \equiv \beta_p;$$

focusing on the pth regression coefficient without loss of generality. It is important to notice that the other regression coefficients are allowed to vary with time. The main reason for developing the efficient estimates and deriving the asymptotics for the cumulatives is that evaluating the two above hypotheses is easy in this framework. Testing the significance of the regression coefficients will equivalently lead to construction of confidence bands. Simultaneous Hall-Wellner $(1-\alpha)$ confidence bands over the period from $[0,\tau]$ are given by

$$\hat{B}_p(t) \pm n^{-1/2} d_\alpha \, \hat{\Phi}_{pp}(\tau)^{1/2} \left(1 + \frac{\hat{\Phi}_{pp}(t)}{\hat{\Phi}_{pp}(\tau)}\right),$$

where $\hat{\Phi}_{pp}(t)$ is the pth diagonal element of $\hat{\Phi}(t)$ and d_α is the $(1-\alpha)$-quantile of $\sup_{t\in[0,1/2]}|B^0(t)|$ with $B^0(t)$ the standard Brownian bridge. This is a simple consequence of the asymptotic properties of the cumulative regression coefficients.

An alternative to the Hall-Wellner band may be constructed using resampling, which is based on obtaining an i.i.d. representation of the estimator. We start by observing that

$$n^{1/2}(\hat{B}(t) - B(t)) = n^{-1/2} \sum_{i=1}^{n} Q_i(t) + o_p(1), \qquad (6.46)$$

where

$$Q_i(t) = \int_0^t (n^{-1} X^T(s) W(s) X(s))^{-1} X_i(s) dM_i(s)$$

and

$$M_i(t) = N_i(t) - \int_0^t Y_i(s) \exp(X_i^T(s)\beta(s)) ds$$

are the basic martingales (Scheike, 2004). The leading term of the right-hand side of (6.46) is, for large n, essentially a sum of independent and identically distributed zero-mean random variables and its covariance may be estimated by

$$\hat{\Phi}(t) = n^{-1} \sum_{i=1}^{n} \hat{Q}_i^{\otimes 2}(t),$$

where

$$\hat{Q}_i(t) = \int_0^t (n^{-1} X^T(s) \hat{W}(s) X(s))^{-1} X_i(s) d\hat{M}_i(s),$$

6.4 Inference for the extended Cox model

with $\hat{M}_i(t)$ obtained by insertion of estimates into $M_i(t)$. If $(G_1, ..., G_n)$ are independent and standard normally distributed, then it can be shown that

$$\Delta_1(t) = n^{-1/2} \sum_{i=1}^{n} \hat{Q}_i(t) G_i$$

has the same limit distribution as $n^{1/2}(\hat{B}(t) - B(t))$. Let the jth component of the kth realization of $\Delta_1(t)$ be denoted as $\Delta_{1,j}^k(t)$.

To test the hypothesis, $H_{02}: \beta_p(t) = \beta_p$, one may then use a simple test statistic depending on $n^{1/2}(\hat{B}(t) - B(t))$ and then approximate its distribution by the resampling approach sketched above. A simple test is based on computing the test statistic

$$n^{1/2} \sup_{t \in [0,\tau]} |\hat{B}_p(t) - \frac{\hat{B}_p(\tau)}{\tau} t|. \tag{6.47}$$

To approximate percentiles for the observed test statistic under the null, compute

$$\sup_{t \in [0,\tau]} |\Delta_{1,p}^k(t) - \frac{\Delta_{1,p}^k(\tau)}{\tau} t|$$

for a large number of realizations $k = 1, \ldots, K$.

Similarly, construction of simultaneous confidence bands and a test for $H_0: \beta_p(\cdot) = 0$, or equivalently $H_0: B_p(\cdot) = 0$, can be based on the maximal deviation test statistic

$$T_{1S} = \sup_{t \in [0,\tau]} |\frac{n^{1/2} \hat{B}_p(t)}{\hat{\Phi}_{pp}^{1/2}(t)}|. \tag{6.48}$$

Percentiles can be approximated from realizations of $\Delta_1(t)$

$$\sup_{t \in [0,\tau]} |\frac{\Delta_{1,p}^k(t)}{\hat{\Phi}_{pp}^{1/2}(t)}|. \tag{6.49}$$

Example 6.4.1 (PBC data. Example 6.0.2 continued)

The estimate of the cumulative regression coefficient for log(bilirubin) can be provided with 95% confidence bands. Figure 6.9 gives the Hall-Wellner band as well as the band based on T_{1S} obtained by the above resampling technique.

```
> plot(fit,xlab="Time (years)",ylab="Cumulative coefficients",
+ sim.ci=2,hw.ci=3,specific.comps=4)
```

logBilirubin

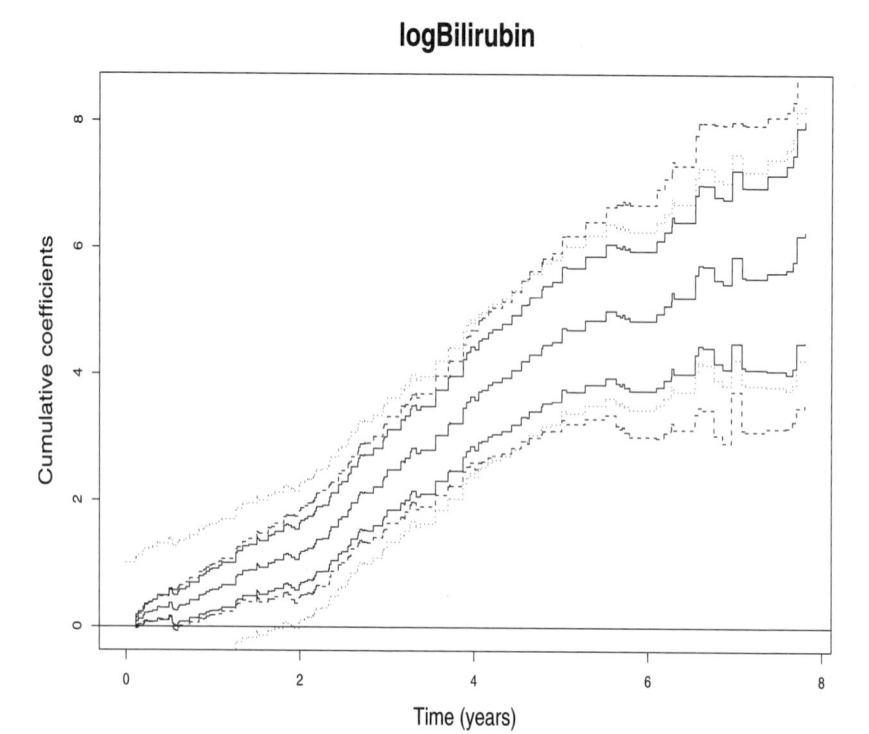

FIGURE 6.9: PBC-data. Estimated cumulative regression function with 95% confidence bands for log(bilirubin). Hall-Wellner band (dotted curves) and simulation based band (broken curves).

Note that the shape of the two confidence bands differ considerably. The Hall-Wellner band being wide initially and narrower later in contrast to the simulation based band. Both bands show, however, that the effect of log(bilirubin) is significant having the constant function 0 outside the bands. The p-values for the simulation based approach for the significance of the individual effects are those reported in the output shown in Example 6.0.2. It is not clear based on Figure 6.9 if the cumulative coefficient is consistent with a constant multiplicative effect or if the corresponding regression coefficient is significantly time-varying. The cumulative coefficient is somewhat flat initially, then steeper in its increase and finally flattening out. The uniform bands depicted in Figure 6.9 cannot be used to test the hypothesis of constant effect because it does not reflect the combined uncertainty about the possible constant effect. To test this hypothesis one may use the Kolmogorov-Smirnov test (6.47) or a Cramér-von Mises type test. First consider the table of test statistics and p-values.

```
Test for time invariant effects
```

logBilirubin

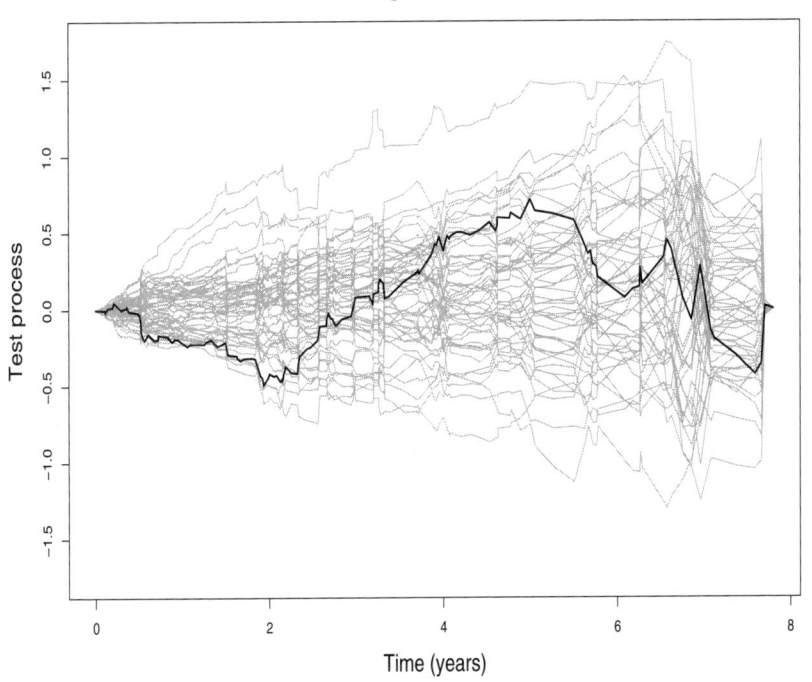

FIGURE 6.10: Test process with 50 simulated processes under the null.

```
                sup| B(t) - (t/tau)B(tau)|  p-value H_0: B(t)=b t
(Intercept)               2.0700                    0.000
Age                       0.0353                    0.940
Edema                     5.4000                    0.000
logBilirubin              0.7170                    0.559
logAlbumin                3.4200                    0.851
logProtime               12.7000                    0.004

                int (B(t)-(t/tau)B(tau))^2dt p-value H_0: B(t)=b t
(Intercept)              1.79e+01                   0.000
Age                      1.29e-03                   0.976
Edema                    7.41e+01                   0.000
logBilirubin             9.16e-01                   0.478
logAlbumin               1.12e+01                   0.943
logProtime               5.28e+02                   0.000

  Call:
timecox(Surv(time/365, status) ~ Age + Edema + logBilirubin +
    logAlbumin + logProtime, pbc, max.time = 8)
```

We see that both the Kolmogorov-Smirnov test and the Cramér-von Mises test lead to very similar p-values, and we see that in the considered model the intercept, edema and log(protime) do have effects that vary significantly with time. A plot of the test process

$$\hat{B}_p(t) - \frac{\hat{B}_p(\tau)}{\tau}t$$

associated with log(bilirubin) along with 50 resampled processes under the model are shown in Figure 6.10. The p-value of the Kolmogorov-Smirnov test is p = 0.55 so we cannot reject the hypothesis of time-invariance. The figure indicates, however, that the observed score process has a somewhat deviating behavior initially, but the supremum test-statistic reflects the behavior around the time-point 6 where there is a lot of variation. This could be investigated further using a variance weighted version of the test statistic, which may be done in timecox using the option weighted.test=1; in this case it does not change our conclusion about the effect of the covariate. □

6.5 A semiparametric multiplicative hazards model

In the previous section we focused on how to investigate whether a specific regression effect is changing with time allowing the other regression coefficients to depend on time. If time-invariance is accepted, then one may want to test the same hypothesis for the remaining variables in the already simplified model. It is therefore of interest to consider the semiparametric model

$$\lambda_i(t) = Y_i(t) \exp(X_i^T(t)\beta(t) + Z_i^T(t)\gamma) \qquad (6.50)$$

where $X_i(t), Z_i(t)$ are predictable bounded covariate vectors of dimension p and q, respectively. The effect of the covariates $X_{i1}(t), \ldots, X_{ip}(t)$ is thus allowed to vary with time while the effect of the covariates $Z_{i1}(t), \ldots, Z_{iq}(t)$ is time-invariant. Define matrices

$$X(t) = (X_1(t), ..., X_n(t))^T$$

and

$$Z(t) = (Z_1(t), ..., Z_n(t))^T.$$

In the following we show how to estimate the unknown quantities and derive the large sample properties of the estimators. To ease notation we show explicit dependence of time in the following only when we wish to emphasize it. For fixed γ the score equation for $\beta(t)$ is

$$X^T\{dN - \lambda dt\} = 0.$$

6.5 A semiparametric multiplicative hazards model

Now, a Taylor expansion around an initial set of estimates $(\tilde{\beta}, \tilde{\gamma})$ gives

$$(\beta - \tilde{\beta})dt = (X^T D X)^{-1} X^T \{dN - \tilde{\lambda}\, dt - DZ(\gamma - \tilde{\gamma})\, dt\} \qquad (6.51)$$

where $D = \tilde{\Lambda}(t) = \mathrm{diag}(\tilde{\lambda}_i)$. The score equation for γ after a Taylor expansion is

$$Z^T \{dN - \tilde{\lambda}\, dt - DX(\beta - \tilde{\beta})dt - DZ(\gamma - \tilde{\gamma})\, dt\} = 0. \qquad (6.52)$$

Inserting (6.51) into (6.52) and solving for γ gives the updating step for γ

$$g_\gamma(\tilde{\gamma}) = \tilde{\gamma} + \left(\int_0^\tau Z^T G D Z\, dt \right)^{-1} \int_0^\tau Z^T G (dN - \tilde{\lambda}\, dt), \qquad (6.53)$$

where

$$G(t) = I - DX(X^T D X)^{-1} X^T.$$

Inserting (6.53) into (6.51) gives the updating step for B:

$$g_B(\tilde{B})(t) = \int_0^t \tilde{\beta}(s)\, ds + \int_0^t (X^T D X)^{-1} X^T \{dN - \tilde{\lambda}\, ds - DZ(g_\gamma(\tilde{\gamma}) - \tilde{\gamma})\, ds\}. \qquad (6.54)$$

Before giving the asymptotic results for the semiparametric model we need some definitions. Let

$$C_1(t) = (n^{-1} \int_0^t Z^T G D Z\, ds)^{-1}, \quad C_2(t) = \int_0^t (X^T D X)^{-1} X^T D Z\, ds$$

with limits in probability $c_1(t), c_2(t)$ respectively, that both exist due to the i.i.d. assumptions combined with existing moments that are uniformly bounded.

Theorem 6.5.1 *Under assumptions similar to those for Theorem 6.3.1 equations (6.53) and (6.54) have $n^{1/2}$-consistent solutions*

$$(g_\gamma(\hat{\gamma}) = \hat{\gamma}, g_B(\hat{B}) = \hat{B})$$

with a probability tending to 1 as $n \to \infty$. Furthermore,

$$n^{1/2}(\hat{\gamma} - \gamma) \xrightarrow{D} V \quad \text{as } n \to \infty,$$

where V is a zero-mean normal with variance Σ, and

$$n^{1/2}(\hat{B} - B) \xrightarrow{D} U \quad \text{as } n \to \infty$$

in $D[0, \tau]^p$, where U is a zero-mean Gaussian process with variance $\Phi(\cdot)$.

6. Multiplicative hazards models

PROOF. We focus only on the distributional properties of the estimators $(\hat{\gamma}, \hat{B})$. Rewriting the expressions for the estimators and using a Taylor-series expansion, we get (suppressing lower order terms)

$$n^{1/2}(\hat{\gamma} - \gamma) = (n^{-1} \int_0^\tau Z^T G D Z\, dt)^{-1} n^{-1/2} \int_0^\tau Z^T G\, dM = C_1(\tau) M_1(\tau),$$

where

$$M_1(t) = n^{-1/2} \int_0^t Z^T G\, dM,$$

and

$$n^{1/2}(\hat{B}(t) - B(t)) = n^{1/2} \int_0^t (X^T D X)^{-1} X^T\, dM$$
$$- n^{1/2} \int_0^t (X^T D X)^{-1} X^T D Z\, ds (\hat{\gamma} - \gamma)$$
$$= M_2(t) - C_2(t) C_1(\tau) M_1(\tau),$$

where

$$M_2(t) = n^{1/2} \int_0^t (X^T D X)^{-1} X^T\, dM.$$

Now, proceeding as in Theorem 6.3.1, it follows that the non-predictable integrands can be replaced by predictable integrands. Therefore, the martingale central limit theorem implies that

$$(M_1, M_2)^T \xrightarrow{D} U = (U_1, U_2) \quad \text{as } n \to \infty$$

in $D[0, \tau]^{(p+q)}$, where U is a zero-mean Gaussian martingale. Thus $n^{1/2}(\hat{\gamma} - \gamma)$ converges in distribution towards a zero-mean normal V with a variance given as the limit in probability of

$$C_1(\tau) \langle M_1 \rangle(\tau) C_1(\tau)^T = (n^{-1} \int_0^\tau Z^T G D Z dt)^{-1} = C_1(\tau),$$

and

$$n^{1/2}(\hat{B}(t) - B(t)) \xrightarrow{D} U_2(t) - c_2(t) c_1(\tau) U_1(\tau),$$

where the covariance function of the right-hand side of (6.5) is given as the limit in probability of

$$\langle M_2(t) - C_2(t) C_1(\tau) M_1(\tau) \rangle$$
$$= \int_0^t (X^T D X)^{-1}\, ds + C_2(t) C_1(\tau) C_2(t)^T + o_p(1)$$

since $\langle M_2, M_1 \rangle(t)$ converges in probability to zero. □

The suggested estimator, $\hat{\gamma}$, for γ is efficient, as its variance attains the variance bound calculated from the efficient influence operator given in Sasieni (1992a).

6.5 A semiparametric multiplicative hazards model

The variances in Theorem 6.5.1 can be estimated by optional variation estimators by noticing that the following martingale decompositions (as in the proof),

$$n^{1/2}(\hat{\gamma} - \gamma) = (n^{-1} \int_0^T Z^T G D Z\, dt)^{-1} n^{-1/2} \int_0^T Z^T G\, dM + o_p(1)$$

and

$$n^{1/2}(\hat{B}(t) - B(t)) = n^{1/2} \int_0^t (X^T D X)^{-1} X^T\, dM$$
$$- n^{1/2} \int_0^t (X^T D X)^{-1} X^T D Z\, ds (\hat{\gamma} - \gamma) + o_p(1).$$

The variance of V is estimated consistently by the (estimated) optional variation process

$$\hat{\Sigma} = C_1(\tau) n^{-1} \int_0^T Z^T G \operatorname{diag}(dN) G Z C_1(\tau)$$

that is asymptotically equivalent to $C_1(\tau)$, and similarly the variance of $n^{1/2}(\hat{B}(t) - B(t))$, $\Phi(t)$, is estimated consistently by the optional variation estimator

$$\hat{\Phi}(t) = n \int_0^t (X^T D X)^{-1} X^T \operatorname{diag}(dN) X (X^T D X)^{-1} + C_2(t) \hat{\Sigma} C_2^T(t)$$

that is asymptotically equivalent to

$$n \int_0^t (X^T D X)^{-1} ds + C_2(t) \hat{\Sigma} C_2^T(t).$$

Example 6.5.1 (PBC data. Example 6.0.2 continued)

In Example 6.0.2 we found that the PBC data were well described by the semiparametric model with constant effects of log(albumin), age and log(bilirubin), and with edema and log(protime) having time-varying effects. The estimates of the parametric terms and their standard errors were found to be

```
Parametric terms :
                    Coef.     SE   Robust SE     z      P-val
const(Age)         0.0377  0.00931   0.00921   4.05   5.2e-05
const(logBilirubin) 0.8210 0.09840   0.08200   8.34   0.0e+00
const(logAlbumin) -2.4500  0.67300   0.60600  -3.64   2.7e-04

   Call:
```

222   6. Multiplicative hazards models

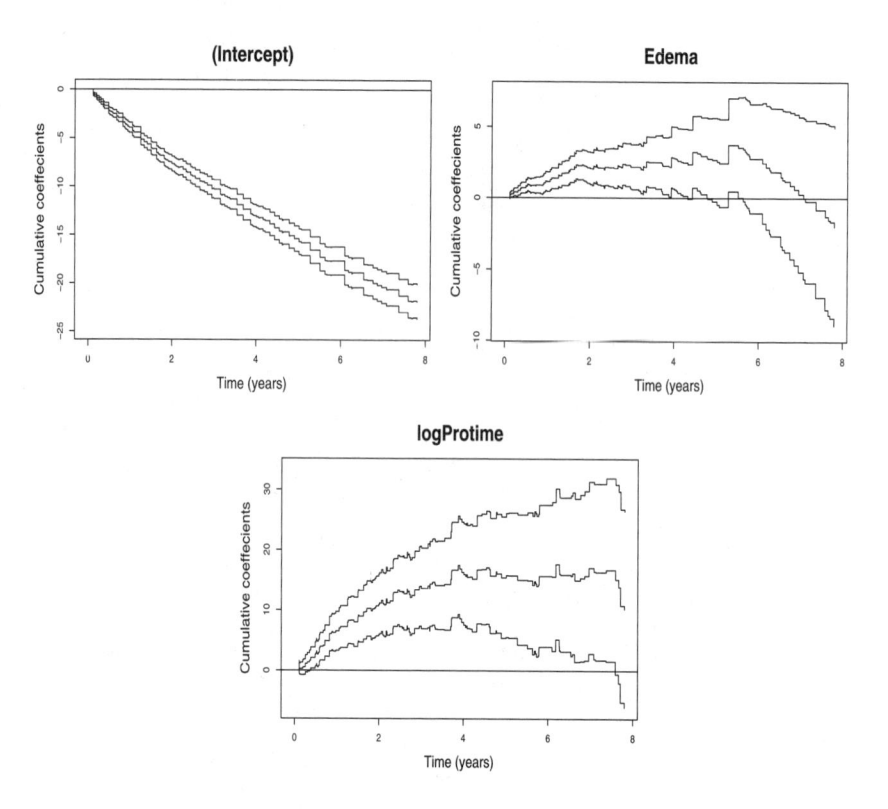

FIGURE 6.11: PBC-data. Estimated cumulative regression coefficients in semiparametric multiplicative risk model along with 95 % confidence intervals.

```
timecox(Surv(time/365, status) ~ const(Age) + Edema +
    const(logBilirubin) + const(logAlbumin) + logProtime, pbc,
    max.time = 8)
```

```
> plot(fit.semi,xlab="Time (years)",ylab="Cumulative coefficient")
```

This gives a much simpler summary of these effects, while the model still allows the needed complexity for the remaining two effects that are shown in Figure 6.11 with 95 % pointwise confidence intervals based on the optional variation formula just given. □

Above we dealt with a particular parameterization of the semiparametric multiplicative intensity model given by (6.50). This parameterization did not specifically include a baseline, although it may be done through a constant among the covariates. In all applications a baseline will be present, and an alternative parameterization, which is standard in the multiplicative setting, is to write this baseline as an explicit nonparametric component of

6.5 A semiparametric multiplicative hazards model

the model
$$\lambda_i(t) = Y_i(t)\lambda_0(t)\exp\{X_i(t)^T\beta(t) + Z_i(t)^T\gamma\}, \tag{6.55}$$

where $X_i(t)$ and $Z_i(t)$ are of dimension p and q, and λ_0 is a baseline intensity function. In the following note we give the similar derivations for this parameterization.

Note. The standard parameterization for semiparametric model.

Establishing the partial likelihood based on the Breslow estimator, first yields the Breslow estimator for $\Lambda_0(t) = \int_0^t \lambda_0(s)ds$ for fixed γ and β

$$\tilde{\Lambda}_0(t) = \int_0^t S_0(s)^{-1}dN.(s).$$

Now, inserting this estimator in the likelihood to obtain a partial likelihood that is Taylor expanded to yield a Newton-Raphson algorithm for estimating γ and $\beta(t)$, we obtain the updating equations

$$\{\beta_{r+1}(t) - \beta_r(t)\}S_{0r}^{-1}dN.(t)$$
$$= \Gamma_r^{-1}\tilde{X}_r^T\left[dN(t) - D\tilde{Z}_r\{\gamma_{r+1} - \gamma_r\}S_{0r}^{-1}dN.(t)\right]$$

and

$$\tilde{Z}_r^T\left[dN(t) - \{D\tilde{X}_r(\beta_{r+1}(t) - \beta_r(t)) - D_r\tilde{Z}_r(\gamma_{r+1} - \gamma_r)\}S_{0r}^{-1}dN.(t)\right] = 0$$

where $\tilde{X}_r = X - \bar{X}_r$, $D_r = \text{diag}\{\phi_{ir}\}$, $\phi_{ir} = \exp(X_i^T\beta_r(t) + Z_i^T\gamma_r)$, $\Gamma_r = \tilde{X}_r^T D\tilde{X}_r$, $\bar{X}_r = S_1^x(t)/S_{0r}^j$, and

$$S_{kr}^x(t) = S_k\{\beta_r, \gamma_r, t\} = \sum_{i=1}^n Y_i \exp\{X_i^T\beta_r(t) + Z_i^T\gamma_r\}X_i^{\otimes k}$$

for $k = 0, 1$, and we define the quantities based on Z similarly. We omitted the time argument from the above equations unless we explicitly wish to emphasize it.

If we solve these equations successively, we obtain

$$\gamma_{r+1} - \gamma_r = \left(\int_0^\tau \tilde{Z}_r^T G_r D_r \tilde{Z}_r \frac{1}{S_0^r}dN.\right)^{-1}\int_0^\tau \tilde{Z}_r^T G_r dN \tag{6.56}$$

where
$$G_r = \{I - D_r\tilde{X}_r(\tilde{X}_r^T D_r \tilde{X}_r)^{-1}\tilde{X}_r^T\}.$$

Using this updated version, γ_{r+1}, we obtain as in the non-parametric case

$$B_{r+1}(t) = \int_0^t \beta_r(t)dt + \int_0^t \Gamma_r^{-1}\lambda_{0r}^{-1}\tilde{X}_r^T\left[dN - D_r\tilde{Z}_r\{\gamma_{r+1} - \gamma_r\}S_{0r}^{-1}dN.\right]. \tag{6.57}$$

The updating step yields an efficient estimator. Iterating yields an estimator of γ and the cumulative regression coefficients. Under weak regularity conditions and with undersmoothing, $\gamma_\infty - \gamma$ is asymptotically normal with a variance that is estimated consistently by

$$C_\gamma(\tau) = \left(\int_0^\tau \tilde{Z}(t)^T G(t) D(t) \tilde{Z}(t) \frac{1}{S_0(t)} dN.(t) \right)^{-1}.$$

Based on $B_\infty(t)$ we may smooth to obtain an estimator of $\beta(s)$ and the cumulative intensity $B_\infty(t)$. It also follows that $B_\infty(t) - \int_0^t \beta(s) ds$ converges towards a Gaussian process with a covariance that is estimated consistently by

$$\int_0^t \Gamma^\infty(s)^{-1} \lambda_0^\infty(s)^{-1} ds + C_1(t) C_\gamma(\tau) C_1(t)^T$$

where $C_1(t) = \int_0^t \Gamma^\infty(s)^{-1} \lambda_0^\infty(s)^{-1} \tilde{X}(s)^T D(s) \tilde{Z}(s) ds$.

The estimation procedure that only involves simple matrix algebra can be written as

Step 1 Start the algorithm with initial estimates of $\beta_r(t)$ and γ_r. Compute the Breslow estimator and smooth to obtain $\lambda_0^r(t)$.

Step 2 Use equation (6.56) to obtain $\gamma_{r+1}(t)$.

Step 3 Use $\gamma_{r+1}(t)$ and equation (6.57) to obtain $B_{r+1}(t)$.

Step 4 Smooth $B_{r+1}(t)$ to obtain an estimate of $\beta^{r+1}(t)$ and return to Step 1.

6.6 Inference for the semiparametric multiplicative model

In this section we outline a test for whether or not an effect of a covariate is time-varying. We consider the semiparametric regression model

$$\lambda_i(t) = Y_i(t) \exp(X_i^T(t)\beta(t) + Z_i^T(t)\gamma)$$

and wish to test the hypothesis $H_0 : \beta_p(t) \equiv \beta_p$ versus the alternative that $\beta_p(t)$ is varying with time. A test for H_0 may be based on the following test process

$$n^{1/2}(\hat{B}_p(t) - \hat{\beta}_p t) \tag{6.58}$$

where $\hat{B}_p(t)$ is the estimator of $B_p(t)$ obtained before simplifying the model, while $\hat{\beta}_p$ is computed under the null hypothesis. It may be shown that (6.58), under the null hypothesis, converges towards a zero-mean Gaussian process. One may then perform a maximal deviation test based on (6.58). The limiting distribution of (6.58) is, however, complicated and the distribution of the maximal deviation test statistic needs to be simulated.

6.6 Inference for the semiparametric multiplicative model

Alternatively, one may use the suggestion by Khmaladze (1981), see Appendix A.

The estimators of the semiparametric model has an i.i.d. representation that may be used for constructing a resampling approach as well as robust standard errors. It may be established that $n^{1/2}(\hat{\gamma} - \gamma)$ is asymptotically equivalent to

$$C_1(\tau) n^{-1/2} \sum_{i=1}^{n} \epsilon_{2i},$$

where

$$\epsilon_{2i} = \int_0^\tau \left(Z_i - (Z^T DX)(X^T DX)^{-1} X_i \right) dM_i.$$

A consistent estimator of the variance of $n^{1/2}(\hat{\gamma} - \gamma)$ is

$$\hat{\Sigma} = n^{-1} \sum_{i=1}^{n} \hat{\epsilon}_{2i}^{\otimes 2}, \tag{6.59}$$

where $\hat{\epsilon}_{2i}$ is defined from ϵ_{2i} by replacing the unknown quantities with their estimates. One may also show that $n^{1/2}(\hat{B}(t) - B(t))$ is asymptotically equivalent to the

$$n^{-1/2} \sum_{i=1}^{n} \epsilon_{3i}(t),$$

where

$$\epsilon_{3i}(t) = \epsilon_{4i}(t) - C_2(t) C_1(\tau) \epsilon_{2i},$$

$$\epsilon_{4i}(t) = \int_0^t (n^{-1} X^T DX)^{-1} X_i dM_i.$$

It can be shown that the variance of $n^{1/2}(\hat{B}(t) - B(t))$ is estimated consistently by

$$\hat{\Phi}(t) = n^{-1} \sum_{i=1}^{n} \hat{\epsilon}_{3i}(t)^{\otimes 2}. \tag{6.60}$$

To make uniform confidence bands and tests one can further show that, if $G_1, ..., G_n$ are independent and standard normally distributed, then

$$\Delta_3(t) = n^{-1/2} \sum_{i=1}^{n} \hat{\epsilon}_{3i}(t) G_i$$

has the same limit distribution as $n^{1/2}(\hat{B}(t) - B(t))$. The construction of uniform confidence bands for $B(t)$ and tests for significance of the nonparametric effects may then be based on replications of $\Delta_3(t)$.

A simple test of the hypothesis of time-invariance, based on $\hat{B}_p(\cdot)$ only, is to compute

$$F_3(\hat{B}_p(\cdot)) = n^{1/2} \sup_{t \in [0,\tau]} |\hat{B}_p(t) - \hat{B}_p(\tau)\frac{t}{\tau}|.$$

The asymptotic properties of this test may be resampled similar to what was done for the Aalen additive model, Chapter 5. We summarize the above results in the below theorem.

Theorem 6.6.1 *Under the conditions of Theorem 6.5.1 and with $G_1, ..., G_n$ independent and standard normally distributed, it follows that*

$$\Delta_2 = C_1(\tau) n^{-1/2} \sum_{i=1}^{n} \hat{\epsilon}_{2i} G_i,$$

$$\Delta_3(\cdot) = n^{-1/2} \sum_{i=1}^{n} \hat{\epsilon}_{3i}(\cdot) G_i,$$

has the same limit distribution as $n^{1/2}(\hat{\gamma} - \gamma, \hat{B}(\cdot) - B(\cdot))$. Further, (6.59) and (6.60) are consistent estimators of the variance of $n^{1/2}(\hat{\gamma} - \gamma)$ and $n^{1/2}(\hat{B}(\cdot) - B(\cdot))$, respectively.

6.7 Estimating the survival function

In Section 7.1.4 we show how to estimate the survival function for an extended version of the Cox model. We here briefly outline how to estimate the survival function for a subject where it is assumed that the hazard is modeled by the semiparametric proportional hazards model

$$\lambda_0(t) = \exp(X_0^T \beta(t) + Z_0^T \gamma)$$

where X_0 and Z_0 are two fixed covariates.

The survival function is then given as

$$S_0(t) = S_0(\beta, \gamma, t) = \exp(-\int_0^t \exp(X_0^T \beta(s) + Z_0^T \gamma) ds)$$

that obviously can be estimated by

$$\hat{S}_0(t) = S_0(\hat{\beta}, \hat{\gamma}, t) = \exp(-\int_0^t \exp(X_0^T \hat{\beta}(s) + Z_0^T \hat{\gamma}) ds).$$

Note that the above integral is easier to compute in the case of the standard parameterization with a baseline function where one does not need to compute a Lebesgue integral.

We now describe how one can construct confidence intervals and a confidence band for the survival function. Using a Taylor series expansion we can approximate the log-survival estimator as follows

$$n^{1/2}(\log(S_0(\hat{B}, \hat{\gamma}, t)) - \log(S_0(B, \gamma, t))) = - \int_0^t \exp(X_0^T \beta(s) + Z_0^T \gamma)$$
$$\left\{ X_0^T d\left\{ n^{1/2}(\hat{B}(s) - B(s)) \right\} + Z_0^T n^{1/2}(\hat{\gamma} - \gamma) ds \right\} + o_p(1).$$

Based on this expansion into the cumulative regression coefficients and the regression coefficients one may now establish a resampling approach to construct an approximate confidence band similarly to what was done for the additive hazards model in Section 5.5.

6.8 Multiplicative rate models

The multiplicative models considered in the previous sections have been specified as intensity models. As noted in Section 5.6 the intensity is equivalent to

$$\lambda(t)dt = E[dN(t)|\sigma(N(s), X(s), Y(s),\ s \in [0, t[)],$$

with $dN(t) = N(t + dt) - N(t)$. The intensity therefore needs to reflect the dependence on the past of $N(t)$, $Y(t)$ and $X(t)$. For recurrent events data it may be an ambitious task to do this modeling. Looking at things in a larger perspective it turns out that even though the model is not the correct intensity an analysis using robust standard errors will still lead to interpretable results if the model is perceived as a model for the rate function. Lin et al. (2000) gave the theory for the Cox rate model building on earlier work by Pepe & Cai (1993), see also Lawless & Nadeau (1995). The results for the rate models are also closely related to the results for misspecified proportional models, see Struthers & Kalbfleisch (1986), Solomon (1984) and in particular Lin & Wei (1989) where robust standard errors were suggested in this context.

We consider the semiparametric model described in Section 6.5. The rate function is thus assumed to be

$$E(\lambda_i(t) \mid Y_i(t), X_i(t), Z_i(t)) = Y_i(t) \exp(X_i(t)^T \beta(t) + Z_i(t)^T \gamma) \quad (6.61)$$

where $X_i(t)$ and $Z_i(t)$ are of dimension p and q, and $Y_i(t)$ is the at risk indicator.

The parameters of the rate model are estimated just as in the intensity context, and when the robust standard errors are used, then the variance estimates given in Section 6.6 are also valid in the rate context and the resampling approach can be applied. To be more specific, the results given in Theorem 6.5.1 and Theorem 6.6.1 still hold, but with γ and B now referring to the rate model (6.61).

6.9 Goodness-of-fit procedures

The extended Cox model (6.31) is very flexible. It is, however, still necessary to investigate the fit of the model. The true model may not be multiplicative and various interactions may have been overlooked. In this section we show how martingale residual techniques may be used to validate the fit of the model. We start by considering

$$M_i(t) = N_i(t) - \int_0^t Y_i(s) \exp(X_i(s)^T \beta(s)) \, ds, \quad i = 1, \ldots, n,$$

and wish to see if estimates thereof have a behavior consistent with the model, where the $M_i(t)$'s are zero-mean martingales (or zero-mean processes in the rate context). The martingales on vector form are estimated by

$$\hat{M}(t) = N(t) - \int_0^t \hat{\lambda}(s) ds$$
$$= M(t) + \int_0^t (\lambda(s) - \hat{\lambda}(s)) ds$$
$$= M(t) - \int_0^t \tilde{W}(\beta(s), s) X(s)(\hat{\beta}(s) - \beta(s)) ds + R(t),$$

where $\tilde{W}(\beta, t) = \operatorname{diag}(Y_i(t) \exp(X_i(t)^T \beta(t)))$, and where the remainder term $R(t)$ is asymptotically negligible. The last integral can be written as

$$\int_0^t W(\beta, s) X(s) d(\hat{B}(s) - B(s)) = \int_0^t W(\beta, s) X(s) A^{-1}(s) X^T(s) dM(s)$$
$$+ o_p(n^{-1/2})$$

using the martingale representation for $n^{1/2}(\hat{B}(t) - B(t))$. Combining the two expression we get that

$$\hat{M}(t) = \tilde{M}(t) + o_p(n^{-1/2}),$$

where

$$\tilde{M}(t) = \int_0^t G(s) dM(s)$$

with

$$G(t) = I - W(\beta, t) X(t) A^{-1}(t) X^T(t).$$

Note that this structure resembles that for the residuals of the additive hazards model, see Section 5.7. The structure implies that

$$X^T(t) d\tilde{M}(t) = 0,$$

and for models containing an intercept, a special case of this reads

$$\sum_{i=1}^{n} Y_i(s) d\tilde{M}_i(t) = 0.$$

The $\hat{M}(t)$ residuals only have this property asymptotically:

$$\int_0^t X^T(s) d\hat{M}(s) = o_p(n^{-1/2}).$$

The residuals $\tilde{M}(t)$ may be used as building blocks in goodness-of-fit procedures. This parallels the development for the additive intensity model, Section 5.7.

One use of the residuals is to sum them depending on the level of the covariates (Aalen, 1993). Define therefore a $m \times n$ matrix possibly depending on time: $K(t)$. A typical choice of $K(t)$ is to let it reflect the quartiles of one of the continuous covariates in the model. The cumulative residual process is then defined by

$$M_K(t) = \int_0^t K^T(s) d\tilde{M}(s) = \int_0^t K^T(s) G(s) dM(s).$$

The variance of $M_K(t)$ can be estimated by the optional variation process

$$[M_K](t) = \int_0^t K^T(s) G(s) \text{diag}(dN(s)) K(s) G(s).$$

An alternative variance estimator, implemented in timereg, is the robust variance estimator based on an i.i.d. representation of the cumulative residual processes, similarly to what was done for the additive intensity model.

Now, plotting the observed cumulative residual process $M_K(t)$ with 95% pointwise confidence intervals will give an indication of whether or not the observed residuals are consistent with the model. When a large number of residuals are computed, it is convenient with a p-value to help summarize how serious a departure from the null that is seen. One may therefore compute the supremum of $M_K(t)$ and approximate the quantiles of its limit distribution, under the model, by resampling. Resampling can also be used to construct confidence bands, as we have indicated in previous chapters.

Example 6.9.1 (PBC-data, Example 6.0.2 continued)

We only show the results for log(bilirubin). Similar results can be obtained for the other covariates.

230   6. Multiplicative hazards models

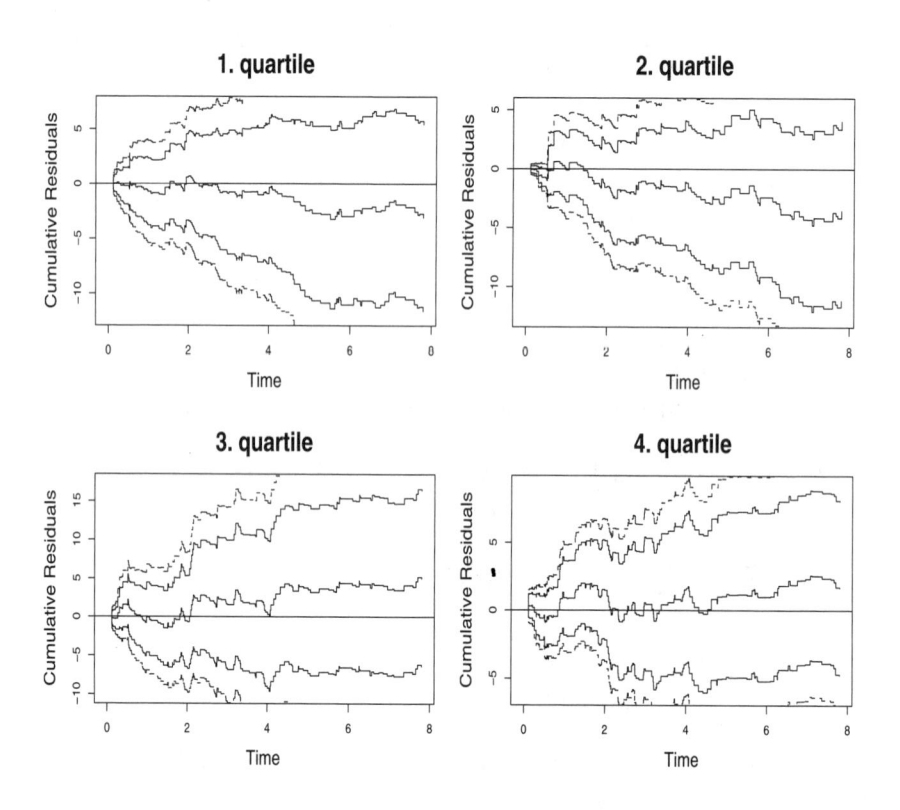

FIGURE 6.12: PBC-data. Observed cumulative residuals with 95% confidence bands (dotted lines) and 95% pointwise confidence intervals (full lines).

```
> fit<-timecox(Surv(time/365,status)~Age+Edema+logBilirubin
+ +logAlbumin+logProtime,max.time=8,pbc,residuals=1,n.sim=0)
Nonparametric Multiplicative Hazard Model
> X<-model.matrix(~-1+cut(Bilirubin,quantile(Bilirubin),
+ include.lowest=T),pbc)
> colnames(X)<-c("1. quartile","2. quartile","3. quartile",
+ "4. quartile");
> resids<-cum.residuals(fit,pbc,X,n.sim=1000);
Cumulative martingale residuals for Right censored survival times
> plot(resids,sim.ci=2)
> summary(resids)
Test for cumulative MG-residuals

Grouped Residuals consistent with model

             sup| hat B(t) |  p-value H_0: B(t)=0
1. quartile         3.229                 0.747
```

6.9 Goodness-of-fit procedures 231

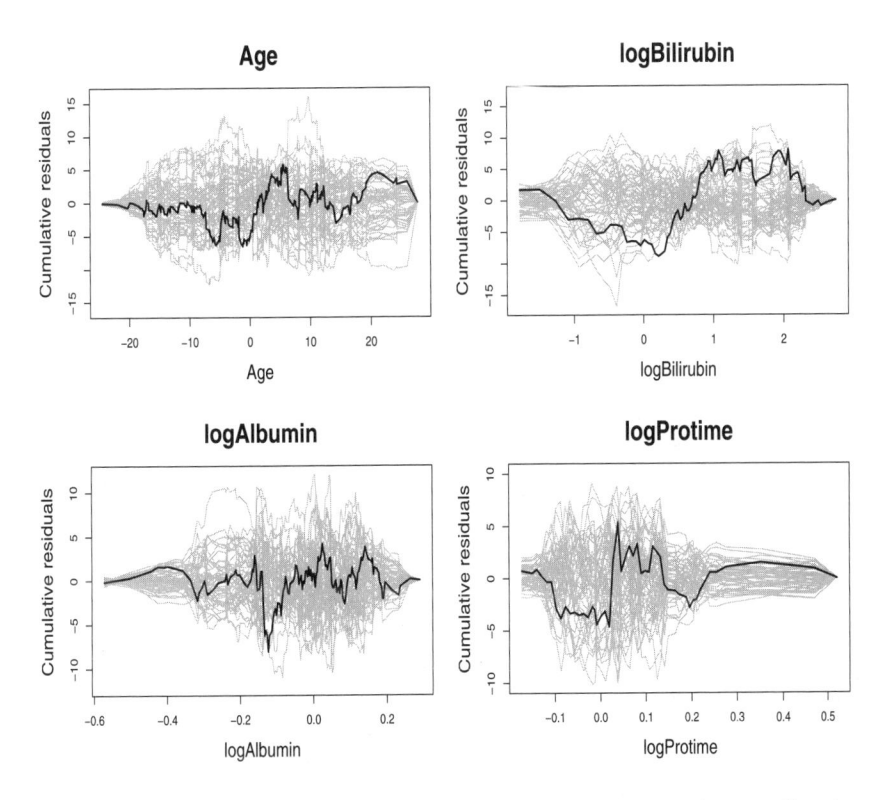

FIGURE 6.13: Observed cumulative residuals with 50 random realizations under the model.

	int (B(t))^2 dt	p-value H_0: B(t)=0
2. quartile	4.773	0.355
3. quartile	5.181	0.635
4. quartile	2.598	0.772

	int (B(t))^2 dt	p-value H_0: B(t)=0
1. quartile	21.567	0.713
2. quartile	45.562	0.384
3. quartile	67.562	0.556
4. quartile	13.534	0.710

The cumulated residuals with 95% confidence intervals and bands, Figure 6.12, show that the effect of log(bilirubin) seems to be well described by the model also supported by the above reported tests. □

These plots are very useful, but it is somewhat inconvenient that one needs to group the continuous covariates. An alternative procedure avoiding this grouping was suggested, as previously mentioned, by Lin et al. (1993) for the Cox model, see Section 6.2. The idea is to cumulate the residuals over

232   6. Multiplicative hazards models

the covariate space as well as over time thus considering the double cumulative processes

$$M_c(t,z) = \int_0^t K_z^T(s) d\tilde{M}(s)$$
$$= \int_0^t K_z^T(s) G(s) dM(s),$$

where $K_z(t)$ is an $n \times 1$ vector with elements

$$I(X_{i1}(t) \leq z) \text{ for } i = 1, .., n$$

focusing here on the first (continuous) covariate denoted X_1. Integrating over the entire time span we get a process in only z

$$M_c(z) = M_c(\tau, z). \tag{6.62}$$

This process can also be written as a sum of i. i. d. components and resampling may thus be used again.

Example 6.9.2 (PBC-data, Example 6.9.1 continued)

We plot the cumulated processes for each of the continuous covariates

```
> fit<-timecox(Surv(time/365,status)~Age+Edema+logBilirubin
+ +logAlbumin+logProtime,max.time=8,pbc,residuals=1,n.sim=0)
Nonparametric Multiplicative Hazard Model
> resids<-cum.residuals(fit,pbc,cum.resid=1)
Cumulative martingale residuals for Right censored survival times
Simulations start N= 500
> plot(resids,score=2);
> summary(resids)
Test for cumulative MG-residuals

Residual versus covariates consistent with model

             sup| hat B(t) |  p-value H_0: B(t)=0
Age                  6.556                  0.714
logBilirubin         8.875                  0.280
logAlbumin           8.049                  0.364
logProtime           5.369                  0.818
```

The output suggests that all cumulated residuals are consistent with the model. Figure 6.13 shows the observed test-process (6.62) with 50 random processes under the model. Note that the summary provided by the p-values might overlook some aspects of the behavior for the log(bilirubin)-covariate. Let us redo the analysis but now with bilirubin included on its original scale.

6.9 Goodness-of-fit procedures 233

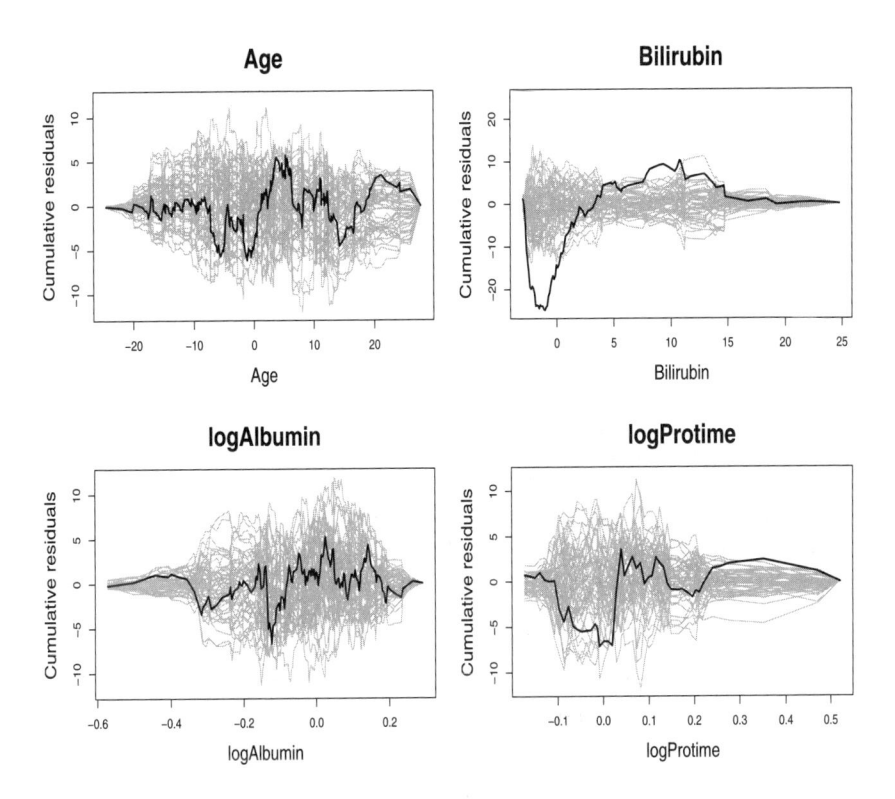

FIGURE 6.14: Cumulative residuals with 50 random realizations under the model.

```
> fit<-timecox(Surv(time/365,status)~Age+Edema+Bilirubin+logAlbumin
+ +logProtime,max.time=8,pbc,residuals=1,n.sim=0)
Nonparametric Multiplicative Hazard Model
> resids<-cum.residuals(fit,pbc,cum.resid=1)
Cumulative martingale residuals for Right censored survival times
Simulations start N= 500
> plot(resids,score=2);
> summary(resids)
Test for cumulative MG-residuals

Residual versus covariates consistent with model

            sup| hat B(t) |  p-value H_0: B(t)=0
Age              6.111               0.686
Bilirubin       24.902               0.000
logAlbumin       6.683               0.602
logProtime       7.136               0.470
```

234   6. Multiplicative hazards models

The output suggests that the model gives a poor fit with respect to effect of the covariate bilirubin. This is supported by Figure 6.14, which gives the cumulated residuals with 50 resampled processes under the model. The behavior of cumulated residual process corresponding to bilirubin is clearly inconsistent with the model. It is thus better to use the extended Cox model with bilirubin included on log-scale. □

6.10 Examples

Below we apply the extended Cox model to the lung cancer data presented in Ying et al. (1995).

Example 6.10.1 (Lung cancer data)

The lung cancer dataset consists of 121 patients with small cell lung cancer. The patients were randomly assigned to one of two treatments: cisplatin followed by etoposide (0); etoposide followed by cisplatin (1). By the end of the study, 47 of the 62 patients on treatment 1 and 51 of the 59 patients on treatment 2 had died. For illustration we fit the extended Cox-model allowing for time-varying effect of the two covariates using the data up to 3 years after beginning of the study. The age variable was centered around its mean before running `timecox`.

```
> fit<-timecox(Surv(times/365,status==1)~trt+age.c,
+ start.time=0,max.time=3,residuals=1,  bandwidth=0.3,n.sim=2000)
Nonparametric Multiplicative Hazard Model
Simulations starts N= 2000
> resids<-cum.residuals(fit,cum.resid=1)
Cumulative martingale residuals for Right censored survival times
Simulations starts N= 500
> plot(resids)
> summary(resids)
Test for cumulative MG-residuals

Residual versus covariates consistent with model

        sup| hat B(t) |  p-value H_0: B(t)=0
age.c         5.215                  0.412
```

The cumulated residuals plotted against the ordered values of age, Figure 6.15, do not appear to be extreme, which is also supported by the above reported supremum test. The fit of the model, see the following output, suggest that there is a time-varying effect (p<0.001) of the treatment while the age effect seems to be constant (p=0.79), see also Figure 6.16. It appears that the risk is higher in treatment group 1 compared to group 0 (keeping age fixed) in the first year or so with no difference thereafter. We can then

6.10 Examples   235

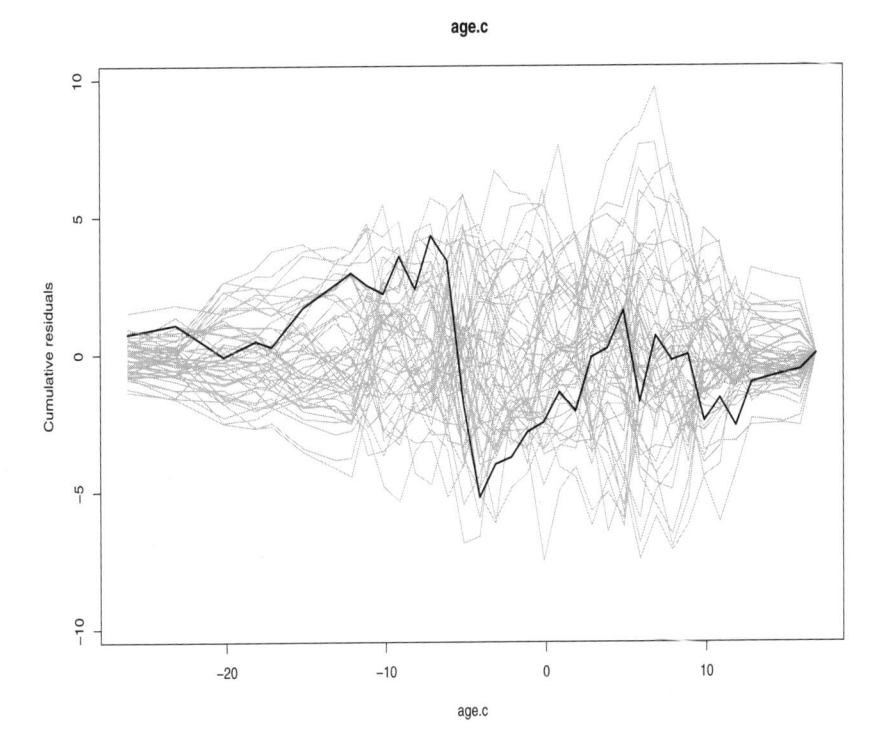

age.c

FIGURE 6.15: Lung cancer data. Cumulated residuals with 50 random realizations under the model.

fit the semiparametric model with constant effect of age, which corresponds to the stratified Cox model. We see from the below output that the age effect is borderline significant with an estimated given by a relative risk of exp(0.021)=1.02 (age is age at entry in years).

```
> summary(fit)
Multiplicative Hazard Model

Test for nonparametric terms

Test for non-significant effects
            sup| hat B(t)/SD(t) | p-value H_0: B(t)=0
(Intercept)            19.30                 0.0000
trt                     5.59                 0.0000
age.c                   3.63                 0.0055
Test for time invariant effects
            sup| B(t) - (t/tau)B(tau)| p-value H_0: B(t)=b t
(Intercept)           0.8660                 0.0005
trt                   1.6200                 0.0000
```

236   6. Multiplicative hazards models

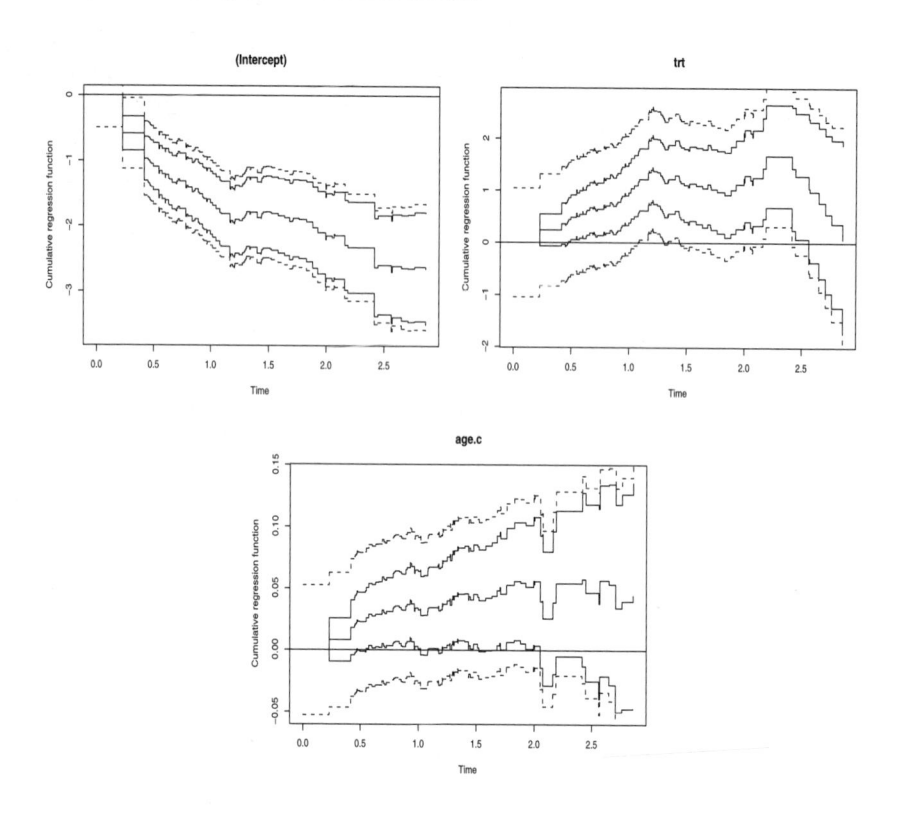

FIGURE 6.16: Lung cancer data. Estimates of cumulative regression coefficients with 95% pointwise confidence intervals (solid lines) and Hall-Wellner confidence band (broken lines).

```
            age.c                      0.0274              0.7910
> fit.semi<-timecox(Surv(times/365,status==1)~trt+const(age.c),
+ start.time=0,max.time=3,residuals=1, bandwidth=0.3,n.sim=2000)
Semiparametric Multiplicative Risk Model
Simulations starts N= 2000
> summary(fit.semi)
Multiplicative Hazard Model

Test for nonparametric terms

Test for non-significant effects
            sup| hat B(t)/SD(t) |  p-value H_0: B(t)=0
(Intercept)           19.8                    0
trt                    5.8                    0
Test for time invariant effects
            sup| B(t) - (t/tau)B(tau)|  p-value H_0: B(t)=b t
(Intercept)          0.874                    0
trt                  1.600                    0
```

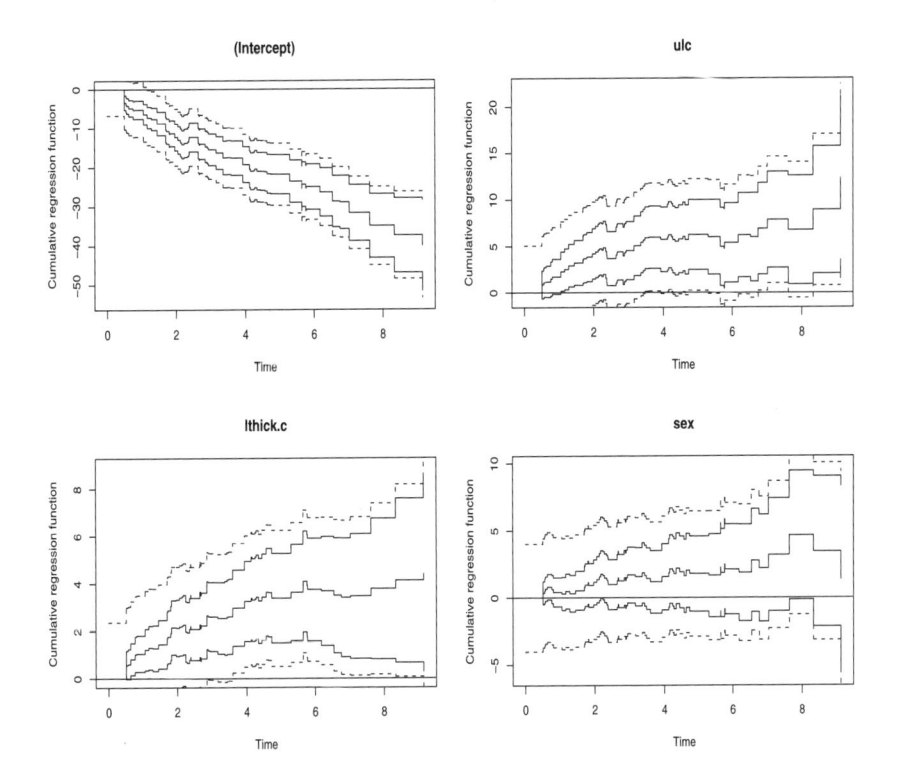

FIGURE 6.17: Melanoma data. Estimates of cumulative regression coefficients with 95% pointwise confidence intervals (solid lines) and Hall-Wellner confidence band (broken lines).

```
Parametric terms :
            Coef.      SE  Robust SE      z   P-val
const(age.c) 0.0206  0.0121     0.0102  1.702  0.0888
```

To further illustrate the use of the extended Cox model we also consider the Melanoma data.

Example 6.10.2 (Melanoma Data)

The data were introduced in Example 3.1.1. Let us fit the extended Cox model to the melanoma data allowing for time-varying effects of sex, ulceration and thickness. The latter covariate was log-transformed and centered around its mean, which seems to be appropriate judging from the below supremum-test with a p-value of 0.21.

```
> fit<-timecox(Surv(days/365,status==1)~ulc+lthick.c+sex,
  residuals=1, bandwidth=0.35,n.sim=2000)
```

238   6. Multiplicative hazards models

```
> resids<-cum.residuals(fit,cum.resid=1)
> plot(fit,hw.ci=2)
> summary(resids)
Test for cumulative MG-residuals

Residual versus covariates consistent with model

          sup| hat B(t) |  p-value H_0: B(t)=0
lthick.c       5.816                 0.212

  Call:
cum.residuals(fit, cum.resid = 1)
> summary(fit)
Multiplicative Hazard Model

Test for time invariant effects
            sup| B(t) - (t/tau)B(tau)|  p-value H_0: B(t)=b t
(Intercept)             4.61                       0.099
ulc                     3.52                       0.191
lthick.c                1.44                       0.049
sex                     3.53                       0.146
```

The test for time-varying effects suggest that the effect of log(thickness) might be time-varying while it is acceptable to assume constant effect of ulceration and sex, see also Figure 6.17. We therefore proceed with the semiparametric model assuming first constant effect of sex, and then of both sex and ulceration:

```
> fit.semi1<-timecox(Surv(days/365,status==1)~ulc+lthick.c+
    const(sex),bandwidth=0.35,n.sim=2000)
> summary(fit.semi1)
Multiplicative Hazard Model

Test for time invariant effects
            sup| B(t) - (t/tau)B(tau)|  p-value H_0: B(t)=b t
(Intercept)             2.83                       0.0715
ulc                     3.13                       0.2230
lthick.c                1.70                       0.0105

Parametric terms :
            Coef.     SE     Robust SE      z      P-val
const(sex)  0.37     0.273      0.252     1.355    0.175

> fit.semi2<-timecox(Surv(days/365,status==1)~const(ulc)+
    lthick.c+const(sex),bandwidth=0.35,n.sim=2000)
Semiparametric Multiplicative Risk Model
Simulations starts N= 2000
> summary(fit.semi2)
Multiplicative Hazard Model
```

6.10 Examples 239

```
Test for time invariant effects
             sup| B(t) - (t/tau)B(tau)|  p-value H_0: B(t)=b t
(Intercept)                       1.46                  0.286
lthick.c                          1.76                  0.001


Parametric terms :
             Coef.    SE      Robust SE      z      P-val
const(ulc)   0.980    0.339   0.292      2.890    0.004
const(sex)   0.395    0.270   0.252      1.462    0.144
```

From these analyses it seems that there is no significant effect of sex while there is a significant higher risk for patients with ulceration with an estimated relative risk of exp(0.98)=2.66. The effect of log(thickness) is time-varying and we see from Figure 6.17 that the effect of this variable diminishes with time. The conclusion about the effect of ulceration depends rather heavily on the considered time span. If we instead consider the survival within the first 6 years, then running a similar analysis as the one above suggests that the effect of ulceration is time-varying:

```
> fit.semi<-timecox(Surv(days/365,status==1)~ulc+lthick.c+
    const(sex),max.time=6,bandwidth=0.35,n.sim=2000)
Semiparametric Multiplicative Risk Model
Simulations starts N= 2000
> summary(fit.semi)
Test for time invariant effects
             sup| B(t) - (t/tau)B(tau)|  p-value H_0: B(t)=b t
(Intercept)                       5.15                 0.0000
ulc                               4.36                 0.0010
lthick.c                          1.17                 0.0805


Parametric terms :
             Coef.    SE      Robust SE      z      P-val
const(sex)   0.388    0.292   0.278      1.328    0.184
```

This logical paradox is a consequence of the simple test for time-varying effects that is used here. First, the supremum test will depend on the considered time range. Secondly, the rough approximation of the constant effect in the semiparametric model by simply using $\hat{B}(\tau)/\tau$ is sensitive to the erratic behavior of $\hat{B}(t)$ in low-information areas. □

6.11 Exercises

6.1 (Equivalence between score test in Cox model and log-rank test)
Consider the situation where we have K groups of right-censored lifetimes with independent censoring. Assume that the conditional hazard function for the ith subject is

$$\alpha_0(t) \exp\Big(\sum_{j=2}^{K} \beta_j X_{ij}\Big),$$

where X_{ij} is the indicator of subject i belonging to group j.

(a) What does $\alpha_0(t)$ describe? Compute the relative risk for two individuals belonging to group 1 and group j, respectively.

(b) Show that the score test of the hypothesis $H_0 : \beta_j = 0$ is the same as the logrank-test.

The logrank-test is thus an optimal test in the case where the Cox model is the underlying true model.

6.2 (Cox's partial likelihood as a marginal likelihood) Let (T_i, X_i), $i = 1, \ldots, n$ be n i.i.d. random variables so that lifetime T_i has conditional hazard function $\alpha_0(t)\exp(\beta X_i)$ given X_i that is assumed to be a scalar. Let $T_{(k)}$, $k = 1, \ldots, n$, denote the ordered values of $T_1, \ldots, T_n$, and let J_k be the item failing at time $T_{(k)}$. In the following things are to be calculated conditional on the covariates so we may think of them as being deterministic.

(a) Show that there is a 1-1 correspondence between

$$(T_1, \ldots, T_n) \quad \text{and} \quad (T_{(1)}, \ldots, T_{(n)}, J_1, \ldots, J_n).$$

In the following we shall thus use the likelihood function $L(\alpha_0, \beta)$ corresponding to observing $(T_{(1)}, \ldots, T_{(n)}, J_1, \ldots, J_n)$. Let

$$\xi_k = (T_{(1)}, \ldots, T_{(k)}, J_1, \ldots, J_k).$$

(b) Show that

$$L(\alpha_0, \beta) = \prod_{k=1}^{n} f^{(k)}_{\xi_{k-1}}(T_{(k)}) \pi^{(k)}_{\xi_{k-1}, T_{(k)}}(J_{(k)}),$$

where $f^{(k)}_{\xi_{k-1}}(t)$ is the conditional density of $T_{(k)}$ given ξ_{k-1} and

$$\pi^{(k)}_{\xi_{k-1}, T_{(k)}}(i) = P(J_k = i \,|\, \xi_{k-1}, T_{(k)}).$$

(c) Compute

$$\prod_{k=1}^{n} \pi^{(k)}_{\xi_{k-1}, T_{(k)}}(J_{(k)}), \quad (6.63)$$

and note that it gives the Cox partial likelihood function.

(d) Show that (6.63) furthermore reduces to the likelihood for observing $J_1, \ldots, J_n$, so that in this case (time-invariant covariates) the Cox partial likelihood is therefore a marginal likelihood.

6.3 Let T_1 and T_2 be independent lifetimes with hazard functions

$$\alpha(t), \quad \theta\alpha(t),$$

respectively, where $\theta > 0$, $\alpha(t) \geq 0$, $t \geq 0$ and $A(t) = \int_0^t \alpha(s)\,ds < \infty$ for all t. Let C_1 and C_2 be independent censoring variables inducing independent censoring, and let $N_j(t) = I(T_j \wedge C_j \leq t, \Delta = 1)$ with $\Delta = I(T_j \leq C_j)$, $j = 1, 2$. Assume we observe in $[0, \tau]$ with τ a deterministic point.

(a) Specify the intensities of $N_j(t)$, $j = 1, 2$.

Assume now that we have n independent copies from the above generic model giving rise to $N_{ji}(t)$, $j = 1, 2$, $i = 1, \ldots, n$. Let $\tilde{\theta}_\tau$ be the solution to

$$0 = \tilde{N}_2(\tau) / \int_0^\tau \frac{\tilde{Y}_2(t)}{\tilde{Y}_1(t) + \theta \tilde{Y}_2(t)} d(\tilde{N}_1(t) + \tilde{N}_2(t))$$

where $\tilde{N}_j(t) = \sum_i N_{ji}(t)$, $\tilde{Y}_j(t) = \sum_i Y_{ji}(t)$, $Y_{ji}(t) = I(t \leq T_{ji} \wedge C_{ji})$, $j = 1, 2$.

(b) Show, for n tending to infinity, that $n^{1/2}(\tilde{\theta}_\tau - \theta)$ converges in distribution towards a zero-mean normal distribution and specify the variance

(c) Let $\beta = \log(\theta)$ and put $\hat{\theta} = \exp(\hat{\beta})$, where $\hat{\beta}$ is the maximum partial likelihood estimator. Compare the asymptotic variance of $n^{1/2}(\hat{\theta} - \theta)$ with that obtained in (c). Is $\hat{\theta}$ different from $\tilde{\theta}_\tau$?

6.4 (One-parameter extension of the Cox-model) Let

$$(T_i, C_i, X_i), \quad i = 1, \ldots, n,$$

be a random sample from the joint distribution of the random variables (T, C, X). Assume that C is independent of (T, X), and that the conditional distribution of T given X has hazard function

$$\alpha(t) = \alpha_0(t) \frac{\exp(\beta^T X)}{(1 + \exp(\beta^T X))^\gamma} \quad (6.64)$$

242   6. Multiplicative hazards models

where the covariate X and its associated regression parameter are assumed to be p-dimensional and γ is an unknown scalar.

(a) Suggest a Cox-score type estimating function for estimation of the unknown the unknown $\theta = (\beta, \gamma)$. We denote the resulting estimator by $\hat{\theta}$.

(b) Derive the limit distribution of $n^{1/2}(\hat{\theta} - \theta)$ (assuming appropriate conditions), and give an estimator of the asymptotic variance-covariance matrix.

(c) Apply the model (6.64) to the melanoma-data with the covariates sex, log(thick) and ulc. Test the hypotheses $H_0 : \gamma = 0$ and $H_0 : \gamma = 1$.

6.5 (Conditional covariate distribution, Xu and O'Quigley (2000))   Let

$$(T_i, C_i, X_i), \quad i = 1, \ldots, n,$$

be a random sample from the joint distribution of the random variables (T, C, X). Assume that C is independent of (T, X), and that the conditional distribution of T given X has hazard function

$$\alpha(t) = \alpha_0(t) \exp(\beta X),$$

where X is assumed to be a one-dimensional continuous covariate with density $g(x)$. Let

$$\pi_i(\beta, t) = Y_i(t) \exp(\beta X_i) / \sum_j Y_j(t) \exp(\beta X_j),$$

where $Y_i(t) = I(t \leq T_i \wedge C_i)$ is the usual at risk indicator function.

(a) Show that the conditional distribution function of X given $T = t$ is consistently estimated by

$$\hat{P}(X \leq z \mid T = t) = \sum_{j : X_j \leq z} \pi_j(\hat{\beta}, t),$$

where $\hat{\beta}$ denotes the maximum partial likelihood estimator of β.

(b) Based on (a) derive an estimator of

$$P(T > t \mid X \in H),$$

where H denotes some subset.

(c) Compute the estimator derived in (b) in the case where $H = \{x\}$.

6.6 (Arjas plot for GOF of Cox model, Arjas (1988)) We shall consider the so-called Arjas plot for goodness-of-fit of the Cox model. For simplicity we consider a two-sample situation. Let $N_i(t)$, $i = 1, \ldots, n$, be counting processes so that $N_i(t)$ has intensity $\lambda_i(t) = Y_i(t)\alpha_0(t)\exp(\beta X_i)$ where $X_i \in \{0, 1\}$. Let

$$N^{(j)}(t) = \sum_i I(Z_i = j)N_i(t), \quad Y^{(j)}(t) = \sum_i I(Z_i = j)Y_i(t), \quad j = 0, 1,$$

and $N(t) = N^{(0)}(t) + N^{(1)}(t)$. The Arjas plot in this situation is to plot

$$\int_0^{T^j_{(m)}} \frac{Y^{(j)}(t)\exp(\hat{\beta}I(j=1))}{Y^{(0)}(t) + Y^{(1)}(t)\exp(\hat{\beta})} dN(t) \tag{6.65}$$

versus m, where $T^j_{(m)}$, $m = 1, \ldots, N^{(j)}(\tau)$, are the ordered jump times in stratum j, $j = 0, 1$.

(a) Argue that the Arjas plot should be approximately straight lines with unit slopes.

Consider now the situation where $\lambda_i(t) = Y_i(t)\alpha_{X_i}(t)$ so that the Cox model may no longer be in force. Here $\alpha_0(t)$ and $\alpha_1(t)$ are two non-negative unspecified functions. The maximum partial likelihood estimator will in this situation converge in probability to β^*, see Exercise 6.7. Let

$$E^{(j)}(t) = \frac{Y^{(j)}(t)\exp(\beta^* I(j=1))}{Y^{(0)}(t) + Y^{(1)}(t)\exp(\beta^*)} dN(t), \quad j = 0, 1.$$

(b) Show that

$$EN^{(1)}(t) = E\int_0^t Y^{(1)}(s)\alpha_1(s)\, ds$$

and

$$EE^{(1)}(t) = E\int_0^t Y^{(1)}(s)\alpha_1(s)f_1(s)\, ds,$$

where

$$f_1(t) = \frac{Y^{(0)}(t)(\alpha_0(t)/\alpha_1(t)) + Y^{(1)}(t)}{Y^{(0)}(t)\exp(-\beta^*) + Y^{(1)}(t)}.$$

Assume that $\alpha_0(t)/\alpha_1(t)$ is increasing in t.

(c) Argue that the Arjas plot for $j = 1$ will tend to be convex and concave for $j = 0$.

6.7 (Misspecified Cox-model, Lin and Wei (1989)) Consider n i.i.d.

$$(N_i(t), Y_i(t), X_i)$$

so that $N_i(t)$ has intensity

$$\lambda_i(t) = Y_i(t)\alpha(t, X_i),$$

where the covariates X_i, $i = 1, \ldots, n$, (p-vectors) are contained in the given filtration and $Y_i(t)$ is the usual at risk indicator. The $N_i(t)$ and $Y_i(t)$ are constructed from lifetime data with right censoring: $N_i(t) = I(T_i \wedge U_i \leq t, \Delta_i = 1)$, $Y_i(t) = I(t \leq T_i \wedge U_i)$ with $\Delta_i = I(T_i \leq U_i)$.

It is not assumed that the intensity is of the Cox-form. Let $\hat{\beta}$ denote the usual Cox partial likelihood estimator under the Cox-model. Struthers & Kalbfleisch (1986) showed that $\hat{\beta}$ is a consistent estimator of β^* where β^* is the solution to the equation $h(\beta) = 0$ with

$$h(\beta) = \int_0^\tau \left(s_1(t) - \frac{s_1(t, \beta)}{s_0(t, \beta)} s_0(t) \right) dt,$$

where $s_j(t) = E(S_j(t))$, $s_j(t, \beta) = E(S_j(t, \beta))$ with

$$S_j(t) = n^{-1} \sum_i X_i^j Y_i(t)\alpha(t, X_i), \quad S_j(t, \beta) = n^{-1} \sum_i X_i^j Y_i(t) \exp(X_i \beta),$$

$j = 0, 1$.

(a) Show under appropriate conditions that $n^{1/2}(\hat{\beta} - \beta^*)$ is asymptotically normal with zero-mean and give a consistent estimator of the covariance matrix.

(b) If the first component of the covariate vector is independent of the other covariates, then show that the Wald-test based on $\hat{\beta}_1$ using the estimator of the covariance matrix derived in (a) is valid for the hypothesis $H_0 : \beta_1 = 0$. (Assume for simplicity that there are no censored observations.)

6.8 (Misspecified Cox-model, Lin (1991)) Consider n i.i.d.

$$(N_i(t), Y_i(t), X_i)$$

so that $N_i(t)$ has intensity

$$\lambda_i(t) = Y_i(t)\alpha(t, X_i),$$

where the covariates X_i, $i = 1, \ldots, n$ (p-vectors) are contained in the given filtration and $Y_i(t)$ is the usual at risk indicator. Consider the following weighted version of the Cox-score

$$U_w(\beta) = \sum_i \int_0^\tau W(t)(X_i - E(\beta, t)) \, dN_i(t),$$

where $W(t)$ is some predictable weight function assumed to converge uniformly in probability to a non-negative bounded function $w(t)$. Let $\hat{\beta}_w$ denote the solution to $U_w(\beta) = 0$.

(a) Show under appropriate conditions that $\hat{\beta}_w$ converges in probability to a quantity β_w that solves the equation $h_w(\beta) = 0$ with

$$h_w(\beta) = \int_0^\tau w(t) \left(s_1(t) - \frac{s_1(t, \beta)}{s_0(t, \beta)} s_0(t) \right) dt$$

using the same notation as in Exercise 6.7.

(b) Let $\hat{\beta}$ denote the usual Cox-estimator. If the Cox-model holds, then show that $n^{1/2}(\hat{\beta}_w - \hat{\beta})$ is asymptotically normal with zero mean and derive a consistent estimator D_w of the covariance matrix.

The test statistic

$$n(\hat{\beta}_w - \hat{\beta}) D_w^{-1} (\hat{\beta}_w - \hat{\beta})$$

is asymptotically χ^2 if the Cox-model holds and may therefore be used as a goodness-of-fit test.

(c) Show that the above test is consistent against any model misspecification under which $\beta_w \neq \beta^*$ or $h_w(\beta^*) \neq 0$, where β^* is the limit in probability of $\hat{\beta}$.

Suppose that X_i, $i = 1, \ldots, n$, are scalars.

(d) If $w(t)$ is monotone, then show that the above test is consistent against the alternative

$$\lambda_i(t) = Y_i(t)\alpha_0(t) \exp(\beta(t) X_i)$$

of time-varying effect of the covariate.

6.9 (Current status data with additive hazards) Let T denote a failure time with hazard function

$$\alpha(t) = \alpha_0(t) + \theta^T X(t)$$

where $X(t)$ is a p-vector of predictable covariates, and $\alpha_0(t)$ and θ are the parameters of interest. Let C denote a random monitoring time with hazard function $\mu(t)$. The observed data consist of $(C, \Delta = I(C \leq T), X_i(\cdot))$. Such data are called current status data since at the monitoring time C it is only known whether or not the event of interest (with waiting time T) has occurred.

(a) Derive the intensity function of the counting process
$$N(t) = \Delta I(C \leq t),$$
which jumps by unity whenever the subject is monitored at time t and found failure-free.

(b) Let $(C_i, \Delta_i, X_i(\cdot))$, $i = 1, \ldots, n$, be n independent replicates of $(C, \Delta = I(C \leq T), X(\cdot))$. Suggest an estimating equation for estimation of the regression parameter θ.

The estimation procedure in (b) is not efficient. Given below is an efficient procedure. Define the following two counting processes,
$$N_{1i}(t) = \Delta_i I(C_i \leq t), \quad N_{2i}(t) = (1 - \Delta_i) I(C_i \leq t).$$

The process N_{1i} jumps by unity when subject i is monitored and failure-free while N_{2i} jumps by unity when subject i is monitored and failure has occurred. Furthermore, let $N_i(t) = N_{1i}(t) + N_{2i}(t)$. The empirical version of the efficient score for θ gives us the score function of interest, namely

$$U(\theta, A) = \sum_{i=1}^{n} \int (X_i - \frac{S_1}{S_0})(\frac{p_i}{1 - p_i} dN_{2i} - dN_{1i}), \tag{6.66}$$

where
$$S_j(t) = \sum_i \frac{p_i}{1 - p_i} Y_i X_i^{\otimes j}, \quad p_i(t, A, \theta) = e^{-A(t) - \theta X_i}$$

and $A(t) = \int_0^t \alpha_0(s) \, ds$. The estimator $\hat{\theta}$ is defined as the solution to the estimated empirical efficient score equation

$$U(\theta, \hat{A}) = 0, \tag{6.67}$$

where $\hat{A}$ is an estimator of A.

(c) Show that (6.66) is a martingale, and that this also true for $U(\theta_0, \hat{A})$, if $\hat{A}$ is a predictable estimator of A.

(d) Derive, under appropriate conditions, the large sample results for $\hat{\theta}$ and give a consistent estimator of the asymptotic variance.

Estimation of θ based on $N_{1i}(t)$, $i = 1, \ldots, n$ was considered by Lin et al. (1998a) while Martinussen & Scheike (2002a) studied estimation of θ based on $(N_{1i}(t), N_{2i}(t))$, $i = 1, \ldots, n$.

6.10 (Covariance for semiparametric multiplicative model)   Assume that i.i.d. subject that all have intensity on the semiparametric multiplicative hazard form
$$\lambda_i(t) = Y_i(t) \exp(X_i(t)^T \beta(t) + Z_i(t)^T \gamma)$$
where $X_i(t)$ and $Z_i(t)$ are predictable covariate vectors of dimension $(p+q)$ is being observed on $[0, \tau]$.

In Theorem 6.5.1 we gave the asymptotic description of the the estimators of γ and $B(t) = \int_0^t \beta(s) ds$. Work out the covariance between the estimators and give a variance estimator based on the underlying optional variation processes.

6.11 (Confidence bands for GOF of Cox's regression model)

(a) Reproduce the output for the "Graphical GOF for Cox's regression model" in Example 6.2.1 and outline the theoretical arguments using the delta-theorem.

To get the covariance matrix for the stratified baseline use the covariance=1 option in the cox.aalen program.

(b) One can also construct confidence bands, outline how this can be done using the i.i.d decomposition of $\hat{\Lambda}_j - \Lambda_j(t)$. To implement it you can see how the resample processes are used in Example 5.5.1.

7
Multiplicative-Additive hazards models

The additive and multiplicative intensity models considered in the two previous chapters postulate different relationships between the hazard and covariates, and sometimes it will not be clear which of the models that should be preferred in a specific application. The models may often be used to complement each other and to provide different summary measures. In some cases, however, covariate effects are best modeled as multiplicative or as additive, and one might then be in a situation where it is best to combine the additive and multiplicative models. The additive and multiplicative intensity models may be combined in various ways to achieve flexible and useful models. We shall here consider two types of models that are based on either adding or multiplying the Cox model and the additive Aalen model. This leads to two somewhat different models, but both being quite flexible and useful. When the basic models are added, it leads to the proportional excess hazard models, where the additive part can be thought of as modeling the baseline mortality while the multiplicative part describes the excess risk due to different exposure levels. Multiplying the two models leads to a model that we term the Cox-Aalen model. For this model some covariate effects are believed to result in multiplicative effects, whereas other effects are better described as additive.

Lin & Ying (1995) considered the following additive-multiplicative intensity model

$$\lambda(t) = Y(t) \left[g(X^T(t)\alpha) + \lambda_0(t)h(Z^T(t)\beta) \right],$$

where $Y(t)$ is the at risk indicator, $(X(t), Z(t))$ is a $q + p$ dimensional covariate vector, (α, β) is a $q+p$ dimensional vector of regression coefficients and $\lambda_0(t)$ is a unspecified baseline hazard. Both h and g are assumed known. This gives a quite flexible framework, but one problem with this model is that only the baseline is time-varying and therefore data with time-varying effects will often not be well described. If additional time-varying effects are included in the model, then it will get added flexibility. It turns out that it is relatively simple to extend the model to deal with time-varying effects such as in the flexible additive-multiplicative intensity model, Martinussen & Scheike (2002b), where the intensity is on the form

$$\lambda(t) = Y(t) \left[X^T(t)\alpha(t) + \rho(t)\lambda_0(t) \exp\{Z^T(t)\beta\} \right], \tag{7.1}$$

where both $Y(t)$ and $\rho(t)$ are at risk (excess risk) indicators, $\alpha(\cdot)$ is a q-vector of time-varying regression functions, $\lambda_0(t)$ is the baseline hazard of the excess risk term, and β is a p-dimensional vector of relative risk regression coefficients. The at risk indicator $\rho(t)$ may be set to $Y(t)$ as in the Lin and Ying model above, but sometimes one will have a baseline group where there is no excess risk. The model is an extension of the Lin and Ying model when $g(x) = x$ and $h(x) = \exp(x)$ and the model is a sum of the additive Aalen model and the Cox model. Sasieni (1996) considered the special case of this model where $X^T(t)\alpha(t)$ is replaced by a known function of $X(t)$. Zahl (2003) illustrated the use of model (7.1) with breast and colon cancer data.

A different way of combining additive and multiplicative models is given by the Cox-Aalen model, Scheike & Zhang (2002), where the intensity is on the form

$$\lambda(t) = Y(t) \left[X^T(t)\alpha(t) \right] \exp(Z^T(t)\beta). \tag{7.2}$$

The Cox-Aalen model allows a flexible (additive) description of covariate effects of $X(t)$ while allowing other covariate effects to act multiplicatively on the intensity. An alternative way of thinking of this model is to consider it as an approximation to the general stratified hazard model

$$\alpha(t, X(t)) \exp(Z^T(t)\beta)$$

suggested by Dabrowska (1997). Compared to the Dabrowska model some structure is introduced to make the estimation easier and to help facilitate the interpretation of the covariate effects.

We start this chapter with studying the Cox-Aalen model (7.2) including prediction of survival accompanied by confidence bands. This material is useful as it generalizes results for the Aalen additive model, the Cox model and also the stratified Cox model. We then turn to the proportional excess model (7.1). Both models may be fitted in R using the `timereg`-package as illustrated in the examples in this chapter.

7.1 The Cox-Aalen hazards model

Dabrowska (1997) studied the so-called smoothed Cox regression model, where the intensity is of the form

$$\lambda(t) = Y(t)\alpha(t, X)\exp(Z^T \beta), \quad (7.3)$$

and where the baseline hazard $\alpha(t, X)$ gives the background intensity for a subject with baseline characteristics X. The second term of the model gives the relative risk of covariates Z. Based on i.i.d. observations, Dabrowska studied the properties of the solution, $\hat{\beta}_S$, to the smoothed partial likelihood score equation

$$\sum_{i=1}^{n} \int_0^\tau \left\{ Z_i - \frac{S_1(X_i, s, \beta)}{S_0(X_i, s, \beta)} \right\} dN_i(s) = 0,$$

where

$$S_k(x, s, \beta) = \sum_{i=1}^{n} K(b, x - X_j) Y_j(s) \exp(Z_i^T \beta) Z_i^{\otimes k},$$

K is a symmetric positive kernel with support $[-1, 1]$, $b > 0$ is a bandwidth and $K(b, s) = K(s/b)$. The estimator of the integrated baseline is

$$\hat{A}(x, t) = \sum_{i=1}^{n} \int_0^t \frac{K(b, x - X_i)}{S_0(x, s, \hat{\beta})} dN_i(s).$$

In the absence of covariates this is the estimator suggested by Beran (1981). If the covariate X vary according to a density and the bandwidth is suitably chosen, Dabrowska showed that the estimator $\hat{\beta}_S$ is efficient and asymptotically normal. The smoothed Cox regression model has not received much attention in practical work although it may be attractive in some situations to avoid specific modeling of the effect of the covariate X. One drawback of the approach is that one needs to choose the smoothing parameter b and that it is difficult to summarize the effect of X. The approach must further be modified if X contains categorical covariates.

A model that also aims at flexible modeling of a covariate dependent baseline and includes other effects as multiplicative effects is the model (7.3) with $\alpha(t, X)$ replaced by an Aalen additive function $X(t)^T \alpha(t)$ that is:

$$\lambda(t) = Y(t) \left\{ X(t)^T \alpha(t) \right\} \exp(Z(t)^T \beta), \quad (7.4)$$

see Scheike & Zhang (2002, 2003) who termed (7.4) as the Cox-Aalen model as it is a mix of these two models. This added regression structure makes estimation and interpretation of covariate effects on the baseline considerably easier at the expense of less flexibility. For many practical purposes this will result in a reasonable compromise between bias and variance. A further practical advantage is that categorical covariates can be handled in the baseline without any special attention.

7.1.1 Model and estimation

Assume that we have n i.i.d. observations (N_i, X_i, Z_i, Y_i) for $i = 1,..,n$, such that the ith counting process, $N_i(t)$, has intensity of the Cox-Aalen form

$$\lambda_i(t) = Y_i(t) \left\{ X_i(t)^T \alpha(t) \right\} \exp(Z_i(t)^T \beta), \tag{7.5}$$

where $Y_i(t)$ is an at risk indicator, $X_i(t)$ and $Z_i(t)$ are predictable bounded covariate vectors of dimensions q and p, respectively, $\alpha(t)$ is a q-dimensional locally integrable function and β is a p-dimensional regression vector. Let

$$N = (N_1, \ldots, N_n)^T, \quad M = (M_1, \ldots, M_n)^T,$$

where $M_i(t) = N_i(t) - \Lambda_i(t)$ with $\Lambda_i(t) = \int_0^t \lambda_i(s) ds$, and define matrices $(n \times q)$

$$Y(\beta, t) = (Y_1(t) \exp(Z_1(t)^T \beta) X_1(t), \ldots, Y_n(t) \exp(Z_n(t)^T \beta) X_n(t))^T$$

and $(n \times p)$

$$Z(t) = (Z_1(t), \ldots, Z_n(t))^T.$$

The log-likelihood function is

$$l(\beta) = \sum_{i=1}^n \int_0^\tau \log \left(Y_i(t) X_i(t)^T dA(t) \exp(Z_i(t)^T \beta) \right) dN_i(t)$$

$$- \sum_{i=1}^n \int_0^\tau Y_i(t) \exp(Z_i(t)^T \beta) X_i(t)^T dA(t),$$

where $A(t) = \int_0^t \alpha(s) \, ds$. The log-likelihood function leads to the score equations for β and $dA(t)$

$$\int Z(t)^T \{dN - Y(\beta, t) dA(t)\} = 0,$$

$$Y(\beta, t)^T W(t) \{dN - Y(\beta, t) dA(t)\} = 0,$$

where $W(t) = \text{diag}(w_i(t))$ with

$$w_i(t) = \frac{Y_i(t)}{\lambda_i(t)} = \frac{Y_i(t) \exp(-Z_i(t)^T \beta)}{X_i(t)^T \alpha(t)},$$

for $i = 1, ..., n$. For known β this leads to the estimator of the cumulative intensity

$$\hat{A}(\beta, t) = \int_0^t Y^-(\beta, s) dN(s),$$

where

$$Y^-(\beta, t) = (Y(\beta, t)^T W(t) Y(\beta, t))^{-1} Y(\beta, t)^T W(t)$$

7.1 The Cox-Aalen hazards model

is a weighted generalized inverse of $Y(\beta,t)$ with the convention that $Y^-(\beta,t)$ is 0 when the above inverse does not exist. Inserting this estimator into the score equation for β gives $U(\beta) = 0$ with

$$U(\beta) = U(\beta, \tau) = \int_0^\tau Z^T(t) G(\beta, t) dN(t), \tag{7.6}$$

where

$$G(\beta, t) = I - Y(\beta, t) Y^-(\beta, t)$$

is the projection onto the orthogonal space spanned by the columns of $Y(\beta,t)$. When we consider the Cox regression model, where

$$Y_i(t) X_i(t)^T \alpha(t) = Y_i(t) \alpha_0(t),$$

then the score function (7.6) reduces to the Cox's partial likelihood score, and then $\alpha_0(t)$ cancels out, and is thus not needed for estimation of β.

Let β_0 denote the true value of β. Simple calculations show that the compensator of $U(\beta_0, t)$ is zero so that

$$U(\beta_0, t) = \int_0^t Z^T(s) G(\beta_0, s) dM(s)$$

is a square integrable martingale. The martingale property of the score function does not depend on the specific choice of the weight matrix $W(t)$ (apart from it being predictable). We can therefore consider the estimating equation $U(\beta) = 0$ for all choices of $W(t)$.

To be able to compute the estimator we need, at least initially, weights that do not depend on the unknown baseline intensities. We use weights of the form

$$w_i(t) = Y_i(t) h_i(t) \exp(-Z_i(t)^T \beta),$$

where $h_i(t)$ $i = 1, ..., n$ are known functions that do not depend on β. A particularly simple choice of the weights that we use as our primary estimator in the remainder is to choose $h_i(t) \equiv 1$ for all i. Define $\hat{\beta}$ as the solution to the score equation

$$U(\beta, \tau) = 0,$$

and estimate $A(t)$ by

$$\hat{A}(\hat{\beta}, t). \tag{7.7}$$

These estimates may now be used to obtain estimates of the maximum likelihood weights. The estimators with the maximum likelihood weights are efficient. Further, since the estimators with estimated maximum likelihood weights have the same properties as the estimators with known weights these estimators are also efficient. For practical purposes, however, it seems sufficient to use the simple initial estimator.

7. Multiplicative-Additive hazards models

Note. The efficiently weighted score equation is an empirical version of the efficient score for the semi-parametric model (Sasieni, 1992b). Suppressing the dependence of time the score for the parametric component can be written as

$$\dot{l}_\beta = \int Z^T dM$$

and similarly the non-parametric components, α, gives a score that when evaluated at $b(t)$ equals

$$\dot{l}_\alpha b = \int b^T Y^T W dM.$$

The efficient score l_β^* for β is of the form

$$\int (Z^T - (b^*)^T Y^T W) dM$$

for some b^* such that l_β^* is orthogonal to $\dot{l}_\alpha b$. This gives that

$$b^* = E((Y^T W Y)^{-1} Y^T Z)$$

and by insertion we get

$$l_\beta^* = \int (Z^T - E((Y^T W Y)^{-1} Y^T Z)^T Y^T W) dM.$$

Now, notice that (7.6) is an empirical version of the efficient score equation.

The derivative of $U(\beta, \tau)$ with respect to β is calculated using matrix derivative rules as in MacRae (1974), see Appendix B. Calculating the derivative of $Y^-(\beta, t)$ with respect to β_j we get

$$\frac{\partial}{\partial \beta_j} Y^-(\beta, t) = -Y^-(\beta, t) \text{diag}(Z_{ij}(t)) Y(\beta, t) Y^-(\beta, t),$$

a $p \times n$ matrix. Note that the particular form of the weight matrix is used actively in the computations of the derivative. The derivative of minus $U(\beta, t)$ is computed to be

$$I(\beta, t) = -\frac{\partial}{\partial \beta} U(\beta, t)$$
$$= \int_0^\tau Z^T(t) \text{diag}(Y(\beta, t) Y^-(\beta, t) dN(t)) Z(t)$$
$$- \int_0^\tau Z^T(t) Y(\beta, t) Y^-(\beta, t) \text{diag}(Y(\beta, t) Y^-(\beta, t) dN(t)) Z(t).$$

7.1.2 Inference and large sample properties

The properties of the suggested estimators are simple to derive using the underlying martingales, and the results may also be extended to the rate function case where the robust standard error estimates are needed.

A Taylor series expansion around the true value of the parameter β_0 yields
$$U(\hat{\beta}, \tau) - U(\beta_0, \tau) = -I(\beta^\star, \tau)(\hat{\beta} - \beta_0),$$
where $\beta^\star$ lies on the line segment between $\hat{\beta}$ and β_0. This implies that
$$(\hat{\beta} - \beta_0) = -I(\beta^\star, \tau)^{-1} U(\beta_0, \tau)$$
if $I(\beta^\star, \tau)$ is invertible. Therefore to show that $n^{1/2}(\hat{\beta} - \beta_0)$ converges in distribution it suffices to show that
$$n^{-1} I(\beta^\star, \tau) \xrightarrow{P} \mathcal{I}(\tau)$$
and that
$$n^{-1/2} U(\beta_0, \tau) \xrightarrow{D} W(\tau),$$
where $\mathcal{I}(\tau)$ is non-singular and $W(t)$ is a Gaussian martingale. The convergence of the score process follows from the martingale central limit theorem.

The optional variation process of the martingale $U(\beta_0, \cdot)$ (and evaluated at τ) is given as
$$[U(\beta_0)](\tau) = \int_0^\tau Z^T(t) G(\beta_0, t) \text{diag}(dN(t)) G(\beta_0, t) Z(t)$$
and may be used as an estimator of its variance with β_0 replaced by $\hat{\beta}$. We denote this expression as $\left[U(\hat{\beta})\right](\tau)$.

Theorem 7.1.1 *Under regularity conditions it follows that $n^{1/2}(\hat{\beta} - \beta_0)$ converges towards a normal distributed variable with zero-mean and a variance that is estimated consistently by*
$$\hat{\Sigma} = n I^{-1}(\hat{\beta}, \tau) [U(\hat{\beta})](\tau) I^{-1}(\hat{\beta}, \tau).$$

For the maximum likelihood weights the variance simplifies since both $I^{-1}(\hat{\beta}, \tau)$ and $[U(\hat{\beta})](\tau)$ estimate the variance of $(\hat{\beta} - \beta_0)$.

For fixed β we let the compensator of $\hat{A}(\beta, t)$ be denoted $A^\star(\beta, t)$. Now, expanding the estimator around β_0 we get that
$$\hat{A}(\hat{\beta}, t) - A(t) = (\hat{A}(\hat{\beta}, t) - \hat{A}(\beta_0, t)) + (\hat{A}(\beta_0, t) - A^\star(\beta_0, t)) + (A^\star(\beta_0, t) - A(t)).$$
The second term on the right-hand side is a martingale and equals
$$M_A(t) = \int_0^t Y^-(\beta_0, s) dM(s),$$

256   7. Multiplicative-Additive hazards models

and the third term represents the bias from the Aalen estimator due to non-invertibility and is asymptotically negligible. Taylor expanding the first term we obtain

$$\hat{A}(\hat{\beta}, t) - \hat{A}(\beta_0, t) = (\hat{\beta} - \beta_0)^T \int_0^t \frac{\partial}{\partial \beta} Y^-(\beta_0, s) dN(s) + R(t),$$

where the remainder term $R(t)$ is asymptotically negligible. Therefore to derive asymptotic properties of $n^{1/2}(\hat{A}(\hat{\beta}, t) - A(t))$, it suffices to show that

$$H(\beta, t) = \int_0^t \frac{\partial}{\partial \beta} Y^-(\beta, s) dN(s) \qquad (7.8)$$

$$= \int_0^t Y^-(\beta, s) \operatorname{diag}(Y(\beta, s) Y^-(\beta, s) dN(s)) Z(s)$$

converges uniformly in probability, that the martingale terms converges jointly in distribution and that the bias term $n^{1/2}(A^\star(\beta_0, t) - A(t))$ converges uniformly to zero in probability.

Theorem 7.1.2 *Under regularity conditions, it follows that $n^{1/2}(\hat{A}(\hat{\beta}, t) - A(t))$ converges in distribution towards a Gaussian process with variance function $\Phi(t)$ that is estimated consistently by*

$$\hat{\Phi}(t) = n \left(\frac{1}{n} H(\hat{\beta}, t)^T \hat{\Sigma} H(\hat{\beta}, t) + [M_A](t) + C(t) \right),$$

where

$$C(t) = H(\hat{\beta}, t)^T I^{-1}(\hat{\beta}, \tau)[U, M_A](t) + [M_A, U](t) I^{-1}(\hat{\beta}, \tau) H(\hat{\beta}, t).$$

The stratified Cox-model is a special case of the Cox-Aalen model, although the estimating equations differ slightly.

The optional variation covariance process, $[U, M_A](t)$, is estimated consistently by

$$\int_0^t \left(Z^T(s) G(\hat{\beta}, s) \right) \operatorname{diag}(dN(s)) \left(Y^-(\hat{\beta}, s) \right)^T,$$

and similarly, $[M_A](t)$ is estimated consistently by

$$\int_0^t \left(Y^-(\hat{\beta}, s) \right) \operatorname{diag}(dN(s)) \left(Y^-(\hat{\beta}, s) \right)^T.$$

For the maximum likelihood weights, the covariance term, $C(t)$, between the two martingales vanishes asymptotically.

When the model is a rate model rather than an intensity model, the estimation is carried out as above but one has to compute robust variance estimators in this case. These derivations are based on an i.i.d. representation

7.1 The Cox-Aalen hazards model

that we also developed for the additive hazards model and the proportional hazards model.

The martingales have increments that can be written as

$$dM_i(t) = dN_i(t) - Y_i(t)\exp(Z_i(t)^T\beta_0)X_i(t)^T dA(t)$$

and estimated by $d\hat{M}_i(t)$ obtained by plugging in the estimates of β_0 and $A(t)$.

The score process evaluated at β_0 can be written as (ignoring lower order terms)

$$U(\beta_0, t) = \sum_{i=1}^{n} \epsilon_{1i}(t), \tag{7.9}$$

where

$$\epsilon_{1i}(t) = \int_0^t \left(Z_i(s) - Z^T(s)Y(\beta_0, s)(Y^T(\beta_0, s)W(s)Y(\beta_0, s))^{-1}X_i(s)^T\right) dM_i(s).$$

It can be shown that the variance of the limit distribution of $n^{1/2}(\hat{\beta} - \beta_0)$ may be estimated consistently by

$$\tilde{\Sigma} = nI^{-1}(\hat{\beta}, \tau)\left\{\sum_{i=1}^{n}\hat{\epsilon}_{1i}^{\otimes 2}(\tau)\right\}I^{-1}(\hat{\beta}, \tau).$$

Similarly, $n^{1/2}(\hat{A}(t) - A(t))$ is asymptotically equivalent to

$$n^{1/2}\sum_{i=1}^{n}\epsilon_{2i}(t), \tag{7.10}$$

where

$$\epsilon_{2i}(t) = \epsilon_{3i}(t) + H^T(\beta_0, t)I(\beta_0, t)^{-1}\epsilon_{1i}(t),$$
$$\epsilon_{3i}(t) = \int_0^t \left(Y^T(\beta_0, s)W(s)Y(\beta_0, s)\right)^{-1} X_i(s)dM_i(s),$$

and where $H(\beta, t)$ was defined in (7.8). Estimates of $\epsilon_{ji}(t)$ for $j = 1, 2, 3$ are obtained by plugging in the estimates of $dM_i(t)$ and β_0, and are denoted $\hat{\epsilon}_{ji}(t)$.

To do inference about the nonparametric components of the model it is very useful that a resampling scheme can approximate the asymptotic distribution of $n^{1/2}(\hat{A}(\hat{\beta}, t) - A(t))$. First, its variance can be estimated consistently by

$$\hat{\Psi}(t) = n\sum_{i=1}^{n}\hat{\epsilon}_{2i}^{\otimes 2}(t).$$

258   7. Multiplicative-Additive hazards models

For $G_1, ..., G_n$ i.i.d. standard normals it follows that the asymptotic distribution of
$$n^{1/2} \sum_{i=1}^{n} \hat{\epsilon}_{2i}(t) G_i$$
is equivalent to the asymptotic distribution of $n^{1/2}(\hat{A}(\hat{\beta}, t) - A(t))$.

This construction may thus be used to implement tests for time-varying effects in the additive part of the model. First, to test if covariate j that is included in the additive part of the model is significant or time-varying, we suggest the two test statistics

$$F_1(\hat{A}_j(\cdot)) = \sup_{t \in [0,\tau]} |\hat{A}_j(t)|$$

and

$$F_2(\hat{A}_j(\cdot)) = \sup_{t \in [0,\tau]} |\hat{A}_j(t) - \frac{\hat{A}_j(\tau)}{\tau} t|.$$

Example 7.1.1 (PBC-data, Cox-Aalen Model)

We consider the PBC data described in Example 1.1.1. We learned from earlier examples, such as Example 6.0.2 and Example 6.2.3, that the effects of edema and protime were not well described by constant proportional effects. We therefore fit a model where these effects are included in the flexible additive part of the Cox-Aalen model, and all other effects are included in the multiplicative part of the model. It is important to recall that the baseline refers to a population where the multiplicative covariates all are zero, and we therefore first center all continuous covariates around their respective averages. The Cox-Aalen model can be fitted using the cox.aalen-function as illustrated below.

```
> fit<-cox.aalen(Surv(time/365,status)~prop(Age)+Edema+
+ prop(logBilirubin)+prop(logAlbumin)+logProtime,
+ max.time=8,pbc)
Cox-Aalen Survival Model
Simulations start N= 500
> summary(fit)
Cox-Aalen Model

Test for Aalen terms
Test for non-significant effects
            sup| hat B(t)/SD(t) | p-value H_0: B(t)=0
(Intercept)              8.45                   0.00
Edema                    2.65                   0.10
logProtime               3.44                   0.01
Test for time-invariant effects
            sup| B(t) - (t/tau)B(tau)|  p-value H_0: B(t)=b t
(Intercept)              0.132                  0.016
```

7.1 The Cox-Aalen hazards model 259

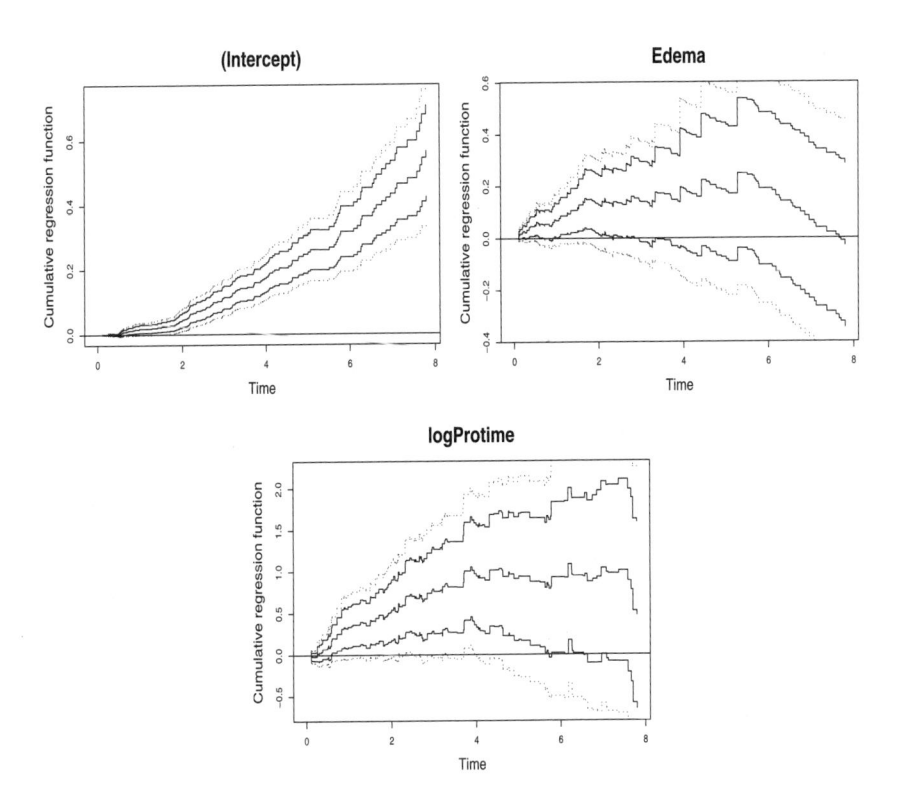

FIGURE 7.1: PBC-data. Estimated cumulative regression functions for additive part of Cox-Aalen model with 95% robust pointwise confidence intervals (solid lines) and 95% simulation based confidence band (broken lines).

```
Edema                              0.269                    0.004
logProtime                         0.821                    0.022

Proportional Cox terms :
                    Coef.        SE  Robust SE  D2log(L)^-1     P-val
prop(Age)          0.0355   0.00747    0.00953      0.00827  2.08e-06
prop(logBilirubin) 0.8000   0.07760    0.08720      0.08660  0.00e+00
prop(logAlbumin)  -2.4600   0.67600    0.64800      0.67500  2.73e-04

Test for Proportionality
                   sup| hat U(t) |  p-value H_0
prop(Age)                  75.700         0.678
prop(logBilirubin)         17.300         0.014
prop(logAlbumin)            0.524         0.998

> plot(fit,robust=2,sim.ci=3)
```

Figure 7.1 shows the estimated cumulative functions for the three additive components of the model with 95% pointwise confidence intervals (broken lines) and 95% confidence band (dotted lines). It is of interest to compare with the similar figure for the semiparametric additive model given in Figure 5.6. The estimates of the Cox-Aalen model differ from the estimates of the additive semiparametric model, and the difference is that we now model age, log(bilirubin), and log(albumin) by multiplicative effects.

To state the practical consequences of these two different models we consider log(albumin). The additive model states that the risk is lowered -0.23 (0.070) for each unit that log(albumin) is higher, and the multiplicative model suggests that the relative risk of log(albumin) is 0.09 ($\exp(-2.46)$), i.e., that the intensity is reduced by 91% for each unit log(albumin) increases. This statement refers to a baseline that varies with edema and the level of log(protime), and this is part of the reason for the different time-varying effects of edema and log(protime). Considering the effect of edema the additive model claims that this effect is independent of the level of albumin whereas the multiplicative models suggests that the effect of edema varies considerably with the level of albumin. We shall later demonstrate that the Cox-Aalen model considered here does not fit the data fully satisfactory. □

7.1.3 Goodness-of-fit procedures

In this section we shall examine if the data are consistent with a specific Cox-Aalen model:

$$\lambda_i(t) = Y_i(t) \left\{ X_i(t)^T \alpha(t) \right\} \exp(Z_i(t)^T \beta).$$

The key is to estimate the underlying martingales

$$M_i(t) = N_i(t) - \int_0^t Y_i(s) \exp(Z_i(s)^T \beta_0) X_i(s)^T dA(s)$$

and see if the their behavior is consistent with that under the model. The martingale vector is estimated by

$$\hat{M}(t) = N(t) - \int_0^t Y(\hat{\beta}, s) Y^-(\hat{\beta}, s) dN(s) = \int_0^t G(\hat{\beta}, s) dN(s),$$

where $G(\hat{\beta}, t) = I - Y(\hat{\beta}, t) Y^-(\hat{\beta}, t)$. Under the Cox and the Aalen model these residuals reduces to the ones considered by Lin et al. (1993) and Aalen (1993), respectively.

7.1 The Cox-Aalen hazards model

Under the Cox-Aalen model the residuals will be asymptotically equivalent to a zero-mean process since

$$\hat{M}(t) = \int_0^t G(\beta_0, s) dM(s)$$
$$+ \int_0^t \left\{ Y(\beta_0, s) Y^-(\beta_0, s) - Y(\hat{\beta}, s) Y^-(\hat{\beta}, s) \right\} dN(s),$$

where the second term can be written as

$$- \int_0^t G(\beta^*, s) \mathrm{diag}\left\{ Y(\beta^*, s) Y^-(\beta^*, s) dN(s) \right\} Z(s)(\hat{\beta} - \beta_0)$$
$$= - \int_0^t G(\beta^*, s) \mathrm{diag}\left\{ Y(\beta^*, s) Y^-(\beta^*, s) dN(s) \right\} Z(s) I^{-1}(\beta^{**}, \tau) U(\beta_0, \tau)$$

with β^* and β^{**} on the line segment between $\hat{\beta}$ and β_0 and interpreted componentwise. The estimated martingale residuals can thus be approximated by

$$\int_0^t G(\beta_0, s) dM(s) + B(\beta_0, t) \int_0^\tau Z^T(t) G(\beta_0, t) dM(t)$$

where $B(\beta_0, t)$ is a $n \times q$ matrix. The last term in the preceding display implies that the estimated martingale residuals do not have independent increments. The variance is, however, easy to estimate.

The behavior of the residuals may be investigated in various ways. One may for example sum the residuals depending on the level of the covariates. Define therefore a $n \times m$ matrix possibly depending on time

$$K(t) = (K_1(t), \ldots, K_n(t))^T.$$

A cumulative residual process is then defined by

$$n^{-1/2} M_K(t) = \int_0^t K^T(s) d\hat{M}(s),$$

which is asymptotically equivalent to

$$n^{-1/2} \int_0^t K^T(s) G(\beta_0, s) dM(s) - B_K(\beta_0, t) U(\beta_0, \tau),$$

where

$$B_K(\beta_0, t) = \int_0^t K^T(s) G(\beta_0, s) \mathrm{diag}\left\{ Y(\beta_0, s) Y^-(\beta_0, s) dN(s) \right\} Z(s) I^{-1}(\beta_0, \tau).$$

262   7. Multiplicative-Additive hazards models

The variance of $M_K(t)$ can be estimated by the optional variation process

$$[M_K](t) = \int_0^t K^T(s)G(\hat{\beta},s)\mathrm{diag}(dN(s))K(s)G(\hat{\beta},s)$$
$$+ B_K(\hat{\beta},t)\left[U(\hat{\beta})\right](\tau)B_K^T(\hat{\beta},t)$$
$$- \int_0^t K^T(t)G(\beta_0,s)\mathrm{diag}(dN(s))G(\beta_0,s)Z(s)B_K^T(\hat{\beta},t)$$
$$- B_K(\hat{\beta},t)\int_0^t Z^T(t)G(\beta_0,s)\mathrm{diag}(dN(s))G(\beta_0,s)K(s).$$

The robust variance estimator that is based on an i.i.d. representation of the cumulative residual processes is derived using the i.i.d. representation of $n^{1/2}(\hat{\beta}-\beta_0)$. It follows that $n^{-1/2}M_K(t)$ is asymptotically equivalent to

$$n^{-1/2}\sum_{i=1}^n \int_0^t \{K_i(s) - K^T(s)Y(\beta_0,s)\left\{Y^T(\beta_0,s)W(s)Y(\beta_0,s)\right\}^{-1}$$
$$\times X_i(s)\}dM_i(s) - n^{-1/2}B_K(\beta_0,t)\sum_{i=1}^n \epsilon_{1i},$$

which may be used for resampling. Plotting the observed cumulative residual process $M_K(t)$ with 95% pointwise confidence intervals will give an indication of whether or not the observed residuals are consistent with the model. One may also compute

$$\sup_{t\in[0,\tau]} |M_{Kj}(t)|, \quad j=1,\ldots,m,$$

and approximate its distribution under the model by resampling. Resampling can also be used to construct confidence bands, as we have indicated in previous chapters.

Example 7.1.2 (PBC-data, Example 7.1.1 continued)

Consider a Cox-Aalen model where the additive part of the model contains the covariates edema, log(bilirubin), log(protime) and the covariates with multiplicative effects are age and log(albumin). To evaluate the fit we grouped all continuous covariates in 4 quartile groups and computed the cumulative martingale residuals for these groups. All variables except log(bilirubin) indicated that the model fitted well. For log(bilirubin) the following supremum test statistics and plots were constructed.

```
> fit<-cox.aalen(Surv(time/365,status)~prop(Age)+Edema+
+ logBilirubin+prop(logAlbumin)+logProtime,max.time=8,pbc,
+ residuals=1,n.sim=0)
Cox-Aalen Survival Model
```

7.1 The Cox-Aalen hazards model

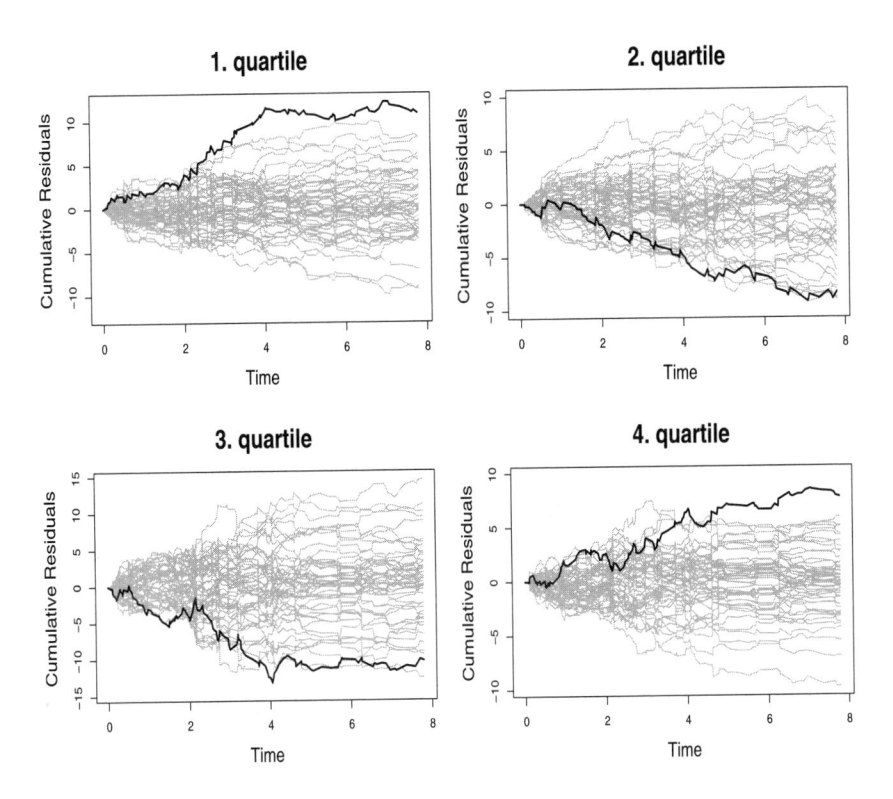

FIGURE 7.2: Observed cumulative martingale residuals for quartiles of bilirubin and 50 random realizations based on model with log(bilirubin).

```
> resids<-cum.residuals(fit,pbc,X,n.sim=1000)
Cumulative martingale residuals for Right censored survival times
> plot(resids,score=T)
> summary(resids)
Test for cumulative MG-residuals

Grouped Residuals consistent with model

             sup| hat B(t) |  p-value H_0: B(t)=0
1. quartile       12.204            0.003
2. quartile        9.196            0.068
3. quartile       13.222            0.035
4. quartile        8.486            0.013

             int ( B(t) )^2 dt p-value H_0: B(t)=0
1. quartile      594.576            0.003
2. quartile      236.869            0.069
3. quartile      594.046            0.036
4. quartile      231.068            0.020
```

264   7. Multiplicative-Additive hazards models

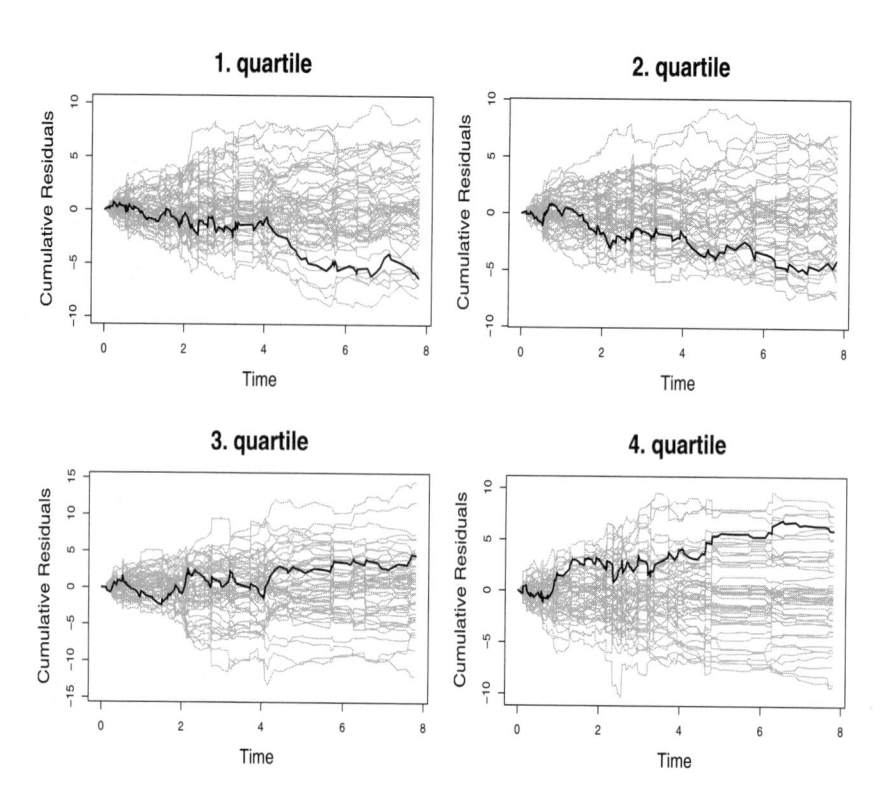

FIGURE 7.3: Observed cumulative martingale residuals for quartiles of bilirubin and 50 random realizations based on model with untransformed version of bilirubin.

The test statistics indicate that there are problems with the fit of the model with respect to log(bilirubin). Figure 7.2 shows the test processes along with 50 random simulations under the model. For low levels of log(bilirubin), for example, the cumulative residual process is too large, thus indicating that the data suggest a higher risk than expected by the model. One may try to remedy this by using, for example, the untransformed version of bilirubin. This was also how bilirubin was used in the additive hazards model.

```
> fit<-cox.aalen(Surv(time/365,status)~prop(Age)+Edema+
+ Bilirubin+prop(logAlbumin)+logProtime,max.time=8,
+ pbc,residuals=1,n.sim=0)
Cox-Aalen Survival Model
> X<-model.matrix(~-1+
+ cut(Bilirubin,quantile(Bilirubin),include.lowest=T),pbc)
> colnames(X)<-c("1. quartile","2. quartile","3. quartile",
+ "4. quartile");
```

7.1 The Cox-Aalen hazards model

```
> resids<-cum.residuals(fit,pbc,X,n.sim=1000)
Cumulative martingale residuals for Right censored survival times
> plot(resids,score=T)
> summary(resids)
Test for cumulative MG-residuals

Grouped Residuals consistent with model

             sup| hat B(t) |  p-value H_0: B(t)=0
1. quartile       6.276               0.249
2. quartile       5.193               0.364
3. quartile       4.592               0.641
4. quartile       6.926               0.141

             int ( B(t) )^2 dt  p-value H_0: B(t)=0
1. quartile       93.677              0.277
2. quartile       67.437              0.340
3. quartile       40.302              0.633
4. quartile      144.889              0.155
```

The output and Figure 7.3 suggest that the untransformed version of bilirubin leads to an acceptable fit. Note, that the model now slightly overestimates the risk for the low levels of bilirubin. □

To evaluate the goodness of fit of the covariates included in the multiplicative part of the model we consider the cumulative score processes. The observed normed score process is given as $n^{-1/2}U(\hat{\beta},t)$ and its asymptotic distribution is equivalent to the asymptotic distribution of

$$n^{-1/2} \sum_{i=1}^{n} \left(\hat{\epsilon}_{1i}(t) + I(\hat{\beta},t)I^{-1}(\hat{\beta},\tau)\hat{\epsilon}_{1i}(\tau) \right) G_i$$

where $G_1, ..., G_n$ are independent standard normals. A test for the proportionality of the jth covariate of the proportional part of the model may be constructed by considering

$$\sup_{t\in[0,\tau]} |U_j(\hat{\beta},t)|, \quad j=1,\ldots,p.$$

Example 7.1.3 (PBC-data, Example 7.1.1 continued)

In Example 7.1.1 we considered the Cox-Aalen model with edema and log(protime) in the additive part of the model and with log(bilirubin), log(albumin) and age in the multiplicative part. Part of the output contained information about the score processes of the relative risk parameters of the model and these can be plotted by the command:

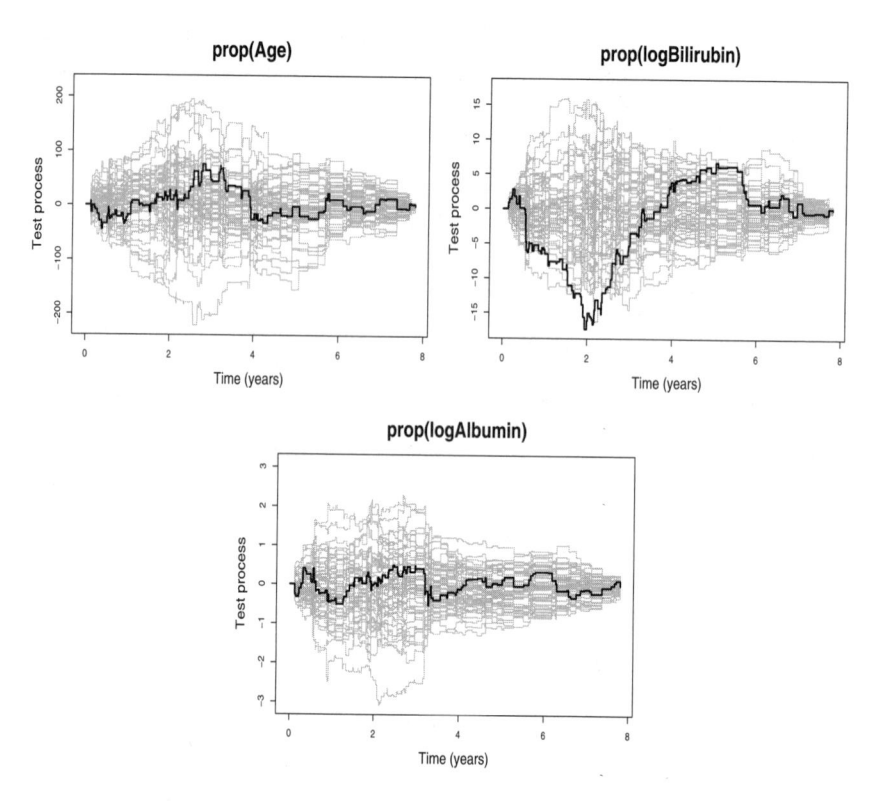

FIGURE 7.4: PBC-data. Score processes for multiplicative part of Cox-Aalen model with 50 random realizations under the model.

```
> plot(fit,score=T,xlab="Time (years)")
```

Figure 7.4 indicates that log(bilirubin) does not fit particularly well when included in the multiplicative part of the model, and the p-value in the output (0.01) also suggests that the fit is not completely satisfactory.

□

7.1.4 Estimating the survival function

After fitting a model and learning about covariates effects one will often summarize the consequences of various covariate combinations by computing the estimated survival function. Below we describe how to estimate the survival function and supply it with pointwise confidence intervals and a confidence band.

Assume that a subject with covariates X_0 and Z_0, that do not depend on time for simplicity, have hazard function

$$\lambda_0(t) = (X_0^T \alpha(t)) \exp(Z_0^T \beta).$$

7.1 The Cox-Aalen hazards model

The survival probability is then given as

$$S_0(t) = S_0(A, \beta, t) = \exp(-X_0^T A(t) \exp(Z_0^T \beta))$$

that can be estimated consistently by

$$\hat{S}_0(t) = S_0(\hat{A}, \hat{\beta}, t) = \exp(-X_0^T \hat{A}(t) \exp(Z_0^T \hat{\beta})).$$

It is a consequence of the asymptotic properties of $n^{1/2}(\hat{A} - A, \hat{\beta} - \beta)$ and the functional delta method applied to the continuous functional S_0 defined above that $n^{1/2}(\hat{S}_0 - S_0)$ converges towards a zero-mean Gaussian process V with variance function Q. A Taylor series expansion yields that (ignoring lower order terms)

$$n^{1/2}(S_0(\hat{A}, \hat{\beta}, t) - S_0(A, \beta, t)) = -S_0(A, \beta, t)$$
$$n^{1/2}\left\{\exp(Z_0^T \beta) X_0^T (\hat{A}(t) - A(t)) + X_0^T A(t) \exp(Z_0^T \beta) Z_0^T (\hat{\beta} - \beta)\right\}. \tag{7.11}$$

There exists a martingale decomposition that leads to an optional variation based estimator of the variance of $\hat{S}_0(t) - S_0(t)$, but we here omit this formula and instead specify an i.i.d. decomposition that can be used to estimate the variance and to construct a confidence band.

We derived in the previous section that $n^{1/2}(\hat{\beta} - \beta, \hat{A} - A)$ was asymptotically equivalent to the processes

$$\Delta_1 = n^{1/2} I(\beta_0, \tau)^{-1} \sum_{i=1}^{n} \hat{\epsilon}_{1i} G_i,$$

$$\Delta_2(t) = n^{1/2} \sum_{i=1}^{n} \hat{\epsilon}_{2i}(t) G_i,$$

where $G_1, ..., G_n$ are independent standard normals. Therefore applying the functional delta method to these asymptotically equivalent processes leads to a resampling version of the survival function estimator. The term

$$n^{1/2} \exp(Z_0^T \beta) X_0^T (\hat{A}(t) - A(t)) + n^{1/2} X_0^T A(t) \exp(Z_0^T \beta) Z_0^T (\hat{\beta} - \beta)$$

is asymptotically equivalent to

$$n^{1/2} \sum_{i=1}^{n} \epsilon_{4i}(t),$$

where

$$\epsilon_{4i}(t) = \exp(Z_0^T \beta) X_0^T \epsilon_{2i}(t) + X_0^T A(t) \exp(Z_0^T \beta) Z_0^T I(\beta_0, \tau)^{-1} \epsilon_{1i}.$$

268   7. Multiplicative-Additive hazards models

Define

$$\hat{\epsilon}_{4i}(t) = \exp(Z_0^T \hat{\beta}) X_0^T \hat{\epsilon}_{2i}(t) + X_0^T \hat{A}(t) \exp(Z_0^T \hat{\beta}) Z_0^T I(\beta_0, \tau)^{-1} \hat{\epsilon}_{1i}.$$

It can be derived that under regularity conditions $n^{1/2}(\hat{S}_0 - S_0)$ has the same asymptotic distribution as

$$\Delta_S(t) = S_0(t) n^{1/2} \sum_{i=1}^{n} \hat{\epsilon}_{4i}(t) G_i, \qquad (7.12)$$

and it also follows that

$$\hat{Q}(t) = n \hat{S}_0^2(t) \sum_{i=1}^{n} \hat{\epsilon}_{4i}^2(t),$$

is a consistent estimator of the variance of $n^{1/2}(\hat{S}_0 - S_0)$. Therefore an approximate $(1-\alpha)$ confidence band is on the form

$$\hat{S}_0(t) \pm n^{-1/2} C_\alpha \hat{Q}^{1/2}(t),$$

where C_α is the $(1-\alpha)$-quantile of

$$\sup_{t \in [0,\tau]} |\frac{\Delta_S^k(t)}{\hat{Q}^{1/2}(t)}|$$

for $\Delta_S^k(t)$ is the kth resampled process for $k = 1, \ldots, K$.

Example 7.1.4 (Survival estimation for PBC data)

We fitted a Cox-Aalen model to the PBC data with edema, log(protime) and bilirubin in the additive part of the model and with age and log(albumin) as parametric relative risk terms. We start by obtaining the estimated and an i.i.d. representation, and then compute the approximate constant that yields an 95% confidence band based on resampling as described above. We estimate the survival function for a subject with or without edema and with average levels of all continuous covariates.

```
> fit<-cox.aalen(Surv(time/365,status)~prop(Age)+Edema+
+ Bilirubin+prop(logAlbumin)+logProtime,max.time=8,pbc,
+ n.sim=0,resample.iid=1)
Cox-Aalen Survival Model
> # fit$B.iid and fit$gamma.iid contains i.i.d. representation
> x0<-c(1,0,0,0); z0<-c(0,0);
> RR<-exp(sum(z0 * fit$gamma))
> delta<-matrix(0,144,418);
> for (i in 1:418) {delta[,i]<-RR * (x0 %*% t(fit$B.iid[[i]]))+
+ RR * (x0 %*% t(fit$cum[,-1])) * sum(z0*fit$gamma.iid[i,]);}
```

7.1 The Cox-Aalen hazards model   269

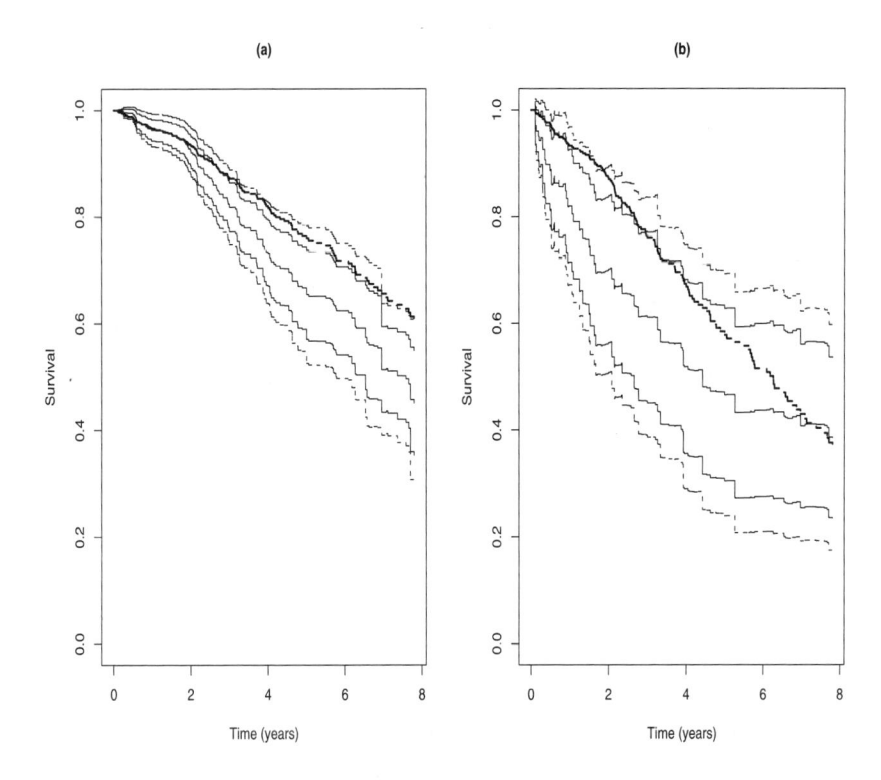

FIGURE 7.5: Survival estimates for specific covariates with 95% pointwise confidence intervals (solid lines), 95% confidence band (broken lines), Cox regression estimate (thick line). Subject without edema (a) and with edema (b) and average level of the other continuous covariates as described in text.

```
> S0<-c(exp(- RR*(x0 %*% t(fit$cum[,-1]))))
> se<-apply(delta^2,1,sum)^.5
> ### pointwise confidence intervals
> plot(fit$cum[,1],S0,type="s",ylim=c(0,1),xlab="Time (years)",
+ ylab="Survival"); title(main="(a)")
> lines(fit$cum[,1],S0-1.96*S0*se,type="s");
> lines(fit$cum[,1],S0+1.96*S0*se,type="s")
> ### uniform confidence bands
> mpt<-c()
> for (i in 1:500) {
+ g<-rnorm(418); pt<-abs(delta %*% g)/se;  mpt<-c(mpt,max(pt[-1]));}
> Cband<-percen(mpt,0.95);
> lines(fit$cum[,1],S0-Cband*S0*se,lty=2,type="s");
> lines(fit$cum[,1],S0+Cband*S0*se,lty=2,type="s")
> # Cox regression estimate
> coxfit<-cox.aalen(Surv(time/365,status)~prop(Age)+prop(Edema)+
```

270   7. Multiplicative-Additive hazards models

```
+ prop(Bilirubin)+prop(logAlbumin)+prop(logProtime),max.time=8,
+ pbc,n.sim=0)
Cox-Aalen Survival Model
> cox.surv<-list(time=coxfit$cum[,1],surv=exp(-coxfit$cum[,2]))
> lines(cox.surv$time,cox.surv$surv,type="s",lwd=2,lty=2)
```

The Cox estimate of the survival function is not particularly close to the estimate based on the Cox-Aalen model. For a subject without edema the Cox estimate works initially but is off for long term survival, (Figure 7.5 (a)), and in contrast is off initially for subjects with edema but ends up alright for long term survival (Figure 7.5 (b)). □

7.1.5 Example

Below we show a worked example of how to use the Cox-Aalen model based on the TRACE data (Jensen et al., 1997). See Example 5.8.1 for a brief introduction to the TRACE data.

Example 7.1.5 (TRACE Data)

We learned from Example 5.8.1 based on the additive model that the covariate vf had a strongly time-varying additive effect, chf and age seemed also to have time-varying effects, but the remaining effects were reasonably well summarized by constant excess risk. In the additive model, age had to enter the model on exponential scale.

In this example we use the entire data set with all 1877 survival times. To start we fit a stratified Cox model where the baseline is allowed to depend on the status of vf. For this model we find that there are problems with the proportionality of the model with regard to chf indicating that the model fit is not satisfactory. Figure 7.6 (a) shows the score function for the stratified Cox model for the chf covariate, and the output gives a p-value for chf at around 0.01.

We also fitted the Cox-Aalen model with vf and chf in the additive part of the model and for this model the score functions did not indicate any dramatic lacking fit. Figure 7.6 (b) shows the diabetes component of the score function that showed the worst behavior, see also the below reported tests for proportionality.

```
> age.m<-TRACE$age-mean(TRACE$age)
> fit<-cox.aalen(Surv(time,status==9)~prop(diabetes)+chf
+ +vf+prop(sex)+prop(age.m),TRACE,max.time=7)
Cox-Aalen Survival Model
Simulations start N= 500
> summary(fit)
Cox-Aalen Model
```

7.1 The Cox-Aalen hazards model   271

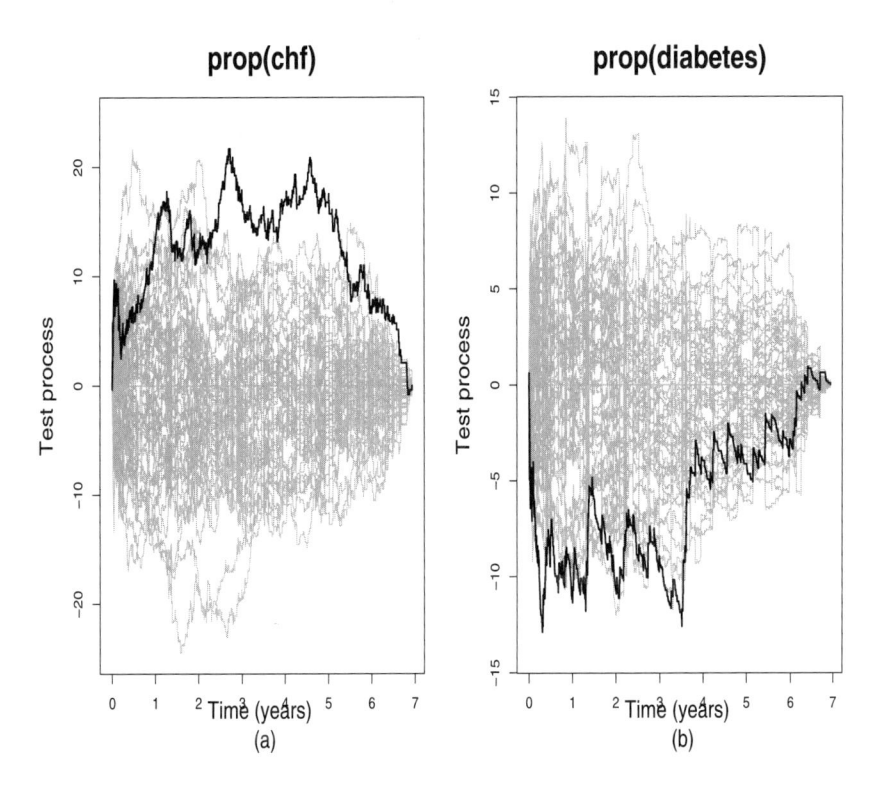

FIGURE 7.6: Score function for selected components with 50 random realizations under the model: (a) for stratified Cox model based on vf; (b) for Cox-Aalen model with both vf and chf in additive part.

```
Test for Aalen terms
Test for non-significant effects
            sup| hat B(t)/SD(t) |  p-value H_0: B(t)=0
(Intercept)           11.90                   0
chf                    8.69                   0
vf                     6.05                   0
Test for time-invariant effects
            sup| B(t) - (t/tau)B(tau)|  p-value H_0: B(t)=b t
(Intercept)          0.0308                   0.068
chf                  0.0966                   0.000
vf                   0.3690                   0.000

Proportional Cox terms :
               Coef.      SE Robust SE D2log(L)^-1     z    P-val
prop(diabetes) 0.5400 0.09550   0.08640     0.09460  5.65 1.61e-08
prop(sex)      0.1760 0.07170   0.07150     0.07130  2.45 1.44e-02
prop(age.m)    0.0583 0.00397   0.00384     0.00375 14.70 0.00e+00
```

272   7. Multiplicative-Additive hazards models

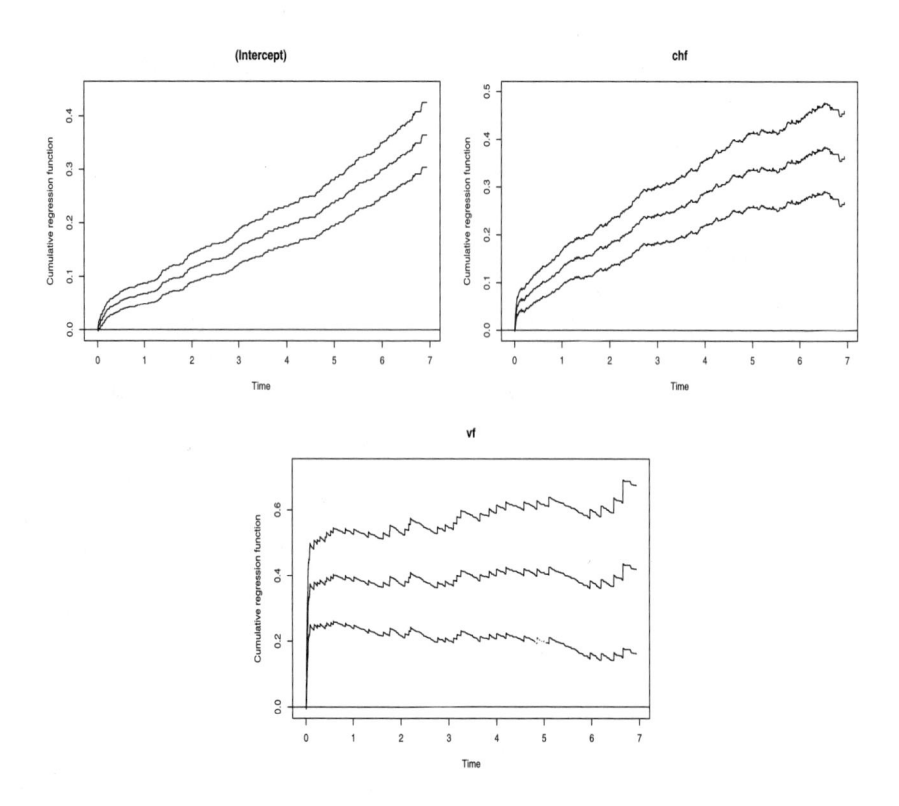

FIGURE 7.7: Estimated cumulative regression functions with 95% pointwise confidence intervals.

```
Test for Proportionality
                sup| hat U(t) |   p-value H_0
prop(diabetes)         12.90              0.090
prop(sex)               7.73              0.918
prop(age.m)           156.00              0.908

> plot(fit)
```

The additive effects of vf and chf both reveal that their effects are strongly time-varying with a much stronger initial effect that wears off for both conditions, and for vf in particular where it vanishes after approximately 2 months, see Figure 7.7. The model fit gives relative risk parameters that are pretty consistent with those of the standard Cox regression model, but as we shall show below the survival estimates differ considerably from those obtained from a Cox regression model where the baseline is stratified depending on vf.

7.2 Proportional excess hazards model

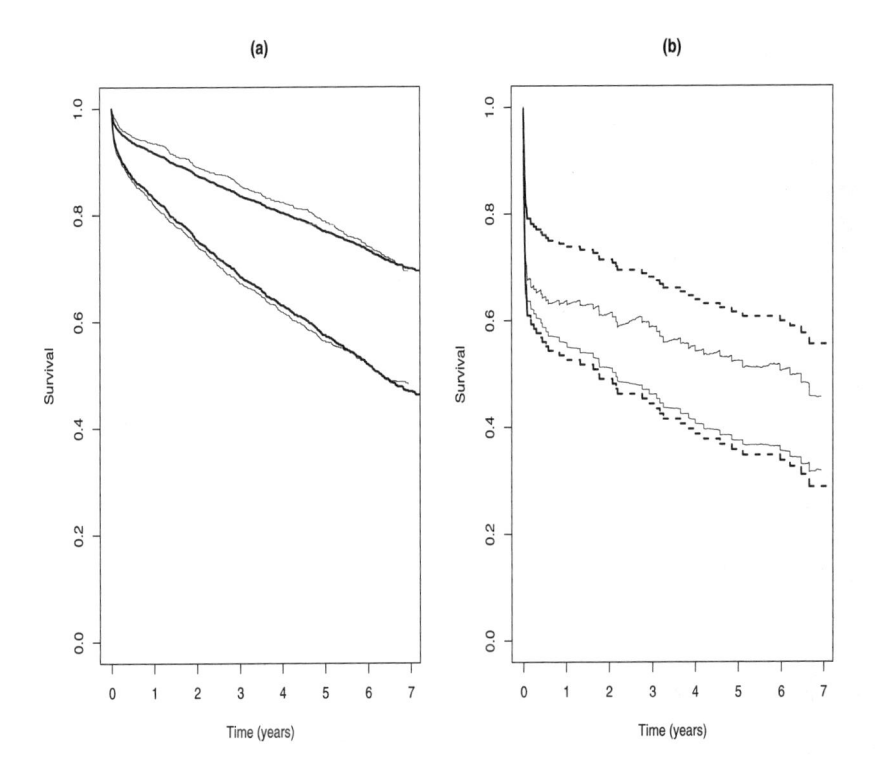

FIGURE 7.8: Survival predictions for Cox-Aalen model (thin lines) with vf and chf in additive part and Cox model (thick lines) with vf stratified baseline. Females with average age, without diabetes and with or without both chf and vf. (a) is without vf and (b) is with vf.

For comparison we compare the fit of the model with that of a standard Cox regression model. The survival estimates are for a female without diabetes and with average age, and for four different combinations of vf and chf. Figure 7.8 (a) shows the computed survival for subject without vf condition, and here the Cox model fits rather well for both subjects with and without the chf condition, respectively. Similarly, Figure 7.8 (b) gives predicted survival for subject with vf condition, and here the Cox model fits only well for subjects with chf condition. □

7.2 Proportional excess hazards model

Sasieni (1996) studied the so-called proportional excess hazards model where the intensity is

$$\lambda(t) = Y(t) \left\{ \alpha(t, X) + \lambda_0(t) \exp\left(Z^T \beta_0\right) \right\}, \tag{7.13}$$

274   7. Multiplicative-Additive hazards models

where the off-set $\alpha(t, X)$ is the background rate of mortality in a control population (defined by X) and is assumed to be known. The second term of the model, which is described by the Cox model, is the excess risk for an "exposed" individual with covariates Z. Sasieni (1996) derived efficient estimators for the unknown parameters β_0 and $\Lambda_0(t) = \int_0^t \lambda_0(s)\, ds$. In some situations, however, the background mortality may not be known. A typical example of this is dose-response trials with animals. Martinussen & Scheike (2002b) considered such a dataset concerning mortality of ticks. The ticks were treated with different doses of the entomopathogenic fungus *Metarhizium anispliae*. Besides zero dose, the doses 10^7, 10^8 and 10^9 (spores/ml) were applied. For such a dataset, the background mortality needs to be estimated from the study population itself. This is possible if we assume that the intensity for the ith individual is

$$\lambda_i(t) = Y_i(t) X_i^T(t) \alpha(t) + \rho_i(t) \lambda_0(t) \exp\{Z_i^T(t)\beta_0\}, \qquad (7.14)$$

where $X_i(t)$ and $Z_i(t)$ are covariates of dimensions q and p, respectively. The unknown parameters of (7.14) are β_0 and $\psi(t) = (\alpha(t), \lambda_0(t))$ where $\psi(t)$ is allowed to depend on time. Note that the known background mortality rate $\alpha(t, X)$ of (7.13) is replaced by an Aalen additive model term. In the dose-response example, $Y_i(t)$ is the general at-risk indicator while $\rho_i(t)$ is zero for the group of ticks which did not receive the dose and one otherwise if the tick is at risk at time t. For the sake of generality, however, we only assume that $Y_i(t)$ and $\rho_i(t)$ are locally bounded predictable processes. Zahl (2003) have used the model to describe mortality in various cancer studies.

7.2.1 Model and score equations

Assume that we have n i.i.d. observations $(N_i, Y_i, \rho_i, X_i, Z_i)$ for $i = 1, ..., n$ observed over some time-interval $[0, \tau]$ such that the ith counting process, $N_i(t)$, has intensity (7.14). Let

$$N = (N_1, \ldots, N_n)^T \quad M = (M_1, \ldots, M_n)^T,$$

where $M_i(t) = N_i(t) - \Lambda_i(t)$ with $\Lambda_i(t) = \int_0^t \lambda_i\, dt$. We suppress the dependence of time unless we explicitly whish to emphasize it. Further, let

$$X = (Y_1 X_1, \ldots, Y_n X_n)^T, Z = (\rho_1 Z_1, \ldots, \rho_n Z_n)^T$$

and $\phi_i = \phi_i(\beta) = \rho_i \exp(Z_i^T \beta)$, $\phi = \phi(\beta) = (\phi_1, ..., \phi_n)^T$, $\Phi = \Phi(\beta) = \mathrm{diag}(\phi_i)$, $W = \mathrm{diag}(w_i)$, $V = \mathrm{diag}(v_i)$, $w = (w_1, \ldots, w_n)^T$ and $v = (v_1, \ldots, v_n)^T$, where $w_i = 1/\lambda_i$ and $v_i = \lambda_0 w_i$. When $\lambda_i(t) = 0$, we put $w_i = 0$.

The score equations for the unknown parameters are given by

$$\int Z^T \Phi V \left\{ dN - \tilde{X} d\Psi(t) \right\} = 0, \qquad (7.15)$$

$$\tilde{X}^T W (dN(t) - d\Psi(t)) = 0, \qquad (7.16)$$

where $\tilde{X} = (X, \phi)$, $\Psi(t) = \int_0^t \psi(s)\, ds$, and with $\psi(t) = (\alpha(t), \lambda_0(t))^T$. The score equations are simply the derivatives of the likelihood with respect to β and $d\psi(t)$. Solving the score equation (7.16) for $d\Psi(t)$ for known β gives

$$\hat{\Psi}(t, \beta) = \int_0^t (\tilde{X}^T W \tilde{X})^{-1} \tilde{X}^T W \, dN(s). \tag{7.17}$$

Insert now (7.17) into the score for β and obtain

$$\int_0^\tau Z^T \Phi V \{I - \tilde{X}(\tilde{X}^T W \tilde{X})^{-1} \tilde{X}^T W\} dN = 0. \tag{7.18}$$

One could then solve (7.18) to obtain $\hat{\beta}$ and then insert this into (7.17) to obtain $\hat{\Psi}(t) = \hat{\Psi}(t, \hat{\beta})$. These estimators are of course not real estimators as they depend on W and V, which in turn depend on the true intensity. It turns out that these estimators are efficient and that this also holds when W and V are replaced by uniformly consistent estimates.

Note. The weighted score equations (7.18) form an empirical version of the efficient score for the semiparametric model (Sasieni, 1992b; Bickel et al., 1993). The score for the parametric component can be written as

$$l_\beta = \int Z^T \Phi V \, dM,$$

and similarly the nonparametric component, ψ, gives a score which when evaluated at $b(t)$ equals

$$l_\psi b = \int b^T \tilde{X}^T W \, dM.$$

The efficient score l_β^* for β is of the form

$$\int \{Z^T \Phi V - (b^*)^T \tilde{X} W\} dM$$

for some b^* such that l_β^* is orthogonal to $l_\psi b$. This gives that

$$(b^*)^T = E\{(\tilde{X}^T W \tilde{X})^{-1} \tilde{X}^T V \Phi Z\}.$$

Note that (7.18) is an empirical version of the efficient score equation since

$$\int_0^\tau Z^T \Phi V \{I - \tilde{X}(\tilde{X}^T W \tilde{X})^{-1} \tilde{X}^T W\} dN$$
$$= \int_0^\tau Z^T \Phi V \{I - \tilde{X}(\tilde{X}^T W \tilde{X})^{-1} \tilde{X}^T W\} dM.$$

We here suggest using unweighted estimators where the efficient weight-matrices, W and V, are set equal to I. But before doing so, let us take a

276   7. Multiplicative-Additive hazards models

closer look at the above estimators to see the resemblance with the usual Cox and Aalen estimators. Let

$$H = I - X(X^TWGX)^{-1}X^TWG, \quad G = I - \phi(\phi^TW\phi)^{-1}\phi^TW.$$

Using the fact that

$$GH = I - \tilde{X}(\tilde{X}^TW\tilde{X})^{-1}\tilde{X}^TW, \tag{7.19}$$

we may rewrite the two components of (7.17) as a weighted Aalen estimator for the additive components

$$\hat{A}(t,\beta) = \int_0^t \{X^TWGX\}^{-1}X^TWG\,dN(s), \tag{7.20}$$

and a Breslow-type estimator for the cumulative baseline

$$\hat{\Lambda}_0(t,\beta) = \int_0^t \frac{\sum_{i=1}^n w_i\phi_i d\tilde{N}_i(s)}{\sum_{i=1}^n w_i\phi_i \exp(Z_i^T\beta)}, \tag{7.21}$$

where $\tilde{N} = HN$. The score equation for β may be rewritten as

$$U(\beta) = \sum_{i=1}^n \int \left\{ Z_i - \frac{\sum_j w_j\phi_j Z_j \exp(Z_j^T\beta)}{\sum_j w_j\phi_j \exp(Z_j^T\beta)} \right\} v_i\phi_i\,d\tilde{N}_i(t) = 0. \tag{7.22}$$

The resemblance of (7.21) and (7.22) to the usual Breslow estimator and Cox-score equation is clear. Instead of using the response $N(t)$ directly, however, it is transformed to the residual space spanned by the design of the additive components. In the case where

$$\lambda_i(t) = Y_i(t)\lambda_0(t)\exp\{Z_i(t)^T\beta_0\},$$

that is the Cox model, equation (7.21) reduces to the Breslow estimator and equation (7.22) gives the Cox score function when the weights, $w_i = w_i(\beta_0)$, are considered as functionals of β rather than fixed at β_0.

The score equations can be solved when $(WX, W\phi(\beta), V\Phi(\beta)Z)$ has full rank, so that even when $X = Z$ the model may be identifiable. This seems like an appealing approach to make goodness-of-fit procedures for Cox's regression model but in practice the model is hard to identify when $X = Z$.

7.2.2 Estimation and inference

Now let us turn to the unweighted estimators, which may be computed directly from the data. They are obtained first by solving (7.18) with $V = W = I$. Denote this solution by $\tilde{\beta}$. The estimator of Ψ is next obtained

7.2 Proportional excess hazards model

from (7.17) using $\tilde{\beta}$ and setting $W = I$. Denote this estimator by $\tilde{\Psi}(t)$, so $\tilde{\Psi}(t) = \hat{\Psi}(t \mid \tilde{\beta}, W = I)$. Setting $V = W = I$ in (7.18) gives

$$\tilde{U}(\beta) = \int Z^T \Phi (I - \tilde{X}(\tilde{X}^T \tilde{X})^{-1} \tilde{X}^T) \, dN(t)$$
$$= \int Z^T \Phi \tilde{H} \, dN(t) = \int Z^T \Phi G_1 H_1 \, dN(t), \qquad (7.23)$$

where

$$\tilde{H} = (I - \tilde{X}(\tilde{X}^T \tilde{X})^{-1} \tilde{X}^T), \quad H_1 = I - X(X^T G_1 X)^{-1} X^T G_1,$$
$$G_1 = I - \phi(\phi^T \phi)^{-1} \phi^T.$$

Above, we have used the result that $G_1 H_1 = \tilde{H}$. Define $\tilde{H}_1$, $\tilde{G}_1$ and $\tilde{\Phi}$ as H_1, G_1 and Φ, with ϕ replaced by $\tilde{\phi} = \phi(\tilde{\beta})$.

Before stating the asymptotic results for $\tilde{\beta}$ we specify the derivate of the score. The derivative of $\tilde{U}$ with respect to β is given by

$$\tilde{I}(\beta) = \int Z^T (\Phi H_1^T \frac{dG_1}{d\beta})\{H_1 dN(t) \otimes I_q\}$$
$$- \int Z^T \frac{d\Phi}{d\beta} G_1 \{H_1 dN(t) \otimes I_q\},$$

where

$$\frac{dG_1}{d\beta} = -\left\{ \left(\frac{1}{\phi^T \phi} \frac{d\phi}{d\beta} - \frac{\phi}{(\phi^T \phi)^2} \frac{d\phi^T \phi}{d\beta} \right)(\phi^T \otimes I_q) + \frac{\phi}{\phi^T \phi} \frac{d\phi^T}{d\beta} \right\}.$$

This is a consequence of the matrix derivative rules given in Appendix B. Define

$$\tilde{\mathcal{D}}(\tilde{\beta}) = \int Z^T \tilde{\Phi} \tilde{G}_1 \tilde{H}_1 \mathrm{diag}\{dN(t)\} \tilde{H}_1^T \tilde{G}_1^T \tilde{\Phi} Z.$$

Theorem 7.2.1 *Under regularity conditions, it follows that* $n^{\frac{1}{2}}(\tilde{\beta} - \beta_0)$ *converges in distribution to a zero-mean normal with covariance matrix that is consistently estimated by the sandwich estimator*

$$n \tilde{I}(\tilde{\beta})^{-1} \tilde{\mathcal{D}}(\tilde{\beta}) \tilde{I}(\tilde{\beta})^{-1}.$$

PROOF. We have

$$\tilde{U}(\beta_0) = \int Z^T \Phi G_1(\beta_0) H_1(\beta_0) \, dN(t)$$
$$= \int Z^T \Phi G_1(\beta_0) H_1(\beta_0) \{X dA(t) + \phi(\beta_0) d\Lambda_0(t) + dM(t)\}$$
$$= \int Z^T \Phi G_1(\beta_0) H_1(\beta_0) dM(t)$$

278   7. Multiplicative-Additive hazards models

since $H_1(\beta_0)X = 0$, $H_1(\beta_0)\phi(\beta_0) = \phi(\beta_0)$ and $G_1(\beta_0)\phi(\beta_0) = 0$. The proposed estimating equation therefore has mean zero for the true value of the parameter. By use of Lenglart's inequality it may be seen that $\tilde{I}(\beta_0)$ converges in probability to

$$\int Z^T \Phi G_1 H_1 \Phi Z \, d\Lambda_0,$$

which is a negative semidefinite matrix. Consistency now follows by standard arguments.

The proof of asymptotic normality follows from a Taylor series expansion of $\tilde{U}(\cdot)$ around β_0 and evaluated at $\tilde{\beta}$:

$$n^{1/2}(\tilde{\beta} - \beta_0) = \{n^{-1}\tilde{I}(\beta^*)\}^{-1} n^{-1/2} \int_0^t Z^T \Phi G_1 H_1 \, dM(s),$$

for some β^* on the line segment between $\tilde{\beta}$ and β_0. □

To give the asymptotic properties of the estimator for the nonparametric components of the model $\tilde{\Psi}(t)$ we define

$$C_1(t) = \int_0^t (\tilde{X}^T(\tilde{\beta})\tilde{X}(\tilde{\beta}))^{-1} \tilde{X}^T(\tilde{\beta}) \tilde{\Phi} Z d\tilde{\Lambda}_0(s),$$

where $\tilde{\Lambda}_0(t)$ is the appropriate component of $\tilde{\Psi}(t)$.

Define

$$M_1(t) = \{n^{-1}\tilde{I}(\beta_0)\}^{-1}$$
$$\times n^{-1/2} \int_0^t Z^T \left(I - \tilde{X}(\beta_0)\left\{\tilde{X}^T(\beta_0)\tilde{X}(\beta_0)\right\}^{-1} \tilde{X}^T(\beta_0)\right) dM(s),$$

$$M_2(t) = n^{\frac{1}{2}} \int_0^t \left\{\tilde{X}^T(\beta_0)\tilde{X}(\beta_0)\right\}^{-1} \tilde{X}^T(\beta_0) \, dM(s).$$

In the following theorem we let $[M_2](t)$ denote the optional variation process evaluated in $\hat{\beta}$, and similarly for the other estimated quadratic (co)-variation processes.

Theorem 7.2.2 *Under regularity conditions, $n^{\frac{1}{2}}\{\tilde{\Psi}(t) - \Psi(t)\}$ converges in distribution to a zero-mean Gaussian process with a covariance function that is estimated consistently by*

$$[M_2](t) - \{[M_2, M_1](t)C_1(t)^T + C_1(t)[M_1, M_2](t)\} + C_1(t)[M_1](\tau)C_1(t)^T.$$

PROOF. Since $\phi(\beta_0) = \phi(\tilde{\beta}) + \Phi^* Z(\tilde{\beta} - \beta_0)$, where $\Phi^* = \text{diag}\{\phi(\beta^*)\}$ and β^* is on the line segment between $\tilde{\beta}$ and β, it follows that

$$n^{\frac{1}{2}}\{\tilde{\Psi}(t) - \Psi(t)\} = C_1^*(t) n^{\frac{1}{2}}(\tilde{\beta} - \beta_0)$$
$$+ n^{\frac{1}{2}} \int_0^t \left\{\tilde{X}(\beta_0)^T \tilde{X}(\beta_0)\right\}^{-1} \tilde{X}(\beta_0)^T \, dM(s)$$
$$= C_1^*(t) M_1(\tau) + M_2(t) + o_p(1),$$

where
$$C_1^*(t) = \int_0^t \left\{ \tilde{X}(\beta_0)^T \tilde{X}(\beta_0) \right\}^{-1} \tilde{X}(\beta_0)^T \Phi^* Z \lambda_0(s) \, ds.$$

As $n \to \infty$ $C_1^*(t)$ converges in probability for each t. By the martingale central limit theorem, it may furthermore be shown that (M_1, M_2) converges in distribution to a Gaussian martingale $U = (U_1, U_2)$ with mean zero, and the result follows. □

Again it is convenient to have an i.i.d. representation of the above limit distributions to, for example, construct confidence bands. The score process evaluated at β_0 and viewed as process in t, $\tilde{U}(\tilde{\beta}_0, t)$, can be written as

$$n^{-1/2} \tilde{U}(\beta_0) = n^{-1/2} \sum_{i=1}^n \epsilon_{1i}(t) + o_p(1),$$

where

$$\epsilon_{1i}(t) = \int_0^t \left\{ \rho_i Z_i - E[\rho_1 Z_1 \tilde{X}_1^T(\beta_0)] E[Y_1 \tilde{X}_1(\beta_0) X_1^T(\beta_0)^T]^{-1} X_i(\beta_0) \right\} dM_i. \tag{7.24}$$

It can be shown that the variance of the limit distribution of $n^{1/2}(\tilde{\beta} - \beta_0)$ may be estimated consistently by the (robust) estimator

$$n \tilde{I}(\tilde{\beta})^{-1} \left\{ \sum_{i=1}^n \hat{\epsilon}_{1i}^{\otimes 2}(\tau) \right\} \tilde{I}(\tilde{\beta})^{-1},$$

where $\hat{\epsilon}_{1i}(t)$ is given by (7.24) with insertion of estimates

$$d\hat{M}(t) = dN(t) - \tilde{X}(t, \tilde{\beta}) d\tilde{\Psi}(t).$$

Also, $n^{1/2}(\tilde{\Psi}(t) - \Psi(t))$ is asymptotically equivalent to

$$n^{1/2} \sum_{i=1}^n \epsilon_{2i}(t), \tag{7.25}$$

where

$$\epsilon_{2i}(t) = \epsilon_{3i}(t) + n^{-1} c_1(t) \mathcal{I}(\beta_0)^{-1} \epsilon_{1i}(t),$$
$$\epsilon_{3i}(t) = n^{-1} \int_0^t \left\{ (E[Y_1 \tilde{X}_1(\beta_0) X_1^T(\beta_0)^T])^{-1} X_i(\beta_0) \right\} dM_i,$$

with $c_1(t)$ and $\mathcal{I}(\beta_0)$ the limits in probability of $C_1(t)$ and $n^{-1}\tilde{I}(\beta_0)$, respectively. Estimates of $\epsilon_{ji}(t)$, denoted $\hat{\epsilon}_{ji}(t)$, for $j = 1, 2, 3$ are obtained by replacement of the limits (in probability) by their empirical counterparts and by plugging in the estimates of $dM_i(t)$ and β_0. One consequence of this i.i.d. representation is that a consistent estimate of the variance (function) $\Upsilon(t)$ of $n^{1/2}(\tilde{\Psi}(\tilde{\beta},t) - \Psi(t))$ is given by $\hat{\Upsilon}(t)$, where

$$\hat{\Upsilon}(t) = n^{-1} \sum_{i=1}^{n} \hat{\epsilon}_{2i}^{\otimes 2}(t).$$

To do inference about the nonparametric components of the model it is very useful that a resampling scheme can approximate the asymptotic distribution of $n^{1/2}(\tilde{\Psi}(\tilde{\beta},t) - \Psi(t))$. For $G_1, ..., G_n$ i.i.d. standard normals it can be shown that the asymptotic distribution of $n^{1/2}(\tilde{\Psi}(\tilde{\beta},t) - \Psi(t))$ is equivalent to the asymptotic distribution of

$$n^{-1/2} \sum_{i=1}^{n} \hat{\epsilon}_{2i}(t) G_i.$$

This may be used to construct Hall-Wellner type confidence bands by resampling of the distribution

$$\sup_{t \leq \tau} \left| n^{1/2} (\tilde{\Psi}_k(\tilde{\beta},t) - \Psi_k(t)) \frac{\Upsilon_{kk}^{-1/2}(\tau)}{1 + \Upsilon_{kk}(t)/\Upsilon_{kk}(\tau)} \right|$$

giving the (approximate) $(1-\alpha)$-quantile d_α. The approximate $(1-\alpha)$ Hall-Wellner confidence band for $\Psi(t)$ is given by

$$\tilde{\Psi}_k(\tilde{\beta},t) \pm d_\alpha n^{-1/2} \hat{\Upsilon}_{kk}^{1/2}(\tau) \left(1 + \frac{\hat{\Upsilon}_{kk}(t)}{\hat{\Upsilon}_{kk}(\tau)} \right).$$

7.2.3 Efficient estimation

One may construct efficient estimators $\hat{\beta}$ and $\hat{\Psi}(t)$ on the basis of the unweighted estimators $\tilde{\beta}$ and $\tilde{\Psi}(t)$. This may be done as follows.

(i) Obtain $\tilde{\beta}$ and $\tilde{\Psi}$ as outlined above.

(ii) Use a predictable kernel smoother to estimate ψ and obtain estimates of the efficient weights $\hat{V}$ and $\hat{W}$.

(iii) Obtain the efficient estimates using (7.17) and (7.18) with $\hat{V}$ and $\hat{W}$ in place of V and W.

In the following we derive the large sample properties of these estimators. Using similar arguments as McKeague & Sasieni (1994), it turns out that the asymptotic properties of $\hat{\beta}$ and $\hat{\Psi}(t)$ is unaffected by a replacement of $(\hat{V}, \hat{W})$ with (V, W). We may hence derive the asymptotic properties of $\hat{\beta}$

7.2 Proportional excess hazards model

and $\hat{\Psi}(t)$ using fixed weights. Let $\hat{\Phi}$, $\hat{G}$ and $\hat{H}$ be defined as Φ, G and H with β replaced by $\hat{\beta}$, and let

$$I(\beta) = \frac{dU(\beta)}{d\beta}.$$

By applying the matrix derivative rules to $U(\beta)$ we find that

$$I(\beta) = \int \left[Z^T \frac{d\Phi}{d\beta} \{VGHdN(t) \otimes I_q\} + Z^T \Phi H^T V \frac{dG}{d\beta} \{HdN(t) \otimes I_q\} \right],$$

where

$$\frac{dG}{d\beta} = -\left[\frac{1}{\phi^T W \phi} \frac{d\phi}{d\beta} - \frac{\phi}{(\phi^T W \phi)^2} \{ \frac{d\phi^T}{d\beta}(W\phi \otimes I_q) + \phi^T W \frac{d\phi}{d\beta} \} \right] (\phi^T W \otimes I_q)$$
$$- \frac{\phi}{\phi^T W \phi} \frac{d\phi^T}{d\beta}(W \otimes I_q).$$

Using (7.19), we have that

$$U(\beta_0) = \int Z^T \Phi V G H \, dM(t).$$

Theorem 7.2.3 *Under regularity conditions, $n^{\frac{1}{2}}(\hat{\beta} - \beta_0)$ converges in distribution to a zero-mean normal with a covariance matrix which is the limit in probability of*

$$\left(n^{-1} \int Z^T \Phi V G H \Phi Z \lambda_0 \, dt \right)^{-1}$$

and which is consistently estimated by

$$nI(\hat{\beta})^{-1}$$

or by the optional variation

$$n \int Z^T \hat{\Phi} V \hat{G} \hat{H} \, diag(dN) (V \hat{G} \hat{H})^T \hat{\Phi} Z.$$

PROOF. By use of Lenglart's inequality, it may be seen that $n^{-1}I(\beta_0)$ has the same limit in probability as

$$\int n^{-1} \lambda_0 Z^T \Phi H^T W \frac{dG}{d\beta} [H\{XdA(t) + \phi(\beta_0)\lambda_0 \, dt\} \otimes I_q]. \qquad (7.26)$$

After some matrix algebra it may be seen that (7.26) reduces to

$$n^{-1} \int Z^T \Phi V G H \Phi Z \lambda_0 \, dt.$$

282   7. Multiplicative-Additive hazards models

We also have that

$$\left\langle \int Z^T \Phi V G H \, dM(t) \right\rangle = \int Z^T \Phi V G H W^{-1} (WGH)^T \Phi Z \lambda_0 \, dt$$
$$= \int Z^T \Phi V G H \Phi Z \lambda_0 \, dt$$

since $(WGH)^T = WGH$ and $(GH)^2 = GH$. The asymptotic variance is therefore given as the limit in probability of

$$\{n^{-1} I(\hat{\beta})\}^{-1} \left\langle n^{-1/2} \int Z^T \Phi V G H \, dM(t) \right\rangle \{n^{-1} I(\hat{\beta})\}^{-1}$$
$$= \left(n^{-1} \int Z^T \Phi V G H \Phi Z \lambda_0 \, dt \right)^{-1}.$$

□

The asymptotic properties of the nonparametric component of the model is given in the following theorem. Define

$$C_2(t) = \int_0^t (\tilde{X}^T(\hat{\beta}) \hat{W} \tilde{X}(\hat{\beta}))^{-1} \tilde{X}^T(\hat{\beta}) \hat{W} \hat{\Phi} Z d\hat{\Lambda}_0(s),$$

where $\hat{\Lambda}_0(t)$ is the appropriate component of $\hat{\Psi}(t)$. Define

$$M_3(t) = \{n^{-1} I(\beta)\}^{-1} n^{-1/2} \int Z^T \Phi V G H \, dM(t),$$
$$M_4(t) = n^{\frac{1}{2}} \int_0^t (\tilde{X}(\beta_0)^T W \tilde{X}(\beta_0)^T)^{-1} \tilde{X}(\beta_0)^T W \, dM(s).$$

Theorem 7.2.4 *Under regularity conditions, $n^{\frac{1}{2}}\{\hat{\Psi}(t) - \Psi(t)\}$ converges in distribution to a zero-mean Gaussian process with covariance function that is estimated consistently by*

$$[M_4](t) - C_2(t)[M_3](\tau) C_2(t)^T.$$

PROOF. Since $\phi(\beta_0) = \phi(\tilde{\beta}) + \Phi^* Z(\tilde{\beta} - \beta_0)$, where $\Phi^* = \text{diag}\{\phi(\beta^*)\}$ and β^* is on the line segment between $\tilde{\beta}$ and β, it follows that

$$n^{\frac{1}{2}}\{\tilde{\Psi}(t) - \Psi(t)\} = C_1^*(t) n^{\frac{1}{2}} (\tilde{\beta} - \beta_0)$$
$$+ n^{\frac{1}{2}} \int_0^t \left\{ \tilde{X}(\beta_0)^T \tilde{X}(\beta_0) \right\}^{-1} \tilde{X}(\beta_0)^T \, dM(s)$$
$$= C_1^*(t) M_1(\tau) + M_2(t) + o_p(1),$$

where

$$C_1^*(t) = \int_0^t \left\{ \tilde{X}(\beta_0)^T \tilde{X}(\beta_0) \right\}^{-1} \tilde{X}(\beta_0)^T \Phi^* Z \lambda_0(s) \, ds.$$

As $n \to \infty$ $C_1^*(t)$ converges in probability for each t. By the martingale central limit theorem, it may furthermore be shown that (M_1, M_2) converges in distribution to a Gaussian martingale $U = (U_1, U_2)$ with mean zero, and the result follows. □

It may be shown that the weighted estimator $(\hat{\beta}, \hat{\Psi}(t))$ is efficient. In practice, however, we recommend to use the simple and unweighted estimators. They seem to be very stable numerically and the loss in efficiency is often very modest. In contrast, it is not always a trivial task to obtain the efficient weights in practice.

7.2.4 Goodness-of-fit procedures

Goodness-of-fit procedures may be developed along the same lines as for the Cox-Aalen model in the previous section. Specifically one may use a cumulative martingale residual process

$$M_K(t) = \int_0^t K^T(t) d\hat{M}(s),$$

where

$$\hat{M}(t) = N(t) - \int_0^t \tilde{X}(\tilde{\beta}, t) d\tilde{\Psi}(t).$$

The score function evaluated at $\tilde{\beta}$ and viewed as a process in t:

$$\tilde{U}(\tilde{\beta}, t) = \int_0^t Z^T \Phi(\tilde{\beta}) \tilde{H}(\tilde{\beta}) dN(t)$$

may also be used to evaluate the fit of the model. By a Taylor expansion it may be written as

$$\tilde{U}(\tilde{\beta}, t) = \int_0^t Z^T \Phi(\beta_0) \tilde{H}(\beta_0) dM(t) \\ - \tilde{I}(\tilde{\beta}, t) \tilde{I}(\tilde{\beta}, \tau)^{-1} \int_0^\tau Z^T \Phi(\beta_0) \tilde{H}(\beta_0) dM(t),$$

where $\tilde{I}(\beta, t)$ is the derivative of $\tilde{U}(\beta, t)$ with respect to β. The asymptotic distribution of the process $\tilde{U}(\tilde{\beta}, t)$ may be resampled by

$$\sum_{i=1}^n \hat{\epsilon}_{1i}(t) G_i - \tilde{I}(\tilde{\beta}, t) \tilde{I}(\tilde{\beta}, \tau)^{-1} \sum_{i=1}^n \hat{\epsilon}_{1i}(\tau) G_i,$$

where $G_1, \ldots, G_n$ are independent standard normals. This enables us to obtain percentiles from the distribution of, for example,

$$\sup_{t \leq \tau} |U(\tilde{\beta}, t)|.$$

284   7. Multiplicative-Additive hazards models

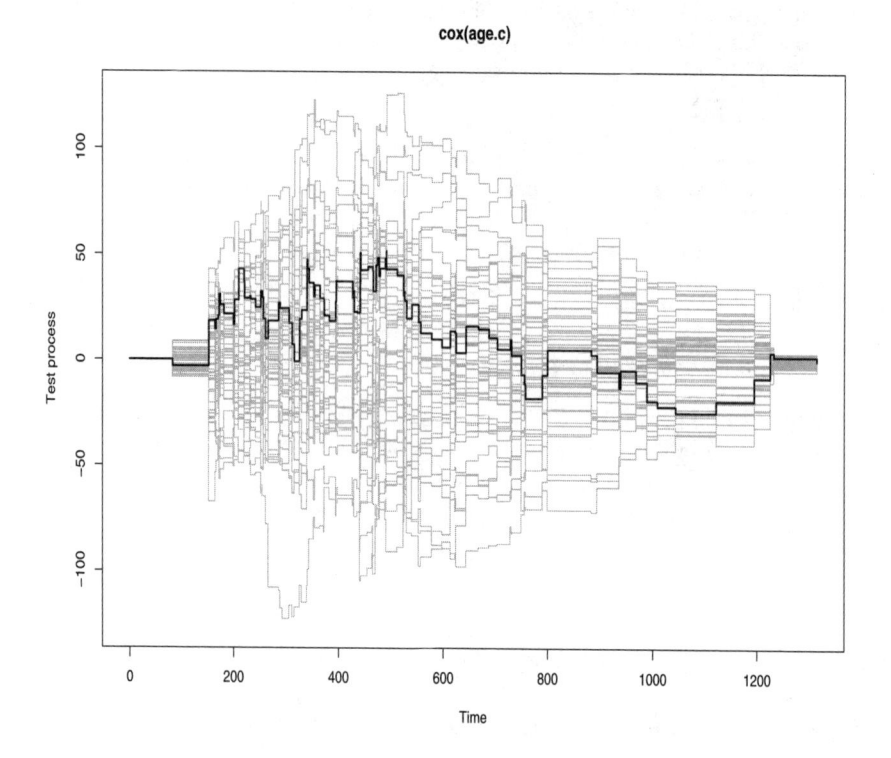

cox(age.c)

FIGURE 7.9: Lung cancer data: Score process along with 50 simulated process under the model (7.27).

7.2.5   Examples

We first give an illustration where the model (7.14) is used as a general flexible additive-multiplicative model.

Example 7.2.1 (Lung cancer data)

We apply the model to the lung cancer data presented in Ying et al. (1995) that we also analyzed by use of the multiplicative hazards model in Example 6.10.1. This dataset consists of 121 patients with small cell lung cancer. The patients were randomly assigned to one of two treatments: cisplatin followed by etoposide (0); etoposide followed by cisplatin (1).

By the end of the study, 47 of the 62 patients on treatment 1 and 51 of the 59 patients on treatment 2 had died. Lin & Ying (1995) noticed that a Cox-model

$$\lambda_i(t) = Y_i(t)\lambda_0(t)\exp\left(\beta_1 X_{i1} + \beta_2 X_{i2}\right),$$

7.2 Proportional excess hazards model

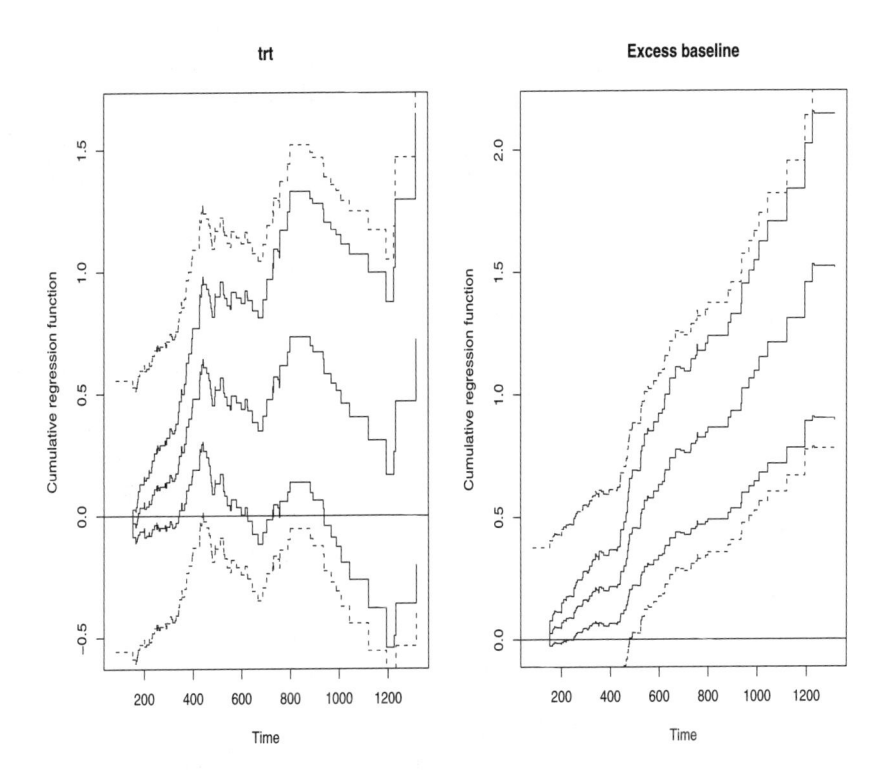

FIGURE 7.10: Lung cancer data. Estimates of $A_0(t)$ (left panel) and $\Lambda_0(t)$ (right panel) with 95% pointwise confidence intervals (full lines) and Hall-Wellner confidence bands (broken lines).

where X_{i1} is 1 if the patient was on treatment 2 and zero otherwise, and X_{i2} is the age of the patient at study entry, did not fit the data very well with respect to treatment.

They proceeded with the following additive-multiplicative model

$$\lambda_i(t) = Y_i(t)(\beta_1 X_{i1} + \lambda_0(t)\exp{(\beta_2 X_{i2})}),$$

and found that $\hat{\beta}_1 =$5.2e-04 (2.6e-04) and $\hat{\beta}_2 = 0.035(0.0174)$. They also indicated, however, that there might be a time-varying effect of the treatment covariate, so it may be more appropriate to apply the more general model

$$\lambda_i(t) = Y_i(t)(\alpha(t) X_{i1} + \lambda_0(t)\exp{(\beta X_{i2})}), \qquad (7.27)$$

which is seen to be of the form (7.14) with $\rho_i = 1$ for all subjects. We fitted this latter model with X_{i2} centered around its mean so that the "excess" hazard rate $\lambda_0(t)$, in this example, corresponds to the hazard rate for an averaged aged patient in treatment group 1. The model is fitted

286   7. Multiplicative-Additive hazards models

using the function `prop.excess`. As illustrated below, one may plot the score process (adhering to the proportional part of the model) along with 50 resampled processes under the model, and also estimated cumulatives with for example Hall-Wellner bands.

```
> age.c<-age-mean(age)
> excess<-1+numeric(n)
> fit<-prop.excess(Surv(times,status==1)~-1+trt+cox(age.c),
  excess=excess,n.sim=2000)
 Proportional Excess Survival Model
 Simulations start N=    2000
> plot(fit,score=T)
> plot(fit,hw.ci=2)
> summary(fit)
 Proportional Excess Survival Model

 Test for non-significant effects

 Test for Aalen terms, H_0: B(t)=0
                 KS-test pval  CM-test pval
 trt                    0.033         0.004
 Excess baseline        0.000         0.000


 Proportional  terms :
              coef se(coef)    z      p
 cox(age.c) 0.0469  0.0288 1.63  0.103

   Call: prop.excess(Surv(times, status == 1) ~ -1 + trt +
      cox(age.c),excess = excess, n.sim = 2000)
```

The score process does not seem extreme in this case as seen in Figure 7.9. The associated Kolmogorov-Smirnov type test based on 2000 simulated processes gives a p-value of 0.74. The unweighted estimates of the cumulatives, $A(t)$ and $\Lambda_0(t)$, are depicted in Figure 7.10, and we see there is an indication of a time-varying effect of the treatment: treatment 1 seems initially to be superior to treatment 2, but a maximal deviation test would not be able to reject the hypothesis of a constant effect. The Kolmogorov-Smirnov test for the hypothesis of no difference between the two treatments gives a p-value of 0.033. □

As mentioned earlier, the model (7.14) may be applied in situations where it is speculated that a certain group of subjects has an excess mortality when compared to a control group. Let us illustrate this with use of the malignant melanoma dataset.

Example 7.2.2 (Survival with malignant melanoma)

We consider the three covariates sex, ulceration and the logarithm of tumor

	Sex (S_i)	Ulceration (U_i)	log(thickness) (LT_i)
$\hat{\beta}$(SEE)	-0.09 (0.47)	-1.46 (0.82)	0.21 (0.51)
$\tilde{\beta}$(SEE)		-1.44 (0.81)	0.21 (0.53)
$\tilde{\beta}$(SEE)		-1.67 (0.79)	

TABLE 7.1: Estimates of β and standard error estimates (SEE) based on model (7.28).

thickness. We hence define LT_i to be the logarithm of tumor thickness for patient i,

$$S_i = \begin{cases} 1 & \text{if patient } i \text{ is a man} \\ 0 & \text{if patient } i \text{ is a woman} \end{cases}$$

and

$$U_i = \begin{cases} 1 & \text{if ulceration is not present in the tumor of patient } i \\ 0 & \text{otherwise.} \end{cases}$$

We shall here treat patients with a tumor thickness below a certain cut-point as the "exposed" group. By use of the results in Jespersen (1986), Andersen et al. (1993) found that an optimal breakpoint for the covariate thickness, based on the Cox-model, is 2.1 mm. As an illustration, we consider the group with a possible excess risk as the one consisting of patients with tumor thickness above 2.1 mm. The dataset was first analyzed using the model

$$\lambda_i(t) = Y_i(t)\{\alpha_0(t) + \alpha_1(t)S_i + \alpha_2(t)U_i \\ + \rho_i \lambda_0(t) \exp(\beta_0 S_i + \beta_1 U_i + \beta_2 LT_i)\}, \qquad (7.28)$$

where ρ_i is equal to 1 if the patients tumor thickness is above 2.1 mm, and 0 otherwise:

```
> excess<-0+1*(thick>=210)
> lt<-log(thick)
> ulc0<-(-1)*(ulc-1)
> status[status!=1]<-0
> fit<-prop.excess(Surv(days,status==1)~sex+ulc0+
        cox(sex)+cox(ulc0)+cox(lt),excess=excess,n.sim=2000)
 Proportional Excess Survival Model
 Simulations start N=    2000
> summary(fit)
 Proportional Excess Survival Model
```

288   7. Multiplicative-Additive hazards models

Test for non-significant effects

Test for Aalen terms, H_0: B(t)=0
```
                KS-test pval  CM-test pval
(Intercept)         0.187        0.498
sex                 0.514        0.574
ulc0                0.735        0.893
Excess baseline     0.799        0.772
```

Proportional terms:
```
             coef   se(coef)     z       p
cox(sex)   -0.0877   0.465   -0.189  0.8500
cox(ulc0)  -1.4600   0.822   -1.780  0.0751
cox(lt)     0.2070   0.514    0.403  0.6870
```

The score processes may be plotted as in the previous example, and these give no indication of a poor fit. Based on the estimates of the parametric components given in Table 7.1, it seems reasonable to simplify the model to

$$\lambda_i(t) = Y_i(t)\{\alpha_0(t) + \alpha_1(t)S_i + \alpha_2(t)U_i + \rho_i\lambda_0(t)\exp(\beta U_i)\}.$$

The p-values, based on a Kolmogorov-Smirnov test, for testing the non-parametric components, $\alpha_j(t)$, $j = 0, 1, 2$, equal to zero are 0.095, 0.475, and 0.71. Reducing the model first by setting $\alpha_2(t)$ equal to zero and then also $\alpha_1(t)$ gives us a model with only significant effects:

```
> fit<-prop.excess(Surv(days,status==1)~ cox(ulc0),excess=excess,
  n.sim=2000)
 Proportional Excess Survival Model
 Simulations start N=   2000
> plot(fit,hw.ci=2)
null device
          1
> summary(fit)
Proportional Excess Survival Model
```

Test for non-significant effects

Test for Aalen terms, H_0: B(t)=0
```
                KS-test pval  CM-test pval
(Intercept)         0.002        0.04
Excess baseline     0.000        0.00
```

Proportional terms :
```
             coef   se(coef)     z       p
cox(ulc0)   -1.67    0.794   -2.11  0.0352
```

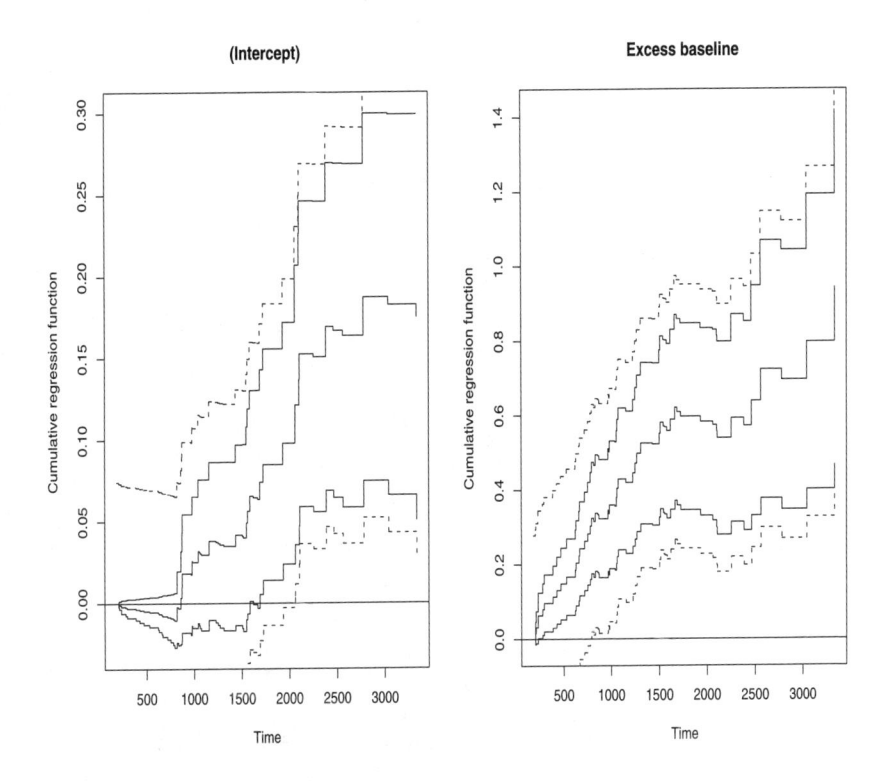

FIGURE 7.11: Melanoma data. Estimates of $A_0(t)$ (left panel) and $\Lambda_0(t)$ (right panel) with 95% pointwise confidence intervals (full lines) and Hall-Wellner confidence bands (broken lines).

corresponding to

$$\lambda_i(t) = Y_i(t)\{\alpha_0(t) + \rho_i\lambda_0(t)\exp(\beta U_i)\}. \tag{7.29}$$

In this model, $\tilde{\beta} = -1.67(0.79)$, and the unweighted estimates of the cumulatives, $A(t)$ and $\Lambda_0(t)$, are displayed in Figure 7.11 together with 95% pointwise confidence intervals (full lines) and Hall-Wellner confidence bands (broken lines). The mortality for patients with a small tumor is described by $\alpha_0(t)$ while $\lambda_0(t)$ describes the excess risk for a patient with tumor thickness above 2.1 mm. in the stratum defined by presence of ulceration. Both of these are clearly significant different from zero. The excess risk is reduced by a factor $\exp(-1.67)$ for patients without ulceration. □

7.3 Exercises

7.1 (Blocked Cox-Aalen) Let $N(t) = I(T \leq t)$ have intensity on the Cox-Aalen form:
$$\lambda(t) = Y(t)(X^T(t)\alpha(t))\exp(Z^T(t)\beta)$$
and assume that n i.i.d. replicas of the model are observed over the time-interval $[0, \tau]$. Some effects are multiplicative and they can thus be interpreted as effect modifiers. The model assumes the effect of X_1 and X_2, say, is modified in the same way by Z. One extension of the model allows different effect modification
$$\lambda(t) = Y(t)\left(\sum_{k=1}^{K} X_k^T(t)\alpha_k(t))\exp(Z^T(t)\gamma_k)\right)$$
where $X = (X_1, X_2, ..., X_K)$ is grouped into K blocks.

(a) By redefining the covariate Z the model can be written as
$$\lambda(t) = Y(t)\left(\sum_{k=1}^{K}(X_k^T(t)\alpha_k(t)\exp(Z_k^T(t)\tilde{\gamma})\right).$$
Specify this construction in detail.

(b) Derive a score equation for $\gamma = (\gamma_1, .., \gamma_K)$ or $\tilde{\gamma}$ in the alternative parametrization.

(c) Make the basic derivations to obtain the asymptotic properties.

7.2 (Cox-Aalen model: Alternative weights) Let $N(t) = I(T \leq t)$ have intensity on the Cox-Aalen form:
$$\lambda(t) = Y(t)(X^T(t)\alpha(t))\exp(Z^T(t)\beta)$$
and assume that n i.i.d. replicas of the model is observed over the time-interval $[0, \tau]$.

(a) Validate that the second derivative $\mathcal{I}$ is on the specified form when $w_i(t) = \exp(-Z_i^T\beta)$.

(b) Compute the score and second derivative in the case where $w_i(t) = 1$.

(c) The optimal weights are
$$w_i(t) = \exp(-Z_i^T\beta)/(X_i^T\alpha(t)).$$
Do a simulation study to learn about the finite sample performance when 1) α is known in the weights; 2) the weights are estimated based on and initial estimator and compare with the suggested weights.

(d) Show that the second derivative converges in probability to a negative definite matrix.

(e) Validate that the optional variation of the score process for β and the second derivative have the same asymptotic limit in the case with optimal weights.

7.3 (Veterans data) Consider the Veterans data available in the survival package in R, see Therneau & Grambsch (2000) for more details.

(a) Analyze the data using the Cox-Aalen model. Focus on the variables celltype, karno and age.

(b) Is treatment significant or time-varying?

(c) Does a Cox regression model provide a reasonable fit?

(d) Does the Cox-Aalen model provide a reasonable fit?

7.4 (Proportional excess model: alternative weights) Let $N(t) = I(T \leq t)$ have intensity on the proportional excess form:

$$\lambda(t) = Y(t)(X^T(t)\alpha(t) + \rho(t)\lambda_0(t)\exp(X^T(t)\beta))$$

and assume that n i.i.d. replicas of the model is observed over the time-interval $[0, \tau]$.

(a) The optimal weights are

$$w_i(t) = 1/\lambda_i(t).$$

Do a simulation study to learn about the finite sample performance when 1) α is known in the weights; 2) the weights are estimated based on and initial estimator and compare with the suggested weights.

(b) Show that the second derivative converges in probability to a negative definite matrix when the optimal weights are used.

(c) Validate that the optional variation of the score process for β and the second derivative have the same asymptotic limit in the case with optimal weights.

(d) Validate equation (7.19).

7.5 (Estimating the survival function) Assume that n i.i.d. replications from the proportional excess model is observed over the time-interval $[0, \tau]$.

(a) Suggest an estimator of the survival function, and derive an optional variation estimator of the variance for $n^{1/2}(\hat{S}_0(t) - S_0(t))$.

(b) Make an i.i.d. decomposition formula for $n^{1/2}(\hat{S}_0(t) - S_0(t))$, and give the recipe for making a 95 % confidence band.

7.6 (Data example) Consider the TRACE data of the timereg package. It may be sensible to work with a smaller sample of this data, for example the first 500 patients. Mortality due to ventricular fibrillation (vf) may be considered as excess risk, and it may relevant to modify this excess risk for gender. Suggest a proportional excess risk model that can be used to describe the excess risk due to vf.

8
Accelerated failure time and transformation models

In the past chapters we have presented various additive and multiplicative hazards models. These models are well suited for regression modeling of survival data, are simple to fit, and can deal with time-varying regression coefficients as well as time-dependent covariates. These models, however, are not the only important models in survival analysis, and in this section we give a brief review of the *accelerated failure time models* and *transformation models*.

To focus ideas, let T be a survival time and Z a covariate vector that does not depend on time. The accelerated failure time model assumes that

$$\log(T) = -Z^T \beta + \varepsilon$$

where β is a set of regression parameters and ε is a residual term with un-specified distribution. Note that the parameter appears to be quite easy to interpret because they directly refer to the level of $\log(T)$, but with censored observations, however, one should be very cautious to interpret them as standard linear regression effects that refers to the mean of $\log(T)$. The model is not quite as easy to fit as the regression models in the previous sections (with censored observations!), and the asymptotics of the estimators is also more difficult to get at, although there recently has been some good advances in making the model more practically applicable. Some important key references are Miller (1976), Buckley & James (1979), Koul et al. (1981), Lai & Ying (1991a), Prentice (1978), Ritov (1990), Tsiatis (1990), Lai & Ying (1991b), Wei et al. (1990); Ying (1993). See also Bagdonavicius & Nikulin (2001) and Kalbfleisch & Prentice (2002) for a summary of these techniques.

Another class of models are the transformation models:

$$h(T) = -Z^T\beta + \varepsilon$$

where the transformation h is now an unspecified monotone transformation while ε is a known error distribution. Special cases are the Cox regression model when ε has an extreme value distribution with distribution function $F(t) = \exp(-\exp(t))$ and the proportional odds model when ε is a standard logistic distribution. Some authors have dealt with this model quite generally by inverse probability weighting techniques (Cheng et al., 1995, 1997; Fine et al., 1998; Cai et al., 2000). A drawback of the inverse probability weighting technique is that the censoring distribution needs to be estimated. Alternatively, as we shall do here, one may consider an estimating equations approach, as in for example Bagdonavicius & Nikulin (1999) and the recent Chen et al. (2002). For a detailed treatment see the book Bagdonavicius & Nikulin (2001). The transformation model has some advantages, and has proved its relevance in the two special cases mentioned above, but for other choices of ε the regression coefficients are more difficult to interpret because they refer to the scale given by the unknown h.

8.1 The accelerated failure time model

The accelerated failure time (AFT) model simply makes a linear regression for the log-transformed event time, $\log(T)$, given a p-dimensional covariate $Z = (Z_1, ..., Z_p)$ such that

$$\log(T) = -Z^T\beta + \varepsilon \tag{8.1}$$

where $\beta = (\beta_1, ..., \beta_p)$ is a p-dimensional regression parameter, and ε is unspecified. This specification leads to the hazard function for T given Z:

$$\lambda(t) = \lambda_0(t\exp(Z^T\beta))\exp(Z^T\beta), \tag{8.2}$$

where $\lambda_0(t)$ is the hazard associated with the unspecified error distribution $\exp(\varepsilon)$. We see that the covariates acts multiplicatively on time so that their effect is to accelerate or decelerate time to failure relative to $\lambda_0(t)$. Note that when there are censorings present one should be very careful interpreting β as in the standard linear regression case where β gives the effect of Z on the mean of $\log(T)$. Let C be the censoring time for T, and put $\tilde{T} = T \wedge C$ and $\Delta = I(T \leq C)$. We now consider (8.2) as our basic model for the intensity of the counting process $N(t) = I(\tilde{T} \leq t)\Delta$ constructed by observing the possibly right-censored event time. The intensity is thus assumed to be $Y(t)\lambda(t)$ with $Y(t) = I(t \leq \tilde{T})$ being the at risk indicator.

Assume that n i.i.d. counting processes are being observed subject to this generic hazard model. We thus consider $N(t) = (N_1(t), ..., N_n(t))$ the n-

8.1 The accelerated failure time model

dimensional counting process of all subjects. Define also the time-transformed counting process

$$N^*(t) = (N_1(t\exp(-Z_1^T\beta)),..,N_n(t\exp(-Z_n^T\beta)))$$

with associated at risk process $Y_i^*(t,\beta) = Y_i(t\exp(-Z_i^T\beta))$, $i = 1,\ldots,n$. The time-transformation for each counting process is useful because the intensity of $N_i(t\exp(-Z_i^T\beta))$ is

$$\lambda_i^*(t) = Y_i^*(t)\lambda_0(t),$$

which immediately suggest that $\Lambda_0(t) = \int_0^t \lambda_0(s)ds$ should be estimated by the Breslow-type estimator

$$\hat{\Lambda}_0(t,\beta) = \int_0^t \frac{1}{S_0^*(s,\beta)} dN_{\cdot}^*(s) \tag{8.3}$$

where $dN_{\cdot}^*(t) = \sum_{i=1}^n dN_i^*(t)$, and

$$S_0^*(t,\beta) = \sum_{i=1}^n Y_i^*(t,\beta)$$

if β were known. Let us now turn to estimation of β. The efficient score function for β is

$$\sum_{i=1}^n \int_0^\infty \frac{\partial}{\partial \beta}(\lambda_i(t,\beta))\lambda_i^{-1}(t,\beta)\left(dN_i(t) - Y_i(t)\lambda_i(t)dt\right) \tag{8.4}$$

$$= \sum_{i=1}^n \int_0^\infty \left(\frac{\lambda_0'(t\exp(Z_i^T\beta))t\exp(Z_i^T\beta)}{\lambda_0(t\exp(Z_i^T\beta))} + 1\right) Z_i(dN_i(t) - Y_i(t)\lambda_i(t)dt)$$

$$= \sum_{i=1}^n \int_0^\infty \left(\frac{\lambda_0'(u)u}{\lambda_0(u)} + 1\right) Z_i(dN_i^*(u) - Y_i^*(u,\beta)d\Lambda_0(u)),$$

and inserting $d\hat{\Lambda}_0(u,\beta)$ for $d\Lambda_0(u)$ gives

$$U_W(\beta) = \sum_{i=1}^n \int_0^\infty W(u)Z_i \left(dN_i^*(u) - \frac{Y_i^*(u,\beta)}{S_0^*(u,\beta)} dN_{\cdot}^*(u)\right)$$

$$= \sum_{i=1}^n \int_0^\infty W(u)\left(Z_i - E^*(u,\beta)\right) dN_i^*(u), \tag{8.5}$$

where

$$S_1^*(u,\beta) = \sum_{i=1}^n Y_i^*(u,\beta)Z_i, \quad E^*(u,\beta) = \frac{S_1^*(u,\beta)}{S_0^*(u,\beta)},$$

and
$$W(u) = \left(\frac{\lambda_0'(u)u}{\lambda_0(u)} + 1\right) \tag{8.6}$$

is the efficient weight function. The score function can also be written on the (log)-transformed time scale

$$U_{\tilde{W}}(\beta) = \sum_{i=1}^{n} \int_{-\infty}^{\infty} \tilde{W}(t) \left(Z_i - E^*(e^t, \beta)\right) dN_i^*(e^t)$$

$$= \sum_{i=1}^{n} \int_{-\infty}^{\infty} \tilde{W}(t) \left(Z_i - \tilde{E}(t - Z_i^T\beta, \beta)\right) d\tilde{N}_i(t - Z_i^T\beta), \tag{8.7}$$

where $\tilde{N}_i(t) = I(\log(\tilde{T}_i) \leq t)\Delta_i$, $\tilde{Y}_i(t) = I(t \leq \log(\tilde{T}_i))$,

$$\tilde{E}(t,\beta) = \sum_{i=1}^{n} Z_i \tilde{Y}_i(t) / \sum_{i=1}^{n} \tilde{Y}_i(t), \quad \tilde{W}(t) = \frac{\lambda_{0\varepsilon}'(t)}{\lambda_{0\varepsilon}(t)},$$

with $\lambda_{0\varepsilon}(t)$ the hazard function for ε.

We cannot use (8.5) directly for estimation purposes since the weight function $W(u)$ involves the unknown baseline hazard function $\lambda_0(u)$ and its derivative $\lambda_0'(u)$. These can be estimated and inserted into (8.5) but it is not recommendable since it is hard to get reliable estimates of especially $\lambda_0'(t)$. A way around this is to take (8.5) and replacing the weight function $W(u)$ with one that can be computed as for example $W(u) = 1$ or $W(u) = n^{-1}S_0^*(u, \beta)$ referred to as the log-rank and Gehan weight functions, respectively.

Note. The classical way of arriving at (8.7) with $\tilde{W}$ just being any weight function is as follows (Tsiatis, 1990). If we want to test the hypothesis, $\beta = 0$, then a class of linear rank tests can be written as

$$\sum_{i=1}^{n} \int_{0}^{\infty} W(t)(Z_i - \tilde{E}(t))d\tilde{N}_i(t)$$

with W being some weight function. Generalizing this test statistic to test the hypothesis $\beta = \beta_0$ is done by replacing $\log(\tilde{T}_i)$ with $\log(\tilde{T}_i) + Z_i^T\beta_0$, which leads to (8.7). So it is natural to choose the estimator of β_0 as the β that minimizes (8.7).

A practical complication is that the score function $U_W(\beta)$ is a step function of β so $U_W(\beta) = 0$ may not have a solution. The score function may furthermore not be component-wise monotone in β. It is actually monotone in each component of β if the Gehan-weight is chosen (Fygenson & Ritov, 1994). The estimator $\hat{\beta}$ is usually chosen as the one which minimizes $\|U_W(\beta)\|$.

It has been established under regularity conditions that $n^{1/2}(\hat{\beta} - \beta)$ is asymptotically zero-mean normal with covariance matrix $A_W^{-1} B_W A_W^{-1}$, where A_W and B_W are the limits in probability of

$$\frac{1}{n}\sum_{i=1}^{n}\int_0^\infty W(u)\,(Z_i - E^*(u,\beta))^{\otimes 2}\left(\frac{\lambda_0'(u)u}{\lambda_0(u)} + 1\right) dN_i^*(u),$$

$$\frac{1}{n}\sum_{i=1}^{n}\int_0^\infty W(u)^2\,(Z_i - E^*(u,\beta))^{\otimes 2}\,dN_i^*(u)$$

respectively (Tsiatis, 1990; Ying, 1993). It is seen that A_W and B_W coincide in the case where $W(u)$ is taken as the efficient weight function (8.6). The asymptotic covariance matrix depends on λ_0', which is difficult to estimate. One may, however, apply a resampling technique avoiding estimation of λ_0', see Lin et al. (1998b) and Jin et al. (2003)

Chen & Jewell (2001) considered the interesting variant of (8.2):

$$\lambda(t) = \lambda_0(t\exp(Z^T\beta_1))\exp(Z^T\beta_2), \tag{8.8}$$

which contains both the proportional hazards model ($\beta_1 = 0$), the accelerated failure time model ($\beta_1 = \beta_2$), and for $\beta_2 = 0$ what is called the accelerated hazards model (Chen & Wang, 2000). Chen & Jewell (2001) suggested estimating equations for estimation of $\beta = (\beta_1, \beta_2)$ and showed for the resulting estimator, $\hat{\beta}$, that $n^{1/2}(\hat{\beta}-\beta)$ is asymptotically zero-mean normal with a covariance that also involves the unknown baseline hazard (and its derivative). They also suggested an alternative resampling approach for estimating the covariance matrix (attributed to Eugene Huang) without having to estimate the baseline hazard function or its derivative. With these tools at hand one may then investigate whether it is appropriate to simplify (8.8) to either the Cox-model or the AFT-model.

Note. There exists other ways of estimating the regression parameters β of the AFT-model, which build more on classical linear regression models estimation (Buckley & James, 1979). Starting with (8.1), let $V = \log(T)$, $U = \log(C)$ and $\tilde{V} = V \wedge U$, and write model (8.1) as

$$V = -\beta_0 - Z^T\beta + \varepsilon$$

assuming that ε is independent of $Z = (Z_1, \ldots, Z_p)^T$ and has zero mean. If V was not right-censored, then it is of course an easy task to estimate the regression parameters. The idea is therefore to replace V with a quantity that has the same mean as V, and which can be computed based on the right-censored sample. With

$$V^* = V\Delta + (1-\Delta)E(V\,|\,V > U, Z),$$

and $\Delta = I(V \leq U)$, then $E(V^*\,|\,Z) = E(V\,|\,Z)$. Still, V^* is not observable but it can be estimated as follows. Since

$$E(V\,|\,V > U, Z) = -Z^T\beta + \frac{\int_{U+Z^T\beta}^\infty v\,dF(v)}{1 - F(U+Z^T\beta)}$$

with F the distribution of $V + Z^T\beta$, one can construct the so-called synthetic data points:

$$\hat{V}_i^*(\beta) = V_i\Delta_i + (1 - \Delta_i)\left(-Z_i^T\beta + \frac{\int_{U_i+Z_i^T\beta}^{\infty} v d\hat{F}(v)}{1 - \hat{F}(U_i + Z_i^T\beta)}\right),$$

where $\hat{F}$ is the Kaplan-Meier estimator based on $(\tilde{V}_i + Z_i^T\beta, \Delta_i)$, $i = 1, \ldots, n$. One may then estimate the parameters from the normal equations leading to the following estimating equation for the regression parameter vector β:

$$\sum_{i=1}^{n}(\hat{V}_i^*(\beta) + Z_i^T\beta)(Z_i - \overline{Z}) = 0, \tag{8.9}$$

where $\overline{Z} = n^{-1}\sum_i Z_i$. Equation (8.9) needs to be solved iteratively if it has a solution. The large sample properties of the resulting estimator were studied by Ritov (1990). Equation (8.9) can also be written as, with $S(v) = v$,

$$U_S(\beta) = \sum_{i=1}^{n}\left(\Delta_i S(U_i + Z_i^T\beta) + (1 - \Delta_i)\frac{\int_{U_i+Z_i^T\beta}^{\infty} S(v) d\hat{F}(v)}{1 - \hat{F}(U_i + Z_i^T\beta)}\right)(Z_i - \overline{Z})$$
$$= 0, \tag{8.10}$$

that may derived from a likelihood principle; the efficient choice of $S(v)$ being $S(v) = f'(v)/f(v)$ with $f(v) = F'(v)$ the density function. Ritov (1990) also established an asymptotic equivalence between the two classes of estimators given by (8.7) and (8.10). He showed that for any $S(\cdot)$ in (8.10) there exist a $\tilde{W}(\cdot)$ so that $U_{\tilde{W}}(\beta) = U_S(\beta)$, and vice versa. Explicit expressions of the relations between $S(\cdot)$ and $\tilde{W}(\cdot)$ was also given by Ritov (1990).

8.2 The semiparametric transformation model

The transformation model also makes a linear regression for the event time, T, on a scale given by the *unknown* strictly increasing function h given a p-dimensional covariate $Z = (Z_1, ..., Z_p)$ such that

$$h(T) = -Z^T\beta + \varepsilon, \tag{8.11}$$

where $\beta = (\beta_1, ..., \beta_p)$ is a p-dimensional regression parameter, and the residual ε has a *known distribution* with distribution function F_ε, say. If $S(t|Z)$ denotes the conditional survival function of T given Z then we may also write model (8.11) as

$$S_\varepsilon^{-1}(S_Z(t)) = h(t) + Z^T\beta,$$

8.2 The semiparametric transformation model

where $S_\epsilon(t) = 1 - F_\epsilon(x)$. The hazard function for T given Z is

$$\lambda(t) = \lambda(t, Z) = \{\frac{\partial}{\partial t}h(t)\}\lambda_\epsilon(Z^T\beta + h(t)),$$

where $\lambda_\epsilon(t)$ is the hazard function associated with ϵ.

In the following we prefer to reparameterize the model and write it as

$$G(T) = \exp(-Z^T\beta)\exp(\epsilon) \tag{8.12}$$

where $G = \exp(h)$ is a strictly increasing positive function such that $G(0) = 0$ and $\lim_{t\to\infty} G(t) = \infty$. Let $g(t) = G'(t)$ denote the derivative of $G(t)$. The hazard of T given Z can now be written as

$$\lambda(t) = g(t)\exp(Z^T\beta)\lambda_0(\exp(Z^T\beta)G(t)), \tag{8.13}$$

where $\lambda_0(t)$ is the hazard associated with $\exp(\epsilon)$.

When ϵ has the extreme value distribution then $\exp(\epsilon)$ is standard exponentially distributed ($\lambda_0(t) = 1$), and the hazard function (8.13) is then the Cox regression model with cumulative baseline hazard function $G(t)$.

In the case of the standard logistic distribution as the error distribution, $F(x) = \exp(x)/(1+\exp(x))$, we see that

$$\text{logit}(1 - S_Z(t)) = \log(G(t)) + Z^T\beta \tag{8.14}$$

and the model is therefore in this situation referred to as the proportional odds model. The survival function and hazard function (8.13) are

$$S(t) = S(t|Z) = \frac{1}{1 + G(t)\exp(Z^T\beta)}; \quad \lambda(t) = \frac{g(t)}{\exp(-Z^T\beta) + G(t)}.$$

The *relative risk* for two individual with covariates Z_1 and Z_2, respectively, is

$$\text{RR}(t) = \frac{\lambda(t, Z_2)}{\lambda(t, Z_1)} = \frac{\exp(-Z_1^T\beta) + G(t)}{\exp(-Z_2^T\beta) + G(t)}$$

with $\text{RR}(0) = \exp((Z_2 - Z_1)^T\beta)$ and $\lim_{t\to\infty}\text{RR}(t) = 1$ so the model results in what is referred to as converging hazards. This is an appealing property of the model, as converging hazards are encountered in many practical settings.

We now take (8.13) as our basic model for the intensity of the associated counting process. Assume that n i.i.d. counting processes, representing survival times with independent censoring, are being observed subject to this generic hazard model. We thus consider $N(t) = (N_1(t), .., N_n(t))$ the n-dimensional counting process of all subjects with intensity $\lambda(t) = (Y_1(t)\lambda_1(t), ..., Y_n(t)\lambda_n(t))$, where $Y_i(t)$, $i = 1, \ldots, n$, are the at-risk indicators. We use $M_i(t)$, $i = 1, \ldots, n$, to denote the associated counting process martingales.

8. Accelerated failure time and transformation models

The martingale decomposition of $dN.(t)$ reads

$$dN.(t) = S_0(t,\beta,G)dG(t) + dM.(t),$$

where

$$S_0(t,\beta,G) = \sum_{i=1}^{n} Y_i(t)\exp(Z_i^T\beta)\lambda_0(\exp(Z_i^T\beta)G(t-))$$

writing $G(t-)$ to stress the needed predictability of the intensities. Based on this decomposition it seems natural to estimate $G(t)$ by the following Breslow-type estimator (keeping β fixed)

$$\tilde{G}(t,\beta) = \int_0^t \frac{1}{S_0(s,\beta,\tilde{G})} dN.(s). \tag{8.15}$$

Equation (8.15) gives a recursive way of computing $\tilde{G}(t,\beta)$ starting with $\tilde{G}(0,\beta) = 0$.

Estimation of β may be based on the (partial) likelihood function

$$\prod_{i=1}^{n}\prod_{t\geq 0} \left[Y_i(t)\exp(Z_i^T\beta)dG(t)\lambda_0(\exp(Z_i^T\beta)G(t-))\right]^{\Delta N_i(t)}$$

$$\times \exp\left\{-\int_0^\infty Y_i(t)\exp(Z_i^T\beta)\lambda_0(\exp(Z_i^T\beta)G(t-))dG(t)\right\}.$$

The idea is now to replace $dG(t)$ with $d\tilde{G}(t,\beta)$ and $G(t)$ with $\tilde{G}(t,\beta)$, which leads to

$$\prod_{i=1}^{n}\prod_{t\geq 0} \left\{Y_i(t)\exp(Z_i^T\beta)d\tilde{G}(t,\beta)\lambda_0(\exp(Z_i^T\beta)G(t-))\right\}^{\Delta N_i(t)},$$

where we have dropped terms not depending on β. The derivative with respect to β of the log of this (pseudo) profile-likelihood is

$$\tilde{U}(\beta) = \sum_{i=1}^{n}\int_0^\infty \left\{\frac{\dot{w}_i(t,\beta,\tilde{G})}{w_i(t,\beta,\tilde{G})} - \frac{S_1(t,\beta,\tilde{G})}{S_0(t,\beta,\tilde{G})}\right\} dN_i(t), \tag{8.16}$$

where

$$w_i(t,\beta,\tilde{G}) = \exp(Z_i^T\beta)\lambda_0(\exp(Z_i^T\beta)\tilde{G}(t-,\beta)),$$

$$\dot{w}_i(t,\beta,\tilde{G}) = \frac{\partial}{\partial\beta}w_i(t,\beta,\tilde{G}) \quad \text{and} \quad S_1(t,\beta,\tilde{G}) = \frac{\partial}{\partial\beta}S_0(t,\beta,\tilde{G}).$$

When computing the derivative of w_i with respect to β one should remember that $\tilde{G}$ is also a function of β. When $\lambda_0(t) = 1$, (8.16) reduces to the usual Cox score function, and for the proportional odds model one obtains

$$\sum_{i=1}^{n}\int_0^\infty \left\{\frac{Z_i\exp(-Z_i^T\beta) - \frac{\partial}{\partial\beta}\tilde{G}(t-,\beta)}{\exp(-Z_i^T\beta) + \tilde{G}(t-,\beta)} - \frac{S_1(t,\beta,\tilde{G})}{S_0(t,\beta,\tilde{G})}\right\} dN_i(t) = 0.$$

8.2 The semiparametric transformation model

We denote minus the derivative of $\tilde{U}(\beta)$ (8.16) with respect to β by

$$I(\beta) = I(\tau, \beta) = -\frac{\partial}{\partial \beta}\tilde{U}(\beta).$$

Let $\hat{\beta}$ be the root of $\tilde{U}(\beta) = 0$ and use β_0 and G_0 for the true values of β and G. The estimator $\hat{\beta}$ is called the modified partial likelihood estimator. One may show (under some regularity conditions) that $n^{1/2}(\hat{\beta} - \beta_0)$ is asymptotically zero-mean normal with covariance matrix that is consistently estimated by

$$\{n^{-1}I\}^{-1}(\hat{\beta})\hat{\Sigma}\{n^{-1}I\}^{-1}(\hat{\beta}), \tag{8.17}$$

where an expression for $\hat{\Sigma}$ is given below in (8.18). Further, to estimate $G_0(t)$ one may use the estimator $\hat{G}(t) = \tilde{G}(\hat{\beta}, t)$. It can also be shown that $n^{1/2}(\hat{G}(t) - G_0(t))$ converges to a Gaussian process with a variance that can be estimated by formula (8.19) below. Further, to get a uniform confidence band one may resample the residuals. In the below note, some of the basic steps in the derivation of the asymptotic properties of these estimators are given, following Bagdonavicius & Nikulin (1999).

Note. Asymptotic properties for the modified partial likelihood estimators. Let $s_0(t, \beta_0)$ and $s_1(t, \beta_0)$ denote the limits in probability of the quantities $n^{-1}S_0(t, \beta_0)$ and $n^{-1}S_1(t, \beta_0)$, respectively. We start by making the observation that (up to $o_p(1)$)

$$n^{1/2}(\tilde{G}(t, \beta_0) - G_0(t)) = n^{-1/2}\int_0^t \frac{1}{n^{-1}S_0(s, \beta_0, \tilde{G})}dM_\bullet(s)$$
$$+ n^{1/2}\int_0^t \frac{S_0(s, \beta_0, G_0) - S_0(s, \beta_0, \tilde{G})}{S_0(s, \beta_0, \tilde{G})}dG_0(s).$$

Note that the first term, by the martingale CLT, can be shown to converge to a Gaussian martingale process $V(t)$ with variance $\sigma^2(t) = \int_0^t s_0^{-1}(t)dG_0$. The difference in the last integral of the above display can be Taylor expanded (up to $o_p(1)$)

$$n^{-1/2}(S_0(t, \beta_0, \tilde{G}) - S_0(t, \beta_0, G_0)) = n^{-1}S_0^*(t, \beta_0)$$
$$n^{1/2}(\tilde{G}(t-, \beta_0) - G_0(t-)),$$

where we define

$$S_j^*(t, \beta_0) = \sum_{i=1}^n Y_i(t)\left\{\frac{\dot{w}_i(t, \beta_0, \tilde{G})}{w_i(t, \beta_0, \tilde{G})}\right\}^j \exp(2Z_i^T\beta_0)\dot{\lambda}_0(\exp(Z_i^T\beta_0)G_0(t-))$$

for $j = 1, 2$ with $\dot{\lambda}_0(t) = \frac{\partial}{\partial t}\lambda_0(t)$. Define also the limit in probability of $S_0^*(t, \beta_0)/S_0(t, \beta_0)$ by $e^*(t, \beta_0) = s_0^*(t, \beta_0)/s_0(t, \beta_0)$, where $s_0^*(t, \beta_0)$ is the limit in probability of $n^{-1}S_0^*(t, \beta_0)$.

302   8. Accelerated failure time and transformation models

This implies that $n^{1/2}(\tilde{G}(t,\beta_0) - G_0(t))$ converges in distribution to a process $W(t)$ that satisfies the integral equation

$$W(t) = -\int_0^t e^*(u,\beta_0)W(u)dG_0(u) + V(t),$$

which is solved for

$$W(t) = k(t,\beta_0)\int_0^t k^{-1}(u,\beta_0)dV(u),$$

where $k(t,\beta_0) = \exp(-\int_0^t e^*(u,\beta_0)dG_0(u))$.

After this preliminary observation we turn to the modified partial likelihood score $\tilde{U}(\beta)$. The score evaluated at the true point may be decomposed as

$$\tilde{U}(\beta_0) = \sum_{i=1}^n \int_0^\infty \left\{ \frac{\dot{w}_i(t,\beta_0,\tilde{G})}{w_i(t,\beta_0,\tilde{G})} - \frac{S_1(t,\beta_0,\tilde{G})}{S_0(t,\beta_0,\tilde{G})} \right\} dM_i(t)$$

$$+ \sum_{i=1}^n \int_0^\infty \frac{\dot{w}_i(t,\beta_0,\tilde{G})}{w_i(t,\beta_0,\tilde{G})} Y_i(t) \left\{ w_i(t,\beta_0,G_0) - w_i(t,\beta_0,\tilde{G}) \right\} dG_0(t)$$

$$+ \int_0^\infty \frac{S_1(t,\beta,\tilde{G})}{S_0(t,\beta_0,\tilde{G})} \left\{ S_0(t,\beta_0,\tilde{G}) - S_0(t,\beta_0,G_0) \right\} dG_0(t).$$

By a Taylor expansion it may be shown that (up to $o_p(1)$)

$$n^{1/2}\left(w_i(t,\beta_0,\tilde{G}) - w_i(t,\beta_0,G_0)\right) =$$
$$\exp(2Z_i^T\beta_0)\dot{\lambda}_0(\exp(Z_i^T\beta_0)G_0(t-))W(t).$$

Define $e(t,\beta) = s_1(t,\beta)/s_0(t,\beta)$,

$$l(t,\beta) = \frac{s_1(t,\beta)s_0^*(t,\beta) - s_0(t,\beta)s_1^*(t,\beta)}{s_0(t,\beta)},$$

$$q(t,\beta) = e(t,\beta) - \frac{1}{k(t,\beta)s_0(t,\beta)}\int_t^\infty l(s,\beta)k(s,\beta)dG_0(s).$$

Then we can write the normed score as (up to an $o_p(1)$ term):

$$n^{-1/2}\tilde{U}(\beta_0) = \int_0^\infty l(t,\beta_0)W(t)dG_0(t)$$
$$+ n^{-1/2}\sum_{i=1}^n \int_0^\infty \left\{ \frac{\dot{w}_i(t,\beta_0,G_0)}{w_i(t,\beta_0,G_0)} - e(t,\beta_0) \right\} dM_i(t)$$
$$= n^{-1/2}\sum_{i=1}^n \int_0^\infty \left\{ \frac{\dot{w}_i(t,\beta_0,G_0)}{w_i(t,\beta_0,G_0)} - q(t,\beta_0) \right\} dM_i(t).$$

This is a sum of i.i.d. terms (or a martingale) and therefore converges to a normal distribution with variance that is consistently estimated by the robust estimator

$$\hat{\Sigma} = n^{-1}\sum_{i=1}^n \left[\int_0^\infty \left\{ \frac{\dot{w}_i(t,\hat{\beta},\tilde{G})}{w_i(t,\hat{\beta},\tilde{G})} - \hat{q}(t,\hat{\beta}) \right\} d\hat{M}_i(t)\right]^{\otimes 2} \quad (8.18)$$

8.2 The semiparametric transformation model

or by the optional variation process

$$n^{-1}\sum_{i=1}^{n}\int_{0}^{\infty}\left\{\frac{\dot{w}_i(t,\hat{\beta},\tilde{G})}{w_i(t,\hat{\beta},\tilde{G})} - \hat{q}(t,\hat{\beta})\right\}^{\otimes 2} dN_i(t),$$

where $\hat{q}(t,\hat{\beta})$ is obtained by replacing unknown quantities by their empirical counterparts. We therefore get that (up to an $o_p(1)$ term)

$$n^{1/2}(\hat{\beta} - \beta_0) = \{n^{-1}I(\hat{\beta})\}^{-1}n^{-1/2}\tilde{U}(\beta_0),$$

and a consistent estimator of the variance of $n^{1/2}(\hat{\beta} - \beta_0)$ is given by (8.17).

Finally, we consider the asymptotic distribution of $\hat{G}(t) = \tilde{G}(t,\hat{\beta})$. It can can be derived that (up to an $o_p(1)$ term)

$$n^{1/2}\left(\hat{G}(t) - G_0(t)\right) = -\int_0^t \frac{S_1(t,\beta_0,\tilde{G})}{S_0(t,\beta_0,\tilde{G})} dG_0(s) n^{1/2}(\hat{\beta} - \beta_0)$$
$$+ k(t,\beta_0)n^{-1/2}\sum_{i=1}^{n}\int_0^t Y_i(s)k^{-1}(s,\beta_0)\frac{1}{s_0(s,\beta_0)}dM_i(s)$$
$$= n^{1/2}\sum_{i=1}^{n} H_i(t,\beta_0),$$

where

$$H_i(t,\beta) = -P(t,\beta_0)I^{-1}(\beta_0)\int_0^\infty Y_i(t)\left[\frac{\dot{w}_i(t,\beta_0,G_0)}{w_i(t,\beta_0,G_0)} - q(t,\beta_0)\right]dM_i(t)$$
$$+ n^{-1}k(t,\beta_0)\int_0^t Y_i(s)k^{-1}(s,\beta_0)\frac{1}{s_0(s,\beta_0)}dM_i(s)$$

with $P(t,\beta_0) = \int_0^t s_1(t,\beta_0)/s_0(t,\beta_0)dG_0$. Let $\hat{H}_i$ denote the estimator of H_i by plugging in the estimates of the unknown quantities. The variance of $\hat{G}(t) - G_0(t)$ may therefore be estimated by

$$\sum_{i=1}^{n} \hat{H}_i^{\otimes 2}(t,\hat{\beta}) \qquad (8.19)$$

or by the estimated optional variation. The entire process has an asymptotic distribution that can be obtained by resampling of the residuals

$$\sum_{i=1}^{n} \hat{H}_i(t,\hat{\beta})D_i,$$

where D_i are independent standard normals.

Note also that the goodness-of-fit of the model may be evaluated by comparing the observed score process versus resampled versions under the model.

Our experience with the modified partial likelihood method is that it performs well in practice. One should note, however, that it does not correspond to the nonparametric maximum likelihood estimator (NPMLE), see Slud & Vonta (2004) and Murphy et al. (1997) for details on the NPMLE for the proportional odds model. The NPMLE is more difficult to implement as no explicit expressions are available.

Yet another procedure is to substitute $d\tilde{G}(t, \beta)$ for $dG(t)$ in the efficient score function for β. The efficient score function for β (assuming that G is known) is

$$\sum_{i=1}^{n} \int_0^\infty \frac{\partial}{\partial \beta}(\lambda_i(t,\beta))\lambda_i^{-1}(t,\beta)\,(dN_i(t) - Y_i(t)\lambda_i(t)dt)$$

$$= \sum_{i=1}^{n} \int_0^\infty \frac{\dot{v}_i(t,\beta,G)}{v_i(t,\beta,G)}\,(dN_i(t) - Y_i(t)v_i(t,\beta,G)dG(t)), \quad (8.20)$$

where

$$v_i(t,\beta,G) = \exp(Z_i^T \beta)\lambda_0(\exp(Z_i^T \beta)G(t-)) \quad \text{and}$$
$$\dot{v}_i(t,\beta,G) = \frac{\partial}{\partial \beta}v_i(t,\beta,G).$$

Now, inserting $\tilde{G}(t,\beta)$ into (8.20) leads to the estimating function for β:

$$\check{U}(\beta) = \sum_{i=1}^{n} \int_0^\infty \frac{\dot{v}_i(t,\beta,\tilde{G})}{v_i(t,\beta,\tilde{G})}\left(dN_i(t) - Y_i(t)v_i(t,\beta,\tilde{G})d\tilde{G}(t,\beta)\right)$$

$$= \sum_{i=1}^{n} \int_0^\infty \left\{\frac{\dot{v}_i(t,\beta,\tilde{G})}{v_i(t,\beta,\tilde{G})} - \frac{\tilde{S}_1(t,\beta,\tilde{G})}{S_0(t,\beta,\tilde{G})}\right\} dN_i(t), \quad (8.21)$$

where

$$\tilde{S}_1(t,\beta,G) = \frac{\partial}{\partial \beta}S_0(t,\beta,G).$$

We see that (8.16) and (8.21) look very similar, the difference being that the derivatives in (8.21) are computed with $G(t)$ fixed, and then $\tilde{G}$ is inserted into these derivatives. Let $\check{\beta}$ denote the solution to $\check{U}(\beta) = 0$ and let $\check{I}(\beta)$ be the derivative of $\check{U}(\beta)$ with respect to β (which we note in passing is not symmetric). Following the above sketch of proof one may show that $n^{1/2}(\check{\beta} - \beta_0)$ is asymptotically zero-mean normal with covariance matrix that is consistently estimated by

$$\check{I}^{-1}(\check{\beta})\check{\Gamma}\check{I}^{-1}(\check{\beta}),$$

where $\check{\Gamma}$ is a consistent estimator of the asymptotic variance of $\check{U}(\beta_0)$.

We end this section by fitting the proportional odds model to the PBC-data.

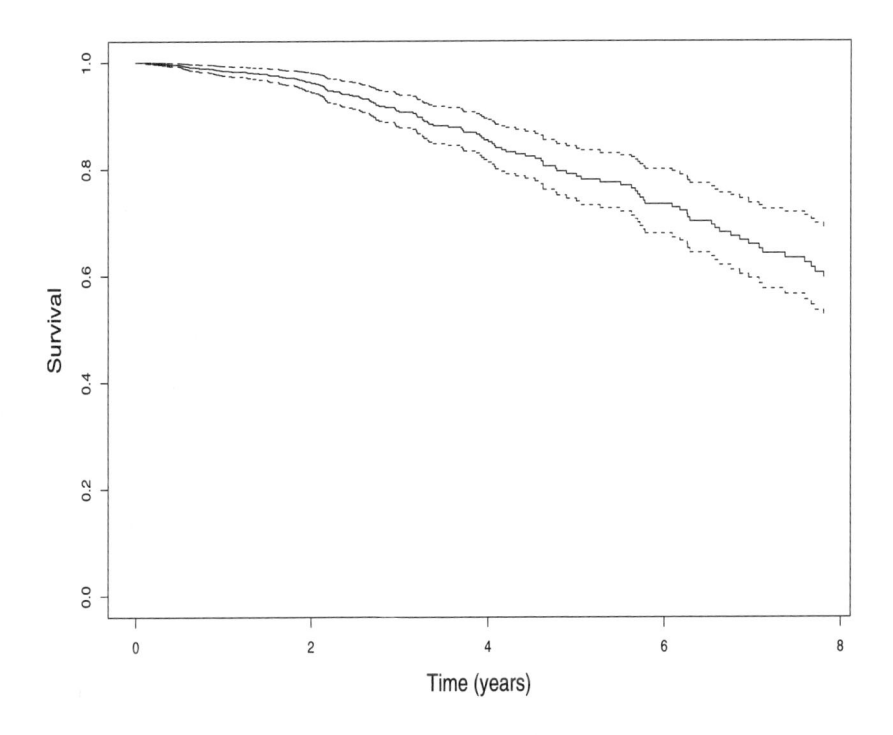

FIGURE 8.1: Estimated survival for proportional odds survival model along with 95% pointwise confidence intervals for subject with average value of all covariates and without edema.

Example 8.2.1 (The PBC data)

We consider the PBC data described in Example 1.1.1, and again wish to study the predictive effect on survival of the following covariates: age, log(albumin), log(bilirubin), edema, log(protime). The proportional odds model (8.14) may be fitted in the `timereg` package using the `prop.odds`-function. The continuous covariates are first centered around their means before fitting the model.

```
> fit<-prop.odds(Surv(time/365,status)~Age+Edema+logBilirubin
+ +logAlbumin+logProtime,pbc,max.time=8)
Proportional odds model
Simulations start N= 500
> summary(fit)
Proportional Odds model

Test for baseline
```

```
Test for non-significant effects
        sup| hat B(t)/SD(t) | p-value H_0: B(t)=0
Baseline                6.74                        0
Test for time-invariant effects
        sup| B(t) - (t/tau)B(tau)| p-value H_0: B(t)=b t
Baseline                0.18                        0.01

Covariate effects
              Coef.      SE  Robust SE  D2log(L)^-1      z   P-val
Age          0.0512  0.0116     0.0124       0.0118   4.41 1.04e-05
Edema        1.2800  0.3570     0.3960       0.3390   3.59 3.31e-04
logBilirubin 1.1200  0.1250     0.1280       0.1250   8.99 0.00e+00
logAlbumin  -2.9500  0.9320     0.9160       0.9250  -3.17 1.53e-03
logProtime   3.9400  1.2600     1.4900       1.3000   3.12 1.78e-03

Test for Goodness-of-fit
             sup| hat U(t) | p-value H_0
Age                  41.100           0.936
Edema                 5.030           0.026
logBilirubin         13.900           0.008
logAlbumin            0.647           0.802
logProtime            1.140           0.038

> S<-1/(1+fit$cum[,2]);
> Su<-1/(1+fit$cum[,2]+1.96*fit$robvar.cum[,2]^.5)
> Sn<-1/(1+fit$cum[,2]-1.96*fit$robvar.cum[,2]^.5)
> plot(fit$cum[,1],S,type="s",ylim=c(0,1),ylab="Survival",
+ xlab="Time (years)")
> lines(fit$cum[,1],Su,lty=2,type="s")
> lines(fit$cum[,1],Sn,lty=2,type="s")
```

The proportional odds effects of the covariates are all significant. We note that the coefficients are somewhat similar to the results of the Cox-model that in this context is equivalent to a cloglog model for the survival, compared to the logit transformation used for the proportional odds model. Patients with edema present, for example, will have an $\exp(1.28) = 3.60$ increased odds compared to patients without edema (keeping everything else fixed).

Figure 8.1 shows the estimated survival functions with 95% pointwise robust confidence intervals for a subject with average values for all covariates and without edema.

The goodness of fit of the proportional odds model is evaluated by considering the score processes $\tilde{U}(\hat{\beta}, t)$ and inspecting their behavior with what should be expected under the model. The above summary and Figure 8.2 (containing the observed score processes and 50 random realizations under the model) suggest that the model does not give a good description

8.2 The semiparametric transformation model

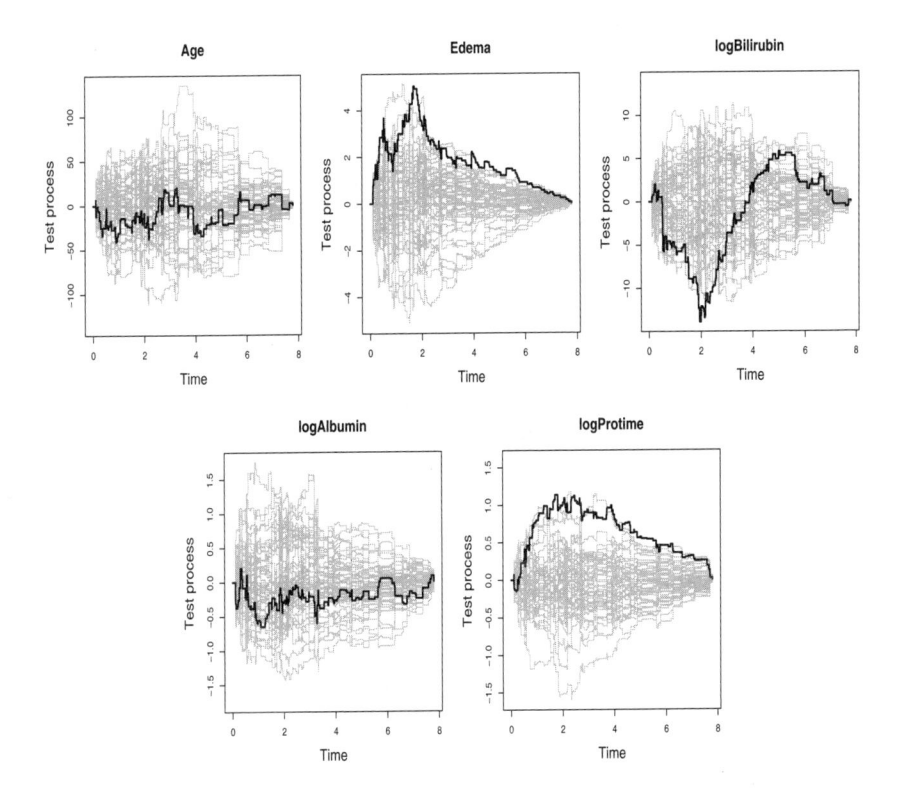

FIGURE 8.2: Score processes, $\tilde{U}(t)$, along with 50 resampled processes under the model.

for edema, log(bilirubin) and log(protime). The plot is obtained by the command

```
> plot(fit,score=1)
```

One way of extending the model is to let the covariates (or some of them) have time-varying effects, which we have studied in detail for the Aalen additive hazards model and the Cox-model. Similar techniques have not yet been developed for the proportional odds model. Recall that the hazard function for the semiparametric proportional odds model is

$$\lambda(t) = \frac{g(t)}{\exp(-Z^T\beta) + G(t)}.$$

One way of extending this model is to allow β to depend on time. We here make an approximation of this by instead letting Z change over time and consider the model

$$\lambda(t) = \frac{g(t)}{\exp(-Z(t)^T \beta) + G(t)}.$$

We here consider the case where edema was allowed to change its effect at time 2 years and again at 4 years (coded with 3 dummy variables Edema02, Edema24, and Edema4).

```
Covariate effects
              Coef.    SE  Robust SE  D2log(L)^-1     z    P-val
Age           0.049  0.012   0.012       0.012     4.083  0.000
Edema02       1.770  0.400   0.409       0.388     2.775  0.006
Edema24       0.415  0.635   0.643       0.622     0.654  0.513
Edema4       -1.338  0.982   1.045       0.941    -1.362  0.173
logBilirubin  1.103  0.123   0.128       0.125     8.967  0.000
logAlbumin   -3.101  0.938   0.911       0.916    -3.305  0.001
logProtime    4.590  1.387   1.513       1.361     3.564  0.000

Test for Goodness-of-fit
             sup| hat U(t) |  p-value H_0
Age              54.776          0.728
Edema02           2.130          0.450
Edema24           0.824          0.816
Edema4            1.046          0.120
logBilirubin     14.574          0.010
logAlbumin        0.449          0.978
logProtime        0.875          0.120
```

We see that presence of edema has a significant effect in an initial phase (first two years) while it seems to be insignificant thereafter. Note also that the model now seems to give a better fit to the data, at least with respect to edema. □

8.3 Exercises

8.1 Consider the accelerated failure time model
$$\log(T) = -Z^T\beta + \varepsilon.$$

(a) Show that T has hazard function
$$\lambda(t) = \lambda_0(t\exp(Z^T\beta))\exp(Z^T\beta),$$
where $\lambda_0(t)$ is the hazard associated with $\exp(\varepsilon)$.

(b) Show that
$$\left(\frac{\lambda_0'(u)u}{\lambda_0(u)}+1\right) = \frac{\lambda_{0\varepsilon}'(\log(u))}{\lambda_{0\varepsilon}(\log(u))},$$
where $\lambda_{0\varepsilon}(t)$ is the hazard function for ε.

(c) Verify the second equality of (8.4).

(d) Show that $U_W(\beta) = U_{\tilde{W}}(\beta)$.

8.2 (Estimating function with Gehan-weight, Jin et al. (2003))

(a) Show that $U_W(\beta)$ given by (8.5) and with $W(t) = G(t) = n^{-1}S_0^*(t,\beta)$, the Gehan-weight, can be written as
$$U_G(\beta) = n^{-1}\sum_{i=1}^{n}\sum_{j=1}^{n}\Delta_i(Z_i - Z_j)I(e_i(\beta) \leq e_j(\beta)),$$
where $e_i(\beta) = \log(\tilde{T}_i) + Z_i^T\beta$ and $\Delta_i I(T_i \leq C_i)$.

(b) Show that $U_G(\beta)$ is the gradient of
$$L_G(\beta) = n^{-1}\sum_{i=1}^{n}\sum_{j=1}^{n}\Delta_i(e_i(\beta) - e_j(\beta))^-,$$
where $a^- = |a|I(a < 0)$, and that $L_G(\beta)$ is a convex function.

8.3 (Extended accelerated failure time model, Chen & Jewell (2001)) Consider the model (8.8)
$$\lambda(t) = \lambda_0(t\exp(Z^T\beta_1))\exp(Z^T\beta_2),$$
and suppose we have n i.i.d. right-censored observations $(\tilde{T}_i, \Delta_i, Z_i)$ from this model. Let $N_i(t) = I(\tilde{T}_i \leq t)\Delta_i$ and $Y(t) = I(t \leq \tilde{T})$.

310   8. Accelerated failure time and transformation models

(a) Argue that a natural estimator of $\Lambda_0(t) = \int_0^t \lambda_0(s)\,ds$ is

$$\hat{\Lambda}_0(t,\beta) = \int_0^t \frac{\sum_{i=1}^n dN_i(u\exp(-\beta_1 Z_i))}{\sum_{i=1}^n Y_i(u\exp(-\beta_1 Z_i))\exp\{(\beta_2-\beta_1)Z_i\}}. \qquad (8.22)$$

(b) Use (8.4) to derive the efficient estimating equations for (β_1,β_2):

$$\sum_{i=1}^n \int_0^\infty W(t,Z_i,\beta)dM_i(t) = 0, \qquad (8.23)$$

where

$$M_i(t) = N_i(t\exp(-\beta_1 Z_i))$$
$$-\int_0^t Y_i(t\exp(-\beta_1 Z_i))\exp\{(\beta_2-\beta_1)Z_i\}d\Lambda_0(t),$$
$$W(t,Z,\beta) = (Z,(\lambda_0'(t)/\lambda_0(t))Z)^T.$$

(c) Use (8.22) to rewrite (8.23) in a form like (8.5).

8.4 (Log-logistic proportional odds model)   Consider the proportional odds model (8.13) so that the baseline survival function (that is all covariate values equal to zero) is assumed to have the structure

$$(1+\exp(\theta)t^\gamma)^{-1},$$

and suppose that the covariate Z is an indicator variable (two groups). We wish to apply this model to a dataset concerning breast cancer reported in Collett (2003). Two groups of women are being compared: women with tumors which were negatively or positively stained with HPA. Positive staining corresponds to a tumor with the potential for metastasis. The data can be found at Dave Collett's homepage: www.personal.rdg.ac.uk.

(a) The appropriateness of the model may be judged by plotting the estimated log-odds (using the Kaplan-Meier estimates) against log(time). Verify this and make the plot for the breast cancer data.

(b) Estimate the parameters of the model for the breast cancer data, and report the estimated odds-ratio along with a 95%-confidence interval comparing the two groups of women (hint: the model may be fitted using the survreg-function in R). Add the straight lines estimates to the plot in (a).

(c) Compare with fit provided by (8.13) without assuming a particular structure of the baseline survival function (use the prop.odds-function).

8.5 (Testing the proportional odds model (Dauxois & Kirmani, 2003))
We shall consider a test for the proportional odds model with Z being an indicator variable. Let $F_j(t)$, $j = 1, 2$ be the two distribution functions of the lifetimes of the two groups, and let $\phi_j(t) = (1 - F_j(t))/F_j(t)$. Under the proportional odds model we have $\phi_2(t) = \theta \phi_1(t)$, which is our null hypothesis. Let

$$\psi_{jk} = \int_{\tau_1}^{\tau_2} k_j(t)\phi_k(t)\,dt, \quad j = 1, 2; k = 1, 2,$$

where τ_1 and τ_2 are some pre-specified timepoints, and k_1 and k_2 are two positive functions such that the ration k_1/k_2 is an increasing function. Let further

$$\gamma(k_1, k_2) = \psi_{11}\psi_{22} - \psi_{12}\psi_{21}.$$

(a) Show that $\gamma(k_1, k_2) = \psi_{11}\psi_{22} - \psi_{12}\psi_{21} = 0$ if and only if the proportional odds model holds.

Let $\tilde{T}_{ij}$, $i = 1, \ldots, n_j$ be independent lifetimes with distribution functions $F_j(t)$, $j = 1, 2$. The lifetime $\tilde{T}_{ij}$ is censored by U_{ij} that are assumed to be i.i.d. and independent of the lifetimes. Put as usual $T_{ij} = \tilde{T}_{ij} \wedge U_{ij}$. Let $\hat{\phi}_j(t)$ be the estimator of $\phi_j(t)$ based on the group specific Kaplan-Meier estimators, and let

$$K_1(t) = \frac{(n_1 + n_2)}{n_1 n_2} \frac{Y_1(t)Y_2(t)}{Y_1(t) + Y_2(t)}, \quad K_2(t) = \frac{Y_1(t)Y_2(t)}{n_1 + n_2}$$

where $Y_j(t) = \sum_i Y_{ij}(t)$ with $Y_{ij}(t) = I(t \le T_{ij})$. Let k_j be the limits in probability of K_j. Finally put

$$\Gamma(K_1, K_2) = \hat{\psi}_{11}\hat{\psi}_{22} - \hat{\psi}_{12}\hat{\psi}_{21},$$

where

$$\hat{\psi}_{kj} = \int_{m_1 \vee \tau_1}^{m_2 \wedge \tau_2} K_j(t)\hat{\phi}_k(t)\,dt$$

with m_1 the largest of the smallest observed lifetimes of the two groups, and m_2 is the smallest of the largest observed lifetimes of the two groups.

(b) Show, under the null and under appropriate conditions, that

$$(n_1 + n_2)^{1/2}(\Gamma(K_1, K_2) - \gamma(k_1, k_2))$$

converges in distribution to a zero mean normal variate U, and derive an expression for $\sigma^2 = \text{Var}(U)$ (hint: Use (4.3) in Chapter 4). Suggest an estimator of σ^2.

(c) Apply the test to the breast cancer data in Exercise (8.4) to investigate whether the proportional odds model is appropriate.

9
Clustered failure time data

In many failure time studies there is a natural clustering of study subjects such that failure times within the same cluster may be correlated. An example is the time to onset of blindness in patients with diabetic retinopathy. Patients were followed over several years and the pair of waiting times to blindness in the left and right eyes, respectively, were observed. In such a study one should expect some correlation between the waiting times within the patients. Here the clustering is due to the patients. The primary interest in this study was to evaluate whether laser treatment could delay onset to blindness. For this purpose one eye of each patient was randomly chosen for laser treatment while the other acted as a control. A second example is given by twin studies. The Danish twin study is analyzed in Hougaard (2000), and here one aim is to study the genetic effect on mortality. This is done by comparing the strength of dependency between the time to death for monozygotic and dizygotic twins, so in this case the focus is on the potential clustering in the data.

For correlated failure time data several issues arise. How should the cluster effect (if present) be modeled? What is the purpose of the study? It may be to compare treatments or to estimate the correlation within clusters, or both! In classical linear models a cluster factor is usually modeled as a random effect. Because of the linear structure of these models, the mean of the response variable is unaltered by adding a random effect. Random effects models also exist for failure time data, where they are denoted frailty models. In these models the random effect (the frailty variable) is typically multiplied on to the intensity function. A convenient mathematical choice of frailty distribution is the gamma distribution, but others exists.

In frailty models, covariate effects are typically specified *conditionally* on the value of the frailty variable, and one could therefore term them conditional models. One should note that the observed intensity will typically be different from the conditional intensity. Thus, a conditional Cox model is for instance only preserved with respect to the observed history in the special case where the multiplicative frailty variable has a positive stable distribution. Frailty models may be used to model different cluster structures and will lead to estimates of subject specific regression effects, that is a comparison of the failure times *within* clusters. They can also provide estimates of random effect parameters describing the correlation between failure times from the same cluster. Frailty models have received a lot of attention in the nineties and are described in detail in Hougaard (2000).

If interest centers on comparing the failure times of individuals *across* clusters it is simpler and more direct to apply so-called *marginal models*, where the covariate effects are specified unconditionally. In fact, for these models, the cluster structure is often ignored when estimating the covariate effects and is only used to derive valid estimates of standard errors to ensure correct inference. This approach is closely linked to the GEE methodology (Liang & Zeger, 1986) and has mostly been considered in the context of proportional (marginal) hazards models. Lee et al. (1992) considered the marginal Cox model and Wei et al. (1989) the marginal stratified Cox model. A detailed asymptotic analysis for these models formulated in a general setting were given by Spiekerman & Lin (1998). Marginal models may be used to estimate marginal regression effects and but also the correlation within clusters. We return to this in Section 9.1.2.

In this chapter we focus almost solely on marginal models and outline how the dynamic models we have considered so far can be extended to a cluster setting. We show how the dynamic additive regression models can be most of the models models presented The marginal models are further easy to use in practice because existing software only needs simple modifications to do correct estimation and inference. Frailty models are only briefly discussed at the end of this chapter; we refer to Hougaard (2000) for a thorough account.

9.1 Marginal regression models for clustered failure time data

The marginal regression models approach for clustered failure time data is well suited for the situation where one aims at estimating regression effects on the population level, and only have to deal with correlation to get correct estimates of the standard errors for the regression effects. In Section 9.1.2 we extend the marginal model approach to also provide estimates of the correlation within clusters.

9.1.1 Working independence assumption

In what follows we describe the so-called working independence assumption approach for marginal proportional hazards models for right-censored survival data. For $k = 1, \ldots, K$, $i = 1, \ldots, n$, let $\tilde{T}_{ik}$ and C_{ik} be the failure and censoring times for the ith individual in the kth cluster and let $X_{ik}(t)$ be a p-vector of covariates. Put

$$\tilde{T}_k = (\tilde{T}_{1k}, \ldots, \tilde{T}_{nk}),\ C_k = (C_{1k}, \ldots, C_{nk}),\ X_k(t) = (X_{1k}(t), \ldots, X_{nk}(t)).$$

We assume that $(\tilde{T}_k, C_k, X_k(\cdot))$, $k = 1, \ldots, K$ are independent and identically distributed variables and these variables follow the model described in the following. The right-censored failure time is denoted $T_{ik} = \tilde{T}_{ik} \wedge C_{ik}$ and as usual we let $Y_{ik}(t) = 1(T_{ik} \geq t)$ and $N_{ik}(t) = 1(T_{ik} \leq t, T_{ik} = \tilde{T}_{ik})$ denote the individual at risk process and counting process, respectively. A marginal model is a model for the intensity of $N_{ik}(t)$ with respect to the marginal filtration

$$\mathcal{F}_t^{ik} = \sigma\{N_{ik}(s), Y_{ik}(s), X_{ik}(s) : 0 \leq s \leq t\}, \tag{9.1}$$

which records information generated by observing the ikth individual only. Such a model could for instance be the Cox model:

$$\lambda_{ik}^{\mathcal{F}_t^{ik}}(t) = Y_{ik}(t)\lambda_0(t)\exp\left(X_{ik}^T(t)\beta\right). \tag{9.2}$$

It is important to note that (9.2) is not the intensity with respect to the observed filtration

$$\mathcal{F}_t = \bigvee_k \mathcal{F}_t^k, \tag{9.3}$$

where

$$\mathcal{F}_t^k = \sigma\{N_{ik}(s), Y_{ik}(s), X_{ik}(s) : i = 1, \cdots n,\ 0 \leq s \leq t\}$$

is the information generated by observing all the individuals in the kth cluster. This limits the scope of martingale calculus. It is, however, still possible to estimate and perform inference about the regression parameter β.

In the following, inference and estimation for (9.2) is reviewed. Had there been independence between subjects within clusters then, to estimate β, we should use the usual Cox-score,

$$U(\beta) = \sum_{k=1}^K \sum_{i=1}^n \int_0^\tau \left(X_{ik}(t) - E^1(t, \beta)\right) dN_{ik}(t),$$

where τ denotes end of observation period, and

$$E^1(t, \beta) = \frac{S_1^1(t, \beta)}{S_0^1(t, \beta)}$$

with

$$S_j^1(t,\beta) = \sum_{k=1}^{K}\sum_{i=1}^{n} Y_{ik}(t) X_{ik}^j(t) \exp\left(X_{ik}^T(t)\beta\right),$$

for $j = 0,1$. In the case of independence $U(\beta_0)$, where β_0 denotes the true parameter, is a martingale and asymptotics may be derived using the central limit theorem for martingales as described in Section 6.1. The so-called working independence estimator of β_0 is $\hat{\beta}_I$ that solves $U(\hat{\beta}_I) = 0$. This will lead to a consistent estimator of β_0, but $U(\beta_0)$ is no longer a martingale and minus the derivative of $U(\beta)$, denoted as $I(\beta)$, cannot be used as tool to estimate the standard errors. However, valid estimated standard errors are easily derived exploiting the independence across clusters by establishing and i.i.d. representation for clusters. Under standard regularity assumptions one may write

$$U(\beta_0) = U(\tau,\beta_0) = \sum_{k=1}^{K}\sum_{i=1}^{n}\int_0^\tau (X_{ik}(t) - e^1(t,\beta_0)) dM_{ik}^1(t) + o_p(K^{1/2})$$

$$= \sum_{k=1}^{K} \epsilon_{1k} + o_p(K^{1/2}), \qquad (9.4)$$

where

$$\epsilon_{1k} = \epsilon_{1k}(\tau) = \sum_{i=1}^{n}\int_0^\tau (X_{ik}(t) - e^1(t,\beta_0)) dM_{ik}^1(t),$$

$e^1(t,\beta_0)$ is the limit in probability of $E^1(t,\beta_0)$, and

$$M_{ik}^1(t) = N_{ik}(t) - \int_0^t \lambda_{ik}^{F^{ik}}(s)\,ds$$

denotes the marginal martingales. The above (9.4) gives the required sum of n i.i.d. random vectors with zero mean. It follows from the multivariate central limit theorem that $K^{-1/2}U(\beta_0)$ is asymptotical normal with zero-mean and covariance matrix $B = E(\epsilon_{1k}\epsilon_{1k}^T)$. By a Taylor series expansion one further gets

$$K^{1/2}(\hat{\beta}_I - \beta_0) = \left(K^{-1}I(\beta^*)\right)^{-1}K^{-1/2}U(\beta_0),$$

where β^* is on the line segment between $\hat{\beta}_I$ and β_0. Since $K^{-1}I(\beta^*)$ converges in probability towards a matrix A, say, $K^{1/2}(\hat{\beta}_I - \beta_0)$ is asymptotically normal with zero-mean and covariance matrix $A^{-1}BA^{-1}$. The covariance matrix is estimated consistently by $\hat{A}^{-1}\hat{B}\hat{A}^{-1}$, where

$$\hat{A} = K^{-1}I(\hat{\beta}_I), \quad \hat{B} = K^{-1}\sum_{k=1}^{K}\hat{\epsilon}_{1k}\hat{\epsilon}_{1k}^T,$$

with

$$\hat{\epsilon}_{1k} = \sum_{i=1}^{n} \int_0^\tau (X_{ik}(t) - E^1(t, \hat{\beta}_I))d\hat{M}_{ik}^1(t),$$

that is based on the subject specific residuals

$$\hat{M}_{ik}^1(t) = N_{ik}(t) - \int_0^t Y_{ik}(t) \exp(\hat{\beta}_I^T X_{ik}(t))d\hat{\Lambda}_{0I}(t, \hat{\beta}_I).$$

In the latter display

$$\hat{\Lambda}_{0I}(t, \beta) = \int_0^t \frac{1}{S_0^1(s, \beta)} dN_{..}(s)$$

denotes the usual (independence) Breslow estimator of the cumulative hazard function $\Lambda_0(t) = \int_0^t \lambda_0(s)ds$. One may furthermore show that

$$K^{1/2}(\hat{\Lambda}_{0I}(t, \hat{\beta}_I) - \Lambda_0(t))$$

converges in distribution to a zero-mean Gaussian process with covariance function $E(\Phi_k(t)^2)$, where

$$\Phi_k(t) = \int_0^t \frac{dM^1_{.k}(s, \beta_0, \Lambda_0)}{s_0^1(s, \beta_0)} - \left(\int_0^t e^1(s, \beta_0)d\Lambda_0(s)\right)^T A^{-1}\epsilon_{1k} \quad (9.5)$$

with $s_0^1(t, \beta_0)$ being the limit in probability of $K^{-1}S_0^1(t, \beta_0)$. The covariance function is consistently estimated by

$$K^{-1} \sum_{k=1}^{K} \hat{\Phi}_k(t)\hat{\Phi}_k(t)^T,$$

where

$$\hat{\Phi}_k(t) = \int_0^t \frac{d\hat{M}^1_{.k}(s, \hat{\beta}_I, \hat{\Lambda}_{0I})}{\frac{1}{K}S_0^1(s, \hat{\beta}_I)} - \left(\int_0^t E^1(s, \hat{\beta}_I)d\hat{\Lambda}_{0I}(s)\right)^T \hat{A}^{-1}\hat{\epsilon}_{1k}. \quad (9.6)$$

Example 9.1.1 (Diabetic retinopathy data)

The purpose of the Diabetic Retinopathy Study was to assess the efficacy of laser photocoagulation treatment in delaying onset of blindness in patients with diabetic retinopathy. In the following we use the subset of 197 patients defined in Huster et al. (1989). One eye of each patient was randomly selected for treatment while the other eye was observed without treatment. The patients were then followed over several years for observation of blindness in the left and right eyes. Besides the treatment variable we also use the explanatory variable `adult` indicating if age at diagnosis of diabetes is above 20 years.

```
> fit<-coxph(Surv(time,status)~adult*trt+cluster(id),
     data=diabetes)
> fit
Call:
coxph(formula = Surv(time, status) ~ adult * trt + cluster(id),
    data = diabetes)

            coef exp(coef) se(coef) robust se      z       p
adult      0.341    1.407    0.199    0.196    1.74  0.0810
trt       -0.425    0.654    0.218    0.185   -2.30  0.0220
adult:trt -0.846    0.429    0.351    0.304   -2.79  0.0053
```

The marginal Cox model analysis is easily carried out in R using coxph with the cluster option. In the present example id is the variable keeping track of the patients. The estimated coefficients and the se(coef) are the same as those obtained if we had run coxph without the cluster option that is assuming independence. The reported so-called robust standard errors are the proper standard errors derived above taking into account that observations within clusters (patients) cannot be taken as independent. Notice that the robust standard errors are smaller in this case than the naive estimates, which is to be expected due to the design of the study with one treated and one un-treated eye for each patient. The treatment appears to be effective with a more pronounced effect for adult onset diabetes than for juvenile diabetes. □

We can do goodness-of-fit testing for the marginal Cox-regression as outlined in the previous chapters, see for example Section 6.2. Let us describe how this proceed focusing on the score process, which among other goodness-of-fit tools were also considered by Spiekerman & Lin (1996). The idea is, just as for the regular Cox model, to derive the asymptotic distribution of the process

$$K^{-1/2}U(t,\hat{\beta}_I),$$

and see whether the it behaves as it should under the assumed model. In the following example we also consider other cumulative sums of residuals that are aimed at validating whether the functional form of the covariates is misspecified and if there are different time-interaction with the level of the covariates.

A Taylor series expansion of $U(t,\hat{\beta}_I)$ around β_0 gives

$$K^{-1/2}U(t,\hat{\beta}_I) = K^{-1/2}U(t,\beta_0) - (K^{-1}I(t,\beta^*))K^{1/2}(\hat{\beta}_I - \beta_0),$$

where $I(t,\beta)$ is the derivative $U(t,\beta)$ with respect to β, and β^* is on the line segment between $\hat{\beta}_I$ and β_0. The right-hand side of the last display can be decomposed into i.i.d. terms,

$$K^{-1/2}U(t,\hat{\beta}_I) = K^{-1/2}\sum_{k=1}^{K}\hat{\epsilon}_{2k}(t) + o_p(1),$$

where
$$\epsilon_{2k}(t) = \epsilon_{1k}(t) - I(t,\beta)I(\tau,\beta)^{-1}\epsilon_{1k}(\tau)$$
and $\hat{\epsilon}_{2k}(t)$ is obtained from $\epsilon_{2k}(t)$ by replacing $e^1(t,\beta)$ with $E^1(t,\beta)$ in the expression for $\epsilon_{1k}(t)$ and also inserting the working independence estimators for β and $\Lambda_0(t)$. One may also show that the limit distribution $W(t)$ of $K^{-1/2}U(t,\hat{\beta}_I)$ may be approximated by generating i.i.d. copies of

$$\hat{W}(t) = K^{-1/2}\sum_{k=1}^{K}\hat{\epsilon}_{2k}(t)G_k,$$

where $G_1,\ldots,G_K$ are independent standard normals. Therefore, we can make a graphical inspection to evaluate if the observed patterns of the co-ordinate processes of $K^{-1/2}U(t,\hat{\beta}_I)$ are consistent with the behavior under the assumed model. We may further approximate the p-value of e.g. the supremum test for the jth coordinate

$$\sup_{t \leq \tau}|K^{-1/2}U_j(t,\hat{\beta}_I)| \tag{9.7}$$

by generating a suitable number of $\sup_{t \leq \tau}|\hat{W}_j(t)|$ to see whether (9.7) is extreme in this distribution.

Example 9.1.2 (Diabetic retinopathy data, continued)

We now check the goodness-of-fit of the marginal Cox model for the Diabetic retinopathy data considered in Example 9.1.1. First we fit the model using the cox.aalen function specifying the cluster structure by setting the cluster variable.

```
> adult.treat<-(diabetes$adult==2)*(diabetes$treat)
> fit<-cox.aalen(Surv(time,status) ~prop(adult)+prop(treat)
+ +prop(adult.treat),diabetes,cluster=diabetes$id,residuals=1)
Cox-Aalen Survival Model
Simulations start N= 500
> summary(fit)
Cox-Aalen Model

Test for Aalen terms
Test for non-significant effects
            sup| hat B(t)/SD(t) |  p-value H_0: B(t)=0
(Intercept)               3.2                    0.012
Test for time-invariant effects
            sup| B(t) - (t/tau)B(tau)|  p-value H_0: B(t)=b t
(Intercept)              0.089                           0.066

Proportional Cox terms :
            Coef.    SE Robust SE D2log(L)^-1     z  P-val
```

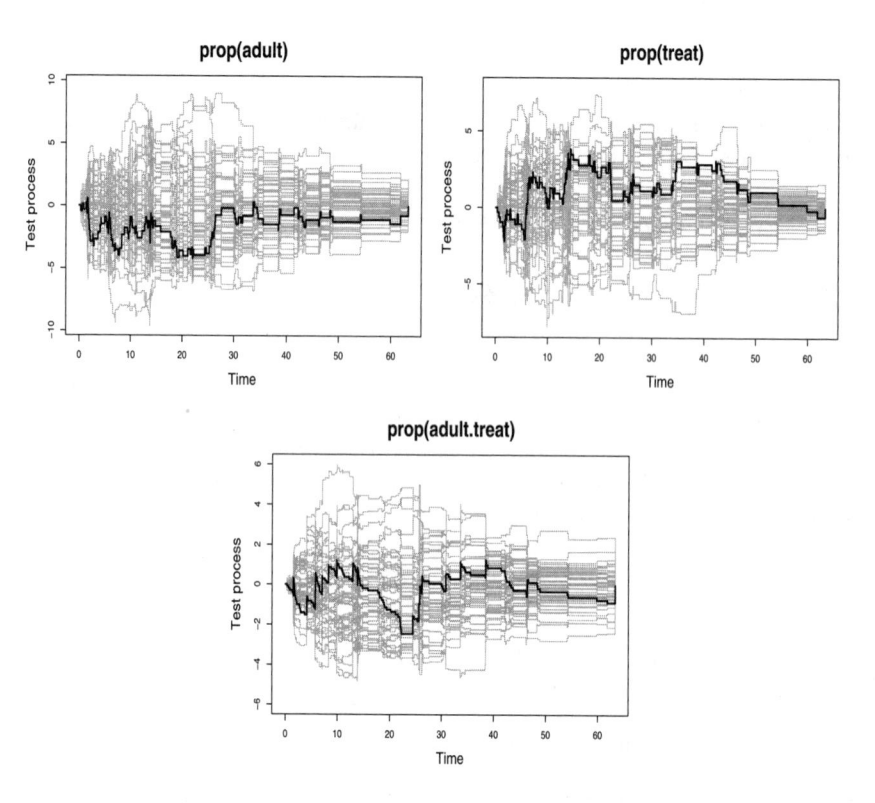

FIGURE 9.1: Diabetic retinopathy data. Cumulative residuals with 50 simulated processes under the model.

```
prop(adult)          0.341 0.199    0.196    0.199  1.71 0.0866
prop(treat)         -0.425 0.217    0.185    0.218 -1.96 0.0505
prop(adult.treat)   -0.846 0.350    0.304    0.351 -2.42 0.0156

Test for Proportionality
                    sup| hat U(t) | p-value H_0
prop(adult)                  4.15         0.696
prop(treat)                  3.80         0.694
prop(adult.treat)            2.45         0.684

> plot(fit,score=2)
```

The output concerning the regression effect differs slightly with the one from the coxph function, which is due to different handling of ties. The output from the cox.aalen function contains the score processes and these are plotted with 50 simulated processes under the model, see Figure 9.1. This indicates that the effects of the covariates are not time-varying and

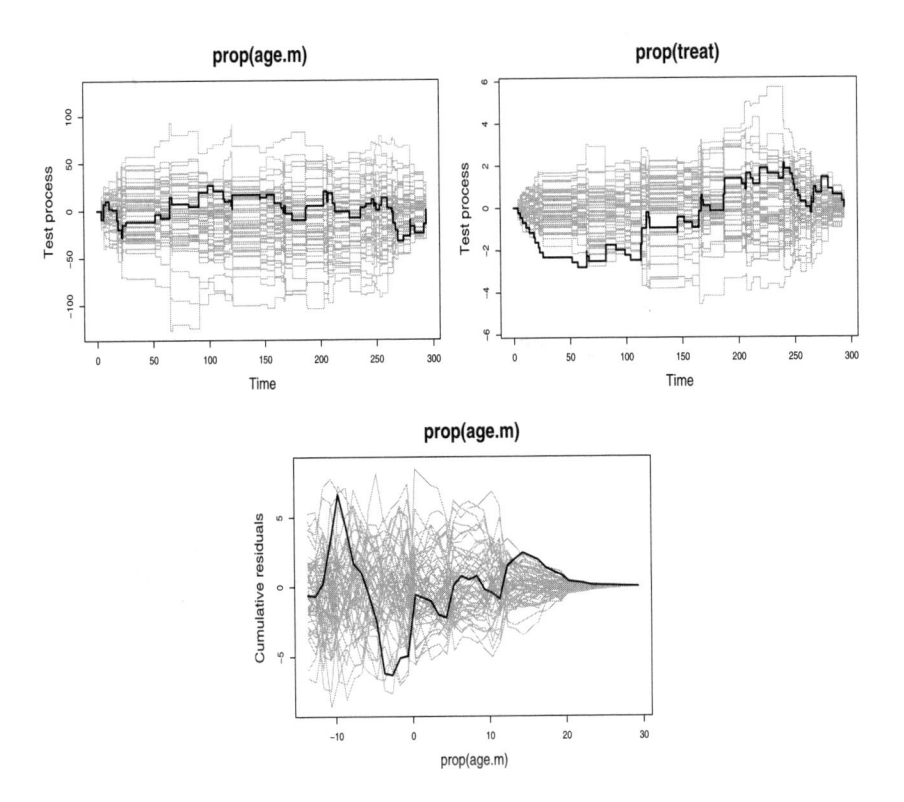

FIGURE 9.2: CGD-data. Cumulative residuals with 50 simulated processes under the model.

that the model seems to fit well, which is also supported by the above reported tests. □

We also illustrate that the residuals in the clustered case may be accumulated versus the continuous covariates to validate the functional form of the covariates.

Example 9.1.3 (CGD-data)

The CGD data are multiple infection data given in Fleming & Harrington (1991). CGD is a disorder characterized by recurrent pyogenic infections. The study was conducted to evaluate a treatment with gamma interferon. Data were collected between 1988 and 1989 and comprised of 128 patients, 63 of these patients received treatment and 65 were placebo treated. In the treatment group 14 patients had more than one event and in the placebo group 30 patients had more than one event. We restrict attention to the first 300 days of follow-up time. and start by considering a simple Cox model with age and treatment as explanatory variables.

9. Clustered failure time data

```
> age.m<-cgd2$age-mean(cgd2$age)
> fit<-cox.aalen(Surv(time,status) ~prop(age.m)+prop(treat),
+ cgd2,cluster=cgd2$id,residuals=1,max.time=300)
Cox-Aalen Survival Model
Simulations start N= 500
> summary(fit)
Cox-Aalen Model

Test for Aalen terms
Test for non-significant effects
            sup| hat B(t)/SD(t) | p-value H_0: B(t)=0
(Intercept)              4.98                       0
Test for time-invariant effects
            sup| B(t) - (t/tau)B(tau)| p-value H_0: B(t)=b t
(Intercept)                    0.0275                  0.062

Proportional Cox terms :
              Coef.     SE Robust SE  D2log(L)^-1       z    P-val
prop(age.m) -0.0337 0.0139    0.0169       0.0143   -2.42 1.53e-02
prop(treat) -1.1900 0.2910    0.3400       0.2890   -4.10 4.05e-05

Test for Proportionality
              sup| hat U(t) | p-value H_0
prop(age.m)           34.50          0.880
prop(treat)            3.04          0.336

> resid.fit<-cum.residuals(fit,cgd2,cum.resid=1)
> plot(resid.fit,score=2)
```

The score processes along with 50 simulated processes under the model are shown in Figure 9.2 upper panel. These indicate that the effects of the covariates are not time-varying and that the model seems to fit reasonably well. Treatment appears, however, to have an effect that is not completely consistent with the proportional hazard assumption, the effect being stronger in the beginning and the end of the period; we describe this in further detail below. Figure 9.2 lower panel shows the residuals cumulated over time and plotted versus the covariate age indicating that the functional representation of age appears to be consistent with the model. The treatment effect, although not significant by the supremum test statistic, shows some time-varying nature. We therefore also fit a stratified proportional hazards model that is a Cox-Aalen survival model.

```
> fit<-cox.aalen(Surv(time,status) ~prop(age.m)+treat,cgd2,
+ cluster=cgd2$id,residuals=1,max.time=300)
Cox-Aalen Survival Model
Simulations start N= 500
> summary(fit)
```

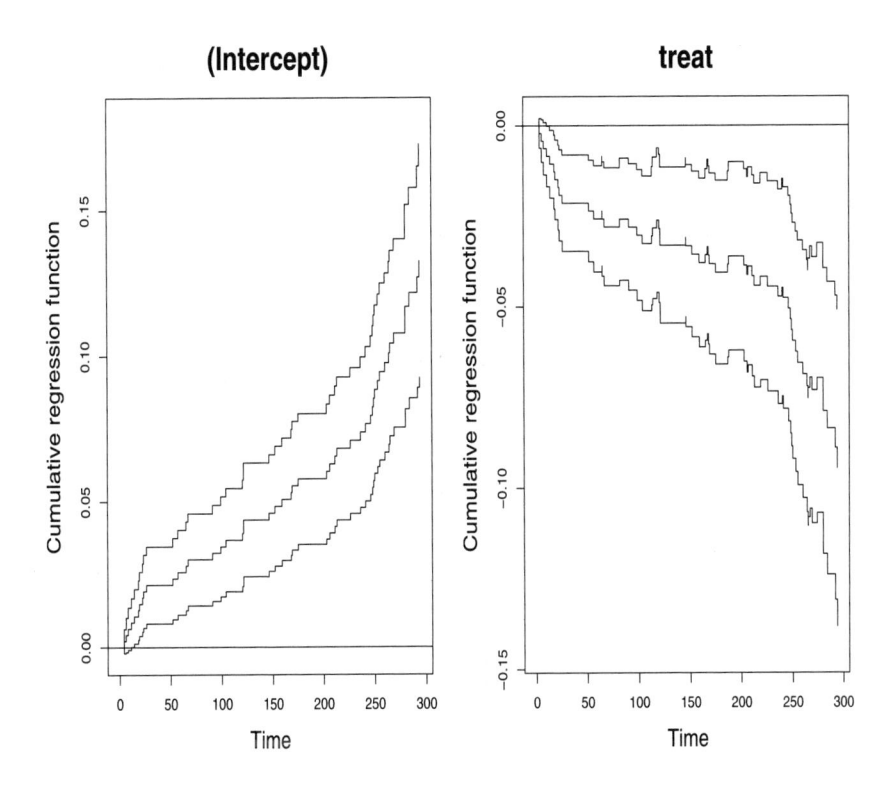

9.1 Marginal regression models for clustered failure time data   323

FIGURE 9.3: CGD-data. Cumulative baseline for placebo and cumulative effect of treatment with 95 % pointwise confidence intervals.

```
Cox-Aalen Model

Test for Aalen terms
Test for non-significant effects
            sup| hat B(t)/SD(t) | p-value H_0: B(t)=0
(Intercept)            5.03                 0.000
treat                  3.37                 0.006
Test for time-invariant effects
            sup| B(t) - (t/tau)B(tau)| p-value H_0: B(t)=b t
(Intercept)            0.0347               0.030
treat                  0.0326               0.058

Proportional Cox terms :
            Coef.    SE Robust SE D2log(L)^-1      z   P-val
prop(age.m) -0.0338 0.0138   0.0168    0.0142  -2.45  0.0145

Test for Proportionality
            sup| hat U(t) | p-value H_0
prop(age.m)         32.6         0.892
```

Figure 9.3 shows the cumulative baseline function for a placebo treated patient and the effect of treatment. The latter suggests a somewhat more pronounced effect of treatment in the first and last part of the time-period being borderline significant (on the additive scale). Note, however, that this test for constant additive effect (constant excess risk) is not equivalent to the test for constant multiplicative effect. □

We finish this section by looking at the marginal additive intensity model. Instead of the Cox model we assume the Aalen additive model for the marginal intensities,

$$\lambda_{ik}^{\mathcal{F}^{ik}}(t) = Y_{ik}(t) X_{ik}^T(t) \beta(t), \qquad (9.8)$$

where $\beta(t)$ is a p-vector of unknown regression functions. A possible intercept term is absorbed into the covariate vector. Let

$$N_k(t) = (N_{1k}(t), \ldots, N_{nk}(t))^T$$

and let $\tilde{X}_k(t)$ be the $n \times p$-matrix with ith row

$$(Y_{ik}(t) X_{ik1}(t), \ldots, Y_{ik}(t) X_{ikp}(t)).$$

Define also ·

$$M_k(t) = N_k(t) - \int_0^t \tilde{X}_k(s) dB(s),$$

where $B(t) = \int_0^t \beta(s)\, ds$ denotes the cumulative coefficients. The ith component of $M_k(t)$, $M_{ik}(t)$ is a (local square integrable) martingale with respect to $\mathcal{F}_t^{ik}$, but $M_k(t)$ is not a martingale with respect to the observed filtration. The (unweighted) working independence estimator of $B(t)$ is

$$\hat{B}(t) = \sum_{k=1}^K \int_0^t [\sum_{k=1}^K \tilde{X}_k^T(s)\tilde{X}_k(s)]^{-1} \tilde{X}_k^T(s) dN_k(s)$$

assuming that the inverses exists. We have that (except for lower order terms)

$$K^{1/2}(\hat{B}(t) - B(t)) = K^{-1/2} \sum_{k=1}^K \int_0^t [K^{-1} \sum_{k=1}^K \tilde{X}_k^T(s)\tilde{X}_k(s)]^{-1} \tilde{X}_k^T(s) dM_k(s)$$

$$= K^{-1/2} \sum_{k=1}^K \epsilon_k(t) \qquad (9.9)$$

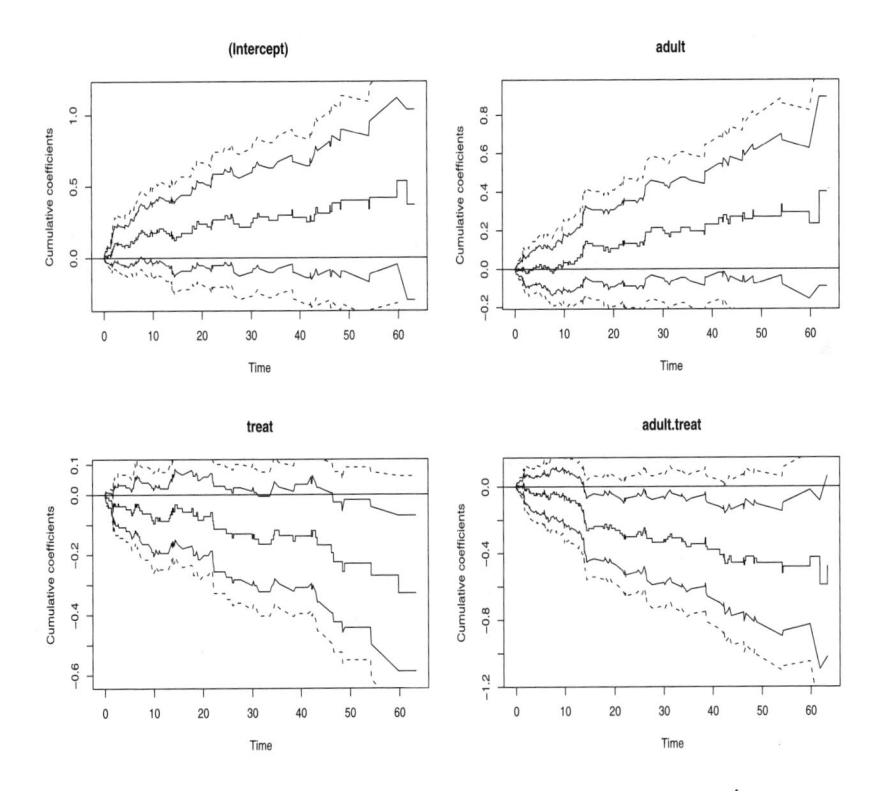

FIGURE 9.4: Diabetes-data. Cumulative regression estimators along with 95% confidence intervals (full lines) and uniform bands (broken lines).

which is essentially a sum of i.i.d. components (replace $K^{-1} \sum_{k=1}^{K} \tilde{X}_k^T(t)\tilde{X}_k(t)$ by its limit in probability). One may also show that (9.9) has the same limit distribution as

$$K^{-1/2} \sum_{k=1}^{K} \hat{\epsilon}_k(t) G_k, \qquad (9.10)$$

where

$$\hat{\epsilon}_k(t) = K^{-1/2} \sum_{k=1}^{K} \int_0^t [K^{-1} \sum_{k=1}^{K} \tilde{X}_k^T(s)\tilde{X}_k(s)]^{-1} \tilde{X}_k^T(s) d\hat{M}_k(s)$$

with

$$\hat{M}_k(t) = N_k(t) - \int_0^t \tilde{X}_k(s) d\hat{B}(s)$$

and $G_1, \ldots G_K$ are independent standard normals. The asymptotic covari-

326   9. Clustered failure time data

ance matrix of $K^{1/2}(\hat{B}(t) - B(t))$ is estimated consistently by

$$K^{-1} \sum_{k=1}^{K} \hat{\epsilon}_k^{\otimes 2}(t)$$

and the representation (9.10) may be used to construct uniform confidence bands. One may derive similar results for the semiparametric version of the marginal additive intensity model, see Exercise 9.1 for a special case. The marginal additive model may be fitted using the cluster-option in the aalen-function. Consider the Diabetic Retinopathy data as an illustration.

Example 9.1.4 (Diabetic retinopathy data. Additive model.)

We wish to fit the marginal additive model to this data using the covariates treatment and the variable adult and the interaction between these two. This model poses no restrictions on the marginal intensities.

```
> adult.treat<-(diabetes$adult==2)*(diabetes$treat)
> fit<-aalen(Surv(time,status) ~adult+treat+adult.treat,
     diabetes,cluster=diabetes$id)
> plot(fit)
> summary(fit)
Additive Aalen Model

Test for nonparametric terms

Test for non-significant effects
            sup| hat B(t)/SD(t) |  p-value H_0: B(t)=0
(Intercept)            2.09                  0.387
adult                  1.86                  0.534
treat                  2.49                  0.180
adult.treat            2.99                  0.057
Test for time invariant effects
            sup| B(t) - (t/tau)B(tau)|  p-value H_0: B(t)=b t
(Intercept)            0.187                 0.791
adult                  0.144                 0.765
treat                  0.101                 0.553
adult.treat            0.154                 0.809

            int (B(t)-(t/tau)B(tau))^2dt  p-value H_0: B(t)=b t
(Intercept)            0.5970                0.669
adult                  0.1610                0.904
treat                  0.0849                0.713
adult.treat            0.4330                0.658
```

We see from Figure 9.4 and from the output that all effects seem to be time-invariant, and that the interaction term is borderline significant. If we fit the model with the effect of the interaction term being constant, we get the following estimate with estimated standard errors:

Parametric terms :

	Coef.	SE	Robust SE	z	P-val
const(adult.treat)	-0.00942	0.00392	0.0034	-2.403	0.0162

giving a p-value of 0.0162. □

9.1.2 Two-stage estimation of correlation

The marginal analysis described in the previous section gives correct inferences, provided of course that the assumed marginal model holds, and will in many cases provide a good starting point when one is dealing with clustered failure time data and is interested in estimating regression effects (on the population level). Sometimes, however, there is also interest in quantifying the correlation structure present in data, which may also be exploited to give a more efficient analysis. Some methods have been suggested to improve on efficiency for the marginal proportional hazards model. Cai & Prentice (1997) suggested an approach similar to the GEE-methodology, that is, they introduce weights into the standard Cox partial score function. Their approach only assumes the marginal Cox model, which is appealing, but the efficiency gain appears to be modest as is also concluded by Cai & Prentice (1995). More importantly perhaps is that the marginal Cox-analysis only provides estimates and inference for the regression parameters (and the cumulative baseline hazard function). Thus if the potential correlation present in data is of interest then one needs another methodology. Frailty models, which we return to in Section 9.2, is one such option. As mentioned previously, these models specify regression effects conditionally on random effects. In this section we continue to model regression effects on the marginals, however, and then either estimate the correlation in a two-step procedure or build a model that contains correlation as well as marginal regression parameters.

One approach to this is the so-called *copula models* (Genest & MacKay, 1986) that for the failure times within a cluster $(\tilde{T}_1, \ldots, \tilde{T}_n)$, say, assume that the joint survival function is given by

$$P(\tilde{T}_1 > t_1, \ldots, \tilde{T}_n > t_n) = C_\theta(S_1(t_1), \ldots, S_n(t_n)),$$

where S_j, $j = 1, \ldots, n$, denotes the marginal survivor functions that may be specified conditionally on covariates. The copula C_θ is a n dimensional survival function with uniform margins and θ is a parameter (possibly a vector). The vector $(\tilde{T}_1, \ldots, \tilde{T}_n)$ is said to come from the C_θ copula. Different C_θ's give different joint distribution but the marginals are unaltered. A special class of copulas is the Archimedean copula model family, where the copulas are on the form

$$C_\theta(u_1, \ldots, u_n) = \phi_\theta(\phi_\theta^{-1}(u_1) + \cdots + \phi_\theta^{-1}(u_n))$$

for some non-negative convex decreasing function ϕ_θ with $\phi_\theta(0) = 1$. Multiplicative random effects models, as for instance the Clayton-Oakes model (Clayton, 1978; Oakes, 1982), constitute an important subclass of copula models, see Exercise 9.2. Estimation in copula models is usually carried out using a two-stage method. The marginal parameters are first estimated using the working independence estimators. In the second stage these estimators are plugged into the likelihood for the dependence parameter(s). Genest & MacKay (1995) and Shih & Louis (1995) used this approach in the situation without covariates and Glidden (2000) generalized the approach to the Clayton-Oakes model with covariates while Andersen (2005) considered general copula models with covariates.

Below we describe the two-stage method for the Clayton-Oakes model with marginal hazards on Cox form. We use the notation introduced in Section 9.1.1. In addition we assume the presence of some (unobserved) random effects V_k, $k = 1, \ldots, K$ in such a way that $(\tilde{T}_k, C_k, X_k(\cdot), V_k)$, $k = 1, \cdots, K$ are i.i.d. variables. Censoring, conditional on V_k and covariates, is assumed to be independent and noninformative on V_k. We also assume that $\tilde{T}_{ik}$, $i = 1, \cdots, n$, are independent variables given $V_k, X_1(\cdot), \cdots, X_n(\cdot)$, and that V_k is a Gamma distributed variate with mean 1 and variance θ^{-1}. Let $T_{ik} = \tilde{T}_{ik} \wedge C_{ik}$, $Y_{ik}(t) = 1(T_{ik} \geq t)$ and $N_{ik}(t) = 1(T_{ik} \leq t, T_{ik} = \tilde{T}_{ik})$ denote the observed failure time, the individual at risk process and the counting process for the ikth individual, respectively. The model is specified by making the assumption that the intensity with respect to the (unobserved) filtration

$$\mathcal{H}_t = \bigvee_k \mathcal{H}_t^k, \qquad (9.11)$$

where

$$\mathcal{H}_t^k = \sigma\{N_{ik}(s), Y_{ik}(s), X_{ik}(s), V_k : i = 1, \cdots n, 0 \leq s \leq t\},$$

is

$$\lambda_{ik}^{\mathcal{H}}(t) = V_k \lambda_{ik}^*(t, \theta, \lambda_0(\cdot)), \qquad (9.12)$$

referred to as the Clayton-Oakes model, and so that the marginal intensities are on Cox form

$$\lambda_{ik}^{\mathcal{F}^{ik}}(t) = Y_{ik}(t)\lambda_0(t) \exp\left(X_{ik}^T(t)\beta\right), \qquad (9.13)$$

where $\mathcal{F}^{ik}$ refers to the marginal filtration, see (9.1). One may then show that the conditional intensity function λ_{ik}^* is

$$\lambda_{ik}^*(t, \theta, \lambda_0(\cdot)) = Y_{ik}(t)\lambda_0(t) \exp(X_{ik}^T(t)\beta)$$
$$\exp(\theta^{-1} \int_0^t \exp(X_{ik}^T(s)\beta^T)\lambda_0(s)ds),$$

9.1 Marginal regression models for clustered failure time data

see Exercise 9.3. It is of interest to find the intensities with respect to the observed filtration $\mathcal{F}_t$ given in (9.3). It can be shown, see Exercise 9.3, that these are

$$\lambda_{ik}^{\mathcal{F}}(t) = Y_{ik}(t)\lambda_0(t)\exp(X_{ik}^T(t)\beta)f_{ik}(t), \qquad (9.14)$$

where

$$f_{ik}(t) = \left(\frac{\theta + N_{\cdot k}(t-)}{\theta}\right)\left(\frac{\exp(\theta^{-1}\int_0^t \lambda_0(s)\exp(X_{ik}^T(s)\beta)ds)}{f_k(t)}\right),$$

$$f_k(t) = 1 + \sum_{j=1}^n (\exp(\theta^{-1}\int_0^{t-} Y_{jk}(s)\lambda_0(s)\exp(X_{jk}^T(s)\beta)ds) - 1).$$

The principle in the two-stage method is to estimate the marginal parameters using the working independence estimators $\hat\beta_I$ and $\hat\Lambda_{0I}(t)$, and then maximize the observed likelihood with respect to the correlation parameter θ replacing β and Λ_0 by their working independence estimators. The observed (partial) log-likelihood function is

$$\sum_{k=1}^K \int_0^\tau \log\left(1 + \frac{N_{\cdot k}(t-)}{\theta}\right)dN_{\cdot k}(t) + \sum_{k=1}^K \sum_{i=1}^n \int_0^\tau \log(Y_{ik}(t)\cdot\tilde\lambda_{ik}(t))dN_{ik}(t)$$

$$- \sum_{k=1}^K [\theta + N_{\cdot k}(\tau)]\log\left(1 + \theta^{-1}\sum_{i=1}^n \int_0^\tau Y_{ik}(t)\cdot\tilde\lambda_{ik}(t)dt\right), \qquad (9.15)$$

where

$$\tilde\lambda_{ik}(t) = \lambda_0(t)e^{X_{ik}^T(t)\beta}\exp(\theta^{-1}\int_0^{t-} e^{X_{ik}^T(s)\beta}\lambda_0(s)ds).$$

Removing terms not depending on θ in (9.15) gives

$$\frac{1}{K}\Big(\sum_{k=1}^K \int_0^\tau \log(1 + \theta^{-1}N_{\cdot k}(t-))dN_{\cdot k}(t) + \sum_{k=1}^K\sum_{i=1}^n \theta^{-1}N_{ik}(\tau)H_{ik}$$

$$- \sum_{k=1}^K (\theta + N_{\cdot k}(\tau))\log(R_k(\theta))\Big), \qquad (9.16)$$

where

$$H_{ik} = \int_0^\tau Y_{ik}(t)e^{X_{ik}^T(t)\beta}d\Lambda_0(t),\quad R_k(\theta) = 1 + \sum_{i=1}^n (\exp(\theta^{-1}H_{ik}) - 1).$$

Now, by replacing H_{ik} with

$$\hat H_{ik} = \int_0^\tau Y_{ik}(t)\exp(X_{ik}^T(t)\hat\beta_I)d\hat\Lambda_{0I}(t)$$

in (9.16), we obtain the pseudo log likelihood for θ, and maximizing this function in θ gives the two-stage estimator of θ. Under some regularity conditions, Glidden (2000) showed consistency and asymptotic normality of this estimator. The two-stage approach is appealing since it has certain robustness properties due to the fact that the components are fitted in two stages. If, however, one has confidence in the model there might be some efficiency gain by fitting the model in one-step based on maximizing the observed likelihood jointly with respect to all parameters $(\beta, \Lambda_0, \theta)$ and this is what we do in the next section.

9.1.3 One-stage estimation of correlation

With a particular choice of the underlying frailty distribution we here outline how to estimate all parameters jointly using this structure more actively, based on an approximation to the true observed likelihood function (Pipper & Martinussen, 2003) for the Clayton-Oakes model with the marginals described by the Cox model as specified by (9.12) and (9.13). The method is quite similar to the modified partial likelihood method applied for the transformation models considered in Chapter 8. Similar methodology can also be used for the marginal additive hazards model, see Pipper & Martinussen (2004).

The observed intensities (9.14) look at first sight rather complicated due to the f_{ik}-term. However, the similarity of the structure to the Cox model can be exploited as we shall see below. Let $M_{ik}(t)$ denote the counting process martingale with respect to the observed filtration, that is,

$$M_{ik}(t) = N_{ik}(t) - \Lambda_{ik}(t),$$

$$\Lambda_{ik}(t) = \int_0^t Y_{ik}(s) \exp(X_{ik}^T(s)\beta) f_{ik}(s) \, d\Lambda_0(s).$$

Further, let

$$S_r(t) = \sum_{i=1}^n \sum_{k=1}^K Y_{ik}(t) (D_{(\beta,\theta)} W_{ik}(t))^{\otimes r} \exp(X_{ik}^T(t)\beta) f_{ik}(t),$$

$$E(t) = \frac{S_1(t)}{S_0(t)}, \quad V(t) = \frac{S_2(t)}{S_0(t)} - (E(t))^{\otimes 2}.$$

The limits in probability of these quantities are denoted by lower case letters and assumed to exist. Here $D_{(\beta,\theta)}$ denotes differentiation with respect to (β, θ), and

$$W_{ik}(t) = X_{ik}^T(t)\beta + \log(f_{ik}(t)).$$

The equation

$$dN_{..}(t) = dM_{..}(t) + S_0(t) d\Lambda_0(t)$$

9.1 Marginal regression models for clustered failure time data

suggests the following Nelson-Aalen type moment estimator of $d\Lambda_0(t)$:

$$d\tilde{\Lambda}_0(t) = \frac{1}{S_0(t)} dN_{..}(t). \tag{9.17}$$

Inserting this into the likelihood function gives

$$L(\beta, \theta, \Lambda_0) = \Big(\prod_{t \leq \tau} \big(\prod_{i,k} (d\tilde{\Lambda}_0(t) \exp(X_{ik}^T(t)\beta) f_{ik}(t))^{\Delta N_{ik}(t)} \big) \Big)$$

$$\times \exp\big(-\int_0^\tau S_0(t, \beta, \theta, \Lambda_0) d\tilde{\Lambda}_0(t)\big)$$

$$\propto \prod_{t \leq \tau} \big(\prod_{i,k} \big(\frac{\exp(X_{ik}^T(t)\beta) f_{ik}(t, \beta, \theta, \Lambda_0)}{S_0(t)} \big)^{\Delta N_{ik}(t)} \big).$$

Now differentiating $\log(L(\beta, \theta, \Lambda_0))$ with respect to (β, θ) gives

$$U(\beta, \theta, \Lambda_0) = \sum_{i,k} \int_0^\tau R_{ik}(t) dN_{ik}(t), \tag{9.18}$$

where $R_{ik}(t) = D_{(\beta,\theta)} W_{ik}(t) - E(t)$. Note that U evaluated at the true point (β_0, θ_0) is a zero-mean martingale with respect to the observed filtration. The above estimating function can not be used directly for estimation of (β, θ), however, since it depends on the unknown Λ_0. One may proceed by either inserting the Breslow estimator (9.17) or the the Breslow estimator under the working independence assumption, $\hat{\Lambda}_{0I}$. The former will give an approach and asymptotics very similar to the modified partial likelihood method used for the transformation models described in Chapter 8. We here focus on the results when using $\hat{\Lambda}_{0I}$. Replacing Λ_0 by $\hat{\Lambda}_{0I}$ in (9.18) the following estimating function for (β, θ) is obtained:

$$U(\beta, \theta, \hat{\Lambda}_{0I}) = \sum_{i=1}^n \sum_{k=1}^K \int_0^\tau \{D_{(\beta,\theta)} W_{ik}(t, \beta, \theta, \hat{\Lambda}_{0I}) - E(t, \beta, \theta, \hat{\Lambda}_{0I})\} dN_{ik}(t). \tag{9.19}$$

The parameter θ represents the degree of dependence with $\theta \to \infty$ giving independence. It is easily seen that the first (vector)-component of (9.19) converges to the usual Cox-score when $\theta \to \infty$, and one should hence expect the suggested procedure to have similar properties as the usual independence procedure when there is a small degree of dependence.

One may show that there exists a unique consistent solution (with probability tending to one) $(\hat{\beta}, \hat{\theta})$ to the estimating equations (9.19) (Pipper & Martinussen, 2003). Moreover, the below asymptotic result holds. Define

332   9. Clustered failure time data

first the following quantities:

$$g(t,s) = E\Big(\frac{1}{K}\sum_{i=1}^{n}\sum_{k=1}^{K}\big(D_{(\beta,\theta)}W_{ik}(t) - e(t)\big) \times$$
$$g_{ik}(t,s)Y_{ik}(t)\exp(X_{ik}^T(t)\beta)\Big),$$

$$g_{ik}(t,s) = \theta^{-1}f_{ik}(t)\Big(\exp(X_{ik}^T(s)\beta)$$
$$- \frac{\sum_{j=1}^{n}\phi_{jk}(s)\exp(\theta^{-1}\int_0^{t-}\phi_{jk}(s)d\Lambda_0(s))}{f_k(t)}\Big),$$

$$\Phi_k = \sum_{i=1}^{n}\int_0^{\tau}\big((D_{(\beta,\theta)}W_{ik}(t,\beta_0,\theta_0,\Lambda_0) - e(t,\beta_0,\theta_0,\Lambda_0)\big)dM_{ik}(t,\beta_0,\theta_0,\Lambda_0)$$
$$-\int_0^{\tau}\int_0^{t-}g(t,s,\beta_0,\theta_0,\Lambda_0)d\Phi_k(s)d\Lambda_0(t),$$

where $\phi_{jk}(t) = Y_{jk}(t)\exp(X_{jk}^T(t)\beta)$ and $\Phi_k(t)$ is defined by (9.5). Finally let I be the limit in probability of $-K^{-1}(D_{\beta,\theta}\dot{U}(\hat{\beta},\hat{\theta},\hat{\Lambda}_{0I}))$.

Proposition 9.1.1 *The normed score* $K^{-1/2}U(\beta_0,\theta_0,\hat{\Lambda}_{0I})$ *converges in distribution to a normal distribution with zero-mean and covariance matrix* $D = E(\Phi_k\Phi_k^T)$. *Furthermore, the random vector*

$$K^{1/2}\big((\hat{\beta},\hat{\theta}) - (\beta_0,\theta_0)\big)$$

converges in distribution to a normal vector with zero-mean and covariance matrix $I^{-1}DI^{-1}$.

PROOF. Straightforward calculations give

$$K^{-1/2}U(\tau,\beta_0,\theta_0,\hat{\Lambda}_{0I}) = K^{-1/2}\sum_{i,k}\int_0^{\tau}R_{ik}(t,\beta_0,\theta_0,\hat{\Lambda}_{0I})dM_{ik}(t,\beta_0,\theta_0,\Lambda_0)$$
$$- K^{-1/2}\sum_{i,k}\int_0^{\tau}D_{(\beta,\theta)}W_{ik}(t,\beta_0,\theta_0,\hat{\Lambda}_{0I})\Big(\frac{S_0(t,\beta_0,\theta_0,\Lambda_0)}{S_0(t,\beta_0,\theta_0,\hat{\Lambda}_{0I})}f_{ik}(t,\beta_0,\theta_0,\hat{\Lambda}_{0I})$$
$$- f_{ik}(t,\beta_0,\theta_0,\Lambda_0)\Big) \times Y_{ik}(t)\exp(X_{ik}^T(t)\beta_0)d\Lambda_0(t).$$

The first term on the right-hand side of the above expression may be written as

$$K^{-1/2}\sum_{i,k}\int_0^{\tau}\big(D_{(\beta,\theta)}W_{ik}(t,\beta_0,\theta_0,\Lambda_0)$$
$$- e(t,\beta_0,\theta_0,\Lambda_0)\big)M_{ik}(dt,\beta_0,\theta_0,\Lambda_0) + o_P(1).$$

9.1 Marginal regression models for clustered failure time data

Taylor expanding around Λ_0 gives that the second term on the right-hand side in the expression for $K^{-1/2}U(\tau,\beta_0,\theta_0,\hat{\Lambda}_{0I})$ can be written as

$$-\int_0^\tau \int_0^{t-} g(t,s,\beta_0,\theta_0,\Lambda_0) dK^{1/2}(\hat{\Lambda}_{0I}-\Lambda_0)(s) d\Lambda_0(t) + o_P(1).$$

Spiekerman & Lin (1998) show that

$$K^{1/2}(\hat{\Lambda}_{0I}(t)-\Lambda_0(t)) = K^{-1/2}\sum_{k=1}^K \Phi_k(t) + o_P(1),$$

uniformly in $t \leq \tau$, where $\Phi_k(t), k = 1,\cdots,K$, are i.i.d. variables given by (9.5). Using this we conclude that

$$K^{-1/2}U(\tau,\beta_0,\theta_0,\hat{\Lambda}_{0I}) = K^{-1/2}\sum_{k=1}^K \Phi_k + o_P(1).$$

The Φ_k, $k=1,\cdots,K$, are i.i.d. zero-mean variables with well defined variance, and hence the central limit theorem gives us the first part of the theorem. The second part follows by Taylor expanding $U(\hat{\beta},\hat{\theta},\hat{\Lambda}_{0I})$ around (β_0,θ_0) and then using standard arguments. $\square$

The covariance matrix may be estimated consistently by

$$\hat{I}^{-1}\hat{D}\hat{I}^{-1},$$

where

$$\hat{I} = \hat{I}(\tau) = \frac{1}{K}\int_0^\tau \hat{V}(t) dN_{..}(t), \quad \hat{D} = \frac{1}{K}\sum_{k=1}^K \hat{\Phi}_k^{\otimes 2}$$

with $\hat{V}(t) = V(t,\hat{\beta},\hat{\theta},\hat{\Lambda}_{0I})$ and

$$\hat{\Phi}_k = \hat{\Phi}_k(\tau) = \sum_{i=1}^n \int_0^\tau \hat{R}_{ik}(t) dM_{ik}(t,\hat{\beta},\hat{\theta},\hat{\Lambda}_{0I}) -$$

$$\int_0^\tau \int_0^{t-} \Big(\frac{1}{K}\sum_{i=1}^n \sum_{k=1}^K \hat{R}_{ik}(t)\hat{g}_{ik}(t,s)Y_{ik}(t)\exp(X_{ik}^T(t)\hat{\beta})\Big) d\hat{\Phi}_k(s) d\hat{\Lambda}_{0I}(t).$$

In the above display, $\hat{\Phi}_k(t)$ is given by (9.6), $\hat{R}_{ik}(t)$ and $\hat{g}_{ik}(t,s)$ are given by $R_{ik}(t)$ and $g_{ik}(t)$ with unknown parameters replaced by their estimates.

Example 9.1.5 (Diabetic retinopathy data)

Using the marginal proportional hazards model we found a significant interaction between treatment and age of onset of diabetes. Rerunning the marginal Cox analysis on the 83 patients with adult diabetes gives an estimated treatment effect of -1.29 with 95% confidence interval $(-1.78,-0.80)$

based on the robust standard errors. Using the above model, specified by (9.12) and (9.13), on the same subset of data gives the treatment effect $\hat{\beta} = -1.25$ with 95% confidence interval $(-1.73,-0.77)$, which is seen to be slightly narrower than the confidence interval based on the working independence model. An additional benefit of the random effects model is that we also get an estimate of the dependence within clusters (patients). One way of summarizing the dependence is by Kendall's τ that, for the applied Gamma model, is equal to $1/(1+2\theta)$ with $\tau = 0$ and $\tau = 1$ corresponding to independence and maximal dependence, respectively. By use of $\hat{\theta}$ we get the point estimate 0.32 of Kendall's τ with 95%-confidence interval (0.15,0.62). □

The adequacy of the model, specified by (9.12) and (9.13), may be checked partly by investigating the assumed marginal Cox model as outlined for instance in Section 9.1.1. One may also check the assumed observed model directly for example by the test statistic

$$\sup_{t \leq \tau} |K^{-1/2} U(t, \hat{\beta}_0, \hat{\theta}_0, \hat{\Lambda}_{0I})|.$$

Its distribution may approximated by resampling of $\sup_{t \leq \tau} |\hat{W}(t)|$, where

$$\hat{W}(t) = K^{-1/2} \sum_{k=1}^{K} \left[\hat{\Phi}(t) - \hat{I}(t) \hat{I}(\tau)^{-1} \hat{\Phi}(\tau) \right] G_k,$$

with $G_1, \ldots, G_K$ independent standard normals.

9.2 Frailty models

In this section we briefly describe the traditional frailty model for clustered failure time data. It is sometimes also termed the shared frailty model referring to the cluster specific random effects shared by the individuals within clusters, see below. The notation is as in the previous section where

$$(\tilde{T}_k, C_k, X_k(\cdot), V_k),$$

$k = 1, \cdots, K$ are assumed to be i.i.d. variables. Censoring, conditional on V_k and covariates, is assumed to be independent and noninformative on V_k. Again $\tilde{T}_{ik}$, $i = 1, \cdots, n$, are assumed to be independent variables given $V_k, X_1(\cdot), \cdots, X_n(\cdot)$. Let also $T_{ik} = \tilde{T}_{ik} \wedge C_{ik}$, $Y_{ik}(t) = 1(T_{ik} \geq t)$ and $N_{ik}(t) = 1(T_{ik} \leq t, T_{ik} = \tilde{T}_{ik})$. The frailty variable V_k is often assumed to be gamma distributed with mean one and variance θ^{-1} resulting in the Clayton-Oakes model, but several other suggested distributions exist. The gamma frailty model induces high late dependence while the positive stable model (assuming positive stable distributed frailties) induces high early dependence, see Hougaard (2000) for a detailed description of these two models and several others. Which model to use in practice should of course be guided by the data at hand.

The shared frailty model is specified solely with respect to the (unobserved) filtration $\mathcal{H}_t = \bigvee_k \mathcal{H}_t^k$, where

$$\mathcal{H}_t^k = \sigma\{N_{ik}(s), Y_{ik}(s), X_{ik}(s), V_k : \; i = 1, \cdots n, \; 0 \le s \le t\},$$

and often it is assumed to be a proportional hazards model

$$\lambda_{ik}^{\mathcal{H}}(t) = Y_{ik}(t) V_k \lambda_0(t) \exp(X_{ik}^T(t)\beta). \qquad (9.20)$$

Notice the difference between this model and the model given by (9.12) and (9.13). In the latter case the Cox model is used for the marginals whereas, in (9.20), it is used conditionally on the frailty variable.

Estimation in model (9.20), assuming gamma frailties, is elegantly carried out by use of the EM-algorithm (Dempster et al., 1977) regarding the frailties as unobserved variables corresponding to a Cox-regression analysis in each M-step. Large sample properties of these maximum likelihood estimates are difficult to get at, but has recently been derived by Parner (1998). Martinussen & Pipper (2005) studied a modified likelihood approach for the positive stable frailty model and gave large sample results.

Example 9.2.1 (Diabetic retinopathy data)

We here fit the shared frailty model with gamma distributed frailties to the Diabetic Retinopathy data.

```
> fit<-coxph(Surv(time,status)~adult*trt+frailty(id),
        data=diabetes)
> fit
Call:
coxph(formula = Surv(time, status) ~ adult * trt + frailty(id),
    data = diabetes)

              coef  se(coef)  se2    Chisq    DF    p
adult        0.397   0.259   0.205    2.35   1.0  0.1300
trt         -0.506   0.225   0.221    5.03   1.0  0.0250
frailty(id)                         122.54  88.6  0.0098
adult:trt   -0.985   0.362   0.355    7.41   1.0  0.0065

Iterations: 6 outer, 25 Newton-Raphson
      Variance of random effect= 0.926   I-likelihood = -847
```

The model can be fitted in R using `coxph` with the `frailty` option. However, the se's for the regression parameters in the printout are obtained assuming that θ is fixed rather than a parameter to be estimated, and should hence be interpreted with caution. □

The interpretation of the regression parameters β as log relative risks is *conditionally* on the unobserved random effect. These parameters may be of interest when one wants to compare treatments within clusters. The unconditional model is generally not a proportional hazards model. It may be instructive to derive the relationship between conditional hazard and the marginal hazard assuming multiplicative frailty effect. To be explicit, assume that the marginal and conditional intensities are

$$\lambda_{ik}^{\mathcal{F}^{ik}}(t) = \lambda_{ik}(t), \quad \lambda_{ik}^{\mathcal{H}}(t) = V_k \lambda_{ik}^*(t),$$

where we assume that $\lambda_{ik}^*(t)$ is predictable with respect to the marginal filtration. One may show that the relationship between the above two intensities is

$$\lambda_{ik}(t) = Y_{ik}(t)(-\lambda_{ik}^*(t))(D\log\phi_\theta)(\int_0^{t-} \lambda_{ik}^*(s)\,ds),$$

$$\lambda_{ik}^*(t) = Y_{ik}(t)(-\lambda_{ik}(t))\exp\left(-\int_0^t \lambda_{ik}(s)\,ds\right)(D\phi_\theta^{-1})(\exp\left(-\int_0^t \lambda_{ik}(s)\,ds\right)),$$

see Exercise 9.3.

Example 9.2.2 (Conditional proportional hazards model)

In this example we wish to investigate the marginal intensity under a conditional proportional intensity model. For ease of notation we drop subscripts referring to individuals and clusters. Assume that $\lambda^*(t)$ (dropping here subscript ik) is a proportional hazards intensity: $Y(t)\lambda_0(t)\exp(X^T\beta)$. Let us compute the marginal intensities under different frailty distributions. Consider first the gamma model, that is, V is gamma distributed with mean 1 and variance θ^{-1}. The Laplace transform is $\phi_\theta(t) = (1+\theta t)^{-1/\theta}$ giving rise to the marginal intensity

$$Y(t)\lambda_0(t)\exp(X^T\beta)\frac{1}{1+\theta\Lambda^*(t)}$$

with $\Lambda^*(t) = \int_0^t \lambda^*(s)\,ds$. If the covariate-vector is one-dimensional then the relative risk in the unconditional model is

$$\exp(\beta)\left(\frac{1+\theta\Lambda_0(t)}{1+\exp(\beta)\theta\Lambda_0(t)}\right), \tag{9.21}$$

where $\Lambda_0(t) = \int_0^t \lambda_0(s)\,ds$. The relative risk based on the unconditional model is seen to depend on time and hence the proportional hazards assumption of the Cox model is no longer in play. It is equal to $\exp(\beta)$ at time $t=0$ and tends to 1 as time increases giving what converging hazards as was also the case for the proportional odds model in Chapter 8, see also Exercise 9.6. If we instead use the positive stable model, that is,

9.2 Frailty models

assume that V follows a positive stable distribution with Laplace transform $\phi_\theta(t) = \exp(-t^\theta)$, $0 < \theta \leq 1$, then the marginal intensity is

$$Y(t)\theta\lambda_0(t)\Lambda_0(t)^{\theta-1}\exp(\theta X^T\beta),$$

so here we still have a Cox model with the regression parameter attenuated by the amount θ.

We see for both the gamma and positive stable model that the regression effect is attenuated in terms of a smaller relative risk assuming without loss of generality that $\beta > 0$. One might ask whether this holds true in general. This is actually so. Assume that V is a positive stochastic variable with Laplace transform $\phi_\theta(t)$, that the covariate is one-dimensional, and that $\beta > 0$. The relative risk in the marginal model is

$$\exp(\beta)\frac{(D\log\phi_\theta)(\exp((X+1)\beta)\Lambda_0(t))}{(D\log\phi_\theta)(\exp(X\beta)\Lambda_0(t))} = \exp(\beta)k(t),$$

and we see that $k(t) \leq 1$ if and only if $(D\log\phi_\theta)(\exp((X+1)\beta)\Lambda_0(t)) \leq (D\log\phi_\theta)(\exp(X\beta)\Lambda_0(t))$. The latter inequality holds if $\log(\phi_\theta)$ is convex, which is the case since

$$D^2\log(\phi_\theta)(t) = E(V^2 h(t,V)) - E(Vh(t,V))^2 \geq 0$$

with $h(t,V) = \exp(-tV)/E(\exp(-tV))$. $\square$

Above, the relationship between the conditional and marginal intensities was given. One may also establish the relationships between these and the intensity with respect to the observed filtration containing $\mathcal{F}_t$. One gets for instance that the relationship between the marginal intensity and the observed intensity is

$$\lambda_{ik}^{\mathcal{F}} = \lambda_{ik}^{\mathcal{F}_{ik}}(t)f_{ik}(t), \qquad (9.22)$$

where

$$f_{ik}(t) = -\exp(-\int_0^t \lambda_{ik}^{\mathcal{F}_{ik}}(s)\,ds)(D\phi_\theta^{-1})(\exp(-\int_0^t \lambda_{ik}^{\mathcal{F}_{ik}}(s)\,ds))E(V_k \mid \mathcal{F}_{t-})$$

with

$$E(V_k \mid \mathcal{F}_{t-}) = -\frac{(D^{N_{\cdot k}(t-)+1}\phi_\theta)(\sum_i \phi_\theta^{-1}(\int_0^t \lambda_{ik}^{\mathcal{F}_{ik}}(s)\,ds))}{(D^{N_{ik}(t-)}\phi_\theta)(\sum_i \phi_\theta^{-1}(\int_0^t \lambda_{ik}^{\mathcal{F}_{ik}}(s)\,ds))}.$$

If one wishes to build the model based on the marginal intensities (e.g. a proportional intensity model), then (9.22) gives the observed intensity, which opens the route for doing likelihood inference.

9.3 Exercises

9.1 (Marginal additive intensity model) Let the situation be as in Section 9.1.1, but where the marginal intensities are assumed to be

$$\lambda_{ik}^{\mathcal{F}^{ik}}(t) = Y_{ik}(t)(\beta(t) + \gamma^T X_{ik}(t)), \tag{9.23}$$

where $\beta(t)$ is a (local integrable) scalar function of time and γ is p-vector of unknown regression coefficients. Let $B(t) = \int_0^t \beta(s)\, ds$.

(a) Verify that the (unweighed) working independence estimator of γ is

$$\hat{\gamma} = [\sum_{k=1}^K \sum_{i=1}^n \int_0^\tau Y_{ik}(t)\{X_{ik}(t) - \overline{X}(t)\}^{\otimes 2}\, dt]^{-1}$$

$$\times [\sum_{k=1}^K \sum_{i=1}^n \int_0^\tau \{X_{ik}(t) - \overline{X}(t)\}dN_{ik}(t)],$$

which is the solution to $U(\gamma) = 0$ with

$$U(\gamma) = \sum_{k=1}^K \sum_{i=1}^n \int_0^\tau \{X_{ik}(t) - \overline{X}(t)\}\{dN_{ik}(t) - Y_{ik}(t)\gamma^T X_{ik}(t)dt\}.$$

In the above displays,

$$\overline{X}(t) = \frac{\sum_{k=1}^K \sum_{i=1}^n Y_{ik}(t) X_{ik}(t)}{\sum_{k=1}^K \sum_{i=1}^n Y_{ik}(t)}.$$

The (unweighted) estimator of $B(t)$ is

$$\hat{B}(t, \hat{\gamma}) = \sum_{k=1}^K \sum_{i=1}^n \int_0^t \frac{1}{\sum_{k=1}^K \sum_{i=1}^n Y_{ik}(s)} dN_{ik}(s) - \hat{\gamma}^T \int_0^t \overline{X}(s)\, ds.$$

(b) Derive the asymptotic distribution (K tending to infinity) of

$$K^{1/2}(\hat{\gamma} - \gamma)$$

and give a consistent estimator of the asymptotic variance-covariance matrix.

(c) Give an i.i.d. representation of

$$K^{1/2}(\hat{B}(t, \hat{\gamma}) - B(t)) \tag{9.24}$$

that may be used for resampling to approximate the limit distribution of (9.24).

9.2 (Multiplicative random effects hazards models as a copula) Let V denote a non-negative random variate with Laplace transform $\phi(v)$. Assume that the failure times $\tilde{T}_1, \ldots, \tilde{T}_n$ are conditional independent given V with conditional hazards
$$V\lambda_j(t), \quad j = 1, \ldots, n.$$

(a) Show that the joint survival function and the marginal survivor functions are related as follows:
$$P(\tilde{T}_1 > t_1, \ldots, \tilde{T}_n > t_n) = \phi(\phi^{-1}(S_1(t_1)) + \cdots + \phi^{-1}(S_n(t_n))),$$
where $S_1, \ldots, S_n$ denote the marginal survivor functions.

The Clayton-Oakes model (Clayton, 1978; Oakes, 1982) is such a multiplicative random effects model with V gamma distributed with mean 1 and variance θ^{-1}.

(b) Show that the corresponding copula for this model is
$$C_\theta(u_1, \ldots, u_n) = \left(u_1^{-1/\theta} \cdots + u_n^{-1/\theta} - (n-1)\right)^{-\theta}, \quad \theta > 0.$$

9.3 (Relationship between marginal, observed and conditional intensities) Let
$$T_{ik} = \tilde{T}_{ik} \wedge C_{ik}, \quad Y_{ik}(t) = 1(T_{ik} \geq t) \text{ and } N_{ik}(t) = 1(T_{ik} \leq t, T_{ik} = \tilde{T}_{ik})$$
denote the observed failure time, the individual at risk process and the counting process for the ith individual in the kth cluster, $i = 1, \ldots, n$ and $k = 1, \ldots, K$. Assume the presence of some (unobserved) random effects V_k, $k = 1, \ldots, K$ in such a way that
$$(\tilde{T}_k, C_k, X_k(\cdot), V_k), \quad k = 1, \cdots, K,$$
are i.i.d. variables, where
$$\tilde{T}_k = (\tilde{T}_{1k}, \ldots, \tilde{T}_{nk}), \quad C_k = (C_{1k}, \ldots, C_{nk}), \quad X_k(t) = (X_{1k}(t), \ldots, X_{nk}(t))$$
with $X_{ik}(\cdot)$ denoting the ikth covariate process. Censoring, conditional on V_k and covariates, is assumed to be independent and noninformative on V_k, the distribution of the latter having density p_θ and Laplace transform ϕ_θ. Assume also that failure times $\tilde{T}_{ik}$, $i = 1, \cdots, n$, are independent variables given $V_k, X_1(\cdot), \cdots, X_n(\cdot)$.

9. Clustered failure time data

We shall now study the relationship between the marginal, observed and conditional intensity of $N_{ik}(t)$. Assume that $N_{ik}(t)$ has intensity

$$\lambda_{ik}^{\mathcal{H}}(t) = V_k \lambda_{ik}^*(t),$$

with respect to the conditional (unobserved) filtration (9.11) so that $\lambda_{ik}^*(t)$ is predictable with respect to the marginal filtration $\mathcal{F}_t^{ik}$, see (9.1). Denote the marginal intensity of $N_{ik}(t)$ by

$$\lambda_{ik}^{\mathcal{F}^{ik}}(t) = \lambda_{ik}(t)$$

where $\mathcal{F}^{ik}$ refers to the marginal filtration.

(a) Show that likelihood based on the $\mathcal{H}_{t-}$-filtration is

$$p_\theta(V_k) \prod_{s<t} (V_k \lambda_{ik}^*(s))^{\Delta N_{ik}(s)} \exp\left(-V_k \int_0^{t-} \lambda_{ik}^*(s)\,ds\right)$$

giving that

$$E(V_k \mid \mathcal{F}_{t-}^{ik}) = -\frac{(D^{N_{ik}(t-)+1}\phi_\theta)(\int_0^{t-} \lambda_{ik}^*(s)\,ds)}{(D^{N_{ik}(t-)}\phi_\theta)(\int_0^{t-} \lambda_{ik}^*(s)\,ds)},$$

which reduces to $-(D \log \phi_\theta)(\int_0^{t-} \lambda_{ik}^*(s)\,ds)$ when $Y_{ik}(t) = 1$ where $D^j g$ means the jth derivative of the function g.

(b) Derive the relationships

$$\lambda_{ik}(t) = Y_{ik}(t)(-\lambda_{ik}^*(t))(D \log \phi_\theta)(\int_0^{t-} \lambda_{ik}^*(s)\,ds),$$

$$\lambda_{ik}^*(t) = Y_{ik}(t)(-\lambda_{ik}(t)) \exp\left(-\int_0^t \lambda_{ik}(s)\,ds\right)$$

$$\times (D\phi_\theta^{-1})(\exp(-\int_0^t \lambda_{ik}(s)\,ds)).$$

We shall now also consider the intensity of $N_{ik}(t)$ with respect to the observed filtration $\mathcal{F}_t$, see (9.3).

(c) Show that observed intensity is related to the marginal intensity as

$$\lambda_{ik}^{\mathcal{F}} = \lambda_{ik}^{\mathcal{F}^{ik}}(t) f_{ik}(t),$$

where

$$f_{ik}(t) = -\exp(-\int_0^t \lambda_{ik}^{\mathcal{F}^{ik}}(s)\,ds)$$

$$\times (D\phi_\theta^{-1})(\exp(-\int_0^t \lambda_{ik}^{\mathcal{F}^{ik}}(s)\,ds)) E(V_k \mid \mathcal{F}_{t-})$$

with
$$E(V_k \mid \mathcal{F}_{t-}) = -\frac{(D^{N_{\cdot k}(t-)+1}\phi_\theta)(\sum_i \phi_\theta^{-1}(\int_0^t \lambda_{ik}^{\mathcal{F}_{ik}}(s)\,ds))}{(D^{N_{ik}(t-)}\phi_\theta)(\sum_i \phi_\theta^{-1}(\int_0^t \lambda_{ik}^{\mathcal{F}_{ik}}(s)\,ds))}.$$

9.4 (Two-stage method) Verify the expressions (9.15) and (9.16).

9.5 (Two-stage estimation in copula models, Andersen (2005)) We shall consider the two-stage method for copula models. To simplify notation we consider the case where $n = 2$, that is two subjects in each cluster. Let $(\tilde{T}_{1k}, \tilde{T}_{2k})$ and (C_{1k}, C_{2k}) denote the paired failure times and censoring times for pair $k = 1,\ldots,K$. We observe $T_{ik} = \tilde{T}_{ik} \wedge C_{ik}$ and $\Delta_{ik} = I(T_{ik} = \tilde{T}_{ik})$. Let X_{ik} covariate vector for ikth subject and assume that $(\tilde{T}_{1k}, \tilde{T}_{2k})$ and (C_{1k}, C_{2k}) are conditionally independent given the covariates. Let $S(t_{1k}, t_{2k})$ be the joint survival function for pair k, which is specified via the marginal survival function through the copula C_θ.

(a) Show that the partial log-likelihood function can be written as

$$\sum_{k=1}^K \Delta_{1k}\Delta_{2k} \log\{\frac{\partial^2}{\partial T_{1k}\partial T_{2k}} S(T_{1k}, T_{1k})\}$$
$$+ \Delta_{1k}(1 - \Delta_{2k}) \log\{\frac{-\partial}{\partial T_{1k}} S(T_{1k}, T_{1k})\}$$
$$+ (1 - \Delta_{1k})\Delta_{2k} \log\{\frac{-\partial}{\partial T_{2k}} S(T_{1k}, T_{1k})\}$$
$$+ (1 - \Delta_{1k})(1 - \Delta_{2k}) \log\{S(T_{1k}, T_{1k})\}.$$

Consider now the situation where the marginal hazards are specified using the Cox model,
$$\alpha_{ik}(t) = \lambda_0(t) \exp(X_{ik}^T \beta).$$
We estimate the β and $\Lambda_0(t) = \int_0^t \lambda_0(s)\,ds$ using the working independence estimators of Section 9.1.1 (first stage). Let U_θ denote the derivative with respect to θ of the partial log-likelihood function. At the second stage we estimate θ as the solution to
$$U_\theta(\theta, \hat{\beta}, \hat{\Lambda}_{0I}) = 0.$$

(b) Write $K^{-1/2} U_\theta(\theta, \hat{\beta}_i, \hat{\Lambda}_{0I})$ as
$$\sum_{k=1}^K \Phi_k + o_p(1),$$
where $\Phi_1,\ldots,\Phi_K$ are i.i.d. terms (hint: use a Taylor expansion and the corresponding representation of the working independence estimators).

342   9. Clustered failure time data

(c) Under appropriate conditions, derive the asymptotic distribution of
$$K^{1/2}(\hat{\theta} - \theta)$$
as K tends to infinity. Give also the asymptotic variance and an estimator thereof.

9.6 (Converging hazards) Let $N(t) = I(\tilde{T} \wedge C \leq t, \tilde{T} \leq C)$ and let X denote a covariate vector. Consider the situation described in the beginning of Example 9.2.2, where $N(t)$ has conditional intensity
$$VY(t)\lambda_0(t)\exp(X^T\beta)$$
given V, that is gamma distributed with mean one and variance θ^{-1}. As usual $Y(t) = I(t \leq \tilde{T} \wedge C)$ denotes the at risk indicator.

(a) Verify that the marginal intensity is
$$Y(t)\frac{\lambda_0(t)\exp(X^T\beta)}{1+\theta\exp(X^T\beta)\Lambda_0(t)} = Y(t)\alpha_X(t), \qquad (9.25)$$
which is a hazard from the Burr distribution.

The hazard $\alpha_X(t)$ converges with time, but to zero rather than to an arbitrary baseline hazard. This led Barker & Henderson (2004) to suggest the following class of hazard models. Partition X into X_1 and X_2, and suppose that
$$\alpha_X(t) = \frac{\exp(X_1^T\beta_1 + X_2^T\beta_2)\exp(\gamma\Lambda_0(t))}{1+\exp(X_2^T\beta_2)(\exp(\gamma\Lambda_0(t))-1)}\lambda_0(t), \qquad (9.26)$$
where γ is an unknown scalar parameter.

(b) Observe the following points.

- At baseline, $X_1 = X_2 = 0$, $\alpha_X(t) = \lambda_0(t)$;
- If $\gamma = 0$, then the model reduces to the Cox model with covariates (X_1, X_2); if $\beta_1 = 0$ then the model reduces to the Burr model with covariate X_2;
- As t tends to infinity, $\alpha_X(t)$ converges to $\exp(X_1^T\beta_1)\lambda_0(t)$, rather than zero.

Suppose now that we have n i.i.d. observations from the generic model given by (9.26).

(c) Use a modified likelihood approach similar to the one applied for the proportional odds model in Chapter 8 to construct an estimating equation for $\phi = (\gamma, \beta_1, \beta_2)$,
$$U(\phi) = 0,$$
and an estimator of $\Lambda_0(t)$, $\hat{\Lambda}_0(t, \hat{\phi})$, where $\hat{\phi}$ satisfies $U(\hat{\phi}) = 0$.

9.3 Exercises

(d) Derive, under suitable conditions, the asymptotic properties of the estimators defined in (c).

9.7 (Checking the gamma assumption, Glidden (1999)) Consider the Clayton-Oakes described in Section 9.1.2 so that

$$\lambda_{ik}^{\mathcal{H}}(t) = Y_{ik}(t) V_k \lambda^*(t)$$

where $\lambda^*(t)$ is deterministic function, V_k is gamma distributed with mean one and variance θ^{-1}, and so that

$$\lambda_{ik}^{\mathcal{F}^{ik}}(t) = Y_{ik}(t) \lambda_0(t)$$

with $\lambda_0(t)$ being a deterministic function.

(a) Show that the conditional mean of V_k given the observed filtration $\mathcal{F}_{t-}$ is

$$\psi_k(t) = E(V_k \mid \mathcal{F}_{t-}) = \frac{1 + \theta^{-1} N_{\cdot k}}{R_k(t, \theta)},$$

where

$$R_k(t, \theta) = 1 + \sum_{i=1}^n \theta^{-1} \int_0^t Y_{ik}(s) \lambda^*(s) \, ds.$$

Express $R_k(t,\theta)$ as a function of $\Lambda_0(t) = \int_0^t \lambda_0(s)\,ds$: $R_k(t,\theta,\Lambda_0)$. Under the assumed model $\psi_1(t), \ldots, \psi_K(t)$ are i.i.d. with mean one. Let

$$W_n(t) = K^{-1/2} \sum_{k=1}^{K} (\psi_k(t) - 1).$$

(b) Show that $W_n(t)$ may rewritten as

$$W_n(t) = K^{-1/2} \sum_{k=1}^{K} \int_0^t H_k(s) \, dM_k(s),$$

where

$$H_k(t) = \frac{\theta^{-1}}{R_k(t,\theta,\Lambda_0)}, \quad M_k(t) = N_{\cdot k} - \sum_{i=1}^n \int_0^t \psi_k(s-) Y_{ik}(s) \lambda^*(s) \, ds,$$

and conclude that $W_n(t)$ is a $\mathcal{F}_t$-martingale.

(c) Suggest estimators $\hat{\theta}$ and $\hat{\Lambda}_0(t)$ for θ and $\Lambda_0(t)$, respectively.

(d) Use the estimators constructed in (c) to estimate $W_n(t)$ by $\hat{W}_n(t)$, say. Is $\hat{W}_n(t)$ a $\mathcal{F}_t$-martingale?

A resampling technique can be developed to approximate the limit distribution of $\hat{W}_n(t)$, which then can be used to study whether the observed $\hat{W}_n(t)$ is extreme in this distribution. One may for example construct a supremum test.

9.8 (EM-algorithm for gamma frailty model) Consider the setup of Section 9.2. Devise the E- and M-step of the EM-algorithm for the model (9.20) where it is assumed that V_k is gamma distributed with mean one and variance θ^{-1}.

9.9 (Discrete time survival data) Time to pregnancy that is preferably counted in the number of menstrual cycles it takes for a couple to achieve pregnancy (TTP) should be analyzed by discrete time survival models, as in Scheike & Jensen (1997) and Scheike et al. (1999).

The basic set-up is as follows. T_i is a discrete time TTP that is modeled by the discrete time hazard probability

$$\lambda_i(t) = P(T_i = t | T_i \geq t) = h^{-1}(X_i(t)^T \beta) \tag{9.27}$$

where h is a link function and $X_i(t) = X_{it}$ are possibly time-dependent covariates for subject i. Assume that we observed n independent survival times from this model, with possible right censoring. We shall here consider the cloglog link $h(t) = \log(-\log(t))$ and the special case where

$$\beta = (\gamma_1, ..., \gamma_m, \alpha_1, ..., \alpha_q)$$

where $m, q > 0$, and

$$X_{it}^T \beta = \gamma_t + X_i^T \alpha.$$

Then the probability function and the survival probability are given by the following expressions:

$$\begin{aligned} P(T_i = t) &= \lambda_i(t) \prod_{j=1}^{t-1}(1 - \lambda_i(j)) \tag{9.28} \\ &= \lambda_i(t) \exp(-\sum_{j=1}^{t-1} \exp(X_{ij}^T \beta)) \\ &= \exp(-F_i(t-1)) - \exp(-F_i(t)), \end{aligned}$$

where

$$F_i(t) = \sum_{j=1}^{t} \exp(X_{ij}^T \beta),$$

with the definition $F_i(0) = 0$, and it follows that

$$P(T_i \geq t) = \exp(-F_i(t-1)).$$

(a) Write down the likelihood for right-censored survival data from this model. How can maximization be implemented on the computer, by for example Fisher scoring.

(b) Now assume that given an unobserved random effect R_i, the conditional hazard for T_i is

$$\lambda_i(t|R_i) = 1 - \exp\left(-\exp(R_i + X_{it}^T \beta)\right). \tag{9.29}$$

Assume that $U_i = \exp(R_i)$ is gamma distributed with mean 1 and variance ν, and work out the marginal probabilities for T_i, and the marginal hazard probability. Note, that the frailty variance can be identified in the presence of covariates.

(c) Now, assume that two TTP's are given to each i (couple), T_{i1} and T_{i2}, and are observed in succession and that given R_i the TTP's are independent with hazard given by (9.29). Work out the hazard rate for T_{i2} given either T_{i1} or $T_{i1} > C_{i1}$ and use this to write down the likelihood for T_{i1} and T_{i2} with possible right-censoring.

(d) Modify the above to deal with left truncation.

(e) Now, assume that T_{i1} and T_{i2} have marginal models, i.e., models for the observed (population) hazards, given by

$$\text{cloglog}(\lambda_i^p(t)) = X_{ipt}^T \beta, \quad p = 1, 2. \tag{9.30}$$

To model the association we assume that underlying these marginal models is a frailty model such that given R_i the waiting times are given by the hazards

$$\text{cloglog}(\lambda_i^p(t)) = \alpha_{ip}(t) + R_i, \quad p = 1, 2, \tag{9.31}$$

where $U_i = \exp(R_i)$ is gamma distributed with mean 1 and variance ν.

Work out an expression for $\alpha_{ip}(t)$ such that the marginal models are given by (9.30).

(f) Discuss the difference between the two frailty models described above. How is the frailty variance identified in the models?

10
Competing Risks Model

The competing risks models is concerned with failure time data, where each subject may experience one of K different types of failures. Mathematically speaking it is a special case of the marked point process setup, but this observation does not add much to the understanding of the underlying problems and practical matters that need to be resolved when dealing with competing risks data. Competing risks data are encountered, for example, when medical studies are designed to learn about the effect of various treatments aimed at a particular disease. For the melanoma data the primary interest was on the effect of the treatment (removal of the tumor) on the mortality from malignant melanoma. Some of the patients died of causes not related to the disease, however.

In the following we introduce some notation to construct models for competing risks data. Let T denote the failure time and ε a stochastic variable that registers the type of death, $\varepsilon \in \{1, ..., K\}$. One way of describing a model for competing risks data is to specify the intensities for the counting processes $N_k(t) = I(T \leq t, \varepsilon = k)$, $k = 1, ..., K$, registering the failures of type k. This is done via the so-called cause specific hazard functions:

$$\alpha_k(t) = \lim_{\Delta t \to 0} \frac{P(t \leq T < t + \Delta t, \varepsilon = 1 \mid T \geq t)}{\Delta t}, \quad k = 1, ..., K.$$

With $Y(t)$ denoting the at risk indicator, allowing for right censoring and left-truncation, we assume that

$$\lambda_k(t) = Y(t)\alpha_k(t), \quad k = 1, ..., K,$$

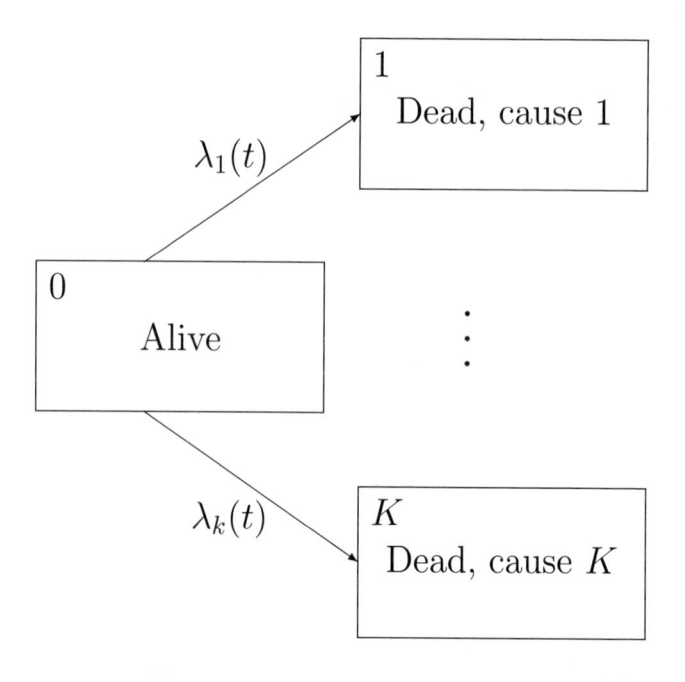

FIGURE 10.1: Competing risks model. Each subject may die from k different causes

are the intensities associated with the K-dimensional counting process $N = (N_1, ..., N_K)^T$ and define its compensator

$$\Lambda(t) = (\int_0^t \lambda_1(s)ds, ..., \int_0^t \lambda_K(s)ds)^T,$$

such that $M(t) = N(t) - \Lambda(t)$ becomes a K-dimensional (local square integrable) martingale. A competing risks model can thus be described by specifying all the cause specific hazards. The model can be visualized as shown in Figure 10.1, where a subject can move from the "alive" state to death of one of the K different causes.

Based on the cause specific hazards various consequences of the model can be computed. One such summary statistic is the *cumulative incidence function*, or cumulative incidence probability, for cause $k = 1, .., K$, defined as the probability of dying of cause k before time t

$$P_k(t) = P(T \leq t, \varepsilon = k) = \int_0^t \alpha_k(s)S(s-)ds, \qquad (10.1)$$

where $S(t) = P(T > t)$ is the survival function. The survival function is expressed in terms of the hazards as

$$S(t) = \exp(-\int_0^t \alpha.(s)ds)$$

with the total hazard

$$\alpha.(t) = \sum_{k=1}^{K} \alpha_k(t).$$

As is clear from (10.1), the cumulative incidence function for cause 1, say, depends on the other cause specific hazard functions, which may speak for another approach, see Section 10.3.

In this chapter we shall focus on different approaches for estimating the cumulative incidence probability. One approach is based on estimating the cause specific hazards and then either use the above formula to estimate P_k or the product limit estimator (Aalen, 1978a; Aalen & Johansen, 1978; Fleming, 1978b,a; Andersen et al., 1993). Alternatively one may estimate the cumulative incidence probability directly by the subdistribution approach (Pepe, 1991; Gray, 1988; Fine & Gray, 1999; Scheike & Zhang, 2004).

Example 10.0.1 (Melanoma data.)

For the Melanoma data the interest lies in studying the effect of various factors on time to death of malignant melanoma after removal of tumor. The study was closed end of 1977, the number of deaths caused by malignant melanoma in the considered period being 57, 14 died from other causes and the remaining 134 patients were censored at the closure of the study since they were still alive at that point in time. We now estimate the cumulative incidence function based on the techniques described in the next section. The estimates can be obtained using the cmprsk R-library of Robert Gray.

```
> data(melanom);attach(melanom)
> status.i<-status;status.i[status==2]<-0
> status.i[status==3]<-1;status.i[status==1]<-2
>
> fit<-cuminc(days/365,status.i)
> plot(fit$"1 2"$time,fit$"1 2"$est,ylim=c(0,1),
+ xlim=c(0,8),xlab="Time (years)",
+ ylab="Probability",type="s")
> se<-fit$"1 2"$var^.5; up<-fit$"1 2"$est+1.96*se;
> low<-fit$"1 2"$est-1.96*se
> lines(fit$"1 2"$time,up,type="s");
> lines(fit$"1 2"$time,low,type="s");
```

350   10. Competing Risks Model

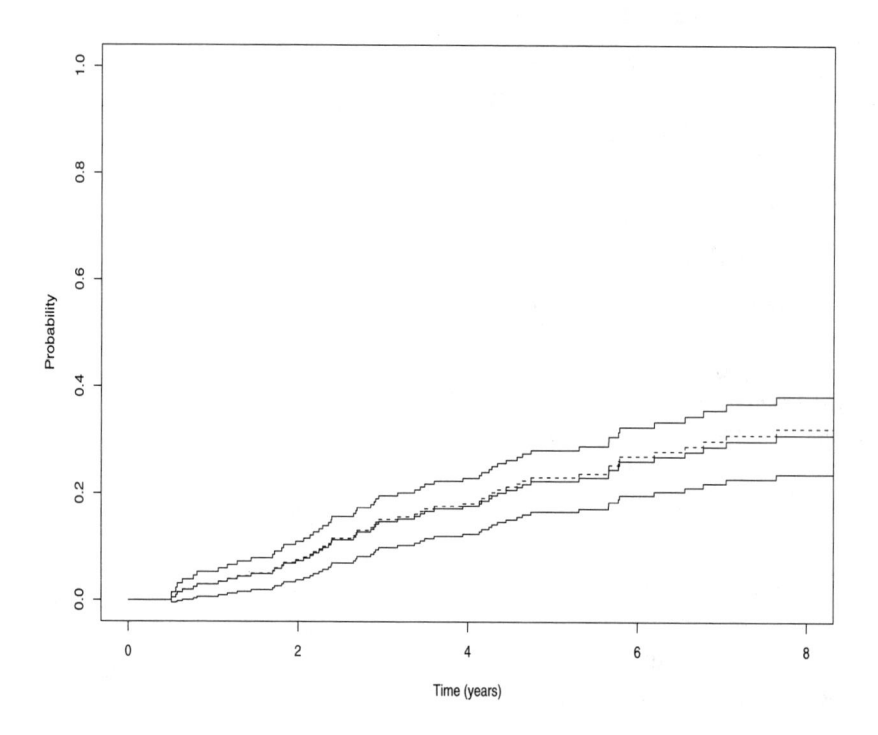

FIGURE 10.2: Melanoma data. Cumulative incidence probability function along with 95% pointwise confidence intervals for cause 1 (malignant melanoma, full lines) and $1 - S_1(t)$ (see text, broken line).

Inspection of Figure 10.2 suggest that the probability of dying of malignant melanoma before 8 years after surgery is 0.22; in contrast the number $1 - S_1(t)$ (dotted line) that is 0.24 when evaluated at 8 years. Here

$$S_1(t) = \prod_{s \leq t} \left(1 - \Delta \hat{A}_1(s)\right),$$

is the Kaplan-Meier where all deaths with respect to other causes are considered as censorings. This number is often computed and used in the cause specific hazards setting but has no simple interpretation as a probability except for very special cases. Note that $S_1(t)$ is a consistent estimator of $\exp(-A_1(t))$. Therefore $1 - S_1(t)$ will only equal the probability of dying of cause 1 before time t

$$\int_0^t \alpha_1(s) \exp(-A_1(s) - A_{-1}(s)) ds$$

when $A_{-1}(t) = \sum_{k=2}^{K} A_k(t)$ equals 0, see also Exercise 10.1.

For the melanoma data S_1 and P_1 only differ marginally because the cause specific hazard related to the other causes is quite small. □

10.1 Product limit estimator

We start this section by considering a simple direct estimator of the cumulative incidence probability in the case where there are no covariates. We wish to estimate the cumulative incidence curve for cause 1 that can be written as

$$P_1(t) = \int_0^t \alpha_1(s)S(s-)ds = \int_0^t S(s-)dA_1(s) = \int_0^t \exp(-A.(s-))dA_1(s),$$

where

$$A_k(t) = \int_0^t \alpha_k(s)\,ds, \quad k=1,\ldots,K,$$

and

$$A.(t) = \sum_{k=1}^K A_k(t).$$

An estimate of $P_1(t)$ is then obtained by estimating the cause specific cumulative baselines by their respective Nelson-Aalen estimators, and the survival function $S(t)$ by the Kaplan-Meier estimator.

To look more closely at the properties of the simple estimator suggested above we assume that n i.i.d. K dimensional counting processes $(N_{i1},...,N_{iK})$ with at risk indicators $Y_i(t)$ are being observed from the competing risks model. Focusing on the cumulative incidence function for cause 1 we denote

$$N_{i,-1}(t) = \sum_{k=2}^K N_{ik}(t), \quad N_{\cdot 1}(t) = \sum_{i=1}^n N_{i1}(t),$$

$$N.(t) = N._{-1}(t) + N._1(t),$$

and the total number of subjects at risk at time t by

$$Y.(t) = \sum_{i=1}^n Y_i(t).$$

We have the decomposition

$$dN_{ik}(t) = Y_i(t)dA_k(t) + dM_{ik}(t),$$

where the $M_{ik}(t)$'s are martingales with respect to the *observed* filtration, which immediately suggest that the cumulative intensities can be estimated by the Nelson-Aalen estimator

$$\hat{A}_k(t) = \int_0^t \frac{J(s)}{Y_\cdot(s)} dN_{\cdot k}(s),$$

where $J(t) = I(Y_\cdot(t) > 0)$ with the convention that $0/0 = 0$. These estimators may also be derived as maximum likelihood estimators, see Exercise 10.2.

Let $\hat{S}(t)$ be the Kaplan-Meier estimator:

$$\hat{S}(t) = \prod_{s \leq t} \left(1 - \frac{\Delta N_\cdot(s)}{Y_\cdot(s)}\right),$$

where $\Delta f(t) = f(t) - f(t-)$ for a function f. This leads to the estimator of $P_1(t)$:

$$\hat{P}_1(t) = \int_0^t \hat{S}(s-) d\hat{A}_1(s).$$

To get the asymptotic variance of $n^{1/2}(\hat{P}_1(t) - P_1(t))$ one may apply the functional delta-method by noting that $\hat{P}_1(t)$ is asymptotically equivalent to

$$H(\hat{A}_1, \hat{A}_2) = \int_0^t \prod_{u \in)0,s]} \left\{1 - d\left(\hat{A}_1(u) + \hat{A}_2(u)\right)\right\} d\hat{A}_1(s), \qquad (10.2)$$

considering here the case with only two causes of death. See Andersen et al. (1993) for more details about the functional H and its derivative on the relevant functional space. It can be derived that $n^{1/2}(\hat{P}_1(t) - P_1(t))$ is asymptotically equivalent to a Gaussian martingale with zero mean and a variance that is consistently estimated by

$$n(\int_0^t \hat{S}^2(s-) \left\{\hat{P}_1(t) - \hat{P}_1(s)\right\}^2 \frac{J(s)}{Y_\cdot^2(s)} dN_\cdot(s)$$

$$+ \int_0^t \hat{S}^2(t-) \left\{1 - 2\left[\hat{P}_1(t) - \hat{P}_1(s)\right]\right\} \frac{J(s)}{Y_\cdot^2(s)} dN_{\cdot 1}(s)). \qquad (10.3)$$

Alternatively, one may derive the asymptotic properties of the estimator by recognizing it as an Aalen-Johansen product limit estimator. The product integration estimator, or the product limit estimator, and the elegant theory for such structures can be used to estimate transition probabilities for any multi-state model, but we here only consider the competing risk model. The transition probabilities in the competing risk model can be written on matrix form $P(s,t) = (P_{i,j}(s,t)$ for $i,j \in \{0, 1, ..., K\}$, where $P_{i,j}(s,t)$ denotes the probability of moving from state i at time s to state j at time t. In the competing risks model $P_{0,i}(0,t)$ for $i = 0, 1, ..., K$ are the

10.1 Product limit estimator

cumulative incidence probabilities and $P_{0,0}(0,t)$ is simply the probability of surviving beyond time t, $S(t)$. Similarly as above we define $P_i = P_{0,i}$ for $i = 1, ..., K$.

Below follows some general formulas for how one can compute the transition probabilities for a multi-state model. These are then specialized to the competing risks model when specifying the underlying Nelson-Aalen estimates. The transition probability matrix can be written as

$$P(0,t) = \prod_{s \in]0,t]} (I + dA(s)),$$

where A is the matrix of cumulative intensities with $A_{0,k} = \int_0^t \alpha_k(s)ds$, $k = 1, ..., K$, and $A_{k,k} = -\sum_{j \neq k} A_{k,j}$ for $k = 0, 1, ..., K$; and all other cumulatives are zero. Define also the equivalent transitions intensities $\alpha_{0,k}(s) = \alpha_k(s)$ for $k = 1, ..., K$, and minus the intensity out of state k $\alpha_{k,k}(s) = -\sum_{j \neq k} \alpha_{k,j}(s)$ for $k = 0, 1, ..., K$, and let all other transitions intensities by zero.

This suggests, with an estimator $\hat{A}$ of A, that we can estimate $P(0,t)$ by

$$\hat{P}(0,t) = \prod_{s \in [0,t]} \left(I + d\hat{A}(s) \right), \tag{10.4}$$

which is referred to as the product-limit estimator of $P(0,t)$. To estimate A we use the Nelson-Aalen estimator. By looking at the estimators more closely it follows that the two estimators (10.2) and (the relevant part of) (10.4) are equivalent. Therefore the variance for (10.2) follows from the general expression for the product integration estimator that we give below.

Define $A_{j,k}^*(t) = \int_0^t J(s)\alpha_{j,k}(s)ds$, organize these in the matrix A^*, and define

$$P^*(0,t) = \prod_{s \in [0,t]} (I + dA^*(s)).$$

Then it follows from the properties of product integration, see Gill & Johansen (1990), that

$$\hat{P}(0,t) - P^*(0,t) = \int_0^t \hat{P}(0, s-) d\left(\hat{A} - A^*\right)(s) \hat{P}^*(s,t),$$

which is a product of matrices integrated over time. This equation implies that

$$\hat{P}(0,t) P^*(0,t)^{-1} - I = \int_0^t \hat{P}(0, s-) d\left(\hat{A} - A^*\right)(s) \hat{P}^*(0,s)^{-1},$$

and since $\hat{A} - A^*$ is a martingale the asymptotic properties follows from the martingale central limit theorem, similarly to the derivations for the

10. Competing Risks Model

Kaplan-Meier estimator. One obvious consequence is that the estimator is unbiased in the sense that

$$E(\hat{P}(0,t)P^*(0,t)^{-1}) = I.$$

For a general multi-state model the (co)variance of the matrix valued estimates in $\hat{P}$ becomes a $K^2 \times K^2$ matrix, and to calculate each of the covariate terms one must keep track of the appropriate terms if for example the optional variation estimator is used. Let $\text{cov}(\hat{P}(0,t))$ be the covariance of the $K^2 \times 1$ vector with the columns of $\hat{P}$ stacked on top of each other. Then a consistent estimator of $\text{cov}(\hat{P}(0,t))$ is

$$\int_0^t \hat{P}^T(s,t) \otimes \hat{P}(0,s) d[\hat{A} - A^*](s) \hat{P}(s,t) \otimes \hat{P}^T(0,s).$$

Reading the formula for the special terms we have interest in for the competing risks model we find that the covariance between $P_{0,i} - P_{0,i}^*$ and $P_{0,j} - P_{0,j}^*$ for $i, j = 0, ..., K$ can be estimated by

$$\sum_{l=1}^K \int_0^t \hat{P}_{0,0}^2(0,s)(\delta_{lj} - \hat{P}_{0,j}(s,t))(\delta_{lr} - \hat{P}_{0,r}(s,t)) \frac{J(s)}{Y_\cdot^2(s)} dN_{\cdot l}(s)$$

using $\delta_{uv} = I(u = v)$, thus leading to the variance estimates

$$\int_0^t \left\{ \hat{P}_{0,0}(0,s)\hat{P}_{0,j}(s,t) \right\}^2 \frac{J(s)}{Y_\cdot^2(s)} dN_\cdot(s)$$
$$+ \int_0^t \hat{P}_{0,0}^2(s) \left\{ 1 - 2\hat{P}_{0,j}(s,t) \right\} \frac{J(s)}{Y_\cdot^2(s)} dN_{\cdot,j}(s)$$

for $j = 1, ..., K$.

Let us consider the situation where the cause-specific hazards depend on covariates so that for example the hazard for cause k for subject i given covariates relevant for cause k, $\tilde{X}_{ik}$ (of dimension p), is on Cox form

$$\alpha_k(t) = \alpha_{0k}(t) \exp(\tilde{X}_{ik}^T \beta_k).$$

In the latter display β_k are the relative risk regression coefficients related to cause k, $\alpha_{0k}(t)$ is the baseline function for cause k, and $\tilde{X}_{ik}$ denotes a cause specific version of the covariates, which gives a great deal of flexibility. This model can be written with a common set of relative risk parameters if the covariates are stacked. With the appropriate choice of X_{ik} we can write the model as

$$\alpha_k(t) = \alpha_{0k}(t) \exp(X_{ik}^T \beta).$$

In the case where all causes depend on the same covariates in the same functional form, $\tilde{X}_{ik} = X_i$, and the relative risk parameters are different

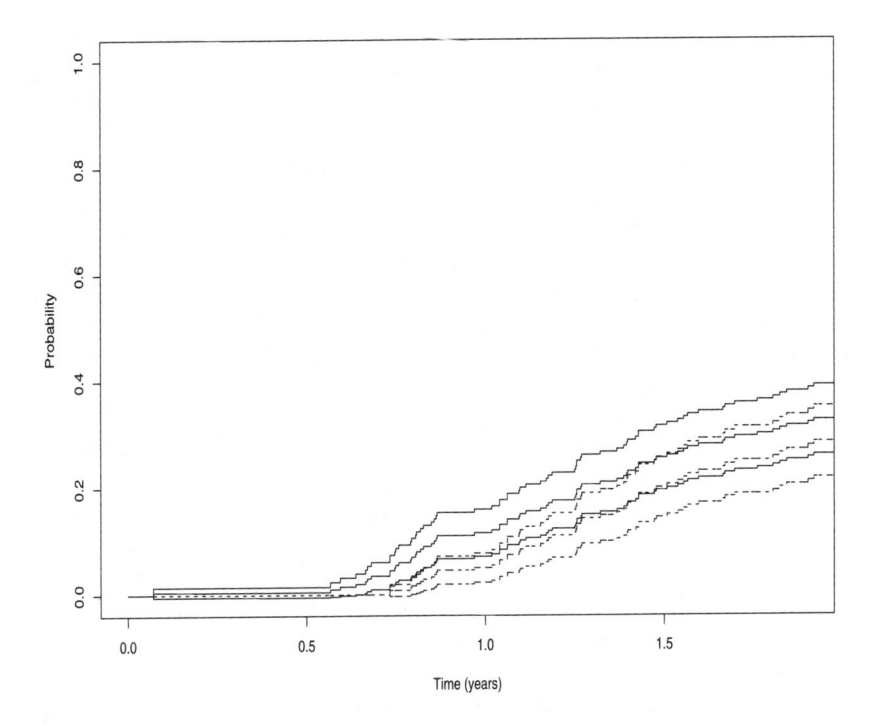

FIGURE 10.3: Mouse Leukemia data. Cumulative incidence probability along with 95% pointwise confidence intervals for thymic leukemia data without covariates (full lines) and with covariates (MHC=1, Sex=2,Color=1, Antibody=50,Virus=8000) (broken lines).

then $X_{ik} = (I(k=1)X_i^T, ..., I(k=K)X_i^T)^T$ is a covariate vector of dimension Kp and $\beta = (\beta_1^T, ..., \beta_K^T)^T$ is the regression coefficient vector with β_k the p dimensional regression effect for cause k.

One may now estimate the relative risk parameters and the cumulative baseline functions for all cause specific hazards and combine these as above to estimate the cumulative incidence function by for example the product limit estimator. This is simply a matter of noting that the cumulative hazard for cause k given covariates X is estimated by

$$\hat{A}_{0k}(t) \exp(X_k^T \hat{\beta}),$$

where X_k is the stacked version of the X covariate that reflects the cause specific version of the covariates and then the product limit estimator may be applied to estimate the cumulative incidence function given X_k: $P_1(t|X_k)$. We illustrate these estimators in the following example.

Example 10.1.1 (Mouse Leukemia data)

Consider the mouse leukemia data given in Kalbfleisch & Prentice (2002) where the effect of various genetic and viral factors on the development of leukemia is studied. The data comprise 204 mice and the covariates that we consider here are MHC phenotype (1 and 2), Sex (1=male, 2=female), Coat color (1 and 2), antibody level in percent (Antibody) and virus level (Virus). The different causes of death were thymic leukemia (1), nonthymic leukemia (2), nonleukemia and no other tumors (3), unknown (4), other tumors (5), and accidental death (6). We here consider just the thymic leukemia as the cause of death of interest and group all other causes into one group (2). We used a SAS-macro developed by Rosthøj et al. (2004) to compute the cumulative incidence curves.

First we show the simple product limit estimator with 95% confidence intervals (full lines) in Figure 10.3. For comparison we also computed a covariate based cumulative incidence probability function correcting for all covariates. The product limit estimator based on different Cox regression models for the cause of interest and other causes are shown with 95% pointwise confidence intervals (broken lines) in Figure 10.3 and computed for a MHC=1, Sex=2, color=1, antibody=50 and virus=8000.

Figure 10.3 clearly illustrates that the predictions of the probability of dying of thymic leukemia is much lower for a subject with the specified covariates than the overall probability. It is hard, however, to precisely summarize the importance of covariate effects apart from computing the cumulative incidence probability for various combinations of the covariates. We address how to summarize covariate effects in the two coming sections.

□

Note, that any regression model may in principle be applied to model the cause specific hazards and many models have been used: Shen & Cheng (1999) studied the predicted cumulative incidence function based on a proportional hazards model; Cheng et al. (1998) considered the semiparametric additive risk model; Scheike & Zhang (2003) used the Cox-Aalen survival model. We consider the Cox-Aalen model in further detail in the next section.

10.2 Cause specific hazards modeling

In this section we show how to estimate the cumulative incidence function based on cause specific hazards modeling, and how to derive the asymptotic properties of the estimators. We use the Cox-Aalen model because the obtained formulas generalize both those obtained based on the Cox regression model and those based on the Aalen additive hazards model. We also show

10.2 Cause specific hazards modeling

how to get uniform confidence band for the cumulative incidence function based on a resampling technique.

Assume that we have underlying covariates $\tilde{X}$. The cause specific hazards for the kth cause is modeled as

$$\lambda_k(t|X_k, Z_k) = \left[X_k^T \alpha(t)\right] \exp(Z_k^T \beta).$$

with $\alpha(t) = (\alpha_1(t), ..., \alpha_p(t))$ and $\beta = (\beta_1, ..., \beta_p)$ and where we have a cause specific version of the covariates, as at the end of the previous section, such that X_k and Z_k are of dimension p and q, respectively. Note that one possible submodel allows all cause specific hazards to have different regression effects and the same partitioning of the covariates into X with additive effects and Z with multiplicative effects such that $\lambda_k(t|X, Z) = \left[X^T \alpha_k(t)\right] \exp(Z^T \beta_k)$.

Let

$$(N_{i1}(t), \ldots N_{iK}), \quad i = 1, \ldots, n,$$

be n independent counting processes of dimension K with intensities

$$\lambda_{ik}(t) = Y_i(t)\lambda_k(t|X_{ik}, Z_{ik}),$$

where $Y_i(t)$ is 0 or 1 indicating whether the individual is at risk at time t. Let $\Lambda_{ik}(t) = \int_0^t \lambda_{ik}(s)ds$ so that $M_{ik}(t) = N_{ik}(t) - \Lambda_{ik}(t)$ are martingales. Let further

$$N_k(t) = (N_{1k}(t), \ldots, N_{nk}(t))^T$$

be a n-dimensional counting process, with compensator

$$\Lambda_k(t) = (\Lambda_{1k}(t), \ldots, \Lambda_{nk}(t))^T$$

and with

$$M_k(t) = (M_{1k}(t), \ldots, M_{nk}(t))^T$$

the n-dimensional martingale for the k specific cause. Let $N(t)$ be the $n \cdot K$ dimensional counting process defined as

$$N(t) = (N_1^T(t), ..., N_K^T(t))^T,$$

and define its compensator and the resulting martingale similarly. Organize the cause specific covariates into matrices $X_k(t)$ (with rows $Y_i(t)X_{ik}$) and $Z_k(t)$ (with rows $Y_i(t)Z_{ik}$) and stack these into matrices $X(t)$ (of dimension $nK \times p$) and $Z(t)$ (of dimension $nK \times q$). Define the generalized inverse

$$Y^-(t) = Y^-(\beta, t) = \left[X^T(t)\text{diag}\left\{\exp(Z(t)\beta)\right\} X(t)\right]^{-1} X^T(t)$$

where $\exp(b) = (\exp(b_1), \ldots \exp(b_r))^T$ for a $r \times 1$-vector b. We estimate β as the solution to the score equation (see Section 7.1 for details)

$$U(\beta, \tau) = \int_0^\tau \left[Z^T(t) - Z^T(t)Y(\beta, t)Y^-(\beta, t)\right] dN(u) = 0,$$

and estimate $A(t) = \int_0^t \alpha(u)du$ by

$$\widehat{A}(t) = \int_0^t Y^-(\hat{\beta}, u)dN(u).$$

The derivative of minus the score function is given by

$$\mathcal{I}(\beta, \tau) = \int_0^\tau Z^T(t)\text{diag}(Y(\beta, t)Y^-(\beta, t)dN(t))Z(t)$$
$$- \int_0^\tau Z^T(t)Y(\beta, t)Y^-(\beta, t)\text{diag}\left\{Y(\beta, t)Y^-(\beta, t)dN(t)\right\}Z(t).$$

To predict the cumulative incidence function for a subject with covariates (x, z) we define

$$\Lambda(t|x, z) = \sum_{k=1}^K \Lambda_k(t|x_k, z_k) = \sum_{k=1}^K \int_0^t \lambda_k(s|x_k, z_k)ds$$
$$S(t|x, z) = P(T > t|x, z) = \exp\left\{-\Lambda(t|x, z)\right\}.$$

Then the conditional cumulative incidence function for the kth cause is defined as

$$P_k(t|x, z) = P(T \le t, \varepsilon = k|x, z) = \int_0^t S(s|x, z)\lambda_k(s|x_k, z_k)ds,$$

where ε represents the type of failure.

We estimate the cumulative incidence function by plugging in the estimates of the cause specific Cox-Aalen models:

$$\widehat{\Lambda}(t|x_k, z_k) = \sum_{k=1}^K \widehat{\Lambda}_k(t|x_k, z_k) = \sum_{k=1}^K \int_0^t \exp(z_k^T \hat{\beta}) x_k^T d\widehat{A}(s)$$
$$\widehat{S}(t|x, z) = \exp(-\widehat{\Lambda}(t|x, z))$$

giving

$$\widehat{P}_k(t|x, z) = \int_0^t \widehat{S}(s-|x, z)d\widehat{\Lambda}_k(s|x_k, z_k), \tag{10.5}$$

where $\widehat{S}(t-|x, z)$ is the left-continuous version of $\widehat{S}(t|x, z)$. The estimator (10.5) is a functional of $\widehat{A}$ and $\hat{\beta}$ and the asymptotic properties can therefore be derived from those of the underlying model. In the below note we give some of the main derivations that lead to a relatively simple estimator of the variance given in (10.6). As we have seen, cause specific hazards modeling and estimation can be employed to estimate the cumulative incidence function of interest $P_1(t|x, z)$, say. It is important to notice, however,

10.2 Cause specific hazards modeling

that we need to model and perform estimation also for the other cause specific hazards $\lambda_k(t)$, $k = 2, \ldots, K$, that may be of no interest. If the target for the analysis is the cumulative incidence function, then the subdistribution approach described in the next section is more direct and it does not need modeling for the other causes. The downside of the subdistribution approach is that modeling of the censoring distribution is required.

Note. Large sample properties, see also Exercise 10.6.

The basic properties of the parameters of the Cox-Aalen can be found in Section 7.1 but we here briefly summarize these (up to $o_p(n^{-1/2})$) in this slightly different set-up. It follows that

$$n^{1/2}(\hat{\beta} - \beta_0) = n^{1/2}\mathcal{I}^{-1}(\beta_0, \tau) \sum_{i=1}^{n} W_{1i}(\tau) + o_p(1),$$

$$n^{1/2}(\widehat{A}(\hat{\beta}, t) - A(t)) = n^{1/2} \sum_{i=1}^{n} W_{2i}(t) + o_p(1),$$

where

$$W_{1i}(\tau) = \sum_{k=1}^{K} \int_0^\tau (Z_{ik}(s)$$
$$- Z^T(s) Y(\beta_0, s) \left[X^T(t) \text{diag}\{\exp(Z(s)\beta)\} X(t) \right]^{-1} X_{ik}(s)^T) dM_{ik}(s),$$

and

$$W_{2i}(t) = W_{3i}(t) - H(\beta_0, t) \mathcal{I}(\beta_0, \tau)^{-1} W_{1i}(\tau),$$

$$W_{3i}(t) = \sum_{k=1}^{K} \int_0^t \left[X^T(s) \text{diag}\{\exp(Z(s)\beta)\} X(s) \right]^{-1} X_{ik}(s) dM_{ik}(s),$$

and with

$$H(\beta, t) = \int_0^t Y^-(\beta, s) \text{diag}(Y(\beta, s) Y^-(\beta, s) dN(s)) Z(s).$$

Further (up to $o_p(1)$),

$$n^{1/2}(\widehat{S}(t|x, z) - S(t|x, z)) = -S(t|x, z) n^{1/2} \left\{ \sum_{k=1}^{K} \widehat{\Lambda}_k(t|x, z) - \Lambda_k(t|x, z) \right\}$$

$$= -S(t|x, z) n^{1/2} \sum_{i=1}^{n} \left\{ \sum_{k=1}^{K} W_{4i}(t|x, z, k) \right\},$$

since $n^{1/2}(\hat{\Lambda}_k(t|x, z) - \Lambda_k(t|x, z))$ is asymptotically equivalent to

$$n^{1/2} \sum_i W_{4i}(t|x, z, k)$$

with

$$W_{4i}(t|x,z,k) = \exp\{Z_k^T \beta_0\} X_k^T A(t) Z_k^T \mathcal{I}^{-1}(\beta_0, \tau) W_{1i}(\tau)$$
$$- \exp\{Z_k^T \beta_0\} X_k^T H(\beta_0, t) \mathcal{I}^{-1}(\beta_0, \tau) W_{1i}(\tau) + \exp\{Z_k^T \beta_0\} X_k^T W_{3i}(t),$$

by a Taylor series expansion of $\Lambda_k(t) = \exp(Z_k^T \beta) X_k^T B(t)$.

Now, considering the cumulative incidence function using partial integration we can write $\widehat{P}_k(t|x,z) - P_k(t|x,z)$ (up to $o_p(n^{-1/2})$) as

$$\int_0^t \widehat{S}(u|x,z) d\left\{\widehat{\Lambda}_k(u|x,z) \Lambda_k(u|x,z)\right\}$$
$$+ \int_0^t \left\{\widehat{S}(u|x,z) - S(u|x,z)\right\} d\Lambda_k(u|x,z)$$
$$= \int_0^t \left(1 - \sum_{l \neq k} P_l(u|x,z)\right) d\widetilde{M}_{k,\Lambda}(u|x,z) - P_k(t|x,z) \int_0^t \sum_{l=1}^K d\widetilde{M}_{l,\Lambda}(u|x,z)$$
$$+ \int_0^t P_k(u|x,z) \sum_{l \neq k} d\widetilde{M}_{l,\Lambda}(u|x,z),$$

where $\widetilde{M}_{k,\Lambda}(u|x,z) = \widehat{\Lambda}_k(t|x,z) - \Lambda_k(t|x,z)$ was decomposed into the form $M(t) + B(t)M(\tau)$ above. One can therefore give an optional variation based estimator of the variance of $\widehat{P}_k(t|x,z) - P_k(t|x,z)$ (see Scheike & Zhang (2003)), but we here for simplicity give an estimator based on the i.i.d. representation.

Note that $n^{1/2}\left(\widehat{P}_k(t|x,z) - P_k(t|x,z)\right)$ is asymptotically equivalent to

$$n^{1/2} \sum_{i=1}^n W_{k,5i}(t|x,z),$$

where

$$W_{k,5i}(t|x,z) = \int_0^t \left(1 - \sum_{l \neq k} P_l(u|x,z)\right) dW_{k,4i}(u|x,z)$$
$$- P_k(t|x,z) \sum_{l=1}^K W_{l,4i}(t|x,z) + \int_0^t P_k(u|x,z) \sum_{l \neq k} dW_{l,4i}(u|x,z).$$

Define its estimate $\widehat{W}_{k,5i}(t|x,z)$ by plugging in estimates of the unknown quantities.

Then the variance of $n^{1/2}\left(\widehat{P}_k(t|x,z) - P_k(t|x,z)\right)$ can be consistently estimated by

$$\widehat{\sigma}^2_{P_k}(t|x,z) = n \sum_{i=1}^n \left(\widehat{W}_{k,5i}(t|x,z)\right)^2. \tag{10.6}$$

Again, the confidence band for the predicted cumulative incidence function $P_k(t|x,z)$ can be constructed using the resampling approach based on

$$\sum_{i=1}^{n} G_i \hat{W}_{k,5i}(t|x,z)$$

where $G_1, ..., G_n$ are i.i.d. standard normals.

10.3 Subdistribution approach

The aim of the subdistribution approach is to express the effects of covariates directly on the cumulative incidence function

$$P_1(t|X) = P(T \leq t, \varepsilon = 1|X),$$

here focusing on cause 1. This is done via the *subdistribution hazard function* $\lambda_1^\star(t|X)$ that is the function so that

$$P_1(t|X) = 1 - \exp(-\int_0^t \lambda_1^\star(s|X)\,ds).$$

Equivalently,

$$\lambda_1^\star(t;|X) = -\frac{d}{dt}(\log\{1 - P_1(t|X)\})$$
$$= \lim_{\Delta t \to 0} \frac{P(t \leq T < t + \Delta t, \varepsilon = 1 \,|\, (T \geq t) \cup (T \leq t, \varepsilon \neq 1), X)}{\Delta t}.$$

One may also think of $\lambda_1^\star(t|X)$ as the hazard function of

$$T^\star = T \times I(\varepsilon = 1) + \infty \times I(\varepsilon \neq 1),$$

which has distribution function equal to $P_1(t|X)$, $t < \infty$, and a point mass at $t = \infty$. This is seen by noticing that

$$P(T^\star > t|X) = P(T > t|X) + P_2(t|X) + ... + P_K(t|X) = 1 - P_1(t|X).$$

Subdistribution hazards was originally considered by Gray (1988), see also Pepe (1991). Fine & Gray (1999) gave estimators and large sample properties in the case, where the Cox model is assumed for the subdistribution hazard corresponding to cause 1.

We assume that the subdistribution hazard is on the Cox-Aalen form

$$\lambda_1^\star(t|x,z) = [X^T \alpha(t)] \exp(Z^T \beta),$$

where we have partitioned the covariates into X and Z. We then cover both the additive and multiplicative models.

362   10. Competing Risks Model

If there is no censoring of the survival time, then $N_1(t) = I(T \leq t, \varepsilon = 1)$ has compensator

$$\int_0^t Y(s) \lambda_1^\star(s|x, z) \, ds$$

with respect to the filtration

$$\sigma(N_1(s), X, Z; s \leq t),$$

where $Y(t) = 1 - N_1(t-)$, see Exercise 10.4. Note that $Y(t) = 1$ as long as the subject has not failed due to cause 1 before time t; that is, the subject stays "at risk" even if it has failed from a cause different from 1. The unknown parameters of the Cox-Aalen model for the subdistribution hazards may thus (in the case of no censoring) be estimated as outlined in Section 7.1 with the appropriate at risk indicators as outlined above. In the case of censoring, one can apply the inverse probability censoring weighting, see for example Horvitz & Thompson (1952) and Robins & Rotnitzky (1992). This technique is based on estimating the probability of being censored for each subject and then correcting the score equation by inverse weighting with these probabilities.

We assume for simplicity that the censoring variable C is independent of both the survival time T and the covariates X, Z, but the below formulas may be extended by modeling of the censoring distribution given X, Z. Let

$$N_{i1}(t) = I(T_i \leq t, \varepsilon_i = 1), \ Y_i(t) = 1 - N_{i1}(t-), \ G_c(t) = P(C \geq t),$$

and let $\widehat{G}_c$ be the Kaplan-Meier estimator of G_c. Note that $N_i(t)$ and $Y_i(t)$ typically will not be fully observed when there is censoring, and that the at risk indicator is 1 as long as no type 1 event has occurred. We assume that we observe n i.i.d. subjects from this generic model. Further define

$$r_i(t) = I(C_i \geq T_i \wedge t),$$

that is one when the subject is un-censored. Note that if $r_i(t) = 1$, then $N_i(t)$ and $Y_i(t)$ are computable up to time t, and if $r_i(t) = 0$, then individuals are observed up to time C_i; thus $N_i(t)$ and $Y_i(t)$ are not observable. However, $r_i(t)N_i(t)$ and $r_i(t)Y_i(t)$ are always computable.

Define a time-dependent weight function

$$w_i(t) = r_i(t) \widehat{G}_c(t) / \widehat{G}_c(T_i \wedge t)$$

and define the $(n \times p)$-matrix $Y_w(\beta, t)$ with ith row

$$w_i(t) Y_i(t) \exp\left\{Z_i(t)^T \beta\right\} X_i(t)$$

for $i = 1, \ldots, n$. Let

$$Z(t) = (Z_1(t), \ldots, Z_n(t))^T, \ X(t) = (X_1(t), \ldots, X_n(t))^T,$$

and
$$Y_w^-(\beta,t) = \left(Y_w(\beta,t)^T W_A(t) Y_w(\beta,t)\right)^{-1} Y_w(\beta,t)^T W_A(t),$$
be a weighted generalized inverse of $Y_w(\beta,t)$. The weight matrix $W_A(t)$ is a $n \times n$-matrix with diagonal elements
$$w_i^A(t) = w_i^{-1}(t) Y_i(t) \exp\{-Z_i(t)^T \beta\}.$$
With the convention that $0/0 = 0$ such that the effect of $w_i^A(t)$ is that it cancels out $w_i(t)\exp(Z_i(t)^T\beta)$.

We estimate $\hat{\beta}$ as the solution to the estimating equation $U(\hat{\beta},\tau) = 0$, where
$$U(\beta,\tau) = \int_0^\tau \left(Z(t)^T - Z(t)^T Y_w(\beta,t) Y_w^-(\beta,t)\right) \operatorname{diag}(w_i(t)) dN(t),$$
$$= \sum_{i=1}^n \int_0^\tau V_i^w(\beta,t) w_i(t) dN_i(t)$$
with τ the end of study time and
$$V_i^w(\beta,t) = Z_i(t) - Z(t)^T Y_w(\beta,t) \left(Y_w(\beta,t)^T W_A(t) Y_w(\beta,t)\right)^{-1} X_i(t).$$
The derivative of minus the score function is given as
$$\mathcal{I}(\beta,t) = -\frac{\partial}{\partial \beta} U(\beta,t)$$
$$= \int_0^t Z^T(u) \operatorname{diag}\left(Y_w(\beta,u) Y_w^-(\beta,u) dN_w(t)\right) Z(u)$$
$$- \int_0^t Z^T(u) Y_w(\beta,u) Y_w^-(\beta,u) \operatorname{diag}\left(Y_w(\beta,u) Y_w^-(\beta,u) dN_w(u)\right) Z(u),$$
where $N_w(t) = \operatorname{diag}(w_i(t)) N(t)$.

It can be shown that $n^{1/2}(\hat{\beta} - \beta_0)$ is asymptotically normal with an asymptotic variance that is consistently estimated by
$$\widehat{\Sigma} = n \left(\mathcal{I}(\hat{\beta},\tau)\right)^{-1} \left(\sum_{i=1}^n \widehat{W}_{5i}^{\otimes 2}\right) \left(\mathcal{I}(\hat{\beta},\tau)\right)^{-1},$$
where $\widehat{W}_{5i}$ is given by the below (10.8). We estimate $A(t) = \int_0^t \alpha(s) ds$ by
$$\widehat{A}(\hat{\beta},t) = \int_0^t Y_w^-(\hat{\beta},s) dN_w(s).$$
Similarly, it can be shown that $n^{1/2}\left(\widehat{A}(\hat{\beta},t) - A(t)\right)$ converges in distribution towards a Gaussian process with variance that may be estimated consistently by
$$\hat{\Phi}(t) = n \sum_{i=1}^n \widehat{W}_{6i}^{\otimes 2}(t),$$

where $\widetilde{W}_{6i}(t)$ is given below by (10.9). The i.i.d. decomposition leading to the above variance estimators is more complicated than the one for the standard Cox-Aalen model because of the estimated weights that give an additional variance term.

The cumulative incidence function $P_1(t|X, Z)$ may then be estimated by

$$\widehat{P}_1(t|X, Z) = 1 - \exp\left\{-\int_0^t \exp\{Z^T\hat{\beta}\} X^T d\widehat{A}(\hat{\beta}, s)\right\},$$

and it may be shown that $n^{1/2}\left(\widehat{P}_1(t|X, Z) - P_1(t|X, Z)\right)$ converges towards a Gaussian process with a variance that can be consistently estimated by

$$\hat{\sigma}_{P_1}^2(t|X, Z) = n\sum_{i=1}^n \widehat{W}_{7i}(t|X, Z)^2,$$

where W_{7i} is defined in (10.12) below. To construct confidence bands one may also use a resampling approach.

Example 10.3.1 (Mouse Leukemia data, continued)

Consider again the mouse leukemia data described in Example 10.1.1, where the effect of various genetic and viral factors on the development of leukemia is studied. We consider thymic leukemia as the cause of death of interest and group all other causes into one group. The subdistribution method is implemented using the Cox-model in the R-package cmprsk. As an illustration we model the subdistribution hazard for thymic leukemia using the Cox model with the covariates Sex (S) (1:female; 0: male), Antibody (A) (1: ≥ 0.5; 0: <0.5) and Virus (V) (1: <10000; 0:≥ 10000). That is the cumulative incidence function is assumed to be

$$P(t|S, A, V) = 1 - \exp\{-\Lambda_0(t)\exp(\beta_S S + \beta_A A + \beta_V V)\}.$$

```
> antibody<-1*(leukdat$antib>=0.5)
> Sex<-leukdat$sex-1
> virusd<-1*(leukdat$virus<10000)
> status1<-leukdat$J
> status1[leukdat$delta==2]<-0
> cov<-as.matrix(cbind(Sex,antibody,virusd))
> fitsub<-crr(leukdat$time/365, status1,cov)
29 cases omitted due to missing values
> print(fitsub)
convergence:   TRUE
coefficients:
[1]   0.09931 -0.45530 -2.34000
standard errors:
[1] 0.2931 0.2977 0.4167
two-sided p-values:
```

10.3 Subdistribution approach

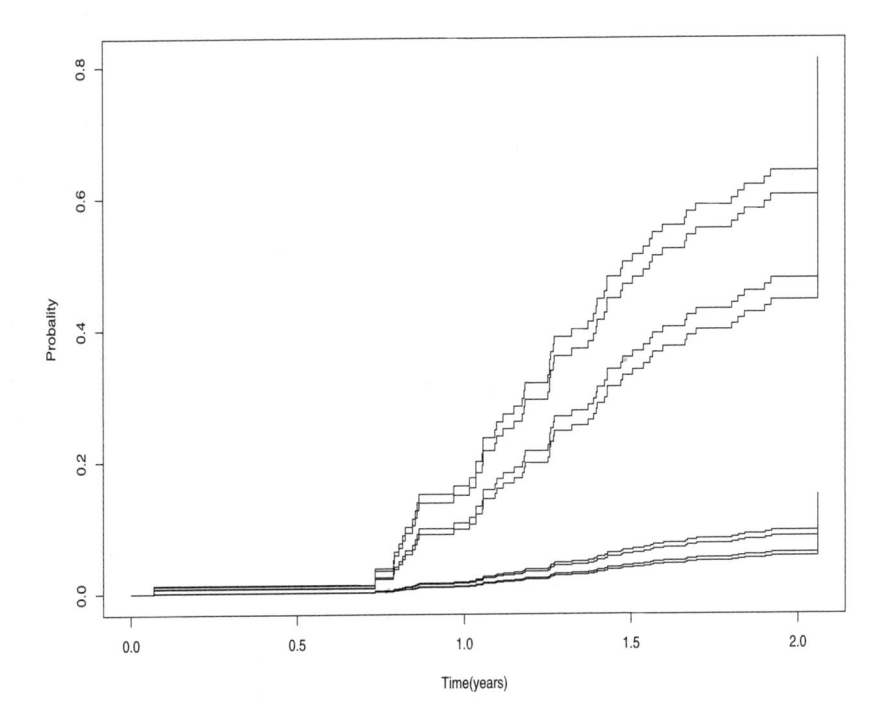

FIGURE 10.4: Mouse Leukemia data. Predicted incidence probability functions based on Cox model for subdistribution hazards (see text).

```
[1] 7.3e-01 1.3e-01 2.0e-08
> P.thymic <- predict(fitsub,rbind(c(1,1,1),c(1,1,0),c(1,0,1),
+                    c(1,0,0),c(0,1,1),c(0,1,0),c(0,0,1),c(0,0,0)))
> plot(P.thymic,lty=1,ylab='Probability',xlab='Time(years)')
```

From this analysis it appears that Virus (dichotomized) is the only important predictor with the above reported p-value. The estimated coefficients with estimated standard errors are $\hat{\beta}_S = 0.099(0.293)$, $\hat{\beta}_A = -0.455(0.298)$, and $\hat{\beta}_V = -2.340(0.417)$. From Figure 10.4 it is seen that the predicted cumulative incidence functions fall in four groups (reflecting the unimportance of the covariate Sex); the upper two groups being those with Virus above 10000. The upper two curves has Virus above 10000 and Antibody below 0.5. □

Note. Subdistribution: large sample properties.

We here give a sketch of how to derive the large sample properties. Many of the considered processes are not martingales and some results must be

10. Competing Risks Model

based on empirical process theory. Martingale asymptotics can nevertheless be invoked in various places. Additional details can be found in Fine & Gray (1999) who studied the Cox model and Scheike & Zhang (2004) who used the Cox-Aalen model.

A Taylor expansion yields

$$n^{1/2}\left(\hat{\beta}-\beta_0\right) \approx \left(n^{-1}\mathcal{I}(\beta_0,\tau)\right)^{-1}\left(n^{-1/2}U(\beta_0,\tau)\right)$$

with $\approx$ (here and in the sequel of this note) indicating that lower order terms are asymptotically negligible. Let $M_i^1(t,\beta_0) = N_i(t) - H_i(t,\beta_0)$, where $\Lambda_i(t,\beta_0) = \int_0^t Y_i(s)\exp(Z_i^T\beta_0)X_i^T(s)dA(s)$ and $A(t) = \int_0^t \alpha(s)ds$. Denote $\widetilde{w}_i(t) = r_i(t)G_c(t)/G_c(T_i \wedge t)$. We then have

$$n^{-1/2}U(\beta_0,\tau)$$

$$= n^{-1/2}\sum_{i=1}^n \int_0^\tau V_i^w(\beta_0,t)w_i(t)dM_i^1(t,\beta_0)$$

$$\approx n^{-1/2}\sum_{i=1}^n \int_0^\tau V_i^w(\beta_0,t)\widetilde{w}_i(t)dM_i^1(t,\beta_0) \qquad (10.7)$$

$$+ n^{-1/2}\sum_{i=1}^n \int_0^\tau \left\{\frac{\widehat{G}_c(t)}{\widehat{G}_c(T_i \wedge t)} - \frac{G_c(t)}{G_c(T_i \wedge t)}\right\} V_i^w(\beta_0,t)r_i(t)dM_i^1(t,\beta_0).$$

Let also $U_i = T_i \wedge C_i$. Note that all $G_c(T_i \wedge t)$ in the above expression can be replaced with $G_c(U_i \wedge t)$ because of $r_i(t)$. Let $\Lambda^C(t)$ be the cumulative hazard function of censoring distribution, define the censoring indicator $\Delta_i = I(T_i \leq C_i)$ and let $N_i^C(t) = I(U_i \leq t, \Delta_i = 0)$ so that

$$M_i^C(t) = N_i^C(t) - \int_0^t I(U_i \geq s)d\Lambda^C(s).$$

Then we have

$$\frac{\widehat{G}_c(t)}{\widehat{G}_c(U_i \wedge t)} - \frac{G_c(t)}{G_c(U_i \wedge t)} \approx -\frac{G_c(t)I(U_i < t)}{G_c(U_i \wedge t)}\sum_{j=1}^n \int_{U_i}^t \frac{dM_j^C(s)}{\sum_k I(U_k \geq s)}.$$

The second term of (10.7) can be approximated by

$$-n^{-1/2}\sum_{i=1}^n \int_0^\tau \frac{G_c(t)I(U_i<t)}{G_c(U_i\wedge t)}$$

$$\times \sum_j \int_{U_i}^t \frac{dM_j^C(s)}{\sum_k I(U_k \geq s)}V_i^w(\beta_0,t)r_i(t)dM_i^1(t,\beta_0)$$

$$\approx n^{-1/2}\sum_{i=1}^n \int_0^\tau \frac{q(t)}{\pi(t)}dM_i^C(t),$$

where

$$q(t) = -\lim_p n^{-1}\sum_{i=1}^n \int_0^\tau V_i^w(\beta_0,s)w_i(s)I(s\geq\!\!> t)I(U_i<s)dM_i^1(s,\beta_0)I(t>U_i),$$

$$\pi(t) = \lim_p n^{-1}\sum_{i=1}^n I(U_i \geq t),$$

10.3 Subdistribution approach

where $\lim_p$ is the limit in probability as n tends to infinity. Define also

$$\hat{\pi}(t) = n^{-1} \sum_{i=1}^{n} I(U_i \geq t)$$

$$\widehat{M}_i^1(t, \beta_0) = N_i(t) - \int_0^t Y_i(s) \exp\left\{Z_i^T(s)\hat{\beta}\right\} X_i^T(s) d\widehat{A}(\hat{\beta}, s),$$

$$\widehat{A}(\hat{\beta}, t) = \int_0^t Y_w^-(\hat{\beta}, s) dN_w(s),$$

$$\widehat{M}_i^C(t) = N_i^C(t) - \int_0^t I(U_i \geq s) d\widehat{\Lambda}^C(s),$$

$$\widehat{\Lambda}^C(t) = \sum_{i=1}^{n} \int_0^t \frac{Y_i(t)}{\hat{\pi}(t)} dN_i^C(t),$$

and where $\hat{q}$ is obtained by using $\widehat{M}_i^1$ and $\hat{\beta}$ in q.

It can be shown that $n^{-1/2} U(\beta_0, \tau)$ converges in distribution to a normal random variable with zero mean and a variance that can be estimated by

$$n^{-1} \sum_{i=1}^{n} \widehat{W}_{5i}^{\otimes 2} = n^{-1} \sum_{i=1}^{n} \left(\hat{\eta}_i + \hat{\psi}_i\right)^{\otimes 2}, \tag{10.8}$$

where

$$\hat{\eta}_i = \int_0^\tau V_i^w(\hat{\beta}, t) w_i(t) d\widehat{M}_i^1(t, \hat{\beta}) \quad \text{and} \quad \hat{\psi}_i = \int_0^\tau \frac{\hat{q}(t)}{\hat{\pi}(t)} d\widehat{M}_i^C(t).$$

The asymptotic variance of $n^{1/2}\left(\hat{\beta} - \beta_0\right)$ can be estimated by

$$\widehat{\Sigma} = n\left(\mathcal{I}(\hat{\beta}, \tau)\right)^{-1} \left(\sum_{i=1}^{n} \widehat{W}_{5i}^{\otimes 2}\right) \left(\mathcal{I}(\hat{\beta}, \tau)\right)^{-1}.$$

Consider

$$n^{1/2}\left(\widehat{A}(\hat{\beta}, t) - A(t)\right) = n^{1/2}\left(\int_0^t Y_w^-(\beta_0, s) dN_w(s) - \int_0^t \alpha(s) ds\right)$$
$$+ n^{1/2} \int_0^t \left(Y_w^-(\hat{\beta}, s) - Y_w^-(\beta_0, s)\right) dN_w(s).$$

The second term on the right-hand side of the above equality is asymptotically equivalent to

$$n^{1/2} \left(\int_0^t \left(\frac{\partial}{\partial \beta} Y_w^-(\beta_0, s)\right) dN_w(s)\right)^T \left(\hat{\beta} - \beta_0\right)$$
$$= n^{1/2} \sum_{i=1}^{n} P_w(\hat{\beta}, t) \mathcal{I}^{-1}(\hat{\beta}, \tau) \widehat{W}_{5i},$$

where

$$P_w(\beta, t) = -\int_0^t Y_w^-(\beta, s) \text{diag}\left(Y_w(\beta, s) Y_w^-(\beta, s) dN_w(s)\right) Z(s),$$

368   10. Competing Risks Model

and the first term is approximated by

$$n^{1/2}\sum_{i=1}^{n}\int_{0}^{t}\left(Y_w^T(\beta_0,s)W_A(s)Y_w(\beta_0,s)\right)^{-1}X_i(s)w_i(s)dM_i^1(s,\beta_0)$$

$$=n^{1/2}\sum_{i=1}^{n}\int_{0}^{t}\left(Y_w^T(\beta_0,s)W_A(s)Y_w(\beta_0,s)\right)^{-1}X_i(s)\widetilde{w}_i(s)dM_i^1(s,\beta_0)$$

$$+n^{1/2}\sum_{i=1}^{n}\int_{0}^{t}\left\{\frac{\widehat{G}_c(s)}{\widehat{G}_c(U_i\wedge s)}-\frac{G_c(s)}{G_c(U_i\wedge s)}\right\}$$

$$\times\left(Y_w^T(\beta_0,s)W_A(s)Y_w(\beta_0,s)\right)^{-1}X_i(s)r_i(s)dM_i^1(s,\beta_0).$$

The term involving the censoring weights may be approximated as before:

$$n^{1/2}\sum_{i=1}^{n}\int_{0}^{\tau}\frac{G_c(t)I(U_i<t)}{G_c(t\wedge U_i)}\sum_{j}\int_{U_i}^{t}\frac{dM_j^C(u)}{\pi(u)}\times$$

$$\left(Y_w^T(\beta_0,t)W_A(t)Y_w(\beta_0,t)\right)^{-1}X_i(t)r_i(t)dM_i^1(t,\beta_0)$$

$$=n^{1/2}\sum_{i=1}^{n}\int_{0}^{\tau}\frac{q_A(t)}{\pi(t)}dM_i^C(t),$$

where

$$q_A(t)=-\lim_{p}n^{-1}\sum_{i=1}^{n}\int_{0}^{\tau}\left(Y_w^T(\beta_0,s)W_A(s)Y_w(\beta_0,s)\right)^{-1}$$

$$\times X_i(s)w_i(s)I(s\geq t)I(U_i<s)dM_i^1(s,\beta_0)I(t>U_i).$$

Denote

$$\widehat{W}_{6i}(t)=P_w(\hat{\beta},t)\mathcal{I}^{-1}(\hat{\beta},\tau)\widehat{W}_{5i}+\widehat{W}_{Ai}(t),\qquad(10.9)$$

with

$$\widehat{W}_{Ai}(t)=\int_{0}^{t}\frac{\widehat{q}_A(s)}{\widehat{\pi}(s)}d\widehat{M}_i^C(s)$$

$$+\int_{0}^{t}\left(Y_w^T(\hat{\beta},s)W_A(s)Y_w(\hat{\beta},s)\right)^{-1}X_i(s)w_i(s)d\widehat{M}_i^1(s,\hat{\beta}),$$

(10.10)

and with $W_{Ai}(t)$ defined similarly. Then $n^{1/2}\left(\widehat{A}(\hat{\beta},t)-A(t)\right)$ converges in distribution towards a Gaussian process with variance that is estimated consistently by

$$\hat{\Phi}(t)=n\sum_{i=1}^{n}\widehat{W}_{6i}^{\otimes 2}(t).$$

10.3 Subdistribution approach

Finally, $n^{1/2}(\widehat{P}_1(t|X,Z) - P_1(t|X,Z))$ is asymptotically equivalent to

$$(1 - P_1(t|X,Z))\left\{\int_0^t \exp(Z^T\beta_0)X^T dA(s) - \int_0^t \exp(Z^T\hat{\beta})X^T d\widehat{A}(\hat{\beta},s)\right\}$$

$$= (1 - P_1(t|X,Z))\left\{\int_0^t \exp(Z^T\beta_0)X^T d\left(\widehat{A}(\beta_0,s) - dA(s)\right)\right\}$$

$$+ (1 - P_1(t|X,Z))$$

$$\left\{\int_0^t \exp(Z^T\hat{\beta})X^T d\widehat{A}(\hat{\beta},s) - \int_0^t \exp\left\{Z^T\beta_0\right\}X^T d\widehat{A}(\beta_0,s)\right\} \quad (10.11)$$

$$\approx n^{1/2}\sum_{i=1}^n W_{7i}(t|X,Z),$$

where

$$W_{7i}(t|X,Z) = (1 - P_1(t|X,Z))\exp(\beta_0^T Z)$$
$$\times \left\{X^T W_{Ai}(t) + \left[(X^T A(t))Z^T + X^T P(\beta_0,t)\mathcal{I}^{-1}(\beta_0,\tau)\right]W_{5i}\right\}. \quad (10.12)$$

and with $\widehat{W}_{7i}(t|X,Z)$ defined by replacing all unknowns with their estimates in (10.12).

10.4 Exercises

10.1 Consider a competing risks situation with cause specific hazards $\lambda_k(t)$, $k = 1, \ldots, K$ without any covariate information. Define

$$\tilde{G}_k(t) = \prod_{s \leq t} \left(1 - \frac{\Delta N_{\cdot k}(s)}{Y_{\cdot}(s)}\right),$$

which could be thought of as a cause specific Kaplan-Meier estimator. Show, however, that it will generally not be a valid estimator of $1 - P_k(t)$.

10.2 (Cause specific hazard modeling) Consider a competing risks model with two causes of death. The model can be described by the two cause specific hazards $\lambda_1(t)$ and $\lambda_2(t)$. Assume that n i.i.d. subjects are observed subject to independent right-censoring. Let $\Lambda_j(t) = \int_0^t \lambda_j(s) ds$ for $j = 1, 2$.

(a) When estimating λ_1 we may treat deaths with respect to cause "2" as independent right censorings even though the causes are not independent.

(b) Construct the likelihood function for estimating λ_1 and λ_2 and suggest an estimator for $\Lambda_1(t)$ and $\Lambda_2(t)$.

10.3 (Cause specific hazard modeling, Kalbfleisch & Prentice (2002)) Consider a competing risks model with two causes of death. Assume that n i.i.d. subjects are observed subject to independent right-censoring such that

$$\lambda_{ji}(t) = \lambda_0(t) \exp(\gamma_j + X_i^T \beta_j),$$

$j = 1, 2$, where X_i denotes a p-vector of covariates for the ith subject, β_j is a p-vector of unknown coefficients, and γ_1 and γ_2 are scalars with $\gamma_1 = 0$.

(a) Derive estimating equations for the parametric components of this model.

(b) Argue that standard software (e.g. coxph) can be used to analyze this model. How should data be organized?

10.4 (Cause specific and subdistribution hazards) Consider a competing risks model with two causes of death and in a situation with no censoring. Let $N_k(t) = I(T \leq t, \varepsilon = k)$ and $Y_k(t) = 1 - N_k(t-)$, $k = 1, 2$. Let $\lambda_1(t)$ and $\lambda_1^*(t)$ be defined by

$$\lambda_1(t) = \lim_{\Delta t \to 0} P(t \leq T < t + \Delta t, \varepsilon = 1 \mid T \geq t)/\Delta t,$$

$$P(T > t, \varepsilon = 1) = \exp(-\int_0^t \lambda_1^*(s) \, ds),$$

that is, the cause specific hazard function and the subdistribution hazard (for cause 1), respectively.

(a) Show that $N_1(t)$ has intensity $I(t \leq T)\lambda_1(t)$ with respect to $\mathcal{F}_t$, where
$$\mathcal{F}_t = \sigma(N_1(s), N_2(s) : s \leq t).$$

(b) Show that $N_1(t)$ has intensity $Y_1(t)\lambda_1^*(t)$ with respect to $\mathcal{F}_t^*$, where
$$\mathcal{F}_t^* = \sigma(N_1(s) : s \leq t).$$

10.5 (Cause specific and subdistribution hazards) Consider a competing risks model with two causes of death. Let
$$\lambda_j(t) = \lambda_{0j}(t) \exp(X^T \beta_j), \qquad (10.13)$$

$j = 1, 2$, where X denotes a p-vector of covariates for the considered subject, β_j is a p-vector of unknown coefficients and $\lambda_{0j}(t)$ denotes the baseline function j.

(a) Assume that the cause specific hazards has the structure (10.13) for $j = 1, 2$. Derive the subdistribution hazard functions.

(b) Assume that the subdistribution hazards has the structure (10.13) for $j = 1, 2$. Derive the cause specific hazard functions.

10.6 (Cause specific hazards: Asymptotics) Consider a competing risks model with two causes of death with the set-up in Section 10.2.

(a) If the martingale asymptotics is applied, the standard errors have a form that is equivalent to nK i.i.d. subjects, although the K causes are not independent. Derive an expression for the optional variation estimator of the standard error for both $\hat{\beta}$ and the cumulative incidence function.

(b) Validate that the i.i.d. representation standard errors have the given form and compare to those given in (a).

(c) Consider the melanoma data, write a program that fits 2 cause specific hazards (melanoma and other) with common regression coefficients for age, ulceration and log(thickness). How does one get the martingale standard errors and the robust standard errors based on the i.i.d. representation?

10.7 (Subdistribution hazard) Consider the Cox-Aalen subdistribution hazards model set-up in Section 10.2.

(a) Show that the weighted score equation for the subdistribution hazard is not on the same form as a weighted version of the score equations for the standard Cox-Aalen model.

(b) The weights
$$\frac{r_i(t)}{G_c(T_i \wedge t)}$$
are justified by having mean 1. We use the weights
$$w_i(t) = r_i(t) \frac{G_c(t)}{G_c(T_i \wedge t)}.$$
How can these by justified? What are the optimal weights if G_c is known?

10.8 (Binomial Regression (Scheike & Zhang, 2005)) We assume as in the previous section, for simplicity, that the censoring variable C is independent of both the survival time T and the covariates X, Z, but the formula may be extended by modeling of the censoring distribution given X, Z. Let $N_i(t) = \mathcal{I}(T_i \leq t, \varepsilon_i = 1)$, $Y_i(t) = 1 - N_i(t^-)$, $G_c(t) = P(C \geq t)$ and $\hat{G}_c$ be the Kaplan-Meier estimator of G_c. Note that $N_i(t)$ and $Y_i(t)$ typically will not be fully observed because of possible censorings. Let also $r_i(t) = \mathcal{I}(C_i \geq T_i \wedge t)$ be the indicator that is one if a subject is uncensored an 0 otherwise. The subdistribution approach can roughly speaking be described as direct modeling of $r_i(t)dN_i(t)$, what we do now is to model the 0/1 response $r_i(t)N_i(t)$ directly.

We shall consider time-varying regression models for the cumulative incidence probability for cause 1 $(P_1(t|X))$
$$h(1 - P_1(t|X)) = -X^T \eta(t), \tag{10.14}$$
where h is some known link function, $X = (1, x_1, \ldots, x_p)^T$ and $\eta(t)$ then give the effects of X on the cumulative incidence curve.

(a) Assume that a underlying subdistribution hazard is additive, what model (10.14) does this lead to. Similarly when the subdistribution is on Cox form.

(b) First assume that all subjects are uncensored. How would you estimate $\eta(t)$? Give an estimating equation.

(c) Now, assume that the censoring distribution is known. Compute the mean of $N_i(t)r_i(t)/G_c(T_i)$ conditional on X_i. Use this to suggest an estimating equation for estimation of $\eta(t)$.

(d) Based on previous questions, suggest an estimating equation based on observed data, and justify that it will lead to sensible estimates.

(e) Given that it can be established that $n^{1/2}(\hat{\eta}(t) - \eta(t))$ converges towards a Gaussian process with a variance that can be estimated by $\hat{\Psi}(t)$, construct a 95 % pointwise confidence interval for $P_1(t, X)$.

(f) Now consider the partially semiparametric model

$$\log(1 - P_1(t|data, X, Z)) = -\left(X^T \eta(t) + g(\gamma, Z, t)\right),$$

where $X = (1, x_1, \ldots, x_p)$ is a $(p+1) \times 1$ vector, g is a known function which is differentiable with respect to γ, Z is a $q_1 \times 1$ vector and γ is a $q_2 \times 1$ vector. How would you estimate the parameters of this model based on estimating equations as above?

11
Marked point process models

In biomedical research one often encounters responses and covariates collected over time for independent subjects. These types of data are called *longitudinal data*. When evaluating the effect of growth-hormones on human growth for example, the typical design consists of following a group of patients with different treatment regimes over time. In this case the response is their height or growth velocity and the purpose of the study may be to describe the treatment effect possibly corrected for other potentially important factors.

Longitudinal data can be described as a marked point process. This is simply a matter of considering the triplets consisting of the responses, the observation times and covariates as a collection of timings and marks (responses and covariates). In this chapter we shall look at models that describe the relationship between a set of covariates and the response. This section is intended as a brief illustration of how models similar to those presented earlier can be formulated as models for the mean of the response in a longitudinal data setting. We shall consider the time-varying additive models where the mean of the responses at time t given covariates can be written as

$$X_\beta^T(t)\beta(t) + X_\gamma^T(t)\gamma,$$

where $X_\beta(t)$ is a p-dimensional time-dependent covariate, $\beta(t)$ is a p-dimensional regression coefficient function of locally integrable functions, $X_\gamma(t)$ is a q-dimensional time-dependent covariate vector and γ is q-dimensional vector of regression coefficients that does not depend on time. Some covariate effects are thus time-varying and others are assumed to be constant. For this model we will show how one can estimate the cumulative regression coefficient functions $B(t) = \int \beta(s)ds$ and the regression coefficients γ using techniques very similar to those applied for the Aalen additive hazards model studied in Chapter 5.

The model where $\gamma = 0$ has been receiving a lot of attention recently, and some key references include Hastie & Tibshirani (1993), Brumback & Rice (1998), Fan & Zhang (1999, 2000b,a), Wu et al. (1998), and Hoover et al. (1998). These papers take a more classical smoothing based approach for estimating the time-varying regression coefficients in contrast to our direct estimation of the cumulative regression coefficients.

Example 11.0.1 (CD4-data)

The AIDS dataset described, for example, in Huang et al. (2002), is a subset from the Multicenter AIDS Cohort Study. The data include the repeated measurements of CD4 cell counts and percentages of 283 homosexual men who became HIV-positive between 1984 and 1991. Details about the design, methods and medical implications of the study can be found in Kaslow et al. (1987). All individuals were scheduled to have their measurements made at semi-annual visits, but, because many individuals missed some of their scheduled visits and the HIV infections happened randomly during the study, there are unequal numbers of repeated measurements and different measurement times per individual.

These data have previously been analyzed by Fan & Zhang (2000a), Wu & Chiang (2000) and Huang et al. (2002) who all considered varying-coefficient models. Their analysis aimed at describing the trend of the mean CD4 percentage depletion over time, and to evaluate the effects of cigarette smoking, pre-HIV infection CD4 percentage and age at infection on mean CD4 percentage after the infection. The model they considered was

$$E(Z(t) \mid X_1, X_2, X_3) = \beta_0(t) + \beta_1(t)X_1 + \beta_2(t)X_2 + \beta_3(t)X_3,$$

where X_1 is 1 or 0 if the individual ever or never smoked cigarettes, respectively, after the HIV-infection; X_2 is the centered age at HIV-infection and X_3 is the centered pre-infection CD4 percentage. □

We now describe how the longitudinal data may be considered as a marked point process. The longitudinal data for the ith subject, $i = 1, \ldots, n$, is denoted by

$$(T_i^k, Z_i^k, X_i(t)) \tag{11.1}$$

where T_i^k is the time-point for the kth measurement Z_i^k of the longitudinal response variable, and $X_i(t)$ is a time-dependent piecewise constant or deterministic (given past information) covariate ($q \times 1$) associated with the ith subject. The covariates can reflect internal information such as the time since the previous measurement and the previous level of response as well

11. Marked point process models 377

as external information in terms of other covariate information such as sex and treatment. We assume that we observe n independent subjects over the time-period $[0, \tau]$ from the generic model described below.

The (T_i^k, Z_i^k) constitutes a marked point process, T_i^k being the kth jump time and Z_i^k the associated mark. The marks (Z_i^k) take their values in the measurable space $(E, \mathcal{E})$ referred to as the mark space. In the longitudinal data setting the mark space is equivalent to $\Re$ with the Borel σ-field.

To each $A_i \in \mathcal{E}$ there is associated a point process

$$N_i(t)(A_i) = \sum_{k \geq 1} 1_{(Z_i^k \in A_i)} 1_{(T_i^k \leq t)},$$

with $N_i(t) = N_i(t)(E)$, $i = 1, \ldots, n$, denoting the basic point processes. The marked point processes can also be identified by their respective induced counting measure $p_i(ds \times dz_i)$ defined by

$$p_i((0, t] \times A_i) = N_i(t)(A_i), \quad A_i \in \mathcal{E}.$$

We consider a history $\mathcal{F}_t = \mathcal{F}_t^1 \vee \cdots \vee \mathcal{F}_t^n$ such that

$$\mathcal{F}_t^i \supset \mathcal{F}_t^{p^i}, \quad t \geq 0,$$

where $\mathcal{F}_t^{p^i}$ is the history generated by the ith marked point process. The $p_i(ds \times dz_i)$ admits the $(P, \mathcal{F}_t)$-intensity kernel $\lambda_t^i(dz_i) = \lambda_i(t)\Phi_t^i(dz_i)$, $i = 1, \ldots, n$, that is, $\lambda_i(t)\Phi_t^i(A_i)$ is the intensity of the point process $N_i(t)(A_i)$, $A_i \in \mathcal{E}$. The history

$$\sigma\{T_i^l, Z_i^l, 1 \leq l \leq k-1; T_i^k; (X_i(t) : t \leq T_i^k)\} \tag{11.2}$$

of all observations up to and including T_i^k is denoted by $\mathcal{F}_{T_i^k-}^i$. An important relation is

$$\Phi_{T_i^k}^i(A_i) = P(Z_i^k \in A_i \mid \mathcal{F}_{T_i^k-}^i),$$

that is, Φ_t^i is the conditional mark distribution given the past up to and including the time-point where the mark is obtained.

The key point of marked point process theory here is that cumulating the responses (and more generally predictable functions of the response) over time gives rise to a martingale decomposition, where the compensator involves the conditional distribution of the responses given the accrued information up to that point in time. To be more specific, let H_i be a $\mathcal{F}_t$-predictable process (determined by the past), see Section 2.4, then the marked point process integral

$$\int_0^t \int_E H_i(s, z_i) p_i(ds \times dz_i),$$

378   11. Marked point process models

which is nothing but the sum

$$\sum_k H_i(T_i^k, Z_i^k) I(T_i^k \le t),$$

may be decomposed as

$$\int_0^t \lambda_i(s) \left(\int_E H_i(s, z_i) \Phi_s^i(dz_i) \right) ds + \int_0^t \int_E H_i(s, z_i) q_i(ds \times dz_i),$$

where $q_i(dt \times dz_i) = p_i(dt \times dz_i) - \lambda_i(t) \Phi_t^i(dz_i) dt$ is a martingale. We assume that the intensity $\lambda_i(t)$ can be written as $Y_i(t) \alpha_i(t)$ where $Y_i(t)$ is an indicator variable keeping track of whether or not subject i is still at study at time t, and $\alpha_i(t)$ is a deterministic function given the accrued information up to time $t-$. This assumption formally restricts the model to measurement times that are varying continuously in time. Although the methodology may be extended to deal with a mix of fixed measurement times and randomly varying measurement times we here consider only the case where the measurement times come from an absolute continuous distribution or at least where it is reasonably such a model as an approximation.

Example 11.0.2 (Two sample situation)

Assume for the moment that we have only one measurement per subject and that they are naturally divided into two groups. Denote data by (Z_{ij}, T_{ij}) where index $j = 1, 2$ identifies group, and $i = 1, ..., n_j$ are the subjects within groups, and $n = n_1 + n_2$ are the total number of subjects. Let

$$E(Z_{ij}|T_{ij} = t) = \int_E z_{ij} \Phi_t^{ij}(dz_{ij}) = \beta_j(t),$$

be the mean value of the response in the jth group at time t. Assume further that there is no difference between the groups with respect to how measurements are sampled over time, and let $\alpha(t)$ denote the sampling hazard. We here initially assume that the sampling hazard is equivalent for the two groups and below return to the situation where the sampling hazard depends on group status and more generally covariates. Suppose we want to test the hypothesis

$$H_0 : \beta_1(t) = \beta_2(t) \quad \text{for all } t.$$

Let $B_{j\alpha}(t) = \int_0^t \beta_j(s) \alpha(s) \, ds$ and $B_\alpha(t) = \int_0^t \beta(s) \alpha(s) \, ds$, where $\beta(t)$ denotes the common value of $\beta_1(t)$ and $\beta_2(t)$ under the hypothesis. Let further

$$Y_{\cdot j}(t) = \sum_{i=1}^{n_j} I(t \le T_{ij})$$

and
$$Y_{\cdot\cdot}(t) = Y_{\cdot 1}(t) + Y_{\cdot 2}(t).$$

We have the decomposition

$$\sum_i \int_E z_{ij} p_{ij}(dt \times dz_{ij}) = \alpha(t) Y_{\cdot j}(t) dB_j(t) + \sum_i \int_E z_{ij} q_{ij}(dt \times dz_{ij}),$$

and under H_0

$$\sum_{i,j} \int_E z_{ij} p_{ij}(dt \times dz_{ij}) = \alpha(t) Y_{\cdot\cdot}(t) dB(t) + \sum_{i,j} \int_E z_{ij} q_{ij}(dt \times dz_{ij})$$

leading to the estimators

$$\hat{B}_{j\alpha}(t) = \sum_i \int_0^t \int_E \frac{z_{ij}}{Y_{\cdot j}(s)} p_{ij}(dt \times dz_{ij}) = \sum_i \frac{Z_{ij}}{Y_{\cdot j}(T_{ij})} I(T_{ij} \le t),$$

$$\hat{B}_\alpha(t) = \sum_{i,j} \int_0^t \int_E \frac{z_{ij}}{Y_{\cdot\cdot}(s)} p_{ij}(dt \times dz_{ij}) = \sum_{i,j} \frac{Z_{ij}}{Y_{\cdot\cdot}(T_{ij})} I(T_{ij} \le t).$$

Let $\tilde{B}_{1\alpha}(t) = \int_0^t J(s) d\hat{B}_\alpha(s)$, $J(t) = I(Y_{\cdot 1}(t) > 0)$. We may now construct test statistics based on

$$R(t) = \int_0^t w(s) \, d(\hat{B}_{1\alpha} - \tilde{B}_{1\alpha})(s),$$

which, under H_0, has compensator

$$\int_0^t w(s) J(s) \alpha(s) dB(s) - \int_0^t w(s) J(s) \alpha(s) dB(s) = 0.$$

In the above two displays, $w(t)$ denotes a weight function. Thus, under H_0,

$$R(t) = \int_0^t w(s) \, d(\hat{B}_{1\alpha} - \tilde{B}_{1\alpha})(s)$$
$$= \sum_i \int_0^t \int_E w(s) J(s) \frac{z_{i1}}{Y_{\cdot 1}(s)} q_{i1}(dt \times dz_{i1})$$
$$- \sum_{i,j} \int_0^t \int_E w(s) J(s) \frac{z_{ij}}{Y_{\cdot\cdot}(s)} q_{ij}(dt \times dz_{ij})$$
$$= M(t),$$

which (properly normed) converges to a Gaussian martingale. The asymptotic variance may be estimated consistently by the quadratic variation process

$$[M](t) = \sum_i w^2(T_{i1})J(T_{i1})(Z_{i1})^2 \left(\frac{1}{Y_{\cdot 1}(T_{i1})} - \frac{1}{Y_{\cdot\cdot}(T_{i1})}\right)^2 I(T_{i1} \leq t)$$
$$- \sum_i w^2(T_{i2})J(T_{i2})(Z_{i2})^2 \frac{1}{Y_{\cdot\cdot}^2(T_{i2})} I(T_{i2} \leq t).$$

A natural test statistic is

$$R^2(\tau)/[M](\tau)$$

which, under H_0, is asymptotically $\chi^2(1)$. One may also perform a supremum test that rejects at level α by

$$\sup_{t \leq \tau} |R(t)[M](\tau)^{1/2}([M](\tau) + [M](t))^{-1}| \geq d_\alpha,$$

where d_α is the $(1-\alpha)$-quantile in the distribution of

$$\sup_{t \in [0,1/2]} |B^0(t)|,$$

see Chapter 2 for selected values of d_α. If the sampling intensities are expected to be different between groups then this should be reflected in the above test statistic. We return to this in Examples 11.1.3 and 11.4.1. □

11.1 Nonparametric additive model for longitudinal data

Consider the situation where several covariates are present, denoted by $X_i(t)$ (q-dimensional) for the ith subject. In the following we develop models for the conditional mean

$$m_i(t) = \int_E z_i \Phi_t^i(dz_i)$$

of the longitudinal response given the accrued information. Throughout it is assumed that the variance function $\sigma^2(t) = \int_E (z_i - m_i(t))^2 \Phi_t^i(dz_i)$ is independent of i. Most of the considered estimators does not utilize this assumption about the variance of the responses, so results are valid even with more flexible models for the variance of the responses.

Our focus is on models that allow for time-dependent effects of the covariates. To enhance estimation and inference some structure on the models is needed and we impose the additive structure:

$$m_i(t) = \beta_0(t) + \beta_1(t)X_{i1}(t) + \cdots + \beta_q(t)X_{iq}(t), \qquad (11.3)$$

11.1 Nonparametric additive model for longitudinal data

where $\beta_0(t), \ldots, \beta_q(t)$ are unspecified locally integrable time-dependent regression functions. The above additive model will often give a good fit to data since it is a first order Taylor expansion of a general conditional mean function around the zero-covariate, but we note that other models may also be relevant, see e.g. Cheng & Wei (2000).

The above conditional mean model may also be written as

$$E\{Z_i(T_i^k) | \mathcal{F}_{T_i^k-}^i\} = \beta_0(T_i^k) + \beta_1(T_i^k)X_{i1}(T_i^k) + \cdots + \beta_q(T_i^k)X_{iq}(T_i^k),$$

where the history we condition on, see (11.2), contains the accrued information about the particular subject up to and including time-point T_i^k. Notice the resemblance of model (11.3) with the Aalen additive model described in Chapter 5. The nice feature of these two models is that the effect of the explanatory variables are allowed to change with time hence accommodating, for example, for a situation where a time-dependent treatment effect is suspected. As is the case for the Aalen additive hazards model it turns out that it is easy to estimate the cumulative regression functions $B(t) = \int_0^t \beta(s) ds$, where $\beta(t) = (\beta_1(t), ..., \beta_q(t))^T$. We shall see in a moment that these appear very naturally in the compensator for a certain marked point process constructed by cumulating the responses over time. To begin with we assume a covariate independent sampling hazard $\alpha(t)$. Cumulating the responses for the ith subject gives the following decomposition

$$\sum_k Z_i^k I(T_i^k \leq t) = \int_0^t \int_E z_i \, p_i(ds \times dz_i)$$

$$= \int_0^t \alpha(s) Y_i(s) m_i(s) \, ds + \int_0^t \int_E z_i \, q_i(ds \times dz_i)$$

$$= \int_0^t \alpha(s) Y_i(s) X_i^T(s) \, dB(s) + \int_0^t \int_E z_i \, q_i(ds \times dz_i),$$

where

$$X_i^T(t) = (1, X_{i1}(t), \ldots, X_{iq}(t))$$

for $i = 1, \ldots, n$. Collecting these n equations in one vector equation, we obtain

$$\int_0^t \int_E D(z) \, p(ds \times dz) = \int_0^t \alpha(s) Y(s) \, dB(s) + \int_0^t \int_E D(z) \, q(ds \times dz) \quad (11.4)$$

where $z = (z_1, \ldots, z_n)$, $D(z) = \text{diag}(z)$,

$$p(dt \times dz) = (p_1(dt \times dz_1), \ldots, p_n(dt \times dz_n))^T,$$

$$q(dt \times dz) = (q_1(dt \times dz_1), \ldots, q_n(dt \times dz_n))^T,$$

and $Y(t) = (Y_{ij}(t))$ is the $n \times (q+1)$-matrix with ith row, $i = 1, \ldots, n$, given by $Y_i(t) X_i^T(t)$.

382   11. Marked point process models

Writing (11.4) on differential form

$$\int_E D(z)\, p(dt \times dz) = \alpha(t) Y(t)\, dB(t) + \int_E D(z)\, q(dt \times dz),$$

where $E(\int_E D(z)\, q(dt \times dz)) = 0$, motivates least squares estimators for $B(t)$ on the form

$$\hat{B}(t) = \int_0^t \int_E \frac{J(s)}{\hat{\alpha}(s)} Y^-(s) D(z)\, p(ds \times dz) \qquad (11.5)$$

where $\hat{\alpha}(t)$ is an estimate of $\alpha(t)$, $Y^-(t)$ is a predictable generalized inverse of $Y(t)$. One choice of generalized inverse is

$$Y^-(t) = (Y(t)^T Y(t))^{-1} Y(t)^T.$$

Using (11.5) we need to specify an estimate of $\alpha(t)$. For simplicity we suggest to use a kernel smoothing estimate, that is, we let

$$\hat{\alpha}(t) = \frac{1}{b_n} \int K\left(\frac{t-s}{b_n}\right) d\hat{A}(s),$$

where $\hat{A}(t) = \int_0^t \frac{1}{Y_\cdot(s)}\, dN_\cdot(s)$, $Y_\cdot(t) = \sum_i Y_i(t)$, $N_\cdot(t) = \sum_i N_i(t)$, K is a bounded kernel function with support $[-1, 1]$, and b_n is the bandwidth. The properties of the estimator (11.5) are stated below.

Theorem 11.1.1 *Assume that $\alpha(t)$ is continuous differentiable and bounded away from zero on $[0, \tau]$, $\hat{\alpha}(t)$ is uniformly consistent and $b_n \to 0$, $n^{1/2} b_n^2 \to 0$. Then, under regularity conditions,*

$$n^{1/2}(\hat{B} - B) \xrightarrow{D} U \quad \text{as } n \to \infty$$

in $D[0, \tau]^{q+1}$, where U is a zero-mean Gaussian martingale with variance function $\Phi(t)$.

PROOF. Let $B^*(t) = \int_0^t J(s) \beta(s)\, ds$. Under the regularity conditions stated in Martinussen & Scheike (2000) it may be seen that $n^{1/2}(\hat{B} - B)$ and $n^{1/2}(\hat{B} - B^*)$ have the same limiting distribution. Now,

$$n^{1/2}(\hat{B} - B^*)(t) = \Delta(t) \qquad (11.6)$$

$$+ n^{1/2} \int_0^t \frac{J(s)}{\hat{\alpha}(s)} \beta(s)\, d(\hat{A}(s) - \tilde{A}(s)),$$

with

$$\Delta(t) = n^{1/2} \int_0^t \frac{J(s)}{\hat{\alpha}(s)} Y^-(s)\, dM(z)(s) - n^{1/2} \int_0^t \frac{J(s)}{\hat{\alpha}(s)} \beta(s)\, d(\hat{A}(s) - A(s))$$

11.1 Nonparametric additive model for longitudinal data

and where $\hat{A}(t) = \int_0^t \frac{1}{Y.(s)} dN.(s)$ and $\tilde{A}(t) = \int_0^t \hat{\alpha}(s) ds$. Interchanging integration order in $\int_0^t \hat{\alpha}(s) ds$ and using a Taylor expansion, it can be seen that

$$\sup_{t \in [0,\tau]} (\hat{A}(t) - \tilde{A}(t)) = O_p(b_n^2).$$

Hence, the last term on the right-hand side of (11.6) converges uniformly to zero in probability. We may write $\Delta(t)$ as

$$\Delta(t) = n^{1/2} \int_0^t \int_E \frac{J(s)}{\hat{\alpha}(s)} Y^-(s)(D(z) - \frac{1}{Y.(s)} Y(s)\beta(s)a)q(ds \times dz) \quad (11.7)$$

where $q(ds \times dz) = (q_1(ds \times dz_1), \ldots, q_n(ds \times dz_n))^T$ and a is the $1 \times n$-vector $(1, \ldots, 1)$. We may replace $\hat{\alpha}(t)$ by $\alpha(t)$ in $\Delta(t)$ and still obtain the same limiting distribution, this is a consequence of for example Lenglart's inequality when we use a predictable version of $\hat{\alpha}$, otherwise the analysis becomes more complicated. The jth component of $\Delta(t)$ may then be written as

$$\Delta_j(t) = \sum_{i=1}^n \int_0^t \int_E n^{-1/2} \frac{J(s)}{\alpha(s)} (V_{ji}(s)z_i - \frac{\beta_j(s)}{n^{-1} Y.(s)}) q_i(ds \times dz_i)$$

$$= \sum_{i=1}^n M_i(H_{ij})(t),$$

where

$$H_{ij}(t, z_i) = n^{-1/2} \frac{J(s)}{\alpha(s)} (V_{ji}(s)z_i - \frac{\beta_j(s)}{n^{-1} Y.(s)})$$

with $V_{ji}(t) = \sum_{l=0}^p (n^{-1} R^{(2)}(t))_{jl}^{-1} Y_{il}(t)$ and with $R^{(2)}(t) = Y^T(t) Y(t)$. To identify the asymptotic variance, we compute the predictable variation process of $\Delta(t)$ (suppressing the dependency of time in the integrands)

$$\langle \Delta_j, \Delta_k \rangle(t) = \sum_{l,m=0}^p \int_0^t \frac{J}{\alpha} (n^{-1} R^{(2)})_{jl}^{-1} (n^{-1} R^{(2)})_{km}^{-1} (n^{-1} \sum_{i=1}^n Y_{il} Y_{im}$$

$$\times (\sum_{f,g=0}^p Y_{if} Y_{ig} \beta_f \beta_g + \sigma^2)) ds - \int_0^t \frac{J \beta_j \beta_k}{\alpha n^{-1} Y.} ds,$$

which converges in probability. We will now turn to the Lindeberg condition in the martingale central limit theorem. The process containing all the jumps of $\Delta_j(t)$ larger in absolute value than ϵ is given by

$$\Delta_{j\epsilon}(t) = \sum_{i=1}^n \int_0^t \int_E \frac{1}{n^{1/2}} \frac{1}{\alpha(s)} (V_{ji}(s)z_i - \frac{\beta_j(s)}{n^{-1} Y.(s)})$$

$$\times I(n^{-1/2} \frac{1}{\alpha(s)} |V_{ji}(s)z_i - \frac{\beta_j(s)}{n^{-1} Y.(s)}| > \epsilon) q_i(ds \times dz_i).$$

The predictable variation process for $\Delta_{je}(t)$ is

$$\langle \Delta_{je}\rangle(t) = \sum_{i=1}^{n} \int_0^t \int_E \frac{1}{n} \frac{Y_i(s)}{\alpha(s)} (V_{ji}(s)z_i - \frac{\beta_j(s)}{n^{-1}Y.(s)})^2$$

$$\times I(n^{-1/2}\frac{1}{\alpha(s)}|V_{ji}(s)z_i - \frac{\beta_j(s)}{n^{-1}Y.(s)}| > \epsilon)\Phi_s^i(dz_i)\, ds$$

and we have to show that $\langle \Delta_{je}\rangle(t) \xrightarrow{P} 0$ as $n \to \infty$.
By applying the elementary inequality

$$(a-b)^2 I(|a-b| > \epsilon) \le 4a^2 I(|a| > \epsilon/2) + 4b^2 I(|b| > \epsilon/2)$$

twice, it may be seen that

$$\langle X_{je}\rangle(t) \le (c_1 G_1^{(n)})^2 16 \int_0^t \frac{1}{\alpha(s)}(\frac{1}{n}\sum_{i=1}^n V_{ji}^2(s))\frac{16}{\epsilon^2}\eta(s)\, ds$$

$$+ 16 \int_0^t \frac{1}{\alpha(s)}(\frac{1}{n}\sum_{i=1}^n V_{ji}^2(s) m_i^2(s)) I(c_2 G_2^{(n)} > \epsilon/4)\, ds$$

$$+ 4 \int_0^t \frac{\beta_j^2(s)}{\alpha(s) n^{-1}Y.(s)} I(n^{-1/2}\frac{1}{\alpha(s)}|\frac{\beta_j(s)}{n^{-1}Y.(s)}| > \epsilon/2)\, ds$$

where c_1 and c_2 are (finite) constants. Again, under regularity conditions, it may be seen that $\langle \Delta_{je}\rangle(t) \xrightarrow{P} 0$ as $n \to \infty$, and this completes the proof. □

The variance-covariance matrix of the limit distribution of $n^{1/2}(\hat{B} - B)$ may be estimated consistently by the quadratic variation process

$$\hat{\Phi}(t) = [\Delta](t),$$

$\Delta(t)$ is the main martingale term of $n^{1/2}(\hat{B}-B)$, see (11.7) above.

We now consider a worked example that illustrates the use of the estimators.

Example 11.1.1 (CD4-data)

Consider the data introduced in Example 11.0.1 on post-infection CD4 percentage. To begin with we consider the conditional mean model

$$m_i(t) = \beta_0(t) + \beta_1(t) X_{i1} + \beta_2(t) X_{i2} + \beta_3(t) X_{i3}(t),$$

where X_1 is smoking, X_2 is age at HIV-infection and $X_3(t)$ is the at time t previous measured response. Both X_2 and X_3 were centered around their respective averages. The above model may be fitted using the function **dynreg** of **timereg** as shown below.

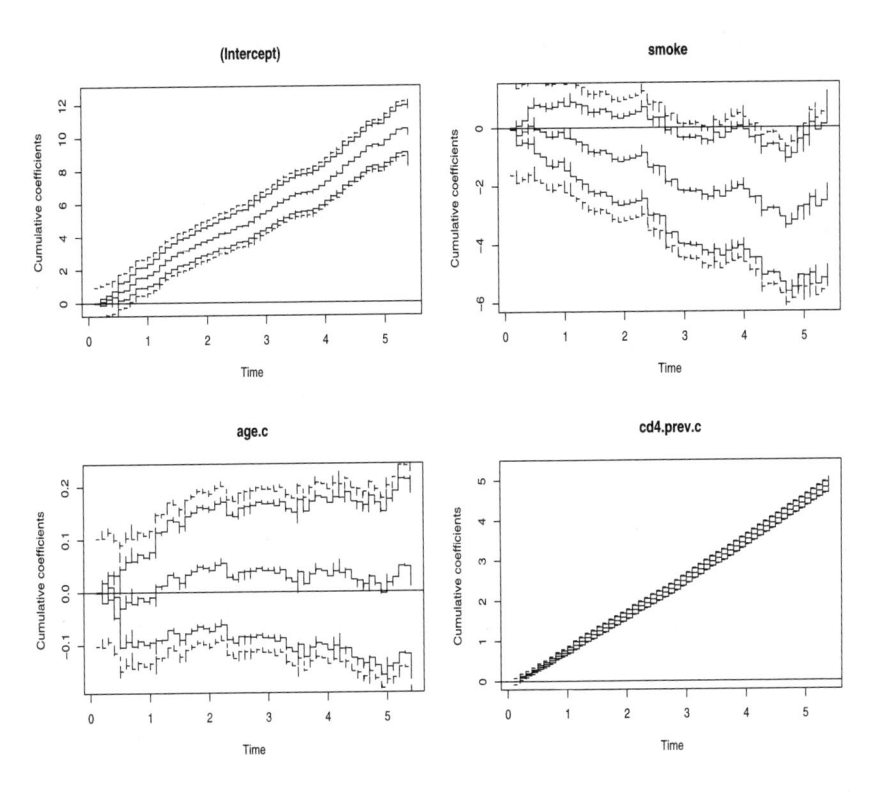

11.1 Nonparametric additive model for longitudinal data

FIGURE 11.1: CD4-data. Estimated cumulative coefficients functions for the baseline CD4 percentage and the effects of smoking, age and previous response. Curves are shown along with 95% pointwise confidence limits and 95% Hall-Wellner bands

```
> age.c<-age-mean(age)
> cd4.prev.c<-cd4.prev-mean(cd4.prev)
> indi<-rep(1,length(cd4$lt))
> fit.cd4<-dynreg(cd4~smoke+age.c+cd4.prev.c,data=cd4,
+ Surv(lt,rt,indi)~+1,start.time=0,max.time=5.5,id=cd4$id,
+ n.sim=500,bandwidth=0.15,meansub=1)
> plot(fit.cd4,hw.ci=2)
```

The plot command gives the estimated cumulatives along with 95% pointwise confidence intervals and the 95% Hall-Wellner band. □

An important technical requirement to obtain the above asymptotic result is that we have to undersmooth when estimating $\alpha(t)$. The optimal bandwidth $b_{n,\mathrm{opt}}$ (for a kernel smoother) is is of order $n^{-1/5}$ such that it balances the effect of the "squared bias term" and the "variance term" of the mean integrated squared error term in an optimal way. We have, however,

386   11. Marked point process models

to require that $n^{1/2}b_n^2 \to 0$ and therefore that b_n converges faster to zero than $b_{n,\text{opt}}$.

Example 11.1.2 (Smoothing and choice of bandwidth)

Consider the standard i.i.d. regression data set-up consisting of i.i.d. samples from the model
$$Z_i = m(T_i) + \epsilon_i$$
where ϵ_i are zero mean with variance σ^2 and T_i is non-negative positive with density $f(s)$. The Nadarya-Watson estimator of m is given as
$$\hat{m}(x) = \frac{\sum_i Z_i K_b(x - T_i)}{\sum_i K_b(x - T_i)},$$
where $K_b(t) = b^{-1} K(t/b)$. Define $H(x) = \int_0^x m(t) dt$ and $\hat{H}(x) = \int_0^x \hat{m}(t) dt$. Scheike & Zhang (1998) showed that if the bandwidth b satisfies that $n^{1/2}b^2 \to 0$ it follows that $n^{1/2}(\hat{H}(x) - H(x))$ converges to a Gaussian martingale with variance function $\Phi(x) = \int_0^x \sigma^2(s)/f(s) ds$.

To estimate $m(x)$ (for twice continuously differentiable m) the asymptotically optimal bandwidth is
$$b(x) = (V(x)/(4L^2(x)))^{1/5} n^{-1/5},$$
where the bias is
$$L(x) = d_K (m''(x) f(x) + 2m'(x) f'(x))/(2f(x))$$
and the variance is
$$V(x) = c_K \sigma^2(x)/f(x),$$
see, e.g., Härdle (1990) or Simonoff (1996) for more details on plug-in bandwidth selection.

In an unpublished report Scheike & Zhang derived the optimal choice of bandwidth for estimation of cumulative regression coefficients. Based on a higher order asymptotic expansion it follows that the optimal bandwidth for estimating $H(x)$ is given as
$$b_H(x) = \left(\frac{V_H(x)}{4L_H^2(x)}\right)^{1/5} n^{-2/5}$$
with
$$L_H(x) = \int_0^s L(s) ds, \quad V_H(x) = c_K \int_0^x \sigma^2(s)/f^2(s) ds.$$
Harboe & Scheike (2001) assumed that the mean of the longitudinal response at time t were on the time-varying regression form $m(t, X) = X^T(t)\beta(t)$ and then estimated $\beta(t)$ by local linear regression techniques

11.1 Nonparametric additive model for longitudinal data

as in Wu et al. (1998). These estimates were then combined to estimate $\hat{B}_S(t) = \int_0^T \hat{\beta}(s)ds$, and a uniform asymptotic description of the estimates of the cumulatives was derived. Optimal bandwidth choice for estimating cumulative time-varying regression coefficients models based on higher order asymptotics should therefore also be possible and should have similar structure to those given in the simple nonparametric regression case. □

In the one-sample situation, that is without any covariates, we get the that the asymptotic variance of $n^{1/2}(\hat{B}(t) - B(t))$ is

$$\int_0^t \frac{\sigma^2(s)}{\alpha(s)y(s)} ds,$$

where $y(t)$ is the limit in probability of $n^{-1}Y.(t)$, just as in the for the nonparametric regression set-up we considered in the previous example.

Considering one component of the cumulative regression functions, $B_j(t)$, say, one may now wish to test if this component is equal to zero. This is done easily through the above Theorem 11.1.1. Let $\hat{\Phi}_{jj}(t)$ denote element (j,j) of $\hat{\Phi}(t)$. A simple test statistic that is useful if B_j is monotone is

$$n^{1/2} \frac{\hat{B}_j(\tau)}{\hat{\Phi}_{jj}^{1/2}(\tau)},$$

which is asymptotically standard normal under the null.

Alternatively, when the studied regression functions are not consistently positive or negative one may use a maximal deviation test statistic of the process

$$\xi_j(t) = \hat{B}_j(t)(\hat{\Phi}_{jj}(\tau))^{1/2}(\hat{\Phi}_{jj}(t) + \hat{\Phi}_{jj}(\tau))^{-1},$$

which converges to a time-changed Brownian bridge. Therefore

$$\sup_{t \in [0,\tau]} |\xi_j(t)|$$

converges to the supremum of the limit distribution.

We now return to the two sample situation in a situation where the sampling intensities may depend on group status. In the following section that extends the models to semiparametric regression models we extend this even further to allow the sampling intensities to depend on covariates.

Example 11.1.3 (Two sample situation (Continued))

Consider the two sample situation described in Example 11.0.2 but now with the complication that the sampling intensities are different in the two groups. Denote them by $\alpha_j(t)$, $j = 1, 2$. We still want to investigate the null

$$H_0: \beta_1(t) = \beta_2(t) \quad \text{for all } t.$$

The decomposition

$$\sum_i \int_E z_{ij} p_{ij}(dt \times dz_{ij}) = \alpha_j(t) Y_{\cdot j}(t) dB_j(t) + \sum_i \int_E z_{ij} q_{ij}(dt \times dz_{ij}),$$

and under H_0

$$\sum_{i,j} \int_E z_{ij} p_{ij}(dt \times dz_{ij}) = (\alpha_1(t) Y_{\cdot 1}(t) + \alpha_2(t) Y_{\cdot 2}(t)) dB(t)$$

$$+ \sum_{i,j} \int_E z_{ij} q_{ij}(dt \times dz_{ij}).$$

lead to the estimators

$$\hat{B}_j(t) = \sum_i \int_0^t \int_E \frac{z_{ij}}{\hat{\alpha}_j(s) Y_{\cdot j}(s)} p_{ij}(dt \times dz_{ij}),$$

$$\tilde{B}(t) = \sum_{i,j} \int_0^t \int_E \frac{z_{ij}}{(\hat{\alpha}_1(s) Y_{\cdot 1}(s) + \hat{\alpha}_2(s) Y_{\cdot 2}(s))} p_{ij}(dt \times dz_{ij}),$$

where $\hat{\alpha}_j(t)$, $j = 1, 2$, are obtained by smoothing the Nelson-Aalen estimators

$$\int_0^t \frac{1}{Y_{\cdot j}(s)} dN_{\cdot j}(t),$$

where $N_{ij}(t) = I(T_{ij} \leq t)$. One may now construct test statistics based on

$$R(t) = \int_0^t w(s) \, d(\hat{B}_1 - \tilde{B}_1)(s),$$

where $w(t)$ denotes a weight function, and $\tilde{B}_1(t) = \int_0^t J(s) d\tilde{B}(s)$ with $J(t) = I(Y_{\cdot 1}(t) > 0)$. We may write

$$\hat{B}_1(t) = \int_0^t J(s) \, dB(s) + \sum_i \int_0^t \int_E \frac{(z_{i1} - \beta(s))}{\hat{\alpha}_1(s) Y_{\cdot 1}(s)} q_{i1}(ds \times dz_{i1}) + O_p(b^2)$$

and

$$\tilde{B}_1(t) = \int_0^t J(s) \, dB(s)$$

$$+ \sum_{i,j} \int_0^t \int_E \frac{(z_{ij} - \beta(s))}{(\hat{\alpha}_1(s) Y_{\cdot 1}(s) + \hat{\alpha}_2(s) Y_{\cdot 2}(s))} q_{ij}(ds \times dz_{ij}) + O_p(b^2).$$

If we choose the bandwidth parameter such that $n^{1/2} b^2$ converges to zero then we may use the above decompositions to show that $R(t)$ (properly normed) converges to a Gaussian martingale. □

11.2 Semiparametric additive model for longitudinal data

The time-varying coefficient model described in the previous section provides a nice graphical summary of the time-dynamics of the covariates and further allow for inference about the covariate effects. It is often of interest, however, to consider semiparametric submodels. A relevant hypothesis about the effect of a given covariate, for example, is whether in fact its effect on the response changes with time or whether it is constant. In any case it is always desirable to try to simplify models to obtain the most precise description of the covariates effects on the response. A natural submodel to consider is therefore

$$m_i(t) = X_{\beta i}^T(t)\beta^T(t) + X_{\gamma i}^T(t)\gamma \tag{11.8}$$

where $\beta(t) = (\beta_1(t), \ldots, \beta_q(t))^T$ are unspecified locally integrable time-dependent regression functions and $\gamma = (\gamma_1, \ldots, \gamma_p)^T$ are unknown parameters. The covariate $X_i(t)$ is thus grouped into two subsets, $X_{\beta i}(t)$, whose effects are allowed to vary with time and $X_{\gamma i}(t)$ whose effects are constant.

In some situations it may further not be reasonable to assume that the sampling intensity for the ith subject $Y_i(t)\alpha(t)$ is independent of covariates. Here one should keep in mind that the intensity is the conditional mean of the increment of the counting process $N_i(t)$ that counts the number of measurements *given* what has been observed so far for that subject. The observed history for some subjects can imply that they are more eligible to being measured. In such situations it may be more appropriate to let the measurement intensity depend on covariates. We start by leaving the intensity totally unspecified and later add some regression structure for the sampling intensities.

The approach is as in the previous sections, that is, we decompose a certain marked point process into its compensator and its martingale. The measurement intensities will show up in the compensator and somehow this should be accounted for when estimating the unknown quantities defining model (11.8).

The ith marked point process $\sum_k Z_i^k I(T_i^k \leq t)$ gives rise to the following decomposition

$$\int_0^t \int_E z_i \, p_i(ds \times dz_i) = \int_0^t \lambda_i(s) m_i(s) \, ds + \int_0^t \int_E z_i \, q_i(ds \times dz_i),$$

and again collecting these n equations into one vector equation and writing it in differential form gives

$$\int_E D(z) \, p(dt \times dz) = \Lambda(t) Y_\beta(t) \, dB(t) + \Lambda(t) Y_\gamma(t)\gamma \, dt$$
$$+ \int_E D(z) \, q(dt \times dz) \tag{11.9}$$

where $\Lambda(t) = \text{diag}(\lambda_i(t))$, $Y_\beta(t) = (Y_1(t)X_{\beta 1}(t), \ldots, Y_n(t)X_{\beta n}(t))^T$, and $Y_\gamma(t)$ are defined similarly. Define also $Y_{\lambda\beta}(t) = \Lambda(t)Y_\beta(t)$, and similarly with $Y_{\lambda\beta}(t)$.

Suppose for a moment that the intensities $\lambda_i(t)$, $i = 1, \ldots, n$, are known. If we further assume that γ is known then an obvious estimator of $B(t)$ based on (11.9) is

$$\hat{B}(\gamma)(t) = \int_0^t \int_E Y_{\lambda\beta}^-(s) D(z) \, p(ds \times dz) - \int_0^t Y_{\lambda\beta}^-(s) Y_{\lambda\gamma}(s) \gamma \, ds,$$

where

$$Y_{\lambda\beta}^-(t) = (Y_\beta^T(t)\Lambda(t)Y_\beta(t))^{-1} Y_\beta^T(t).$$

To obtain an estimator of γ we apply equation (11.9) with $dB(t)$ replaced by $d\hat{B}(\gamma)(t)$ resulting in

$$\tilde{\gamma} = \left(\int_0^\tau Y_\gamma^T(t) H(t) \Lambda(t) Y_\gamma(t) \, dt \right)^{-1} \int_0^\tau \int_E Y_\gamma^T(t) H(t) D(z) \, p(dt \times dz), \tag{11.10}$$

where

$$H(t) = I - Y_{\lambda\beta}(t) Y_{\lambda\beta}^-(t).$$

Note that the estimator of γ may be modified to avoid Lebesgue integration as

$$\int_0^\tau Y_\gamma^T(t) H(t) \Lambda(t) Y_\gamma(t) \, dt \approx \int_0^\tau Y_\gamma^T(t) H(t) \text{diag}(dN(t)) Y_\gamma(t). \tag{11.11}$$

Note also that that $H(t)$ is a projection on the orthogonal space spanned by the columns of $Y_{\lambda\beta}(t)$, and therefore

$$\int_E H(t) D(z) \, p(dt \times dz) = H(t) \Lambda(t) Y_\gamma(t) dt \gamma + \int_E H(t) D(z) \, q(dt \times dz),$$

which shows that difference between $\tilde{\gamma}$ and the true γ is a martingale. Once we have obtained the estimate of γ using (11.10) we may then estimate $B(t)$ by $\hat{B}(\tilde{\gamma})(t)$.

One problem remains, however, since the above estimators depend on the individual sampling intensities, which are unknowns. One option is to build a sufficiently flexible model for the intensities. Note that such a model can be validated separately without involving the longitudinal measurements using the techniques described in the earlier chapters. Martinussen & Scheike (2001) applied the Aalen additive model while Lin & Ying (2001) used the Cox-model. One may also take a fully nonparametric approach as suggested by Sun & Wu (2005). To illustrate how the latter approach works note that $\Lambda(t)$ may be seen as a weight matrix in the above estimators. For example, in the expression for $\tilde{\gamma}$, we may rewrite

$$Y_\gamma^T(t) H(t) \Lambda(t) Y_\gamma(t)$$

11.2 Semiparametric additive model for longitudinal data

as

$$Y_\gamma^T(t)\Lambda(t)Y_\gamma(t) - Y_\gamma^T(t)(Y_\beta^T(t)\Lambda(t)Y_\beta(t))^{-1}Y_\beta^T(t)\Lambda(t)Y_\gamma(t).$$

Terms involving $\Lambda(t)$, such as $Y_\gamma^T(t)\Lambda(t)Y_\gamma(t)$, may then be replaced by kernel estimators as follows:

$$Y_\gamma^T(t)\Lambda(t)Y_\gamma(t) = \sum_i \lambda_i(t) X_{\gamma i}(t) X_{\gamma i}^T(t)$$

$$\approx \sum_i \frac{1}{b}\int K(\frac{t-s}{b}) X_{\gamma i}(s) X_{\gamma i}^T(s) \lambda_i(s)\, ds$$

$$\approx \sum_i \frac{1}{b}\int K(\frac{t-s}{b}) X_{\gamma i}(s) X_{\gamma i}^T(s) dN_i(s),$$

where K denotes a kernel and b a bandwidth. This approach is clearly appealing because it avoids any modeling of the sampling intensities that in this context are nuisance parameters. On the other hand it is our experience that often very simple models will be able to describe the sampling intensities, and the inferred estimators of $(B(t), \gamma)$ may have better small sample properties borrowing strength from the model for the intensities. It remains of course important to validate the intensity model.

Smoothing of the underlying sampling intensities can be avoided at a price, as we indicate in the following example.

Example 11.2.1 (Testing and Estimation without smoothing)

Consider the simple nonparametric regression model with i.i.d. samples from the two sample model

$$Z_{i,j} = m_j(T_{i,j}) + \epsilon_{i,j} \qquad j=1,2$$

where $\epsilon_{i,j}$ are zero mean residuals with variance σ_j^2 and $T_{i,k}$ is positive with density $f_j(s)$. As earlier we let n_j for $j=1,2$ denote the number of observations within each group. Let the ordered design points within each sample and their corresponding response values be denoted $(T_{(i,j)}, Z_{(i,j)})$ $(T_{(i,j)} < T_{(i+1,j)})$.

A Priestley-Chao type estimator of $B_j(x) = \int_0^x m_j(s)ds$ (Priestley & Chao, 1972) is given by

$$\hat{B}_j(t) = \sum_{i=1}^n Z_{(i,j)}(T_{(i,j)} - T_{(i-1,j)}) I(T_{(i,j)} < t) + Z_{(i+1,j)}(t - T_{(i,j)})$$

for $k=1,2$. Let also $n = n_1 + n_2$.

It can be derived (Scheike, 2000) that $n_j^{1/2}(\hat{B}_j(t) - B_j(t))$ converge to a Gaussian martingale process with variance function $2\int_0^x \sigma_j^2(s)/f_j(s)ds$. When the design points are fixed the factor two disappears. The price for not doing smoothing is therefore that the variance is twice as big. Sun & Wu (2003) extended this to the longitudinal data setting and gave a detailed proof. □

In the following we outline the large sample properties of the estimators (11.10) and $\hat{B}(\tilde{\gamma}, t)$ assuming that the measurement intensities may be described by Aalen's additive intensity model. The Aalen additive hazards model assumes that

$$\lambda_i(t) = Y_i(t) X_{\alpha i}^T(t) \alpha(t),$$

where $Y_i(t)$ is the at risk indicator, $\alpha(t) = (\alpha_1(t), \ldots, \alpha_u(t))^T$ is a vector of unspecified locally integrable time-dependent regression functions and $X_{\alpha i}(t)$ are covariates. As mentioned earlier this model will often provide a good fit to data since it is a first order Taylor expansion of the true intensity.

As mentioned earlier, the estimator of γ may be modified avoiding Lebesgue integration leading to

$$\hat{\gamma} = \left(\int_0^\tau Y_\gamma^T(s) \hat{H}(s) \mathrm{diag}(Y_\alpha(s) Y_\alpha^-(s) p(ds \times dz)) Y_\gamma(s) \right)^{-1}$$
$$\times \int_0^\tau \int_E Y_\gamma^T(s) \hat{H}(s) D(z) \, p(ds \times dz)$$

using that $\hat{Y}_{\lambda\gamma}(t) = \mathrm{diag}(Y_\alpha(t) \hat{\alpha}(t)) Y_\gamma(t)$ where for these expressions $\hat{f}(t) = f(\hat{\alpha}, t)$ for a function f of α, and $\hat{\alpha}$ is the estimate of α based on Aalen's model.

The asymptotic distributions of the estimators may now be derived under the regularity conditions stated Martinussen & Scheike (2001). Under these conditions it may be shown that

$$n^{1/2}(\hat{\gamma} - \gamma) = n^{1/2} C_1 \int_0^\tau \int_E H_1(t, z) \, q(dt \times dz) + O_p(n^{1/2} b^2),$$

where

$$C_1 = \left(\int_0^\tau \int_E Y_\gamma^T(t) \hat{H}(t) \mathrm{diag}(Y_\alpha(t) Y_\alpha^-(t) p(dt \times dz)) Y_\gamma(t) \right)^{-1}$$

and

$$H_1(t, z) = Y_\gamma^T(t) \hat{H}(t) \left(D(z) - \mathrm{diag}\left(Y_\beta(t) \beta(t) + Y_\gamma(t) \gamma \right) Y_\alpha(t) Y_\alpha^-(t) \right).$$

Define an estimate $\hat{H}_1(t, z)$ of $H_1(t, z)$ by replacing $\beta(t)$ and γ by their estimates. The variance of the above martingale may be estimated consistently by

$$n C_1^T \int_0^\tau \int_E \hat{H}_2(s, z)^T p(ds \times dz) \hat{H}_2(s, z) C_1.$$

The non-parametric components in the semi-parametric model are asymptotically jointly Gaussian

$$n^{1/2}(\hat{B}(\hat{\gamma})(t) - B(t)) = n^{1/2} \int_0^t \int_E H_2(s,z) q(ds \times dz)$$
$$- \int_0^t \hat{Y}_{\lambda\beta}^-(s) \hat{Y}_{\lambda\gamma}(s) \, ds \, n^{1/2}(\hat{\gamma} - \gamma) + n^{1/2} O_p(b^2),$$

where

$$H_2(t,z) = \hat{Y}_{\lambda\beta}^-(t)\{D(z) - \mathrm{diag}(Y_\beta(t)\beta(t) + Y_\gamma(t)\gamma) \, Y_\alpha(t) Y_\alpha^-(t)\}.$$

Again undersmoothing ($b = o(n^{-1/4})$) is necessary to get the remainder term to disappear asymptotically. Thus implying that $n^{1/2}(\hat{B}(t) - B(t))$ is a Gaussian process (asymptotically) with covariance function that is estimated consistently by (suppressing the dependency on (z,t) in the integrands)

$$\int_0^t \int_E \hat{H}_3^T p(ds \times dz) \hat{H}_3 + C_2(t)^T \left(\int_0^\tau \int_E \hat{H}_2^T p(dt \times dz) \hat{H}_2 \right) C_2(t)$$
$$- C_2(t) \left(\int_0^t \int_E \hat{H}_3^T p(ds \times dz) \hat{H}_2 \right) - \left(\int_0^t \int_E \hat{H}_2^T p(ds \times dz) \hat{H}_3 \right) C_2(t)^T,$$

where $C_2(t) = n \int_0^t \hat{Y}_{\lambda\beta}^-(s)\hat{Y}_{\lambda\gamma}(s) \, ds C_1$.

11.3 Efficient estimation

In the previous section, estimators of the parameters defining the conditional mean of the longitudinal response were developed based on cumulating the response variables over time. Doing so, the unknown parameters appeared in the compensator, and, based on that, natural estimators were developed. In this section we discuss how to obtain more efficient estimators.

Assume that the conditional mean of the response is

$$m_i(t) = X_i^T(t)\beta(t)$$

and that the measurement intensity is

$$\lambda_i(t) = Y_i(t) X_{\alpha i}(t)^T \alpha(t).$$

The estimator suggested in the previous section of $B(t) = \int_0^t \beta(s) \, ds$ is

$$\hat{B}(t) = \int_0^t \int_E \hat{Y}_{\lambda\beta}^-(s) D(z) \, p(ds \times dz).$$

This estimator has good properties after the responses have been subtracted their overall mean, but the estimator is not location-shift invariant. Therefore when the mean of the response is large, one can improve the performance of the estimator by subtracting a quantity from $D(z)$ (the responses). Denote this quantity as $f(t)$ an $n \times n$ matrix. To obtain a zero mean process $\hat{B} - B$, f must satisfy that $f(t)Y_\alpha(t)\alpha(t) = 0$. A natural choice is

$$f(t) = D(E(t))(I - Y_\alpha(t)Y_\alpha^-(t)) \qquad (11.12)$$

where $E(t) = Y_\beta(t)\beta(t)$. Lin & Ying (2001) subtracted $f_{LY}(t)$ defined as $f(t)$ above where $D(E(t))$ is replaced by $D(\bar{Y}(t))$, and where $\bar{Y}(t)$ is the mean of the responses closest in time to t for all subjects. We will proceed with (11.12) but before proposing the estimator, we give some arguments on how the generalized inverse should be chosen. The differential of the marked point process may (asymptotically) be decomposed as

$$\int_E \hat{\Lambda}^{-1}(t)(D(z) - f(t))\, p(dt \times dz)$$

$$\approx Y_\beta(t)\, dB(t) + \int_E \hat{\Lambda}^{-1}(t)(D(z) - D(E(t)))\, q(dt \times dz), \qquad (11.13)$$

where $q(dt \times dz)$ are the basic marked point process martingales. The last term on the right-hand side of (11.13) may be thought of as the error term so an optimal strategy will be to weight with the inverse of the variance of this term when computing the estimator. The variance is given by the predictable variation, which is

$$\hat{\Lambda}^{-1}(t)\Lambda(t)D(\sigma^2(t))\hat{\Lambda}^{-1}(t),$$

where $\sigma^2(t) = (\sigma_1^2(t), ..., \sigma_n^2(t))$ is the variance of the responses. This expression for the variance depends only on the sampling intensities and the variance of the responses. If f is replaced with another function there will be a bias component additional to the variance of the responses.

Supposing variance homogeneity leads to the estimator

$$\hat{B}^*(t) = \int_0^t \int_E \hat{Y}_{\lambda\beta}^-(s)(D(z) - f(s))\, p(ds \times dz), \qquad (11.14)$$

where $\hat{Y}_{\lambda\beta}^-(t) = (Y_\beta^T(t)\hat{\Lambda}(t)Y_\beta(t))^{-1}Y_\beta^T(t)$. If there is different variances across subjects this should be reflected accordingly in the above estimator, but will not be pursued here. The above estimator has a variance that only depends on the design and the residual variation of the responses. The estimator is, however, still only asymptotically location-shift invariant. To get an location-shift invariant estimator we use the asymptotically equivalent estimator to (11.14):

$$\hat{B}(t) = \int_0^t \int_E \hat{Y}_{\lambda\beta}^-(s)(D(z) - D(\tilde{E}(t)))\, p(ds \times dz) + \int_0^t \tilde{\beta}(s)ds, \qquad (11.15)$$

11.3 Efficient estimation

where $\tilde{E}(t) = Y_\beta(t)\tilde{\beta}(t)$ and $\tilde{\beta}(t)$ is an initial estimator of $\beta(t)$. This estimator will typically have better small sample properties than (11.14).

For normally distributed errors one may show that (11.15) is in fact asymptotically efficient. The derivations of this is outlined in the following note.

Note. Normally distributed errors
The estimator (11.15) may be derived from the efficient score approach (Bickel et al., 1993) in the case of normally distributed errors. Assume that the covariates X_i are time independent and that $Z_i \,|\, X_i, T_i = t \sim N(E_i(t), \sigma^2(t))$ with $E_i(t) = X_{\beta i}^T \beta(t)$. Let $\frac{\partial \beta}{\partial \eta}(t) = b(t)$. The normed score operator for β is

$$\dot{l}_\eta(b) = n^{-1} \sum_i \int_0^\tau \int_E \left(\frac{z - X_{\beta i}^T \beta(t)}{\sigma^2(t)} \right) X_{\beta i}^T b(t) p_i(dt \times dz).$$

Given an initial consistent estimator, $\tilde{\beta}(t)$, of $\beta(t)$ we obtain

$$\dot{l}_\eta(b) = n^{-1} \sum_i \int_0^\tau \int_E b^T(t) X_{\beta i} \left(\frac{z - X_{\beta i}^T \tilde{\beta}(t)}{\sigma^2(t)} \right) p_i(dt \times dz)$$
$$- n^{-1} \sum_i \int_0^\tau \sigma^{-2}(t) b^T(t) X_{\beta i} X_{\beta i}^T Y_i(t) \lambda_i(t) dB(t)$$
$$+ n^{-1} \sum_i \int_0^\tau \sigma^{-2}(t) b^T(t) X_{\beta i} X_{\beta i}^T \tilde{\beta}(t) Y_i(t) \lambda_i(t) \, dt + Q$$

where

$$Q = n^{-1} \sum_i \int_0^\tau \int_E \sigma^{-2}(t) b^T(t) X_{\beta i} X_{\beta i}^T (\tilde{\beta}(t) - \beta(t)) q_i(dt \times dz).$$

If either $\tilde{\beta}$ is assumed predictable or of bounded variation it follows by Lenglart's inequality or by Lemma 1 of Spiekerman & Lin (1998) (see Chapter 2) that Q converges to zero in probability. Set $\dot{l}_\eta(b) = 0$ and solve for $\hat{B}(t)$, ignoring the lower order term Q, gives

$$\int_0^\tau b^T(t) \sum_i \sigma^{-2}(t) X_{\beta i} X_{\beta i}^T Y_i(t) \lambda_i(t) d\hat{B}(t)$$
$$= \int_0^\tau b^T(t) \int_E \sum_i X_{\beta i} \left(\frac{z - X_{\beta i}^T \tilde{\beta}(t)}{\sigma^2(t)} \right) p_i(dt \times dz) \qquad (11.16)$$
$$+ \int_0^\tau b^T(t) \sum_i \sigma^{-2}(t) X_{\beta i} X_{\beta i}^T Y_i(t) \lambda_i(t) \tilde{\beta}(t) \, dt.$$

11. Marked point process models

Substituting

$$\hat{B}(t) = \int_0^t \left(\sum_i X_{\beta i} X_{\beta i}^T Y_i(s)\lambda_i(s)\right)^{-1} \left(\int_E \sum_i X_{\beta i}(z - X_{\beta i}^T \tilde{\beta}(s))p_i(ds \times dz)\right.$$
$$\left. + \sum_i X_{\beta i} X_{\beta i}^T Y_i(s)\lambda_i(s)\tilde{\beta}(s)\, ds\right)$$
$$= \int_0^t \int_E (Y_\beta^T \Lambda Y_\beta)^{-1} Y_\beta^T (D(z) - D(\tilde{E}))p(ds \times dz) + \int_0^t \tilde{\beta}(s)\, ds$$

into (11.16) gives a solution for any function b which is equivalent to (11.15) when estimates replace the intensity. We now also compute the information bound for B.

The score operator for β for the generic model is

$$i_n(b) = \int_0^\tau \int_E (\frac{z - X^T\beta(t)}{\sigma^2(t)}) X^T b(t) p(dt \times dz)$$
$$= \int_0^\tau \int_E (\frac{z - X^T\beta(t)}{\sigma^2(t)}) X^T b(t) q(dt \times dz)$$

where we have dropped the subscript β from the design X. The score operator, K, is composed of the two operators $K = LR$:

$$La = \int_0^\tau \int_E (\frac{z - X^T\beta(t)}{\sigma^2(t)}) a(t, X) q(dt \times dz)$$

and $Rb = X^T b$. We need to find the efficient influence operator $K(K^T K)^{-1}$. Since

$$\langle a, L^T Lb \rangle = \langle La, Lb \rangle = E(\int a(T,X)b(T,X)Y(t)\lambda(t)\sigma^{-2}(t)\, dt)$$
$$= E(\int a(T,X)b(T,X)\sigma^{-2}(t)\, dN(t))$$
$$= E(a(T,X)b(T,X)\sigma^{-2}(T)) = \langle a, b\sigma^{-2}\rangle,$$

we have $L^T L = \sigma^{-2} I$, and hence $K(K^T K)^{-1} = \sigma^2 LR(R^T R)^{-1}$. Also, since

$$\langle Rb, c \rangle = E(X^T b(T) c(T, X))$$
$$= E(b^T(T) E(Xc(T,X)\,|\,T)) = \langle b, E(Xc(T,X)\,|\,T)\rangle,$$

the adjoint operator R^T is given by $R^T c(T) = E(Xc(T,X)\,|\,T)$. Therefore

$$R^T Rb(t) = E(XX^T b(t)\,|\,T = t) = E(XX^T\,|\,T = t)b(t),$$

which implies

$$(R^T R)^{-1} b(t) = [E(XX^T\,|\,T = t)]^{-1} b(t).$$

We have now calculated the efficient influence operator $K(K^T K)^{-1}$ and it only remains to evaluate the operator at the gradient of B. Proceeding as Sasieni (1992b), it is seen that efficient influence operator should be evaluated at the scalar function $h(\cdot) = 1_{[0,t]}(\cdot)/f_T(\cdot)$ where f_T denotes the marginal density function of T. The efficient covariance function is thus given by

$$\langle K(K^T K)^{-1} h \rangle = \langle h, \sigma^2(\cdot)(R^T R)^{-1} h \rangle$$
$$= \int_0^t (\sigma^2(s)/f_T(s))[E(XX^T \mid T = s)]^{-1} ds$$
$$= \int_0^t \sigma^2(s)[E(\lambda(s)XX^T Y(s))]^{-1} ds \quad (11.17)$$

since $E(XX^T \mid T = t)f_T(t) = E(\lambda(t)XX^T Y(t))$.

For the semiparametric model

$$m_i(t) = X_{\beta i}^T(t)\beta(t) + X_{\gamma i}^T(t)\gamma$$

the improved estimators are also one-step type estimators. Let $(\tilde{\beta}(t), \tilde{\gamma})$ denote the preliminary estimators. The parametric part of the model is estimated by

$$\hat{\gamma} = C_1 \int_0^\tau \int_E \hat{Y}_{\lambda\gamma}^T(s) G(s) \hat{\Lambda}^{-1}(s)(D(z) - D(\tilde{E}(s))) \, p(ds \times dz) + \tilde{\gamma}, \quad (11.18)$$

where

$$G(t) = I - Y_\beta(t) Y_\beta^-(t)), \quad Y_\beta^-(t) = (Y_\beta^T(t) \hat{\Lambda}(t) Y_\beta(t))^{-1} Y_\beta^T(t),$$

and $\tilde{E}(t) = X_{\beta i}^T(t)\tilde{\beta}(t) + X_{\gamma i}(t)\tilde{\gamma}$ and

$$C_1 = \left(\int_0^\tau \hat{Y}_\gamma^T(s) D(Y_\alpha(s) Y_\alpha^-(s) dN(s)) G(s) Y_\gamma(s) \right)^{-1}. \quad (11.19)$$

The nonparametric component of the model is estimated as

$$\hat{B}(\hat{\gamma})(t) = \int_0^t \int_E Y_\beta^-(s) \hat{\Lambda}^{-1}(s)(D(z) - D(\tilde{E}(s))) \, p(ds \times dz)$$
$$+ \int_0^t \tilde{\beta}(s) ds + C_2(t)(\hat{\gamma} - \tilde{\gamma}).$$

11.4 Marginal models

One key assumption in the above derivation of estimators and for the suggested estimators of their variances in particular was that certain martingales appeared. The martingale structure appeared because the considered mean models where conditional on the entire past available at that point in time. Such an approach may be inappropriate in some situations. For example consider a two sample situation with longitudinal measurements on each subject (more than one measurement per subject). If the primary interest is to compare the profiles of two samples, then the conditional mean of a response (at time t) given the available history is of little use in this respect as it will most likely involve previous observed responses. In this situation one should condition on only a *part* of the history namely the information to which sample the individual belongs to (Pepe & Couper, 1997). Consider therefore the following marginal model:

$$E(Z(t) \mid X_\beta(t), X_\gamma(t)\, Y(t) = 1) = X_\beta^T(t)\beta + X_\gamma^T(t)\gamma, \qquad (11.20)$$

where we only condition on the covariate values at time t and that the subject is at study. A similar approach is taken with respect to the measurement intensity. Aalen's additive model is assumed for the conditional mean of the true intensity given covariates at time t. Letting the intensity of the sampling times for a subject be denoted $\phi(t)$, we assume

$$\lambda(t) = E(\phi(t)|Y(t), X_\beta(t)) = Y(t)X_\alpha^T(t)\alpha(t)$$

with $\alpha(t) = (\alpha_1(t), \ldots, \alpha_u(t))^T$

The primary message of this section is that we compute estimators as if we have conditioned the entire history but inference needs to be carried out differently as we can no longer appeal to martingale calculus.

A key property when developing the estimators in the previous section is that the compensator of the considered marked point processes is a product of a term only involving the measurement intensities and a term only involving the parameters of interest. This structure arises naturally when conditioning on the whole past. To ensure a similar structure now where we only condition on a part of the history we need the following conditional independence assumption

$$\begin{aligned}E(m_i(t)\psi_i(t)|X_{\beta i}(t), Y_i(t)) =\ &E(m_i(t)|X_{\beta i}(t), Y_i(t))\times \\ &E(\psi_i(t)|X_{\beta i}(t), Y_i(t)).\end{aligned} \qquad (11.21)$$

With this assumption

$$E(\int_0^t Y_{\lambda\beta}^-(s)(D(z) - f(s))\, p(ds \times dz)) = E(\int_0^t Y_{\lambda\beta}^-(s)\Psi(s)m(s)ds)$$
$$= E(\int_0^t J(s)\beta(s)ds),$$

where $J(s)$ is one when the inverses can be calculated and zero otherwise. When the level of the response and the sampling intensities are correlated the marginal models will not result in the same product as $\Phi(t)m(t)$. The

11.4 Marginal models

consequence of assumption (11.21) is that when there is some interaction between the sampling times and the responses this interaction must be included among the considered covariates X_β. In other words the partly conditional mean model must be sufficiently large to make the sampling times and the responses conditionally independent.

Under regularity conditions and the above assumption (11.21) it may be shown that $n^{1/2}(\hat{\gamma} - \gamma)$ is asymptotically normal with a covariance matrix that is estimated consistently by

$$n \sum_{i=1}^{n} \epsilon_{1,i}(\tau, \hat{\gamma})^{\otimes 2}$$

where

$$\epsilon_{1,i}(t, \gamma) = \int_0^\tau \int_E Y_i(s)\hat{\lambda}_i(s)(X_{\gamma i}(s) - (\hat{Y}_{\lambda\gamma}(s))^T \hat{Y}_{\lambda\beta}(s))(\hat{Y}_{\lambda\beta}(s))^T \hat{Y}_{\lambda\beta}(s))^{-1}$$
$$\times X_{\beta i}(s))(z - E_i(s))p_i(ds \times dz) \qquad (11.22)$$

with $E_i(t) = X_{\beta i}^T(t)\beta(t) + X_{\gamma i}^T(t)\gamma$.

The asymptotic distribution of $n^{1/2}(\hat{B}(t) - B(t))$ is asymptotically equivalent to

$$n^{1/2} \sum_{i=1}^{n} \epsilon_{2,i}(t, \gamma, B)$$

where

$$\epsilon_{2,i}(t, \gamma, B) = \epsilon_{3,i}(t, \gamma, B) - C_2(t)C_1^{-1}\epsilon_{1,i}(\tau, \gamma),$$
$$\epsilon_{3,i}(t, \gamma, B) = \int_0^\tau \int_E (\hat{Y}_{\lambda\beta}(s))^T \hat{Y}_{\lambda\beta}(s))^{-1} Y_i(s) X_{\beta i}(s) \hat{\lambda}_i^{-1}(s)$$
$$\times (z - E_i(s))p_i(ds \times dz).$$

Therefore, under regularity conditions, it follows that $n^{1/2}(\hat{B}(t) - B(t))$ is a zero mean Gaussian process with a covariance function, that can be estimated consistently by

$$n \sum_i \epsilon_{2,i}^{\otimes 2}(s, \hat{\gamma}, \hat{B})$$

The asymptotic distribution of $n^{1/2}(\hat{B}(t) - B(t))$ is further equivalent to

$$n^{1/2} \sum_{i=1}^{n} \epsilon_{3,i}(t, \hat{\gamma}, \hat{B}) G_i$$

where G_i are independent standard normals. This may be used to implement tests and make uniform confidence bands.

Example 11.4.1 (Two sample situation (Continued))

Consider the two sample situation described in Example 11.0.2 and 11.1.3 in the situation where the sampling intensities are different in the two groups, and now also where there are more than one measurement per subject. Since the interest centers on comparing the longitudinal profiles of the two groups the conditional approach taken in the two earlier examples is not appropriate here as the conditional mean of a response given the history should most likely involve earlier obtained responses.

In this example we hence have that $\beta_j(t)$ and $\alpha_j(t)$, $j = 1, 2$, are the marginal mean functions and rate functions, respectively, but the estimators are as described in Example 11.1.3. Recall that the number of subjects in each group are given as n_1 and n_2, respectively and that $n = n_1 + n_2$ such that $n_j/n \to p_j$ for $j = 1, 2$. We still want to base tests on

$$R(t) = \int_0^t w(s) \, d(\hat{B}_1 - \tilde{B}_1)(s),$$

where

$$\hat{B}_1(t) = \sum_i \int_0^t \int_E \frac{z_{i1}}{\hat{\alpha}_1(s) Y_{\cdot 1}(s)} p_{i1}(dt \times dz_{i1}),$$

$$\tilde{B}_1(t) = \sum_{i,j} \int_0^t \int_E \frac{J(s) z_{ij}}{(\hat{\alpha}_1(s) Y_{\cdot 1}(s) + \hat{\alpha}_2(s) Y_{\cdot 2}(s))} p_{ij}(dt \times dz_{ij}),$$

see Example 11.1.3 for further explanations. The asymptotic distribution hinted at in that example (based on martingale calculus) is, however, no longer appropriate.

To obtain the limit distribution we need essentially an i.i.d. decomposition of the involved processes. The independence across subjects will then give us an estimator of the variance-covariance matrix. Write first

$$n^{1/2}(\hat{B}_1(t) - \int_0^t J(s) dB(s)) = n^{-1/2}$$

$$\sum_i \int_0^t \frac{1}{\hat{\alpha}_1(s) n^{-1} Y_{\cdot 1}(s)} \left(\int_E z_{i1} p_{i1}(dt \times dz_{i1}) - \hat{\alpha}_1(s) Y_{i1}(s) J(s) dB(s) \right).$$

One may show that limit distribution of the quantity in the latter display is unaltered by replacing $\hat{\alpha}_1(t)$ and $n^{-1} Y_{\cdot 1}(t)$ by $\alpha_1(t)$ and $y_1(t)$, respectively, where $y_1(t)$ denotes the limit in probability of $n^{-1} Y_{\cdot 1}(t)$. Doing so we then have the wanted i.i.d. decomposition. Similarly, $n^{1/2}(\tilde{B}_1(t) - \int_0^t J(s) dB(s))$

may be decomposed as

$$n^{-1/2}\sum_i \int_0^t \frac{1}{\hat{f}(s)}\left(\int_E z_{i1}p_{i1}(dt \times dz_{i1}) - \hat{\alpha}_1(s)Y_{i1}(s)J(s)dB(s)\right)$$

$$+n^{-1/2}\sum_i \int_0^t \frac{1}{\hat{f}(s)}\left(\int_E z_{i2}p_{i2}(dt \times dz_{i2}) - \hat{\alpha}_2(s)Y_{i2}(s)J(s)dB(s)\right),$$

where $\hat{f}(t) = \hat{\alpha}_1(t)n^{-1}Y_{\cdot 1}(t) + \hat{\alpha}_2(t)n^{-1}Y_{\cdot 2}(t)$. Again we may replace $\hat{\alpha}_j(t)$ and $n^{-1}Y_{\cdot j}(t)$ by $\alpha_j(t)$ and $y_j(t)$, $j = 1, 2$. We therefore have the following i.i.d. decomposition

$$n^{1/2}(\hat{B}_1(t) - \tilde{B}_1(t)) = \sum_{i,j} Q_{ij}(t), \qquad (11.23)$$

where $Q_{ij}(t) = Q_{ij}(t, \alpha_1, \alpha_2, y_1, y_2, dB^*)$ with $B^*(t) = \int_0^t J(s)dB(s)$. The variance-covariance matrix of the right-hand side of (11.23) may therefore be estimated by

$$\sum_{i,j} \hat{Q}_{ij}^{\otimes 2}(t),$$

where $\hat{Q}_{ij}(t) = Q_{ij}(t, \hat{\alpha}_1, \hat{\alpha}_2, n^{-1}Y_{\cdot 1}, n^{-1}Y_{\cdot 2}, d\tilde{B})$. □

Example 11.4.2 (CD4-data)

Consider the data introduced in Example 11.0.1 on post-infection CD4 percentage. We consider the marginal model

$$m_i(t) = \beta_0(t) + \beta_1(t)X_{i1} + \beta_2(t)X_{i2} + \beta_3(t)X_{i3},$$

where X_1 is smoking, X_2 is age at HIV-infection, X_3 is the pre-HIV infection CD4 percentage. Both X_2 and X_3 were centered around their respective averages. Before analyzing the above marginal mean model we take a look at the sampling rates, considering the model

$$\lambda_i(t) = \tilde{\beta}_0(t) + \tilde{\beta}_1(t)X_{i1} + \tilde{\beta}_2(t)X_{i2} + \tilde{\beta}_3(t)X_{i3},$$

which is analyzed in R as follows (running 2000 simulations to get variance estimates).

```
> age.c<-age-mean(age)
> precd4.c<-precd4-mean(precd4)
> rate.fit<-aalen(Surv(lt,rt,indi)~smoke+age.c+precd4.c,data=cd4,
start.time=0,max.time=5.5,id=cd4$id,n.sim=2000)
> plot(rate.fit,sim.ci=2)
```

11. Marked point process models

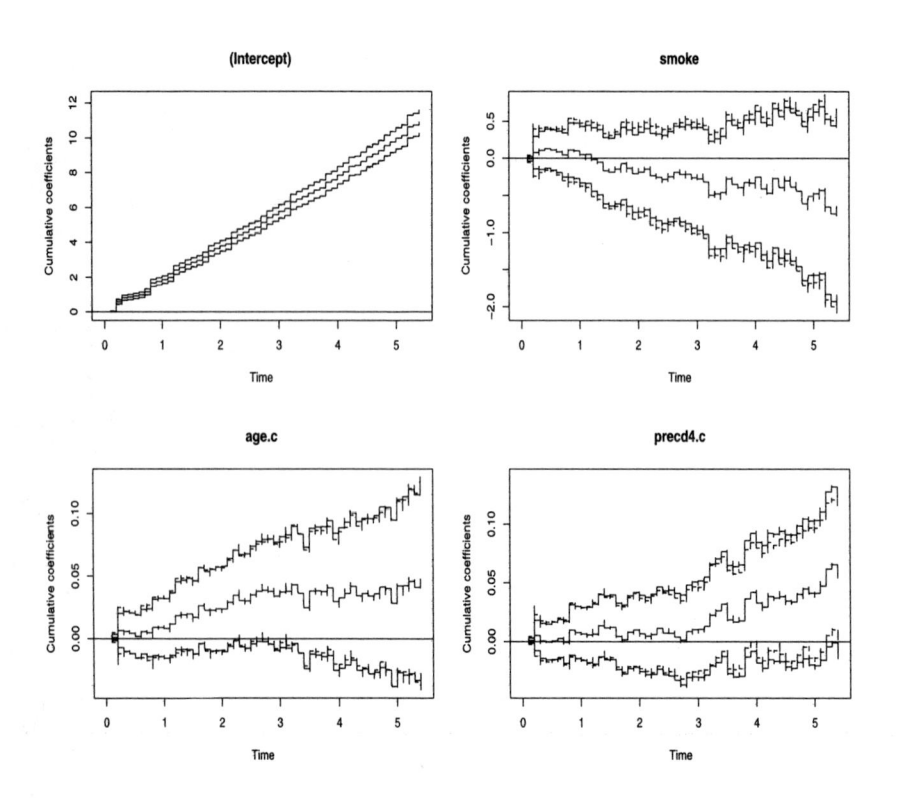

FIGURE 11.2: CD4-data. Estimated cumulative rate coefficients functions for the baseline CD4 percentage and the effects of smoking, age and pre-HIV infection CD4 percentage. Curves are shown along with 95% pointwise confidence limits and a 95% simulation bazsed band

It is seen from Figure 11.2 that there is little indication of any covariate dependency of the rate function, and we proceed with the ordinary Aalen multiplicative model. We turn to the marginal mean model using the Aalen multiplicative model for the rates.

```
> mfit.cd4<-dynreg(cd4~smoke+age.c+precd4.c,data=cd4,
+ Surv(lt,rt,indi)~+1,start.time=0,max.time=5.5,
  id=cd4$id,n.sim=2000,bandwidth=0.2)
Nonparametric Additive Model
Simulations starts N= 2000
> summary(fit.cd4)
> plot(mfit.cd4)


Test for time invariant effects:
            sup| B(t) - (t/tau)B(tau)|   p-value H_0: B(t)=b t
(Intercept)                      9.610                  0.0000
smoke                            4.920                  0.0510
```

11.4 Marginal models

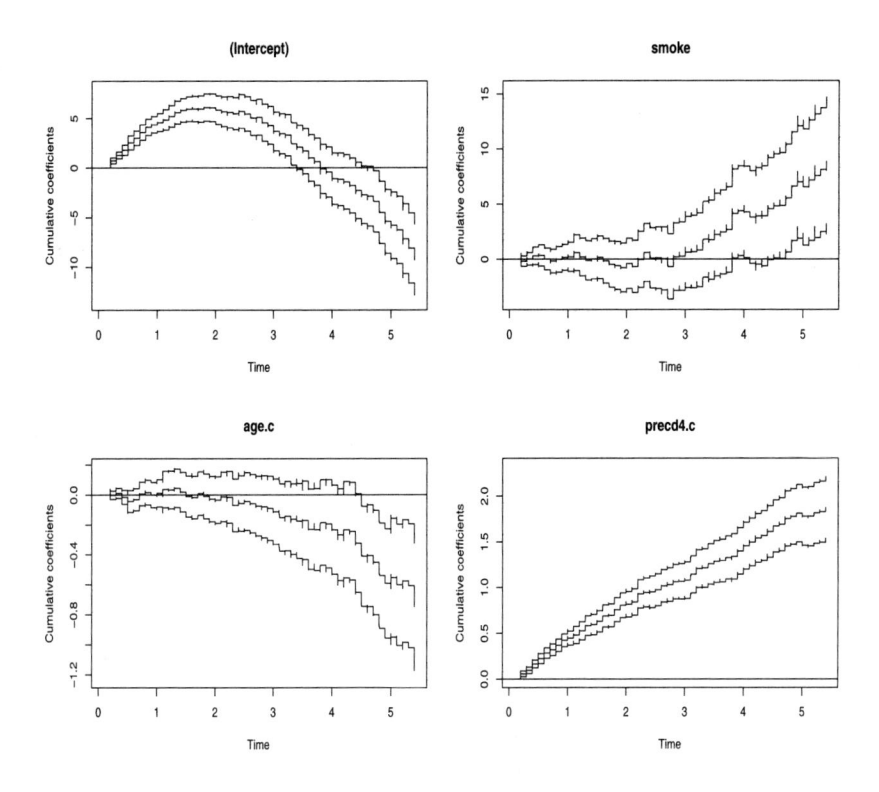

FIGURE 11.3: CD4-data. Estimated cumulative coefficients functions for the baseline CD4 percentage and the effects of smoking, age and pre-HIV infection CD4 percentage. Curves are shown along with 95% pointwise confidence limits

```
age.c                              0.335                  0.0615
precd4.c                           0.195                  0.2640
```

Figure 11.3 and the above tests for time-invariance indicate that it seems appropriate to consider the following semi-parametric model

$$m_i(t) = \beta_0(t) + \beta_1(t)X_{i1} + \beta_2(t)X_{i2} + \gamma_2 X_{i3},$$

with constant effect of pre-HIV infection CD4 percentage.

```
> mfit1.cd4<-dynreg(cd4~smoke+age.c+const(precd4.c),data=cd4,
      Surv(lt,rt,indi)~+1,start.time=0,max.time=5.5,
      id=cd4$id,n.sim=2000,bandwidth=0.2)
> summary(mfit1.cd4)
Test for time invariant effects:
           sup| B(t) - (t/tau)B(tau)|  p-value H_0: B(t)=b t
(Intercept)               9.45                  0.0000
smoke                     5.08                  0.0285
```

```
age.c                              0.40                    0.0170

  Parametric terms :  const(precd4.c)
                Coef.      SE   Robust SE       z   P-val
const(precd4.c)  0.363   0.0305     0.0654    1.190  0.234
```

This suggest that there is a significant indication of the effect of smoking and age being time-varying while there is significant constant effect of pre-HIV infection CD4 percentage with point estimate 0.363 (0.065). There appear to be no effect of smoking the first three years or so and then those who ever smoked seem to have a higher CD4 cell percentage, see Figure 11.3. The age effect generally decreases and is more pronounced as time proceeds. □

To give a further illustration of the methodology we now consider the CSL-data.

Example 11.4.3 (CSL-data)

The CSL1 study were conducted by the Copenhagen Study Group for Liver Diseases (Schlichting et al., 1983). This was a randomized clinical trial where the patients were given either prednisone or placebo. During the period 1962-69, 532 patients with histologically verified liver cirrhosis were included in the trial. In 488 patients the initial biopsy could later be re-evaluated, and we consider only data for these patients. The patients were followed from the date of entry into the trial to death or the closing date of the study, 1 September, 1974. A number of clinical and biochemical variables were registered during the study period. As an illustration, we focus on the variable prothrombin index, which is a measurement of coagulation factors II+VII+X produced by the liver. The range of the prothrombin index in the present dataset is from 6 to 176, where a prothrombin index above 70% is "normal". The number of measurements of prothrombin index for the subjects varies from 1 to 18. The time period that we consider here is the first three years after treatment, which include 70% of the measurements.

It was planned to take measurements at entry, three, six and twelve months after start of treatment and thereafter once a year. Nevertheless, the observed measurement-times cover the whole period. We start by considering a marginal nonparametric model for the current prothrombin index, including sex, age, treatment and a baseline prothrombin index as covariates. Before running the marginal mean model we consider the rate function using the covariates listed above.

```
rate.fit<-aalen(Surv(lt,rt,indi)~treat+prot.base+sex+age,data=csl,
       start.time=0, max.time=3,n.sim=2000)
> summary(rate.fit)
Additive Aalen Model
```

11.4 Marginal models

```
Test for nonparametric terms

Test for non-significant effects
          sup| hat B(t)/SD(t) | p-value H_0: B(t)=0
(Intercept)           22.90                  0.000
treat                  1.73                  0.848
prot.base              4.73                  0.000
sex                    1.41                  0.970
age                    3.48                  0.021

Test for time invariant effects
          sup| B(t) - (t/tau)B(tau)| p-value H_0: B(t)=b t
(Intercept)          1.62000                    0.000
treat                0.23000                    0.220
prot.base            0.00546                    0.115
sex                  0.11600                    0.963
age                  0.00875                    0.562
```

All effects appear to be constant or insignificant. One may in fact reduce the model to include only age and the baseline prothrombin measurement giving the below output, which shows that the effect of these two is significant.

```
rate.fit<-aalen(Surv(lt,rt,indi)~const(prot.base)+const(age),
        data=csl,start.time=0, max.time=3,n.sim=2000)
> summary(rate.fit)
Parametric terms :
                   Coef.      SE   Robust SE        z    P-val
const(prot.base) -0.00528  0.00196   0.00106   -26.938   0.000
const(age)        0.00873  0.00441   0.00226     1.979   0.048
```

We then proceed with the marginal mean model with the rate depending on age and prot.base:

```
> mfit.csl<-dynreg(prot~treat+prot.base+sex+age,data=csl,
        Surv(lt,rt,indi)~const(prot.base)+const(age),
        start.time=0,max.time=3,id=csl$id,
        bandwidth=0.2,meansub=1,n.sim=2000)
> plot(mfit.csl)
> summary(mfit.csl)
Dynamic Additive Regression Model

Test for time invariant effects:
          sup| B(t) - (t/tau)B(tau)| p-value H_0: B(t)=b t
(Intercept)           7.350                    0.2630
treat                 8.420                    0.0015
prot.base             0.123                    0.1090
sex                   2.540                    0.8750
age                   0.211                    0.6000
```

406   11. Marked point process models

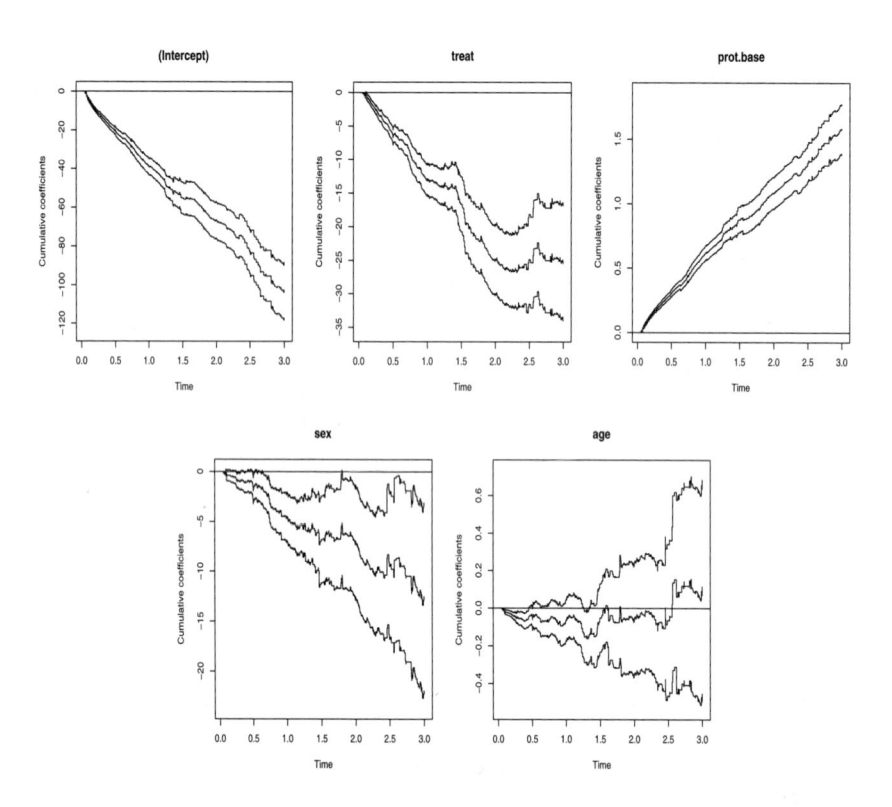

FIGURE 11.4: CSL-data. Estimated cumulative regression functions along with 95% pointwise confidence intervals.

As seen from the above output and Figure 11.4 it seems as the effect of treatment is time-arying while the effect of the remaining covariates is constant.

```
> mfit2.csl<-dynreg(prot~treat+const(prot.base)+const(sex)+
          const(age),data=csl,Surv(lt,rt,indi)~
          const(prot.base)+const(age),start.time=0,
          max.time=3,id=csl$id,bandwidth=0.2,meansub=1,
          n.sim=2000)
> plot(mfit2.csl)
> summary(mfit2.csl)
Dynamic Additive Regression Model

  Nonparametric terms : (Intercept) treat
Test for nonparametric terms
Test for non-significant effects:
           sup| hat B(t)/SD(t) | p-value H_0: B(t)=0
(Intercept)                21.80                   0
treat                       8.19                   0
```

11.4 Marginal models   407

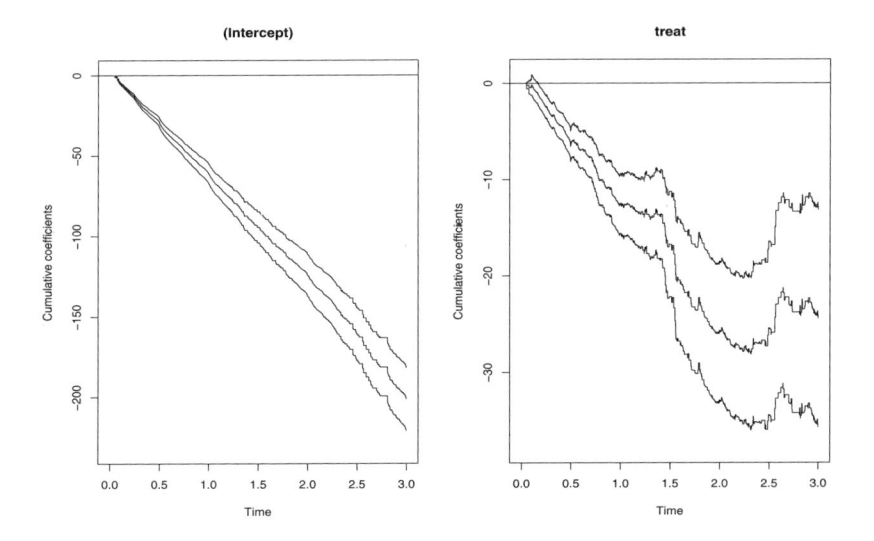

FIGURE 11.5: CSL-data. Estimated cumulative regression functions along with 95% pointwise confidence intervals.

```
Test for time invariant effects:
               sup| B(t) - (t/tau)B(tau)|  p-value H_0: B(t)=b t
(Intercept)                        9.85                    0e+00
treat                             10.10                    5e-04

Parametric terms :  const(prot.base) const(sex) const(age)
                    Coef.     SE   Robust SE       z    P-val
const(prot.base)   0.5880  0.0286     0.0418  20.559    0.000
const(sex)        -4.7100  1.2100     1.7100  -3.897    0.000
const(age)        -0.0525  0.0605     0.0853  -0.867    0.386
```

We conclude that there is significant effect of sex, the baseline prothrombin index and treatment. The men have a lower prothrombin index, the point estimate is −4.71 with standard error 1.71. The effect on the prothrombin index of treatment clearly changes with time. In the two first years or so there seems to be a beneficial effect of prednisone. The effect then levels off and there is even an indication of an adverse effect of prednisone thereafter, see Figure 11.5 □

11.5 Exercises

11.1 (Regression data. Goodness-of-fit.) Consider a sample (X_i, Z_i), $i = 1, \ldots, n$, of n i.i.d. regression data with Z_i being the (one-dimensional) response and X_i the (one-dimensional) regressor. Let

$$E(Z_i \mid X_i = x) = \phi(x)$$

and assume that X_i has an absolute continuous distribution on $[0, \infty)$ with hazard function $\alpha(x)$. Assume also that $\int_0^x \alpha(v)\phi(v)\, dv < \infty$ for all x.

(a) Write $Z_i I(X_i \leq x)$ as a marked point process integral and give its compensator.

(b) Suggest an estimator of $A(x) = \int_0^x \alpha(v)\, dv$ and of $\alpha(x)$. The latter we denote by $\hat{\alpha}(x)$.

(c) Argue that a sensible estimator of $\Phi(x) = \int_0^x \phi(v)\, dv$ is

$$\hat{\Phi}(x) = \sum_{i=1}^n \frac{Z_i I(X_i \leq x)}{\hat{\alpha}(X_i) Y.(X_i)},$$

where $Y.(x) = \sum_{i=1}^n Y_i(x)$ with $Y_i(x) = I(x \leq X_i)$.

We shall now consider the parametric model

$$\phi(x, \theta) = g(x)^T \theta,$$

where $g(x) = (g_1(x), \ldots, g_p(x))^T$ is a vector of known functions of x and θ is a p-vector of unknown parameters.

(d) Give the compensator of $\sum_{i=1}^n g(X_i) Z_i I(X_i \leq x)$. Argue that this leads naturally to the estimator

$$\hat{\theta} = \left(\int_0^\infty Y.(x) g(x) g(x)^T d\hat{A}(x) \right)^{-1} \sum_{i=1}^n \int_0^\infty \int_E g(x_i) z_i p_i(dx_i \times dz_i),$$

and that this estimator is nothing but the usual least squares estimator

$$\left(\sum_{i=1}^n g(X_i) g(X_i)^T \right)^{-1} \sum_{i=1}^n g(X_i) Z_i.$$

As

$$M(x) = \sum_{i=1}^n Z_i I(X_i \leq x) - \int_0^x Y.(v) g(u)^T dA(u) \theta$$

is a martingale it seems natural to base a goodness-of-fit test for fit of the assumed parametric model on the process

$$M_{\text{res}}(x) = \sum_{i=1}^n Z_i I(X_i \leq x) - \int_0^x Y.(v) g(u)^T d\hat{A}(u) \hat{\theta}.$$

(e) Find (under appropriate conditions) the asymptotic distribution of the process $n^{-1/2}M_{\text{res}}(x)$ assuming that the above parametric model holds. Is the limit process a Gaussian martingale?

(f) Try to use the Khmaladze transformation (see Appendix A) on the above goodness-of-fit process so that the obtained limit process is a Gaussian martingale.

11.2 (Simple marked point process) Consider a marked point-process with induced counting process $N(t)$ with intensity $\lambda(t)$ and with marks distribution given by

$$Z_k = m(\theta_0, \theta_1, T_k) + \epsilon_k,$$

where $m(\theta_0, \theta_1, T_k) = \theta_0 + \theta_1 T_k$, T_k denotes the kth jump time and ϵ_k is a standard normal.

(a) What is the compensator of the marked point process?

(b) What is the compensator of the derived marked point process

$$\int_0^t \int_E (z - m(\theta_0, \theta_1, s))^2 p(dz \times ds)?$$

(c) Now assume that n i.i.d. subjects from the above generic model is being observed. Estimate the parameters by least squares and sketch a proof for asymptotic normality and consistency of the estimators.

Appendix A
Khmaladze's transformation

In the sequel we review, based on Martinussen & Skovgaard (2002), how certain processes may be transformed to Gaussian martingales. The technique is originally developed in Khmaladze (1981), where strict proofs are given. Let us first consider the prototype example of a (time-transformed) Brownian bridge before we turn to the general formulation. Let $B(t) = H(t) - \beta t$, where $H(t)$ is a Gaussian martingale on $[0,1]$ with variance function $\mathrm{var} H(t) = \int_0^t a(s)^{-1} ds$. The quantity β may be stochastic such as $\beta = H(1) - H(0)$ corresponding to the Brownian bridge case. We seek a linear transformation of the process B to a Gaussian martingale. Furthermore we can make the term βt vanish by this transformation. The transformation to the new process $\tilde{B}$ is given as

$$\tilde{B}(t) = B(t) - \int_0^t \left(\int_s^1 a(u)\, du \right)^{-1} \int_s^1 a(u)\, dB(u)\, ds, \qquad (\text{A.1})$$

which is a Gaussian martingale with the same variance function as H. The idea behind this result of Khmaladze is described below. But first a direct calculation shows that $\tilde{H} = \tilde{B}$ (with $\tilde{H}(t)$ defined by (A.1) replacing B with H), or in other words that the term βt is killed by the transformation. Thus, in particular, the distribution of $\tilde{B}$ is not affected by β being stochastic, even if it depends on the entire process. More generally let $H(t)$ and $B(t)$ be p-vector processes on $[0, \tau]$ so that that $B(t) = H(t) + g(t)\beta$, where $H(t)$ is a Gaussian martingale, $g(t)$ is a (known) $p \times q$-matrix and β is a q-vector that should be thought of as being random so that B is not Gaussian martingale. Let the variance function H be $\mathrm{var} H(t) = \int_0^t a(s)^{-1} ds$, which

Appendix A. Khmaladze's transformation

is now a $p \times p$-matrix. Then

$$\tilde{H}(t) = H(t) - \int_0^t a^{-1}(s)a(s)g'(s) \left(\int_s^\tau g'(u)^T a(u) a^{-1}(u) a(u) g'(u) \, du \right)^{-1}$$
$$\times \int_s^\tau g'(u)^T a(u) \, dH(u) \, ds$$
$$= H(t) - \int_0^t g'(s) \left(\int_s^\tau g'(u)^T a(u) g'(u) \, du \right)^{-1}$$
$$\times \int_s^\tau g'(u)^T a(u) \, dH(u) \, ds$$

is again a Gaussian martingale with the same variance function, and it is directly verified that $\tilde{H}(t) = \tilde{B}(t)$ for all t, so that any component $g(t)\beta$ is killed by conversion from the process $B(t)$ to $\tilde{B}(t)$. We hence also have that

$$\tilde{B}(t) = B(t) - \int_0^t g'(s) \left(\int_s^\tau g'(u)^T a(u) g'(u) \, du \right)^{-1}$$
$$\times \int_s^\tau g'(u)^T a(u) \, dB(u) \, ds, \qquad (A.2)$$

is a Gaussian martingale with the same variance function as $H(t)$. The transformation of B to $\tilde{B}$ given by (A.2) is what we usually call *Khmaladze's transformation*.

The two key steps in the derivation of the result are a projection followed by a Doob-Meyer decomposition. First the projection, P_L onto the subspace, L, spanned by the columns of $g(t)$ is

$$(P_L H)(t) = g(t) \left(\int_0^\tau g'(s)^T a(s) g'(s) \, ds \right)^{-1} \int_0^\tau g'(s)^T a(s) \, dH(s),$$

where the inverse variance is used as inner product in the definition of the projection. Application of the orthogonal projection $I - P_L$ to $B(t)$ kills the term $g(t)\beta$ and hence gives the same result as when applied to $H(t)$.

Next we need to adjust $(I - P_L)H(t)$ by subtraction of its compensator given the σ-algebra spanned by the original σ-algebra defining the martingale, $\mathcal{F}_t$ say, and $P_L H$. This is done by calculating the martingale increment by subtraction of the conditional expectation,

$$d\tilde{H}(t) = dH(t) - \text{cov}\,(dH(t), Z(t))\,\text{var}(Z(t))^{-1} Z(t),$$

where

$$Z(t) = \int_t^\tau g'(s)^T a(s) \, dH(s)$$

is a non-singular representation of the extra information contained in $P_L H$ relative to the σ-algebra $\mathcal{F}_t$. Note that when we subtract the compensator

Appendix A. Khmaladze's transformation

we should in principle start from the process $(I - P_L)H(t)$ but the term $P_L H(t)$ disappears because it is predictable. The expression for $\tilde{H}$ follows directly by calculation of the covariance and variance above.

That the covariance function for $\tilde{H}$ is the same as that for H may be seen by the following calculation. First write

$$\text{cov}\{\tilde{H}(t_1), \tilde{H}(t_2)\} = \int_0^{t_1} \int_0^{t_2} \text{cov}\{d\tilde{H}(t_1), d\tilde{H}(t_2)\}\, ds_2\, ds_1.$$

For $s_1 < s_2$ we rewrite the integrand as

$$\text{cov}\{d\tilde{H}(s_1), d\tilde{H}(s_2)\} = \text{cov}\{dH(s_1), dH(s_2)\} - \text{cov}\{dH(s_1), b(s_2)Z(s_2)\} - \text{cov}\{b(s_1)Z(s_1), d\tilde{H}(s_2)\},$$

where $b(s)$ equals the non-random regression coefficient

$$\text{cov}\{dg(s), Z(s)\} \text{var}\{Z(s)\}^{-1}.$$

Using the fact that H has independent increments we see that the second term on the right vanishes because $Z(s_2)$ is a linear function of increments of H over the interval (s_2, τ) which is disjoint from $(s_1, s_1 + ds_1)$. To see that also the third term vanishes note that $Z(s_1) = Z(s_2) + U$ where U is a function of increments over the interval (s_1, s_2). By construction $d\tilde{H}(s_2)$ is independent of the "past" and orthogonalized on $Z(s_2)$ thus completing the argument, which applies similarly to $s_2 < s_1$.

Appendix B
Matrix derivatives

In the following we give some convenient formulae for matrix differentiation. The results are taken from MacRae (1974) where additional results and details can be found.

Consider a $m \times n$-matrix Y, which is a function of the $p \times q$-matrix X. The derivative of matrix Y with respect to X is defined to be an $mp \times nq$-matrix of partial derivatives

$$dY/dX = Y \otimes dX,$$

where $\otimes$ denotes the Kronecher product. Hence

$$dY/dX = \begin{pmatrix} dy_{11}/dX & \cdots & dy_{1n}/dX \\ \vdots & \ddots & \vdots \\ dy_{m1}/dX & \cdots & dy_{mn}/dX \end{pmatrix}.$$

The following results can then be shown.

Theorem B.0.1 *Let Y and Z be matrix functions of X, and let the product YZ be defined. Then*

$$d(YZ)/dX = (dY/dX)(Z \otimes I_q) + (Y \otimes I_p)(dZ/dX). \quad \text{(Product rule)}$$

Theorem B.0.2 *Let Y be a nonsingular matrix function of X. Then*

$$d(Y^{-1})/dX = -(Y^{-1} \otimes I_p)(dY/dX)(Y^{-1} \otimes I_q). \quad \text{(Inverse rule)}$$

Appendix C
The Timereg survival package for **R**

This chapter contains a brief description of how to obtain the programs used for the analyses in the book. All programs are available as an add-on-package for the statistical software **R**. The package is available under the general public license (GPL).

The package is available from the Timereg page

http:\\biostat.ku.dk\~ts\timereg.html

where versions for Linux (Unix) and Windows are available.

After downloading the package and following the instructions given on the homepage you should get a library to use within **R**.

We here give a few extra details in the Linux case. If you do not have super-user permissions you might set up your own local library by the commands

```
R CMD INSTALL timereg --library localdir
```

and then inside **R** write

```
> .libPaths("localdir")
> library(timereg)
This is timereg 0.1-2
```

Manual pages from Timereg package

aalen	*Fit additive hazards model*

Description

Fits both the additive hazards model of Aalen and the semi-parametric additive hazards model of McKeague and Sasieni. Estimates are unweighted. Time dependent variables and counting process data (multiple events per subject) are possible.

Resampling is used for computing p-values for tests of time-varying effects.

The modeling formula uses the standard survival modeling given in the **survival package**.

Usage

```
aalen(formula,data=sys.parent(),start.time=0,max.time=0,
robust=1,id=NULL,clusters=NULL,residuals=0,n.sim=1000,
weighted.test=0,covariance=0,resample.iid=0)
```

Arguments

formula	a formula object with the response on the left of a '~' operator, and the independent terms on the right as regressors. The response must be a survival object as returned by the 'Surv' function.
data	a data.frame with the variables.
start.time	start of observation period where estimates are computed.
max.time	end of observation period where estimates are computed. Estimates thus computed from [start.time, max.time]
robust	to compute robust variances and construct processes for resampling. May be set to 0 to save memory.
id	For time-varying covariates the variable must associate each record with the id of a subject.
clusters	cluster variable for computation of robust variances.
n.sim	number of simulations in resampling.

---

[0]Reproduced with permission from the documentation files in the Timereg package

`weighted.test`	to compute a variance weighted version of the test-processes used for testing time-varying effects.
`residuals`	to returns residuals that can be used for model validation in the function cum.residuals
`covariance`	to compute covariance estimates for nonparametric terms rather than just the variances.
`resample.iid`	to return i.i.d. representation for nonparametric and parametric terms.

Details

The data for a subject is presented as multiple rows or "observations", each of which applies to an interval of observation (start, stop]. For counting process data with the)start,stop] notation is used the 'id' variable is needed to identify the records for each subject. The program assumes that there are no ties, and if such are present random noise is added to break the ties.

Value

returns an object of type "aalen". With the following arguments:

`cum`	cumulative time-varying regression coefficient estimates are computed within the estimation interval.
`var.cum`	the martingale based pointwise variance estimates for cumulatives.
`robvar.cum`	robust pointwise variances estimates for cumulatives.
`gamma`	estimate of parametric components of model.
`var.gamma`	variance for gamma.
`robvar.gamma`	robust variance for gamma.
`residuals`	list with residuals.
`obs.testBeq0`	observed absolute value of supremum of cumulative components scaled with the variance.
`pval.testBeq0`	p-value for covariate effects based on supremum test.
`sim.testBeq0`	resampled supremum values.
`obs.testBeqC`	observed absolute value of supremum of difference between observed cumulative process and estimate under null of constant effect.
`pval.testBeqC`	p-value based on resampling.
`sim.testBeqC`	resampled supremum values.

obs.testBeqC.is
: observed integrated squared differences between observed cumulative and estimate under null of constant effect.

pval.testBeqC.is
: p-value based on resampling.

sim.testBeqC.is
: resampled supremum values.

conf.band
: resampling based constant to construct robust 95% uniform confidence bands.

test.procBeqC
: observed test-process of difference between observed cumulative process and estimate under null of constant effect over time.

sim.test.procBeqC
: list of 50 random realizations of test-processes under null based on resampling.

covariance
: covariances for nonparametric terms of model.

B.iid
: Resample processes for nonparametric terms of model.

gamma.iid
: Resample processes for parametric terms of model.

Author(s)

Thomas Scheike

References

Martinussen and Scheike, Dynamic Regression Models for Survival Data, Springer (2006).

Examples

```
library(survival)
data(sTRACE)
# Fits Aalen model
out<-aalen(Surv(time,status==9)~age+sex+diabetes+chf+vf,
sTRACE,max.time=7,n.sim=500)

summary(out)
par(mfrow=c(2,3))
plot(out)

# Fits semi-parametric additive hazards model
out<-aalen(Surv(time,status==9)~const(age)+const(sex)+const(diabetes)+chf
+vf,sTRACE,max.time=7,n.sim=500)

summary(out)
par(mfrow=c(2,3))
plot(out)
```

cd4	*The multicenter AIDS cohort study*

Description

Format

This data frame contains the following columns:

- **obs** a numeric vector. Number of observations.
- **id** a numeric vector. Id of subject.
- **visit** a numeric vector. Timings of the visits in years.
- **smoke** a numeric vector code. 0: non-smoker, 1: smoker.
- **age** a numeric vector. Age of the patient at the start of the trial.
- **cd4** a numeric vector. CD4 percentage at the current visit.
- **cd4.prev** a numeric vector. CD4 level at the preceding visit.
- **precd4** a numeric vector. Post-infection CD4 percentage.
- **lt** a numeric vector. Gives the starting time for the time-intervals.
- **rt** a numeric vector. Gives the stopping time for the time-interval.

Source

MACS Public Use Data Set Release PO4 (1984-1991). See reference.

References

Kaslow et al. (1987), The multicenter AIDS cohort study: rational, organization and selected characteristics of the participants. Am. J. Epidemiology 126, 310–318.

Examples

```
data(cd4)
names(cd4)
```

const	*Identifies parametric terms of model*

Description

Specifies which of the regressors that have constant effect.

Author(s)

Thomas Scheike

cox	*Identifies proportional excess terms of model*

Description

Specifies which of the regressors that lead to proportional excess hazard

Author(s)

Thomas Scheike

cox.aalen	*Fit Cox-Aalen survival model*

Description

Fits an Cox-Aalen survival model. Time dependent variables and counting process data (multiple events per subject) are possible.

Resampling is used for computing p-values for tests of time-varying effects. Test for proportionality is considered by considering the score processes for the proportional effects of model.

The modeling formula uses the standard survival modeling given in the **survival package.**

Usage

```
cox.aalen(formula=formula(data),data=sys.parent(),beta=0,
Nit=10,detail=0,start.time=0,max.time=0,id=NULL,
clusters=NULL,n.sim=500,residuals=0,robust=1,
weighted.test=0,covariance=0,resample.iid=0,weights=NULL)
```

Arguments

formula	a formula object with the response on the left of a '~' operator, and the independent terms on the right as regressors. The response must be a survival object as returned by the 'Surv' function.
data	a data.frame with the variables.
start.time	start of observation period where estimates are computed.
max.time	end of observation period where estimates are computed. Estimates thus computed from [start.time, max.time]
robust	to compute robust variances and construct processes for resampling. May be set to 0 to save memory.
id	For time-varying covariates the variable must associate each record with the id of a subject.
clusters	cluster variable for computation of robust variances.
n.sim	number of simulations in resampling.
weighted.test	to compute a variance weighted version of the test-processes used for testing time-varying effects.
residuals	to returns residuals that can be used for model validation in the function cum.residuals
covariance	to compute covariance estimates for nonparametric terms rather than just the variances.
resample.iid	to return i.i.d. representation for nonparametric and parametric terms.
beta	starting value for relative risk estimates
Nit	number of iterations for Newton-Raphson algorithm.
detail	if 0 no details is printed during iterations, if 1 details are given.
weights	weights for weighted analysis.

Details

The data for a subject is presented as multiple rows or "observations", each of which applies to an interval of observation (start, stop]. For counting process data with the)start,stop] notation is used the 'id' variable is needed to identify the records for each subject. The program assumes that there are no ties, and if such are present random noise is added to break the ties.

Value

returns an object of type "cox.aalen". With the following arguments:

cum	cumulative time-varying regression coefficient estimates are computed within the estimation interval.
var.cum	the martingale based pointwise variance estimates.
robvar.cum	robust pointwise variances estimates.
gamma	estimate of parametric components of model.
var.gamma	variance for gamma.
robvar.gamma	robust variance for gamma.
residuals	list with residuals.
obs.testBeq0	observed absolute value of supremum of cumulative components scaled with the variance.
pval.testBeq0	p-value for covariate effects based on supremum test.
sim.testBeq0	resampled supremum values.
obs.testBeqC	observed absolute value of supremum of difference between observed cumulative process and estimate under null of constant effect.
pval.testBeqC	p-value based on resampling.
sim.testBeqC	resampled supremum values.
obs.testBeqC.is	observed integrated squared differences between observed cumulative and estimate under null of constant effect.
pval.testBeqC.is	p-value based on resampling.
sim.testBeqC.is	resampled supremum values.
conf.band	resampling based constant to construct robust 95% uniform confidence bands.
test.procBeqC	observed test-process of difference between observed cumulative process and estimate under null of constant effect over time.
sim.test.procBeqC	list of 50 random realizations of test-processes under null based on resampling.
covariance	covariances for nonparametric terms of model.
B.iid	Resample processes for nonparametric terms of model.
gamma.iid	Resample processes for parametric terms of model.

`loglike`	approximate log-likelihood for model, similar to Cox's partial likelihood.
`D2linv`	inverse of the derivative of the score function.
`score`	value of score for final estimates.
`test.procProp`	observed score process for proportional part of model.
`pval.Prop`	p-value based on resampling.
`sim.supProp`	re-sampled absolute supremum values.
`sim.test.procProp`	list of 50 random realizations of test-processes for proportionality under the model based on resampling.

Author(s)

Thomas Scheike

References

Martinussen and Scheike, Dynamic Regression Models for Survival Data, Springer (2006).

Examples

```
library(survival)
data(sTRACE)
# Fits Cox model
out<-cox.aalen(Surv(time,status==9)~prop(age)+prop(sex)+
prop(vf)+prop(chf)+prop(diabetes),sTRACE,max.time=7,n.sim=500)

# makes Lin, Wei, Ying test for proportionality
summary(out)
par(mfrow=c(2,3))
plot(out,score=1)

# Fits Cox-Aalen model
out<-cox.aalen(Surv(time,status==9)~prop(age)+prop(sex)+
vf+chf+prop(diabetes),sTRACE,max.time=7,n.sim=500)

# plots the additive part of the model. To obtain more sensible
# plots center covariates in proportional part of model
summary(out)
par(mfrow=c(2,3))
plot(out)
```

csl	CSL liver cirrhosis data

Description

Format

This data frame contains the following columns:

id a numeric vector. Id of subject.

time a numeric vector. Time of measurement.

prot a numeric vector. Prothrombin level at measurement time.

dc a numeric vector code. 0: censored observation, 1: died at eventT.

eventT a numeric vector. Time of event (death).

treat a numeric vector code. 0: active treatment of prednisone, 1: placebo treatment.

sex a numeric vector code. 0: female, 1: male.

age a numeric vector. Age of subject at inclusion time subtracted 60.

prot.base a numeric vector. Prothrombin base level before entering the study.

prot.prev a numeric vector. Level of prothrombin at previous measurement time.

lt a numeric vector. Gives the starting time for the time-intervals.

rt a numeric vector. Gives the stopping time for the time-intervals.

Source

P.K. Andersen

References

Schlichting, P., Christensen, E., Andersen, P., Fauerholds, L., Juhl, E., Poulsen, H. and Tygstrup, N. (1983), The Copenhagen Study Group for Liver Diseases, Hepatology 3, 889–895

Examples

```
data(csl)
names(csl)
```

cum.residuals	Model validation based on cumulative residuals

Description

Computes cumulative residuals and approximative p-values based on resampling techniques.

Usage

```
cum.residuals(object,data=sys.parent(),modelmatrix=0,
cum.resid=0,n.sim=500,weighted.test=1,start.design=1)
```

Arguments

object	an object of class 'aalen', 'timecox', 'cox.aalen' where the residuals are returned ('residuals=1')
data	data frame based on which residuals are computed.
modelmatrix	specifies a grouping of the data that is used for cumulating residuals. Must have same size as data and be ordered in the same way.
n.sim	number of simulations in resampling.
weighted.test	to compute a variance weighted version of the test-processes used for testing constant effects of covariates.
cum.resid	to compute residuals versus each of the continuous covariates in the model.
start.design	if '1' the groupings specified in modelmatrix changes over time, i.e. in the case with time-dependent covariates.

Value

returns an object of type "cum.residuals" with the following arguments:

cum	cumulative residuals versus time for the groups specified by modelmatrix.
var.cum	the martingale based pointwise variance estimates.
robvar.cum	robust pointwise variances estimates of cumulatives.
obs.testBeq0	observed absolute value of supremum of cumulative components scaled with the variance.
pval.testBeq0	p-value covariate effects based on supremum test.
sim.testBeq0	resampled supremum value.

`conf.band`	resampling based constant to construct robust 95% uniform confidence bands for cumulative residuals.
`obs.test`	absolute value of supremum of observed test-process.
`pval.test`	p-value for supremum test statistic.
`sim.test`	resampled absolute value of supremum cumulative residuals.
`proc.cumz`	observed cumulative residuals versus all continuous covariates of model.
`sim.test.proccumz`	list of 50 random realizations of test-processes under model for all continuous covariates.

Author(s)

Thomas Scheike

References

Martinussen and Scheike, Dynamic Regression Models for Survival Data, Springer (2006).

Examples

```
library(survival)
data(sTRACE)
# Fits Aalen model and returns residuals
fit<-aalen(Surv(time,status==9)~age+sex+diabetes+chf+vf,
sTRACE,max.time=7,n.sim=0,residuals=1)

# constructs and simulates cumulative residuals versus age groups
fit.mg<-cum.residuals(fit,sTRACE,
                     model.matrix(~-1+factor(cut(age,4)),sTRACE))

par(mfrow=c(1,4))
# cumulative residuals with confidence intervals
plot(fit.mg);
# cumulative residuals versus processes under model
plot(fit.mg,score=1);
summary(fit.mg)

# cumulative residuals vs. covariates Lin, Wei, Ying style
fit.mg<-cum.residuals(fit,sTRACE,cum.resid=1)

par(mfrow=c(2,4))
plot(fit.mg,score=2)
summary(fit.mg)
```

dynreg	*Fit time-varying regression model*

Description

> Fits time-varying regression model with partly parametric components. Time-dependent variables for longitudinal data. The model assumes that the mean of the observed responses given covariates is a linear time-varying regression model :

$$E(Z_{ij}|X_{ij}(t)) = \beta^T(t)X^1_{ij}(t) + \gamma^T X^2_{ij}(t)$$

> where Z_{ij} is the j'th measurement at time t for the i'th subject with covariates X^1_{ij} and X^2_{ij}. Resampling is used for computing p-values for tests of time-varying effects.

Usage

    dynreg(formula,data=sys.parent(),aalenmod,bandwidth=0.5,
    id=NULL,bhat=NULL,start.time=0,max.time=0,n.sim=500,
    residuals=0,meansub=1,weighted.test=0)

Arguments

formula	a formula object with the response on the left of a '~' operator, and the independent terms on the right as regressors.
data	a data.frame with the variables.
start.time	start of observation period where estimates are computed.
max.time	end of observation period where estimates are computed. Estimates thus computed from [start.time, max.time]
id	For time-varying covariates the variable must associate each record with the id of a subject.
n.sim	number of simulations in resampling.
weighted.test	to compute a variance weighted version of the test-processes used for testing time-varying effects.
residuals	to returns residuals that can be used for model validation in the function 'cum.residuals'.
aalenmod	Aalen model for measurement times. Specified as a survival model (see aalen function).

bandwidth	bandwidth for local iterations. Default is 50% of the range of the considered observation period.
bhat	initial value for estimates. If NULL local linear estimate is computed.
meansub	if '1' then the mean of the responses is subtracted before the estimation is carried out.

Details

The data for a subject is presented as multiple rows or "observations", each of which applies to an interval of observation (start, stop]. For counting process data with the)start,stop] notation is used the 'id' variable is needed to identify the records for each subject. The program assumes that there are no ties, and if such are present random noise is added to break the ties.

Value

returns an object of type "dynreg". With the following arguments:

cum	the cumulative regression coefficients. This is the efficient estimator based on an initial smoother obtained by local linear regression :

$$\hat{B}(t) = \int_0^t \tilde{\beta}(s)ds +$$

$$\int_0^t X^-(Diag(z) - Diag(X^T(s)\tilde{\beta}(s)))dp(ds \times dz),$$

where $\tilde{\beta}(t)$ is an initial estimate either provided or computed by local linear regression. To plot this estimate use type="eff.smooth" in the plot() command.

var.cum	the martingale based pointwise variance estimates.
robvar.cum	robust pointwise variances estimates.
gamma	estimate of semi-parametric components of model.
var.gamma	variance for gamma.
robvar.gamma	robust variance for gamma.
cum0	simple estimate of cumulative regression coefficients that does not use use an initial smoothing based estimate

$$\hat{B}_0(t) = \int_0^t X^- Diag(z) dp(ds \times dz).$$

To plot this estimate use type="0.mpp" in the plot() command.

var.cum0	the martingale based pointwise variance estimates of cum0.
cum.ms	estimate of cumulative regression coefficients based on initial smoother (but robust to this estimator). $$\hat{B}_{ms}(t) = \int_0^t X^-(Diag(z) - f(s))dp(ds \times dz),$$ where f is chosen as the matrix $$f(s) = Diag(X^T(s)\tilde{\beta}(s))(I - X_\alpha(s)X_\alpha^-(s)),$$ where X_α is the design for the sampling intensities. This is also an efficient estimator when the initial estimator is consistent for $\beta(t)$ and then asymptotically equivalent to cum, but small sample properties appear inferior. Its variance is estimated by var.cum. To plot this estimate use type="ms.mpp" in the plot() command.
cum.ly	estimator where local averages are subtracted. Special case of cum.ms. To plot this estimate use type="ly.mpp" in plot.
var.cum.ly	the martingale based pointwise variance estimates.
gamma0	estimate of parametric component of model.
var.gamma0	estimate of variance of parametric component of model.
gamma.ly	estimate of parametric components of model.
var.gamma.ly	estimate of variance of parametric component of model.
gamma.ms	estimate of variance of parametric component of model.
var.gamma.ms	estimate of variance of parametric component of model.
residuals	list of residuals.
obs.testBeq0	observed absolute value of supremum of cumulative components scaled with the variance.
pval.testBeq0	p-value for covariate effects based on supremum test.
sim.testBeq0	resampled supremum values.
obs.testBeqC	observed absolute value of supremum of difference between observed cumulative process and estimate under null of constant effect.
pval.testBeqC	p-value based on resampling.
sim.testBeqC	resampled supremum values.

432   Appendix C.   The Timereg survival package for **R**

`obs.testBeqC.is`
: observed integrated squared differences between observed cumulative and estimate under null of constant effect.

`pval.testBeqC.is`
: p-value based on resampling.

`sim.testBeqC.is`
: resampled supremum values.

`conf.band`
: resampling based constant to construct robust 95% uniform confidence bands.

`test.procBeqC`
: observed test-process of difference between observed cumulative process and estimate under null of constant effect.

`sim.test.procBeqC`
: list of 50 random realizations of test-processes under null based on resampling.

`covariance`
: covariances for nonparametric terms of model.

Author(s)

Thomas Scheike

References

Martinussen and Scheike, Dynamic Regression Models for Survival Data, Springer (2006).

Examples

```
library(survival)
data(csl)
indi.m<-rep(1,length(csl$lt))

# Fits time-varying regression model on time-range from 0 to 3 years.
out<-dynreg(prot~treat+prot.prev+sex+age,csl,
Surv(lt,rt,indi.m)~+1,start.time=0,max.time=3,id=csl$id,
n.sim=500,bandwidth=0.3,meansub=0)
summary(out)
par(mfrow=c(2,3))
plot(out)

# Fits time-varying semi-parametric regression model.
outS<-dynreg(prot~treat+const(prot.prev)+const(sex)+const(age),csl,
Surv(lt,rt,indi.m)~+1,start.time=0,max.time=3,id=csl$id,
n.sim=500,bandwidth=0.3,meansub=0)
summary(outS)
```

melanoma	*The Melanoma Survival Data*

Description

The melanoma data frame has 205 rows and 7 columns. It contains data relating to survival of patients after operation for malignant melanoma collected at Odense University Hospital by K.T. Drzewiecki.

Format

This data frame contains the following columns:

no a numeric vector. Patient code.

status a numeric vector code. Survival status. 1: dead from melanoma, 2: alive, 3: dead from other cause.

days a numeric vector. Survival time.

ulc a numeric vector code. Ulceration, 1: present, 0: absent.

thick a numeric vector. Tumor thickness (1/100 mm).

sex a numeric vector code. 0: female, 1: male.

Source

Andersen, P.K., Borgan Ø., Gill R.D., Keiding N. (1993), *Statistical Models Based on Counting Processes*, Springer-Verlag.

Drzewiecki, K.T., Ladefoged, C., and Christensen, H.E. (1980), Biopsy and prognosis for cutaneous malignant melanoma in clinical stage I. Scand. J. Plast. Reconstru. Surg. 14, 141-144.

Examples

```
data(melanoma)
names(melanoma)
```

mela.pop	*Melanoma data and Danish population mortality by age and sex*

Description

Melanoma data with Danish population mortality rates by age and sex.

Format

This data frame contains the following columns:

id a numeric vector. Gives patient id.

sex a numeric vector. Gives sex of patient.

start a numeric vector. Gives the starting time for the time-interval for which the covariate rate is representative.

stop a numeric vector. Gives the stopping time for the time-interval for which the covariate rate is representative.

status a numeric vector code. Survival status. 1: dead from melanoma, 0: alive or dead from other cause.

age a numeric vector. Gives the age of the patient at removal of tumor.

rate a numeric vector. Gives the population mortality for the given sex and age. Based on Table A.2 in Andersen et al. (1993).

Source

Andersen, P.K., Borgan Ø, Gill R.D., Keiding N. (1993), *Statistical Models Based on Counting Processes*, Springer-Verlag.

Examples

```
data(mela.pop)
names(mela.pop)
```

| plot.aalen | *Plots estimates and test-processes* |

Description

This function plots the non-parametric cumulative estimates for the additive risk model or the test-processes for the hypothesis of time-varying effects with re-sampled processes under the null.

Usage

```
plot.aalen(object,pointwise.ci=1,hw.ci=0,sim.ci=0,robust=0,
specific.comps=FALSE,level=0.05, start.time=0,stop.time=0,
add.to.plot=FALSE,mains=TRUE,xlab="Time",
ylab="Cumulative coefficients",score=FALSE)
```

Arguments

object	the output from the "aalen" function.
pointwise.ci	if >1 pointwise confidence intervals are plotted with lty=pointwise.ci
hw.ci	if >1 Hall-Wellner confidence bands are plotted with lty=hw.ci. Only 0.95 % bands can be constructed.
sim.ci	if >1 simulation based confidence bands are plotted with lty=sim.ci. These confidence bands are robust to non-martingale behaviour.
robust	robust standard errors are used to estimate standard error of estimate, otherwise martingale based standard errors are used.
specific.comps	all components of the model is plotted by default, but a list of components may be specified, for example first and third "c(1,3)".
level	gives the significance level.
start.time	start of observation period where estimates are plotted.
stop.time	end of period where estimates are plotted. Estimates thus plotted from [start.time, max.time].
add.to.plot	to add to an already existing plot.
mains	add names of covariates as titles to plots.
xlab	label for x-axis.

436   Appendix C. The Timereg survival package for **R**

ylab   label for y-axis.

score   to plot test processes for test of time-varying effects along with 50 random realization under the null-hypothesis.

Author(s)

Thomas Scheike

References

Martinussen and Scheike

Examples

```
library(survival)
data(sTRACE)
# Fits Aalen model
out<-aalen(Surv(time,status==9)~age+sex+diabetes+chf+vf,
sTRACE,max.time=7,n.sim=500)

par(mfrow=c(2,3))
# plots estimates
plot(out)
# plots tests-processes for time-varying effects
plot(out,score=TRUE)
```

---

plot.cum.residuals

Plots cumulative residuals

Description

This function plots the output from the cumulative residuals function "cum.residuals". The cumulative residuals are compared with the performance of similar processes under the model.

Usage

```
plot.cum.residuals(object,pointwise.ci=1,hw.ci=0,sim.ci=0,
robust=1, specific.comps=FALSE,level=0.05,start.time=0,
stop.time=0,add.to.plot=FALSE,mains=TRUE,xlab="Time",
ylab ="Cumulative Residuals",ylim=NULL,score=0)
```

Arguments

object   the output from the "cum.residuals" function.

pointwise.ci   if >1 pointwise confidence intervals are plotted with lty=pointwise.ci

`hw.ci`	if >1 Hall-Wellner confidence bands are plotted with lty=hw.ci. Only 95% bands can be constructed.
`sim.ci`	if >1 simulation based confidence bands are plotted with lty=sim.ci. These confidence bands are robust to non-martingale behaviour.
`robust`	if "1" robust standard errors are used to estimate standard error of estimate, otherwise martingale based estimate are used.
`specific.comps`	all components of the model is plotted by default, but a list of components may be specified, for example first and third "c(1,3)".
`level`	gives the significance level. Default is 0.05.
`start.time`	start of observation period where estimates are plotted. Default is 0.
`stop.time`	end of period where estimates are plotted. Estimates thus plotted from [start.time, max.time].
`add.to.plot`	to add to an already existing plot. Default is "FALSE".
`mains`	add names of covariates as titles to plots.
`xlab`	label for x-axis. Default is "Time".
`ylab`	label for y-axis. Default is "Cumulative Residuals".
`ylim`	limits for y-axis.
`score`	if '0' plots related to modelmatrix are specified, thus resulting in grouped residuals, if '1' plots for modelmatrix but with random realizations under model, if '2' plots residuals versus continuous covariates of model with random realizations under the model.

Author(s)

Thomas Scheike

References

Martinussen and Scheike, Dynamic Regression Models for Survival Data, Springer (2006).

Examples

```
library(survival)
data(sTRACE)
# Fits Aalen model and returns residuals
out<-aalen(Surv(time,status==9)~age+sex+diabetes+chf+vf,
sTRACE,max.time=7,n.sim=0,residuals=1)
```

```
# constructs and simulates cumulative residuals versus age groups
out.mg<-cum.residuals(out,sTRACE,
                      model.matrix(~-1+factor(cut(age,4)),sTRACE))

par(mfrow=c(1,4))
# cumulative residuals with pointwise confidence intervals
plot(out.mg);
# cumulative residuals versus processes under model
plot(out.mg,score=1);

# cumulative residuals against covariates Lin, Wei, Ying style
out.mg<-cum.residuals(out,sTRACE,cum.resid=1)
par(mfrow=c(2,4))
plot(out.mg,score=2)
```

---

plot.dynreg   *Plots estimates and test-processes*

Description

This function plots the non-parametric cumulative estimates for the additive risk model or the test-processes for the hypothesis of constant effects with re-sampled processes under the null.

Usage

```
plot.dynreg(object,type="eff.smooth",pointwise.ci=1,hw.ci=0,
sim.ci=0,robust=0, specific.comps=FALSE,level=0.05,
start.time=0,stop.time=0,add.to.plot=FALSE,mains=TRUE,
xlab="Time",ylab="Cumulative coefficients",score=FALSE)
```

Arguments

object	the output from the "dynreg" function.
type	the estimator plotted. Choices "eff.smooth", "ms.mpp", "0.mpp" and "ly.mpp". See the dynreg function for more on this.
pointwise.ci	if >1 pointwise confidence intervals are plotted with lty=pointwise.ci
hw.ci	if >1 Hall-Wellner confidence bands are plotted with lty=hw.ci. Only 0.95 % bands can be constructed.
sim.ci	if >1 simulation based confidence bands are plotted with lty=sim.ci. These confidence bands are robust to non-martingale behavior.

robust	robust standard errors are used to estimate standard error of estimate, otherwise martingale based estimate are used.
specific.comps	all components of the model is plotted by default, but a list of components may be specified, for example first and third "c(1,3)".
level	gives the significance level.
start.time	start of observation period where estimates are plotted.
stop.time	end of period where estimates are plotted. Estimates thus plotted from [start.time, max.time].
add.to.plot	to add to an already existing plot.
mains	add names of covariates as titles to plots.
xlab	label for x-axis.
ylab	label for y-axis.
score	to plot test processes for test of time-varying effects along with 50 random realization under the null-hypothesis.

Author(s)

Thomas Scheike

References

Martinussen and Scheike, Dynamic Regression Models for Survival Data, Springer (2006).

Examples

```
library(survival)
data(csl)
indi.m<-rep(1,length(csl$lt))

# Fits time-varying regression model on time-range from 0 to 3 years.
out<-dynreg(prot~treat+prot.prev+sex+age,csl,
Surv(lt,rt,indi.m)~+1,start.time=0,max.time=3,id=csl$id,
n.sim=500,bandwidth=0.3,meansub=0)

par(mfrow=c(2,3))
# plots estimates
plot(out)
# plots tests-processes for time-varying effects
plot(out,score=TRUE)
```

print.aalen	*Prints call*

Description

   Prints call for object. Lists nonparametric and parametric terms of model

Usage

   `print.aalen(object)`

Arguments

   object   an aalen object

Author(s)

   Thomas Scheike

prop	*Identifies the multiplicative terms in Cox-Aalen model and proportional excess risk model*

Description

   Specifies which of the regressors that belong to the multiplicative part of the Cox-Aalen model or the proportional excess risk model.

Usage

   `see cox.aalen or prop.excess`

Author(s)

   Thomas Scheike

Appendix C. The Timereg survival package for **R**   441

| prop.excess | *Fits Proportional excess hazards model* |

Description

    Fits proportional excess hazards model.

    The models are written using the survival modeling given in the survival package.

Usage

```
prop.excess(formula=formula(data),data=sys.parent(),
excess=1,tol=0.0001,max.time=0,n.sim=1000,alpha=1,frac=1)
```

Arguments

formula	a formula object, with the response on the left of a '~' operator, and the terms on the right. The response must be a survival object as returned by the 'Surv' function.
data	a data.frame with the variables.
excess	specifies for which of the subjects the excess term is present. Default is that the term is present for all subjects.
tol	tolerance for numerical procedure.
max.time	stopping considered time-period if different from 0. Estimates thus computed from [0,max.time] if max.time>0.
n.sim	number of simulations in re-sampling.
alpha	tuning parameter in Newton-Raphson procedure. Value smaller than one may give more stable convergence.
frac	number between 0 and 1. Is used in supremum test where observed jump times t1, ..., tk is replaced by t1, ..., tl with l=round(frac*k).

Details

    The program assumes that there are no ties, and if such are present random noise is added to break the ties.

Value

Returns an object of type "prop.excess". With the following arguments:

cum
: estimated cumulative regression functions. First column contains the jump times, then follows the estimated components of additive part of model and finally the excess cumulative baseline.

var.cum
: robust pointwise variance estimates for estimated cumulatives.

gamma
: estimate of parametric components of model.

var.gamma
: robust variance estimate for gamma.

pval
: p-value of Kolmogorov-Smirnov test (variance weighted) for excess baseline and Aalen terms, H: B(t)=0.

pval.HW
: p-value of supremum test (corresponding to Hall-Wellner band) for excess baseline and Aalen terms, H: B(t)=0. Reported in summary.

pval.CM
: p-value of Cramer von Mises test for excess baseline and Aalen terms, H: B(t)=0.

quant
: 95 percent quantile in distribution of resampled Kolmogorov-Smirnov test statistics for excess baseline and Aalen terms. Used to construct 95 percent simulation band.

quant95HW
: 95 percent quantile in distribution of resampled supremum test statistics corresponding to Hall-Wellner band for excess baseline and Aalen terms. Used to construct 95 percent Hall-Wellner band.

simScoreProp
: observed scoreprocess and 50 resampled scoreprocesses (under model). List with 51 elements.

Author(s)

Torben Martinussen

References

Martinussen and Scheike, Dynamic Regression Models for Survival Data, Springer (2006).

Examples

```
library(survival)
data(melanoma)
attach(melanoma)
lt<-log(thick)         # log-thickness
```

```
excess<-(thick>=210)      # excess risk for thick tumors

# Fits Proportional Excess hazards model
fit<-prop.excess(Surv(days/365,status==1)~sex+ulc+cox(sex)+cox(ulc)
           +cox(lt),excess=excess,n.sim=2000)
summary(fit)
par(mfrow=c(2,3))
plot(fit)
```

---

prop.odds	*Fit Semiparametric Proportional Odds Model*

Description

Fits a semiparametric proportional odds model:

$$logit(1 - S_Z(t)) = log(G(t)) + \beta^T Z$$

where G(t) is increasing but otherwise unspecified. Model is fitted by maximizing the modified partial likelihood. A goodness-of-fit test by considering the score functions is also computed by resampling methods.

The modeling formula uses the standard survival modeling given in the survival package.

Usage

```
prop.odds(formula,data=sys.parent(),beta=0,Nit=10,
detail=0,start.time=0,max.time=0,id=NULL,n.sim=500,
weighted.test=0,profile=1,sym=0)
```

Arguments

formula	a formula object, with the response on the left of a '~' operator, and the terms on the right. The response must be a survival object as returned by the 'Surv' function.
data	a data.frame with the variables.
start.time	start of observation period where estimates are computed.
max.time	end of observation period where estimates are computed. Estimates thus computed from [start.time, max.time]. This is very useful to obtain stable estimates, especially for the baseline.
id	For time-varying covariates the variable must associate each record with the id of a subject.

`n.sim`	number of simulations in resampling.
`weighted.test`	to compute a variance weighted version of the test-processes used for testing time-varying effects.
`beta`	starting value for relative risk estimates
`Nit`	number of iterations for Newton-Raphson algorithm.
`detail`	if 0 no details is printed during iterations, if 1 details are given.
`profile`	if profile is 1 then modified partial likelihood is used, profile=0 fits by simple estimating equation. The modified partial likelihood is recommended.
`sym`	to use symmetrized second derivative in the case of the estimating equation approach (profile=0). This may improve the numerical performance.

Details

The data for a subject is presented as multiple rows or "observations", each of which applies to an interval of observation (start, stop]. The program essentially assumes no ties, and if such are present a little random noise is added to break the ties.

Value

returns an object of type 'cox.aalen'. With the following arguments:

`cum`	cumulative time-varying regression coefficient estimates are computed within the estimation interval.
`var.cum`	the martingale based pointwise variance estimates.
`robvar.cum`	robust pointwise variances estimates.
`gamma`	estimate of proportional odds parameters of model.
`var.gamma`	variance for gamma.
`robvar.gamma`	robust variance for gamma.
`residuals`	list with residuals.
`obs.testBeq0`	observed absolute value of supremum of cumulative components scaled with the variance.
`pval.testBeq0`	p-value for covariate effects based on supremum test.
`sim.testBeq0`	resampled supremum values.
`obs.testBeqC`	observed absolute value of supremum of difference between observed cumulative process and estimate under null of constant effect.
`pval.testBeqC`	p-value based on resampling.

`sim.testBeqC`	resampled supremum values.
`obs.testBeqC.is`	observed integrated squared differences between observed cumulative and estimate under null of constant effect.
`pval.testBeqC.is`	p-value based on resampling.
`sim.testBeqC.is`	resampled supremum values.
`conf.band`	resampling based constant to construct robust 95% uniform confidence bands.
`test.procBeqC`	observed test-process of difference between observed cumulative process and estimate under null of constant effect over time.
`loglike`	modified partial likelihood, pseudo profile likelihood for regression parameters.
`D2linv`	inverse of the derivative of the score function.
`score`	value of score for final estimates.
`test.procProp`	observed score process for proportional odds regression effects.
`pval.Prop`	p-value based on resampling.
`sim.supProp`	re-sampled supremum values.
`sim.test.procProp`	list of 50 random realizations of test-processes for constant proportional odds under the model based on resampling.

Author(s)

Thomas Scheike

References

Martinussen and Scheike, Dynamic Regression Models for Survival Data, Springer (2006).

Examples

```
library(survival)
data(sTRACE)
# Fits Proportional odds model
out<-prop.odds(Surv(time,status==9)~age+diabetes+chf+vf+sex,
sTRACE,max.time=7,n.sim=500)
```

```
summary(out)

par(mfrow=c(2,3))
plot(out,sim.ci=2)
plot(out,score=1)
```

---

summary.aalen   *Prints summary statistics*

Description

Computes p-values for test of significance for nonparametric terms of model, p-values for test of constant effects based on both supremum and integrated squared difference.

Returns parameter estimates and their standard errors.

Usage

```
summary.aalen(aalen.object,digits=3)
```

Arguments

aalen.object   an aalen object.

digits   number of digits in printouts.

Author(s)

Thomas Scheike

Examples

```
library(survival)
data(sTRACE)
# Fits Aalen model
out<-aalen(Surv(time,status==9)~age+sex+diabetes+chf+vf,
sTRACE,max.time=7,n.sim=500)

summary(out)
```

summary.cum.residuals	*Prints summary statistics for goodness-of-fit tests based on cumulative residuals*

Description

Computes p-values for extreme behaviour relative to the model of various cumulative residual processes.

Usage

```
summary.cum.residuals(cum.residuals.object,digits=3
```

Arguments

cum.resids.object
: an cum.residuals object.

digits
: number of digits in printouts.

Author(s)

Thomas Scheike

Examples

```
library(survival)
data(sTRACE)
# Fits Aalen model and returns residuals
out<-aalen(Surv(time,status==9)~age+sex+diabetes+chf+vf,
sTRACE,max.time=7,n.sim=0,residuals=1)

# constructs and simulates cumulative residuals versus age groups
# and versus covariates of model
out.mg<-cum.residuals(out,sTRACE,
modelmatrix=model.matrix(~-1+factor(cut(age,4)),sTRACE),cum.resid=1)

summary(out.mg)
```

timecox	*Fit Cox model with partly time-varying effects.*

Description

Fits proportional hazards model with some effects time-varying and some effects constant. Time dependent variables and counting process data (multiple events per subject) are possible.

Resampling is used for computing p-values for tests of time-varying effects.

The modeling formula uses the standard survival modeling given in the **survival package.**

Usage

```
timecox(formula=formula(data),data=sys.parent(),
start.time=0,max.time=0,id=NULL,clusters=NULL,n.sim=1000,
residuals=0,robust=1,Nit=20,bandwidth=0.5,method="basic",
weighted.test=0,degree=1,covariance=0)
```

Arguments

formula	a formula object with the response on the left of a '~' operator, and the independent terms on the right as regressors. The response must be a survival object as returned by the 'Surv' function.
data	a data.frame with the variables.
start.time	start of observation period where estimates are computed.
max.time	end of observation period where estimates are computed. Estimates thus computed from [start.time, max.time]
robust	to compute robust variances and construct processes for resampling. May be set to 0 to save memory.
id	For time-varying covariates the variable must associate each record with the id of a subject.
clusters	cluster variable for computation of robust variances.
n.sim	number of simulations in resampling.
weighted.test	to compute a variance weighted version of the test-processes used for testing time-varying effects.
residuals	to returns residuals that can be used for model validation in the function cum.residuals
covariance	to compute covariance estimates for nonparametric terms rather than just the variances.
Nit	number of iterations for score equations.
bandwidth	bandwidth for local iterations. Default is 50 % of the range of the considered observation period.
method	Method for estimation. This refers to different parametrizations of the baseline of the model. Options

are "basic" where the baseline is written as $\lambda_0(t) = \exp(\alpha_0(t))$ or the "breslow" version where the baseline is parametrised as $\lambda_0(t)$.

`degree`   gives the degree of the local linear smoothing, that is local smoothing. Possible values are 1 or 2.

Details

The data for a subject is presented as multiple rows or "observations", each of which applies to an interval of observation (start, stop]. When counting process data with the)start,stop] notation is used the 'id' variable is needed to identify the records for each subject. The program assumes that there are no ties, and if such are present random noise is added to break the ties.

Value

Returns an object of type "timecox". With the following arguments:

`cum`	cumulative time-varying regression coefficient estimates are computed within the estimation interval.
`var.cum`	the martingale based pointwise variance estimates.
`robvar.cum`	robust pointwise variances estimates.
`gamma`	estimate of parametric components of model.
`var.gamma`	variance for gamma.
`robvar.gamma`	robust variance for gamma.
`residuals`	list with residuals.
`obs.testBeq0`	observed absolute value of supremum of cumulative components scaled with the variance.
`pval.testBeq0`	p-value for covariate effects based on supremum test.
`sim.testBeq0`	resampled supremum values.
`obs.testBeqC`	observed absolute value of supremum of difference between observed cumulative process and estimate under null of constant effect.
`pval.testBeqC`	p-value based on resampling.
`sim.testBeqC`	resampled supremum values.
`obs.testBeqC.is`	observed integrated squared differences between observed cumulative and estimate under null of constant effect.
`pval.testBeqC.is`	p-value based on resampling.

`sim.testBeqC.is`
: resampled supremum values.

`conf.band`
: resampling based constant to construct robust 95% uniform confidence bands.

`test.procBeqC`
: observed test-process of difference between observed cumulative process and estimate under null of constant effect over time.

`sim.test.procBeqC`
: list of 50 random realizations of test-processes under null based on resampling.

`schoenfeld.residuals`
: Schoenfeld residuals are returned for "breslow" parametrization.

Author(s)

Thomas Scheike

References

Martinussen and Scheike, Dynamic Regression Models for Survival Data, Springer (2006).

Examples

```
library(survival)
data(sTRACE)
# Fits time-varying Cox model
out<-timecox(Surv(time/365,status==9)~age+sex+diabetes+chf+vf,
sTRACE,max.time=7,n.sim=500)

summary(out)
par(mfrow=c(2,3))
plot(out)
par(mfrow=c(2,3))
plot(out,score=TRUE)

# Fits semi-parametric time-varying Cox model
out<-timecox(Surv(time/365,status==9)~const(age)+const(sex)+
const(diabetes)+chf+vf,sTRACE,max.time=7,n.sim=500)

summary(out)
par(mfrow=c(2,3))
plot(out)
```

TRACE	*The TRACE study group of myocardial infarction*

Description

The TRACE data frame contains 1877 patients and is a subset of a data set consisting of approximately 6000 patients. It contains data relating survival of patients after myocardial infarction to various risk factors.

sTRACE is a subsample consisting of 300 patients.

tTRACE is a subsample consisting of 1000 patients.

Format

This data frame contains the following columns:

id a numeric vector. Patient code.

status a numeric vector code. Survival status. 9: dead from myocardial infarction, 0: alive, 7: dead from other causes.

time a numeric vector. Survival time in years.

chf a numeric vector code. Clinical heart pump failure, 1: present, 0: absent.

diabetes a numeric vector code. Diabetes, 1: present, 0: absent.

vf a numeric vector code. Ventricular fibrillation, 1: present, 0: absent.

wmi a numeric vector. Measure of heart pumping effect based on ultrasound measurements where 2 is normal and 0 is worst.

sex a numeric vector code. 1: female, 0: male.

age a numeric vector code. Age of patient.

Source

The TRACE study group.

Jensen, G.V., Torp-Pedersen, C., Hildebrandt, P., Kober, L., F. E. Nielsen, Melchior, T., Joen, T. and P. K. Andersen (1997), Does in-hospital ventricular fibrillation affect prognosis after myocardial infarction?, European Heart Journal 18, 919–924.

Examples

```
data(TRACE)
names(TRACE)
```

Bibliography

AALEN, O. O. (1975). *Statistical inference for a family of counting processes.* PhD thesis, Univ. of California, Berkeley.

AALEN, O. O. (1978a). Nonparametric estimation of partial transition probabilities in multiple decrement models. *Ann. Statist.* **6**, 534–545.

AALEN, O. O. (1978b). Nonparametric inference for a family of counting processes. *Ann. Statist.* **6**, 701–726.

AALEN, O. O. (1980). A model for non-parametric regression analysis of counting processes. In Klonecki, W., Kozek, A., & Rosinski, J., editors, *Lecture Notes in Statistics-2: Mathematical Statistics and Probability Theory*, pages 1–25. Springer-Verlag New York.

AALEN, O. O. (1989). A linear regression model for the analysis of life times. *Statist. Med.* **8**, 907–925.

AALEN, O. O. (1993). Further results on the non-parametric linear regression model in survival analysis. *Statist. Med.* **12**, 1569–1588.

AALEN, O. O. & JOHANSEN, S. (1978). An empirical transition matrix for nonhomogeneous Markov chains based on censored observations. *Scand. J. Statist.* **5**, 141–150.

ANDERSEN, E. W. (2005). Two-stage estimation in copula models used in family studies. *Lifetime Data Anal.* **11**, 333 – 350.

ANDERSEN, P. K., BORGAN, Ø., GILL, R. D., & KEIDING, N. (1993). *Statistical Models Based on Counting Processes.* Springer, New York.

ANDERSEN, P. K. & GILL, R. D. (1982). Cox's regression model for counting processes: A large sample study. *Ann. Statist.* **10**, 1100–1120.

ANDERSEN, P. K. & VÆTH, M. (1989). Simple parametric and nonparametric models for excess and relative mortality. *Biometrics* **45**, 523–535.

ARJAS, E. (1988). A graphical method for assessing goodness of fit in Cox's proportional hazards model. *J. Amer. Statist. Assoc.* **83**, 204–212.

BAGDONAVICIUS, V. & NIKULIN, M. (1999). Generalised proportional hazards model based on modified parital likelihood. *Lifetime Data Anal.* **5**, 329–350.

BAGDONAVICIUS, V. & NIKULIN, M. (2001). *Accelerated life models: Modelling and statistical analysis.* Chapman & Hall, London.

BARKER, P. & HENDERSON, R. (2004). Modelling converging hazards in survival analysis. *Lifetime Data Anal.* **10**, 263–281.

BERAN, R. (1981). Nonparametric regression with randomly censored survival data. Tech. rep., University of California, Berkeley.

BICKEL, P., KLASSEN, C., RITOV, Y., & WELLNER, J. (1993). *Efficient and Adaptive Estimation for Semiparametric Models.* Springer-Verlag New York.

BORGAN, Ø. (1984). Maximum likelihood estimation in parametric counting process models, with applications to censored failure time data. *Scand. J. Statist.* **11**, 1–16. Correction: **11**, 275.

BRÉMAUD, P. (1981). *Point Processes and Queues: Martingale Dynamics.* Springer-Verlag, New York.

BROOKMEYER, R. & GAIL, M. H. (1987). Biases in prevalent cohorts. *Biometrics* **43**, 739–749.

BRUMBACK, B. & RICE, J. (1998). Smoothings spline models for the analysis of nested and crossed samples of curves. *J. Amer. Statist. Assoc.* **93**, 961–994.

BUCKLEY, J. & JAMES, I. R. (1979). Linear regression with censored data. *Biometrika* **66**, 429–436.

CAI, J. & PRENTICE, R. L. (1995). Estimating equations for hazard ratio parameters based on correlated failure time data. *Biometrika* **82**, 151–164.

CAI, J. & PRENTICE, R. L. (1997). Regression estimation using multivariate failure time data and a common baseline hazard function model. *Lifetime Data Anal.* **3**, 197–213.

CAI, T., WEI, L. J., & WILCOX, M. (2000). Semiparametric regression analysis for clustered failure time data. *Biometrika* **87**, 867–878.

CAI, Z. & SUN, Y. (2003). Local linear estimation for time-dependent coefficients in Cox's regression models. *Scand. J. Statist.* **30**, 93–112.

CHEN, K., JIN, Z., & YING, Z. (2002). Semiparametric analysis of transformation models with censored data. *Biometrika* **89**, 659–668.

CHEN, Y. & JEWELL, N. (2001). On a general class of semiparametric hazards regression models. *Biometrika* **88**, 687–702.

CHEN, Y. Q. & WANG, M.-C. (2000). Analysis of accelerated hazards models. *J. Amer. Statist. Assoc.* **95**, 608–618.

CHENG, S. C., FINE, J. P., & WEI, L. J. (1998). Prediction of cumulative incidence function under the proportional hazards model. *Biometrics* **54**, 219–228.

CHENG, S. C. & WEI, L. J. (2000). Inferences for a semiparametric model with panel data. *Biometrika* **87**, 89–97.

CHENG, S. C., WEI, L. J., & YING, Z. (1995). Analysis of transformation models with censored data. *Biometrika* **82**, 835–845.

CHENG, S. C., WEI, L. J., & YING, Z. (1997). Prediction of survival probabilities with semi-parametric transformation models. *J. Amer. Statist. Assoc.* **92**, 227–235.

CLAYTON, D. G. (1978). A model for association in bivariate life tables and its application in epidemiological studies of familial tendency in chronic disease incidence. *Biometrika* **65**, 141–151.

COLLETT, D. (2003). *Modelling Survival Data in Medical Research*. Chapman Hall, London.

COX, D. R. (1972). Regression models and life tables (with discussion). *J. Roy. Statist. Soc. Ser. B* **34**, 187–220.

COX, D. R. (1975). Partial likelihood. *Biometrika* **62**, 269–276.

DABROWSKA, D. M. (1997). Smoothed Cox regression. *Ann. Statist.* **25**, 1510–1540.

DAUXOIS, J.-Y. & KIRMANI, S. N. U. A. (2003). Testing the proportional odds model under random censoring. *Biometrika* **90**, 913–922.

DEMPSTER, A. P., LAIRD, N. M., & RUBIN, D. B. (1977). Maximum likelihood from incomplete data via the EM algorithm. *J. Roy. Statist. Soc. Ser. B* **39**, 1–38. With discussion.

FAN, J. & GIJBELS, I. (1996). *Local Polynomial Modelling and Its Applications*. Chapman Hall London, New York.

FAN, J. & ZHANG, J. (2000a). Statistical estimation in varying-coefficient models. *J. Roy. Stat. Soc. Ser. B* **62**, 303–322.

FAN, J. & ZHANG, W. (1999). Statistical estimation in varying-coefficient models. *Ann. Statist.* **27**, 1491–1518.

FAN, J. & ZHANG, W. (2000b). Simultaneous confidence bands and hypothesis testing in varying-coefficient models. *Scand. J. Statist.* **27**, 715–727.

FINE, J., YING, Z., & WEI, L. J. (1998). On the linear transformation model with censored data. *Biometrika* **85**, 980–986.

FINE, J. P. & GRAY, R. J. (1999). A proportional hazards model for the subdistribution of a competing risk. *J. Amer. Statist. Assoc.* **94**, 496–509.

FLEMING, T. R. (1978a). Asymptotic distribution results in competing risks estimation. *Ann. Statist.* **6**, 1071–1079.

FLEMING, T. R. (1978b). Nonparametric estimation for nonhomogeneous Markov processes in the problem of competing risks. *Ann. Statist.* **6**, 1057–1079.

FLEMING, T. R. & HARRINGTON, D. P. (1991). *Counting Processes and Survival Analysis*. Wiley, New York.

FYGENSON, M. & RITOV, Y. (1994). Monotone estimating equations for censored data. *Ann. Statist.* **22**, 732–746.

GENEST, C. & MACKAY, R. J. (1986). The joy of copulas: Bivariate distributions with uniform marginals. *Amer. Statist.* **40**, 280–283.

GENEST, C. & MACKAY, R. J. (1995). A semiparametric estimation procedure of dependence parameters in multivariate families of distributions. *Biometrika* **82**, 543–552.

GILL, R. D. (1983). Discussion of the papers by Helland and Kurtz. *Bull. Internat. Statist. Inst.* **50**, 239–243.

GILL, R. D. (1985). Discussion of the paper by D. Clayton and J. Cuzick. *J. Roy. Statist. Soc. Ser. A* **148**, 108–109.

GILL, R. D. & JOHANSEN, S. (1990). A survey of product-integration with a view towards application in survival analysis. *Ann. Statist.* **18**, 1501–1555.

GLIDDEN, D. V. (1999). Checking the adequacy of the gamma frailty model for multivariate failure times. *Biometrika* **86**, 381–393.

GLIDDEN, D. V. (2000). A two-stage estimator of the dependence parameter for the Clayton-Oakes model. *Lifetime Data Anal.* **6**, 141–156.

GRAMBSCH, P. M. & THERNEAU, T. M. (1994). Proportional hazards tests and diagnostics based on weighted residuals (corr: 95v82 p668). *Biometrika* **81**, 515–526.

GRAY, R. J. (1988). A class of k-sample tests for comparing the cumulative incidence of a competing risk. *Ann. Statist.* **16**, 1141–1154.

GREENWOOD, M. (1926). The natural duration of cancer. In *Reports on Public Health and Medical Subjects* **33**, pages 1–26. His Majesty's Stationery Office, London.

GREENWOOD, P. E. & WEFELMEYER, W. (1990). Efficiency of estimators for partially specified filtered models. *Stoch. Proc. and their Appl.* **36**, 353–370.

GREENWOOD, P. E. & WEFELMEYER, W. (1991). Efficient estimating equations for nonparametric filtered models. In Prabhu, N. U. & Basawa, I. V., editors, *Statistical Inference in Stochastic Processes*, pages 107–141, New York. Marcel Dekker.

HALL, W. J. & WELLNER, J. A. (1980). Confidence bands for a survival curve from censored data. *Biometrika* **67**, 133–143.

HARBOE, I. S. & SCHEIKE, T. H. (2001). Time-varying coefficient model for longitudinal data: Uniform confidence bands and hypothesis tests applied to growth curves. *unpublished manuscript*.

HARRINGTON, D. P. & FLEMING, T. R. (1982). A class of rank test procedures for censored survival data. *Biometrika* **69**, 133–143.

HASTIE, T. & TIBSHIRANI, R. (1993). Varying-coefficient models. *J. Roy. Stat. Soc. Ser. B* **55**, 757–796.

HÄRDLE, W. (1990). *Applied Nonparametric Regression*. Cambridge University press.

HOOVER, P., RICE, J., WU, C., & YANG, L.-P. (1998). Nonparametric smoothing estimates of time-varying coefficient models with longitudinal data. *Biometrika* **85**, 809–822.

HORVITZ, D. & THOMPSON, D. (1952). A generalization of sampling without replacement from a finite universe. *J. Amer. Stastist. Assoc.* **47**, 663–685.

HOUGAARD, P. (2000). *Analysis of multivariate survival data.* Statistics for Biology and Health. Springer-Verlag, New York.

HUANG, J. Z., WU, C. O., & ZHOU, L. (2002). Varying-coefficient models and basis function approximations for the analysis of repeated measurements. *Biometrika* **89**, 111–128.

HUFFER, F. W. & MCKEAGUE, I. W. (1991). Weighted least squares estimation for Aalen's additive risk model. *J. Amer. Statist. Assoc.* **86**, 114–129.

HUSTER, W. J., BROOKMEYER, R., & SELF, S. G. (1989). Modelling paired survival data with covariates. *Biometrics* **45**, 145–156.

JACOBSEN, M. (1982). *Statistical Analysis of Counting Processes*, volume 12 of *Lecture Notes in Statistics.* Springer-Verlag, New York.

JACOBSEN, M. (1989). Existence and unicity of MLEs in discrete exponential family distributions. *Scand. J. Statist.* **16**, 335–349.

JENSEN, G. V., TORP-PEDERSEN, C., HILDEBRANDT, P., KOBER, L., NIELSEN, F. E., MELCHIOR, T., JOEN, T., & ANDERSEN, P. K. (1997). Does in-hospital ventricular fibrillation affect prognosis after myocardial infarction? *European Heart Journal* **18**, 919–924.

JESPERSEN, N. C. B. (1986). Dichotomizing a continuous covariate in the Cox regression model. Research Report 86/2, Statistical Research Unit, University of Copenhagen.

JIN, Z., LIN, D. Y., WEI, L. J., & YING, Z. (2003). Rank-based inference for the accelerated failure time model. *Biometrika* **90**, 341–353.

JOHANSEN, S. (1978). The product limit estimator as maximum likelihood estimator. *Scand. J. Statist.* **5**, 195–199.

KALBFLEISCH, J. D. & PRENTICE, R. L. (2002). *The Statistical Analysis of Failure Time Data.* Wiley, New York.

KAPLAN, E. L. & MEIER, P. (1958). Non-parametric estimation from incomplete observations. *J. Amer. Statist. Assoc.* **53**, 457–481.

KASLOW, R. A., OSTROW, D. G., DETELS, R., PHAIR, J. P., POLK, B. F., & RINALDO, C. R. (1987). The Multicenter AIDS Cohort Study: rationale, organization and selected characteristics of the participants. *Am. J. Epidem.* **126**, 310–318.

KHMALADZE, E. V. (1981). Martingale approach to the goodness of fit tests. *Theory Probab. Appl.* **26**, 246–265.

KLEIN, J. P. (1992). Semiparametric estimation of random effects using the Cox model based on the EM algorithm. *Biometrics* **48**, 795–806.

KLEIN, J. P. & MOESCHBERGER, M. L. (1997). *Survival Analysis: Techniques for Censored and Truncated Data*. Springer-Verlag Inc.

KOUL, H., SUSARLA, V., & VAN RYZIN, J. (1981). Regression analysis with randomly right censored data. *Ann. Statist.* **9**, 1276–1288.

LAI, T. L. & YING, Z. (1991a). Large sample theory of a modified Buckley-James estimator for regression analysis with censored data. *Ann. Statist.* **19**.

LAI, T. L. & YING, Z. (1991b). Rank regression methods for left-truncated and right-censored data. *Ann. Statist.* **19**.

LAST, G. & BRANDT, A. (1995). *Marked Point Processes on the Real Line. The Dynamic Approach*. Springer-Verlag New York.

LAWLESS, J. F. (1982). *Statistical Models and Methods for Lifetime Data*. Wiley, New York.

LAWLESS, J. F. & NADEAU, C. (1995). Some simple robust methods for the analysis of recurrent events. *Technometrics* **37**, 158–168.

LEE, E. W., WEI, L. J., & AMATO, D. A. (1992). Cox-type regression analysis for large numbers of small groups of correlated failure time observations (disc: P247). In *Survival Analysis*, pages 237–247.

LIANG, K. Y. & ZEGER, S. L. (1986). Longitudinal data analysis using generalized linear models. *Biometrika* **73**, 13–22.

LIN, D. Y. (1991). Goodness of fit for the Cox regression model based on a class of parameter estimators. *J. Amer. Statist. Assoc.* **86**, 725–728.

LIN, D. Y. (1994). Cox regression analysis of multivariate failure time data: The marginal approach. *Statist. Med.* **13**, 2233–2247.

LIN, D. Y., OAKES, D., & YING, Z. (1998a). Additive hazards regression with current status data. *Biometrika* **81**, 289–298.

LIN, D. Y., WEI, L., YANG, I., & YING, Z. (2000). Semiparametric regression for the mean and rate functions of recurrent events. *J. Roy. Stat. Soc. Ser. B* **62**, 711–730.

LIN, D. Y. & WEI, L. J. (1989). The robust inference for the Cox proportional hazards model. *J. Amer. Statist. Assoc.* **84**, 1074–1078.

LIN, D. Y., WEI, L. J., & YING, Z. (1993). Checking the Cox model with cumulative sums of martingale-based residuals. *Biometrika* **80**, 557–572.

LIN, D. Y., WEI, L. J., & YING, Z. (1998b). Accelerated failure time models for counting processes. *Biometrika* **85**, 605–618.

LIN, D. Y. & YING, Z. (1994). Semiparametric analysis of the additive risk model. *Biometrika* **81**, 61–71.

LIN, D. Y. & YING, Z. (1995). Semiparametric analysis of general additive-multiplicative hazard models for counting processes. *Ann. Statist.* **23**, 1712–1734.

LIN, D. Y. & YING, Z. (2001). Semiparametric and nonparametric regression analysis of longitudinal data. *J. Amer. Statist. Assoc.* **96**, 103–126.

LITTLE, R. & RUBIN, D. (1987). *Statistical Analysis with Missing Data*. Wiley , New York.

LYNN, H. (2001). Maximum likelihood inference for left-censored hiv rna data. *Statist. Med.* **20**, 33–45.

MACRAE, E. C. (1974). Matrix derivatives with an application to an adaptive linear decision problem. *Ann. Statist.* **2**, 337–346.

MARTINUSSEN, T. (1997). *Statistical analysis based on incomplete longitudinal data with mortality follow-up*. PhD thesis, Department of Biostatistics, University of Copenhagen.

MARTINUSSEN, T. & PIPPER, C. B. (2005). Estimation in the positive stable shared frailty Cox proportional hazards model. *Lifetime Data Anal.* **11**, 99–115.

MARTINUSSEN, T. & SCHEIKE, T. H. (1999). A semi-parametric additive regression model for longitudinal data. *Biometrika* **86**, 691–702.

MARTINUSSEN, T. & SCHEIKE, T. H. (2000). A non-parametric dynamic additive regression model for longitudinal data. *Ann. Statist.* **28**, 1000–1025.

MARTINUSSEN, T. & SCHEIKE, T. H. (2001). Sampling adjusted analysis of dynamic additive regression models for longitudinal data. *Scand. J. Statist.* **28**, 303–323.

MARTINUSSEN, T. & SCHEIKE, T. H. (2002a). Efficient estimation in additive hazards regression with current status data. *Biometrika* **89**, 649–658.

MARTINUSSEN, T. & SCHEIKE, T. H. (2002b). A flexible additive multiplicative hazard model. *Biometrika* **89**, 283–298.

MARTINUSSEN, T., SCHEIKE, T. H., & SKOVGAARD, I. M. (2002). Efficient estimation of fixed and time-varying covariate effects in multiplicative intensity models. *Scand. J. Statist.* **28**, 57–74.

MARTINUSSEN, T. & SKOVGAARD, I. M. (2002). Goodness-of-fit of semiparametric regression models. Technical report, Royal Veterinary and Agricultural University, Copenhagen.

MARTINUSSEN, T. & SØRENSEN, T. I. A. (1998). Age-dependent U-shaped risk functions and Aalen's additive risk model. *Biometrics* **54**, 989–1001.

McKEAGUE, I. W. (1988). Asymptotic theory for weighted least squares estimators in Aalen's additive risk model. *Contemp. Math.* **80**, 139–152.

McKEAGUE, I. W. & SASIENI, P. D. (1994). A partly parametric additive risk model. *Biometrika* **81**, 501–514.

McKEAGUE, I. W. & UTIKAL, K. J. (1990a). Identifying nonlinear covariate effects in semimartingale regression models. *Probab. Theory and Related Fields* **87**, 1–25.

McKEAGUE, I. W. & UTIKAL, K. J. (1990b). Inference for a nonlinear counting process regression model. *Ann. Statist.* **18**, 1172–1187.

MEYER, P. A. (1976). *Séminaire de Probabilités X.*, volume 511 of *Lecture Notes in Mathematics*, pages 245–400. Springer-Verlag, Berlin.

MILLER, R. G. (1976). Least squares regression with censored data. *Biometrika* **63**, 449–464.

MURPHY, S., ROSSINI, A., & VAN DER VAART, A. (1997). Maximum likelihood estimation in the proportional odds model. *J. Amer. Statist. Assoc.* **92**, 968–976.

MURPHY, S. A. (1993). Testing for a time dependent coefficient in Cox's regression model. *Scand. J. Statist.* **20**, 35–50.

MURPHY, S. A. & SEN, P. K. (1991). Time-dependent coefficients in a Cox-type regression model. *Stochastic Proccess. Appl.* **39**, 153–180.

NÆS, T. (1982). The asymptotic distribution of the estimator for the regression parameter in Cox's regression model. *Scand. J. Statist.* **9**, 107–115.

NELSON, W. (1969). Hazard plotting for incomplete failure data. *J. Qual. Technol.* **1**, 27–52.

NELSON, W. (1972). Theory and applications of hazard plotting for censored failure data. *Technometrics* **14**, 945–965.

NIELSEN, G. G., GILL, R. D., ANDERSEN, P., & SØRENSEN, T. I. A. (1992). A counting process approach to maximum likelihood estimation in frailty models. *Scand. J. Statist.* **19**, 25–43.

OAKES, D. (1982). A model for association in bivariate survival data. *J. Roy. Statist. Soc. Ser. B* **44**, 414–422.

PARNER, E. (1998). Asymptotic theory for the correlated gamma-frailty model. *Ann. Statist.* **26**, 183–214.

PEPE, M. & CAI, J. (1993). Some graphical displays and marginal regression analyses for recurrent failure times and time dependent covariates. *J. Amer. Statist. Assoc.* **88**, 811–820.

PEPE, M. & COUPER, D. (1997). Modelling partly conditional means with longitudinal data. *J. Amer. Statist. Assoc.* **92**, 991–998.

PEPE, M. S. (1991). Inference for events with dependent risks in multiple endpoint studies. *J. Amer. Statist. Assoc.* **86**, 770–778.

PIPPER, C. B. & MARTINUSSEN, T. (2003). A likelihood based estimating equation for the Clayton-Oakes model with marginal proportional hazards. *Scand. J. Statist.* **30**, 509–521.

PIPPER, C. B. & MARTINUSSEN, T. (2004). An estimating equation for parametric shared frailty models with marginal additive hazards. *J. Roy. Statist. Soc. Ser. B* **66**, 207–220.

PONS, O. (2000). Nonparametric estimation in a varying-coefficient Cox model. *Math. Meth. Statist.* **9**, 376–398.

PRENTICE, R. L. (1978). Linear rank tests with right censored data. *Biometrika* **65**, 167–179. Correction **70**,304(1983).

PRIESTLEY, M. B. & CHAO, M. T. (1972). Nonparametric function fitting. *J. Roy. Stat. Soc. Ser. B* **34**, 385–392.

RAMLAU-HANSEN, H. (1983a). The choice of a kernel function in the graduation of counting process intensities. *Scand. Actuar. J.* pages 165–182.

RAMLAU-HANSEN, H. (1983b). Smoothing counting process intensities by means of kernel functions. *Ann. Statist.* **11**, 453–466.

REBOLLEDO, R. (1980). Central limit theorems for local martingales. *Z. Wahrsch. verw. Geb.* **51**, 269–286.

RITOV, Y. (1990). Estimation in a linear regression model with censored data. *Ann. Statist.* **18**, 303–328.

ROBINS, J. M. & ROTNITZKY, A. (1992). Recovery of information and adjustment of dependent censoring using surrogate markers. In *AIDS Epidemiology-Methodological Issues*, pages 24–33.

ROSTHØJ, S., ANDERSEN, P. K., & ABILDSTRØM, S. Z. (2004). SAS macros for estimation of the cumulative incidence function s based on a Cox regressio nmodel for competing risks survival data. *Computer methods and programs in biomedicine* **74**, 69–75.

SASIENI, P. (1992a). Information bounds for the conditional hazard ratio in a nested family of regression models. *J. Roy. Stat. Soc. Ser. B* **54**, 617–635.

SASIENI, P. D. (1992b). Information bounds for the additive and multiplicative intensity models (disc: P263-265). In Klein, J. & Goel, P., editors, *Survival Analysis: State of the Art*, pages 249–263. Klüwer, Dordrecht.

SASIENI, P. D. (1996). Proportional excess hazards. *Biometrika* **83**, 127–141.

SCHEIKE, T. H. (1994). Parametric regression for longitudinal data with counting process measurement times. *Scand. J. Statist.* **21**, 245–263.

SCHEIKE, T. H. (1996). Nonparametric kernel regression when the regressor follows a counting process. *J. Nonparametr. Statist.* **2**, 1–11.

SCHEIKE, T. H. (2000). Comparison of non-parametric regression functions through their cumulatives. *Statist. Probab. Lett.* **46**, 21–32.

SCHEIKE, T. H. (2002). The additive nonparametric and semiparametric Aalen model as the rate function for a counting process. *Lifetime Data Anal.* **8**, 247–262.

SCHEIKE, T. H. (2004). Time-varying effects in survival analysis. In Balakrishnan, N. & Rao, C. R., editors, *Handbook of Statistics 23*, pages 61–85. Elsevier B.V.

SCHEIKE, T. H. & JENSEN, T. K. (1997). A discrete survival model with random effects: An application to time to pregnancy. *Biometrics* **53**, 318–329.

SCHEIKE, T. H. & MARTINUSSEN, T. (2002). Nonparametric and semiparametric dynamic marginal additive regression models. *Research Report, Department of Mathematical Sciences, University of Aalborg* **2002**.

SCHEIKE, T. H. & MARTINUSSEN, T. (2004). On efficient estimation and tests of time-varying effects in the proportional hazards model. *Scand. J. Statist.* **31**, 51–62.

SCHEIKE, T. H., PETERSEN, J. H., & MARTINUSSEN, T. (1999). Retrospective ascertainment of recurrent events: An application to time to pregnancy. *J. Amer. Statist. Assoc.* **94**, 713–725.

SCHEIKE, T. H. & ZHANG, M. (1998). Cumulative regression function tests for longitudinal data. *Ann. Statist.* **26**, 1328–1355.

SCHEIKE, T. H. & ZHANG, M.-J. (2002). An additive-multiplicative Cox-Aalen model. *Scand. J. Statist.* **28**, 75–88.

SCHEIKE, T. H. & ZHANG, M.-J. (2003). Extensions and applications of the Cox-Aalen survival model. *Biometrics* **59**, 1033–1045.

SCHEIKE, T. H. & ZHANG, M.-J. (2004). Predicting cumulative incidence probability: Marginal and cause-specific modelling. *Research Report, Department of Biostatistics, University of Copenhagen* **3**.

SCHEIKE, T. H. & ZHANG, M.-J. (2005). Predicting cumulative incidence probability by direct binomial regression. *Research Report, Department of Biostatistics, University of Copenhagen* **2**.

SCHLICHTING, P., CHRISTENSEN, E., ANDERSEN, P. K., FAUERHOLDT, L., JUHL, E., POULSEN, H., & TYGSTRUP, N. FOR THE COPENHAGEN STUDY GROUP FOR LIVER DISEASES (1983). Identification of prognostic factors in cirrhosis using Cox's regression model. *Hepatology* **3**, 889–895.

SCHOENFELD, D. (1982). Partial residuals for the proportional hazards regression model. *Biometrika* **69**, 239–241.

SCHUMACHER, M. (1984). Two-sample tests of Cramér-von Mises and Kolmogorov-Smirnov type for randomly censored data. *Internat. Statist. Rev.* **52**, 263–281.

SHEN, Y. & CHENG, S. C. (1999). Confidence bands for cumulative incidence curves under the additive risk model. *Biometrics* **55**, 1093–1100.

SHIH, J. H. & LOUIS, T. A. (1995). Inference on association parameter in copula models for bivariate survival data. *Biometrics* **51**, 1384–1399.

SIMONOFF, J. (1996). *Smoothing Methods in Statistics.* Springer-Verlag New York.

SLUD, E. & VONTA, F. (2004). Consistency of the NPML estimator in the right-censored transformation model. *Scand. J. Statist.* **31**, 21–41.

SOLOMON, P. J. (1984). Effect of misspecification of regression models in the analysis of survival data. *Biometrika* **71**, 291–298.

SPIEKERMAN, C. F. & LIN, D. Y. (1996). Checking the marginal Cox model for correlated failure time data. *Biometrika* **83**, 143–156.

SPIEKERMAN, C. F. & LIN, D. Y. (1998). Marginal regression models for multivariate failure time data. *J. Amer. Statist. Assoc.* **93**, 1164–1175.

STRUTHERS, C. A. & KALBFLEISCH, J. D. (1986). Misspecified proportional hazard models. *Biometrika* **73**, 363–369.

SUN, Y. & WU, H. (2003). AUC-based tests for nonparametric functions with longitudinal data. *Statist. Sinica* **13**, 593–612.

SUN, Y. & WU, H. (2005). Semiparametric time-varying coefficient regression model for longitudinal data. *Scand. J. Statist.* **32**, 21–47.

THERNEAU, T. & GRAMBSCH, P. (2000). *Modeling Survival Data: Extending the Cox Model.* Springer-Verlag New York.

TIAN, L., ZUCKER, D., & WEI, L. (2005). On the Cox model with time-varying regression coefficients. *J. Amer. Statist. Assoc.* **100**, 172–183.

TSIATIS, A. A. (1981). A large sample study of Cox's regression model. *Ann. Statist.* **9**, 93–108.

TSIATIS, A. A. (1990). Estimating regression parameters using linear rank tests for censored data. *Ann. Statist.* **18**, 354–372.

VAN DER VAART, A. W. & WELLNER, J. A. (1996). *Weak Convergence and Empirical Processes: With Applications to Statistics.* Springer-Verlag New York.

WEI, L. J. (1984). Testing goodness of fit for proportional hazards model with censored observations. *J. Amer. Statist. Assoc.* **79**, 649–652.

WEI, L. J., LIN, D., & WEISSFELD, L. (1989). Regression analysis of multivariate incomplete failure time data by modeling marginal distributions. *J. Amer. Statist. Assoc.* **84**, 1065–1073.

WEI, L. J., YING, Z., & LIN, D. Y. (1990). Linear regression analysis of censored survival data based on rank tests. *Biometrika* **77**, 845–852.

WINNETT, A. & SASIENI, P. (2001). A note on scaled Schoenfeld residuals for the proportional hazards model. *Biometrika* **88**, 565–571.

WINNETT, A. & SASIENI, P. (2003). Iterated residuals and time-varying covariate effects in Cox regression. *J. Roy. Stat. Soc. Ser. B* **65**, 473–488.

WU, C. & CHIANG, C. (2000). Kernel smoothing on varying coefficient models with longitudinal dependent variable. *Statist. Sinica* **10**, 433–456.

WU, C., CHIANG, C., & HOOVER, D. R. (1998). Asymptotic confidence regions for kernel smoothing of a varying-coefficient model with longitudinal data. *J. Amer. Statist. Assoc.* **93**, 1388–1402.

XU, R. & O'QUIGLEY, J. (2000). Estimating average regression effect under non-proportional hazards. *Biostatistics* **1**, 423–439.

YING, Z. (1993). A large sample study of rank estimation for censored regression data. *Ann. Statist.* **21**.

YING, Z., JUNG, S. H., & WEI, L. J. (1995). Survival analysis with median regression models. *J. Amer. Statist. Assoc.* **90**, 178–184.

ZAHL, P. (2003). Regresion analysis with multiplicative and time-varying additive regression coefficients with examples from breast and colon cancer. *Statist. Med.* **22**, 1113–1127.

ZUCKER, D. M. & KARR, A. F. (1990). Nonparametric survival analysis with time-dependent covariate effects: A penalized partial likelihood approach. *Ann. Statist.* **18**, 329–353.

Index

accelerated failure time model, 294
adapted process, 19
additive Aalen model, 103, *see* additive hazards model
additive hazards model, 103, 205
    additive Aalen model, 108
    clustered data, 324
    definition of, 108
    goodness-of-fit, 151
    inference, 104, 116
    rate model, 149
    resampling inference, 118
    semiparametric version, 104
    survival function estimation, 146
    test for time-varying effects, 116
    TRACE data, 159
additive rate model, 149
    clustered data, 324
    resampling inference, 151
additive-multiplicative hazards model
    Cox-Aalen model, 251
    proportional excess model, 273
attenuation

frailty model, 337

cause specific hazards, 356
censoring, 49
central limit theorem for martingales, 34
clustered survival data, 313
    additive hazards model, 324
    Cox model, 315
    Cox-Aalen model, 322
    frailty model, 334
    goodness-of-fit, 318
    marginal effects, 315
compensator, 21
competing risks model
    cause specific hazards, 351
    cumulative incidence function, 348
    direct binomial approach, 372
    product limit estimator, 351
    subdistribution approach, 361
conditional multiplier central limit theorem, 43
copula models, 327
    Archimedean copula, 327

Index

counting process
  definition of, 23
  intensity process, 24
  likelihood, 62
  multivariate, 25
Cox model, 181
  clustered data, 315
  goodness-of-fit, 193
  misspecified models, 191
  proportional hazards model, 181
  stratified Cox model, 190
  with timevarying effects, 205
Cox-Aalen model, 251
  clustered data, 322
  cumulative residuals, 260
  goodness-of-fit, 260
  resampling inference, 258
  stratified Cox model, 256
  survival function estimation, 266
  TRACE data, 270
Cramér-von Mises test, 39
cumulative incidence function, 348
cumulative residuals
  additive hazards model, 151
  Cox model, 193
  Cox-Aalen model, 260
  multiplicative hazards model, 228
  proportional excess model, 283
current status data, 62

delayed entry, 61
delta-method, 42
discrete time survival model, 344
Doob-Meyer decomposition, 21

estimation
  estimating equations, 70
  maximum likelihood, 62
examples
  Lung cancer data, 234, 284
  Melanoma data, 237
  TRACE data, 7, 159, 270

excess risk
  additive hazards model, 105
exponential distribution, 66

filtering, 51
  independent, 52
  left-censoring, 61
  left-truncation, 59
  noninformative, 64
  progressive type I censoring, 57
  right-censoring, 49
  simple type I censoring, 57
filtration, 19
finite variation process, 21
frailty model, 334
  attenuation, 337
functional delta-method, 42

Gaussian martingale, 34
Gaussian process, 34
Gill's condition, 42
Gompertz distribution, 77
Gompertz-Makeham distribution, 77
goodness-of-fit
  additive hazards model, 151
  clustered survival data, 318
  Cox model, 193
  Cox-Aalen model, 260
  multiplicative hazards model, 228
  proportional excess model, 283
  proportional odds model, 306
Greenwood's formula, 84

hazard function, 23
history
  definition of, 19
  internal history, 19

inference
  additive hazards model, 116
  multiplicative hazards model, 213

innovation theorem, 27
integrable, 20
intensity kernel, 31
intensity process, 24
internal history, 19

Kaplan-Meier estimator, 83
Khmaladze's transformation, 123, 412
Kolmogorov-Smirnov test, 39
Kolmogorov-Smirnov, two sample, 91

left-censoring, 61
left-truncation, 59
Lenglart's inequality, 41
local characteristics, 31
local martingale, 20
local square integrable martingale, 21
locally integrable, 108
log-rank test, 89
    stratified log-rank test, 94
longitudinal data, 375

marginal mean models for longitudinal data, 397
marginal models for survival data, 314
marked point process
    definition of, 30
    intensity kernel, 31
    local characteristics, 31
martingale
    central limit theorem for martingales, 34
    definition of, 20
    Gaussian martingale, 34
    local martingale, 20
    local square integrable martingale, 21
    optional covariation process, 22
    optional variation process, 22
    orthogonal, 21

predictable covariation process, 21
predictable variation process, 21
quadratic covariation process, 22
quadratic variation process, 22
square integrable, 20
misspecified models
    additive hazards models, 133
    Cox model, 191
multiplicative Aalen model, 27
multiplicative hazards model, 175, 205
    goodness-of-fit, 228
    inference, 213
    Lung cancer data, 234
    Melanoma data, 237
    multiplicative rate model, 227
    relative risk, 176
    semiparametric version, 177, 218
    survival function estimation, 226
    test for time-varying effects, 213
multiplicative rate model, 227
multivariate counting process, 25

Nelson-Aalen estimator, 82

occurrence/exposure rate, 66
optional covariation process, 22
optional variation process, 22
orthogonal martingales, 21

partial likelihood, 64
predictable covariation process, 21
predictable process, 21
predictable variation process, 21
product integration estimator, 351
product limit estimator, 351
proportional excess model, 273
    cumulative residuals, 283

goodness-of-fit, 283
  Lung cancer data, 284
  survival function estimation, 292
proportional hazards model, *see* Cox model
proportional odds model, 298
  converging hazards, 299
  goodness-of-fit, 306

quadratic covariation process, 22
quadratic variation process, 22

relative risk, 176
resampling inference
  additive hazards model, 118
  additive rate model, 151
  Cox-Aalen model, 258
  semiparametric additive hazards model, 136
  semiparametric additive rate model, 151
  semiparametric multiplicative hazards model, 224, 226
  semiparametric risk model, 136
right-censoring, 49

smoothed Cox regression model, 251
stochastic process, 19
stopping time, 19
stratified Cox model, 190
stratified log-rank test, *see* log-rank test
stratified tests, 93
subdistribution hazard function, 361
submartingale, 20
survival function
  additive hazards model, 146
  Cox-Aalen model, 266
  multiplicative hazards model, 226
  proportional excess model, 292
  semiparametric additive hazards model, 146

test for time-varying effects
  additive hazards model, 116, 135
  multiplicative hazards model, 213
TRACE data
  additive hazards model, 159
  Cox-Aalen model, 270
  introduction, 7
transformation model, 293, 298
  efficient score, 304
  modified partial likelihood, 300
  nonparametric maximum likelihood, 304

Weibull distribution, 68

Springer
the language of science

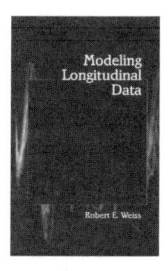

springeronline.com

Modeling Longitudinal Data
Robert E. Weiss

Longitudinal data are ubiquitous across Medicine, Public Health, Public Policy, Psychology, Political Science, Biology, Sociology and Education, yet many longitudinal data sets remain improperly analyzed. This book teaches the art and statistical science of modern longitudinal data analysis. The author emphasizes specifying, understanding, and interpreting longitudinal data models.

2005. 432 p. (Springer Texts in Statsitics) Hardcover ISBN 0-387-40271-3

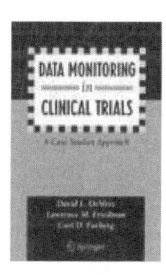

Data Monitoring in Clinical Trials: A Case Study Approach
David DeMets, Curt Furberg, and Lawrence Friedman (Editors)

Randomized clinical trials are the gold standard for establishing many clinical practice guidelines and are central to evidence based medicine. Obtaining the best evidence through clinical trials must be done within the boundaries of rigorous science and ethical principles. One fundamental principle is that trials should not continue longer than necessary to reach their objectives. This book, through a series of case studies presented by many distinguished clinical trial experts, illustrates the complexity of this monitoring process. The editors provide an overview of the process and a summary of a multitude of the lessons learned from the cases presented.

2005. 288 p. Softcover ISBN 0-387-20330-3

Screening
Methods for Experimentation in Industry, Drug Discovery, and Genetics
Angela Dean and Susan Lewis (Editors)

In *Screening*, designed experiments and statistical analyses of the resulting data sets are used to identify efficiently the few features that determine key properties of the system under study. This book brings together accounts by leading international experts that are essential reading for those working in fields such as industrial quality improvement, engineering research and development, genetic and medical screening, drug discovery, and computer simulation of manufacturing systems or economic models.

2006. 280 p. Hardcover ISBN 0-387-28013-8

Easy Ways to Order ▶ Call: Toll-Free 1-800-SPRINGER • E-mail: orders-ny@springer.sbm.com • Write: Springer, Dept. S8113, PO Box 2485, Secaucus, NJ 07096-2485 • Visit: Your local scientific bookstore or urge your librarian to order.